SYNTHETIC REPERTORY
RÉPERTOIRE SYNTHÉTIQUE
SYNTHETISCHES REPERTORIUM

SYNTHETIC REPERTORY

Psychic and General Symptoms
of the Homoeopathic Materia Medica

RÉPERTOIRE SYNTHÉTIQUE

Symptômes Psychiques et Généraux
de la Matière Médicale Homoéopathique

SYNTHETISCHES REPERTORIUM

Gemüts- und Allgemeinsymptome
der Homöopathischen Materia Medica

Published by · Publié par · Herausgegeben von
Dr. med. Horst Barthel, Wilhelmsfeld/Heidelberg

Volume II: General Symptoms
Volume II: Symptômes Généraux
Band   II: Allgemeinsymptome

Dr. med. Horst Barthel, Wilhelmsfeld/Heidelberg

Traduction en Français
Dr. J. Baur, Lyon

2nd revised and improved edition
Deuxième édition révisée, corrigée et augmentée
2., verbesserte und erweiterte Auflage

Karl F. Haug Verlag, Heidelberg

CIP-Kurztitelaufnahme der Deutschen Bibliothek

Synthetic repertory: psychic and general symptoms of the homoeopathic materia medica = Répertoire synthétique = Synthetisches Repertorium / publ. by Horst Barthel. — Heidelberg: Haug

NE: Barthel, Horst [Hrsg.]; 1. PT; 2. PT

Vol. 2. General symptoms/Horst Barthel. Trad. en Français J. Baur — 2. Aufl. — 1982.

ISBN 3-7760-0560-2

2. Auflage 1982

Verlags-Nr. 8201 — ISBN 3-7760-0560-2

Gesamtherstellung: Druckhaus Darmstadt GmbH, Kleyerstr. 9, 6100 Darmstadt

To the master and teacher of homoeopathy Hahnemann's

Dr. med. Jost Künzli von Fimelsberg
St. Gallen

Au grand maître de l'homoéopathie Hahnemannienne

Dr. med. Jost Künzli von Fimelsberg
St. Gallen

Dem Meister und Lehrer der Homöopathie Hahnemanns

Dr. med. Jost Künzli von Fimelsberg
St. Gallen

PREFACE

Over the years the plan to supplement and continue Kent's repertory was influenced by various intermediate concepts and resulted in the present Synthetic Repertory. The resumption of the original title was the result of a threefold synthesis: the supplement from the oldest to the latest homeopathic literature, the register of equivalents and related symptoms, and the composition of individual subjects, as for example, complaints due to psychic trauma.

Progress in homeopathy comes about on the one hand by collecting materia medica and composing it practically for the repertory, and on the other hand by adding symptoms of newly proven drugs. Therefore colleagues are kindly requested by the authors to cooperate with them in increasing the verification of drugs. Furthermore, help is requested in eliminating mistakes carried over from other sources, and others which the authors have overlooked.

The trilinguality brought about problems of translation for the German speaking authors. In most cases the English titles could be used as originally stated. Dr. Pierre Schmidt of Geneva undertook with great competence the very difficult task of translating the mental symptoms. He also translated the preface and the introduction for this volume. In addition the French versions of the third volume were improved by his critical revision. The authors extend to him their warmest thanks for his work in the translation, and are grateful for all the advice and understanding with which Dr. P. Schmidt assisted them in the creation of this work. Dr. Roger Schmidt and Mr. Alain Naude of San Francisco revised the English version of the preface and the introduction for this volume. The authors feel very obliged to them.

Mr. Dr. med. Jacques Baur, Lyon, was not only the translater of all the titles in Vol. II, he also translated the new additional symptoms. We give our special gratitude for his valuable help!

The publishers thank Mr. Dr. med. Jost Künzli von Fimelsberg, St. Gallen, for the permission of printing his supplements in the new edition which he took out of the classic homoeopathic literature into his own Repertory. In that way his long and unprecedented struggle about the sources, especially about Hahnemann's Arzneimittellehren is now made publicly known and available for everyone.

We give our gratitute to Mr. Dr. med. Artur Braun and to cand. med. Klaus-Henning Gypser, for their corrections of Vol. III and we also like to give our thanks to Mr. Martin Weber, Genf, for his help in translating the new french rubrics in Vol. III.

To Dr. Herbert Schindler of Karlsruhe, who contributed significantly to the international nomenclature of homeopathic drugs, the authors are indebted for much information, as well as for the corrections and the final verification of the drug index.

The editors wish to express their thanks to the authors of publications included in this work: to Dr. O. A. Julian of Paris, Dr. J. Mezger † of Stuttgart, Dr. Pierre Schmidt of Geneva, and Dr. J. Stephenson of New York, for their kind permission to use their publications. We wish also to thank the publishers Peyronnet of Paris, Masson of Paris, Roy & Co. of Bombay, and Ternet-Martin of Vienne (Isere).

Dr. E. Fischer, publisher, and Mr. Sieber, production manager, have been responsible for making this book as practical as possible, by responding in the most cooperative manner to all our proposals concerning the book and its printing design. To them we wish to express our special thanks.

INTRODUCTION

The need for the repertory comes from the character of homeopathy itself. Homeopathy means medical action according to the law of similars of Hahnemann (1755–1843): similia similibus curentur. According to this law the drug picture and the characteristic symptoms of the patient have to agree to an optimum degree. Thus we seek the simillimum for the patient.

In the Homeomethodology the homeopathic materia medica is the means by which the results of drug provings and clinical observation of drugs are classified. In practice the choise of a drug needs the classification of drugs according to symptoms. The repertory serves that purpose. The materia medica contains the symptoms of drugs and the repertory relates the drugs to the symptoms. Through the repertory the doctrine of drugs and therapy according to symptoms complement each other.

In the beginning of homeopathy the drug symptoms had already increased to such a degree that it seemed impossible to bear them all in mind. Therefore in 1817 Hahnemann developed the first of his two "symptomdictionaries", which was the first repertory. Compared with the partial information of the materia medica remembered by chance, the repertory permits the choice of a drug through extensive homeopathic knowledge.

Until now almost 110 repertories have been published. The "Repertory of the Homeopathic Materia Medica" by J. T. Kent (1849–1916) is the most appropriate, most complete, and most reliable of all. Kent used older works of the materia medica and clinical observations, but refused numerous insufficiently confirmed symptoms and drugs. Until his death he added by hand into his own copies new symptoms and drugs, and classified them according to his own experience into various degrees.

To keep the repertory continually up to date requires the preservation of symptoms and drugs not listed in Kent's repertory, and also their confirmation by cures. It is also of great importance to make available the primary and repeated provings of younger authors.

Supplements to general and particular symptoms result in a multitude of material which requires a decision as to whether we should limit the number of authors and headings, or whether we should list only the general symptoms. Since the general symptoms will affect the choice of drugs for chronic patients, this Synthetic Repertory is limited to general symptoms. For particulars Kent's "Repertory" is still the best reference book.

According to the hierarchy of general symptoms the Synthetic Repertory is separated into the following three volumes: Vol. I contains the mental symptoms, Vol. II contains the general symptoms in a more selective way. The symptoms for food and drink which in Kent's repertory are separated into different chapters and headings according to aggravation, improvement, aversion and desire, are now summed up in one single heading. Vol. III contains the chapters of sleep symptoms and dreams, as well as the male and female sexual symptoms.

Sources of the Synthetic Repertory

1. KENT, J. T.: Kent's repertory is a climax in the evolution of the repertory because of its extensive contents and logical structure, its moderation between the generalizations and differentiations of tendencies found in other authors, and

finally its reliability and practicability. For more than 70 years it has proven true all over the world; the English version is available in the 6th American and the 3rd Indian edition. There exists a French translation in extracts; a German translation appeared in 1971, in its 2nd edition. The chapters and headings of the above mentioned general symptoms are totally included. Mistakes detected during the last revision were corrected. As further sources Kent's "Lectures on Homeopathic Materia Medica" and "New Remedies" were used.

2. KNERR, C. B.: With his "Guiding Symptoms" C. Hering wrote a classic materia medica of 10 volumes supported by clinical experience. Hering's student Knerr transformed this work into a repertory of two volumes. These detailed empirical data concerning modalities and clinical symptoms are difficult to understand for lack of clarity in the way they are set out; this disadvantage is eliminated in the Synthetic Repertory.

3. VON BOENNINGHAUSEN, C.; BOGER, C. M.: The repertory written by v. Boenninghausen on the advice of Hahnemann was the first repertory to be published, and is still in use. The Synthetic Repertory has used C. M. Boger's English translation and supplement. We have taken into consideration a certain tendency to generalize in this work: the inclusion of modalities into main headings and local symptoms into general symptoms, for instance.

In the 2nd. edition we added symptoms and remedies from C. M. Boger's "Additions to Kent's Repertory" and from his Repertory in "A Synoptic Key of the Materia Medica". By technical reasons we gave all these additions the index number 3.

4. JAHR, G. H. G.: His "Systematic-alphabetic repertory of homeopathic remedy doctrine" which appeared in 1848–49 and is no longer available is noted for its comprehensive listing of symptoms. But because it is split up into synonyms and because of its arrangement it is not practical.

5. GALLAVARDIN, J. P.: In his experience of mental diseases Gallavardin tested and extended the drugs which treat psychiatric patients, which Dulac took from the works of Jahr. The repertory and the materia medica from "Psychisme et Homeopathie", published after the author's death, have been used as sources.

6. STAUFFER, K.: The "Symptom-index" represents Stauffer's vast and critically controlled practical experiences. Apart from verifying drug symptoms it also conveys new additions to the materia medica.

7. SCHMIDT, P.: The supplements by 35 authors to his four repertories of Kent have been integrally included. Further material from the courses of the "Groupement Hahnemannien de Lyon", which have been published in the reports of those meetings, have been included. P. Schmidt obtained his homeopathic knowledge in direct line from Kent, and was instructed by Kent's collaborators in the technical details of establishing the repertory. This, and his 50 years of practical experience, have given him the authority to classify higher grades, and to introduce the fourth grade of drugs in the case of several symptoms. This fourth grade of drugs has been especially useful to him whenever there have been no differentiating symptoms allowing him to consider other drugs under the same heading.

8. BOERICKE, O. E.: The materia medica of W. Boericke, which has been widely used in the English-speaking world, was transcribed into a repertory by O. E. Boericke. It has the advantage of presenting a great many new drugs in English. However, it does not contain a list of drug abbreviations, and there are mistakes

in the nomenclature of the drugs and the symptom complex. Its classification is not always consistent.

9. STEPHENSON, J.: This work, which is laid out as clearly as Kent's repertory, contains drug provings of the years 1924–59, which originate especially from the English and German-speaking countries.

10. MEZGER, J.: The symptoms of 35 reproven or new drugs have been taken from his critical work "Gesichtete Homeopathische Arzneimittellehre" (Selected Homeopathic materia medica).

11. ALLEN, T. F.: The ten volumes of the "Encyclopedia of Pure Materia Medica", which only contain pure drug symptoms, have a two-volume index, "A General Symptom Register of the Homeopathic Materia Medica", of which pertinent parts were added to the Synthetic Repertory. They provide access to the older proven symptoms for future verification. They also contain numerous rare remedies.

12. CLARKE, J. H.: His "A Clinical Repertory to the Dictionary of Materia Medica" from his three-volume materia medica, remaining to this day one of the best, reports mainly clinical indications and rare drugs.

13. The most recent drug provings published in various journals.

14. JULIAN, O. A.: His "Matière Médicale d'Homéothérapie" of 1971 is up to the present day the most complete summary of drug provings in the international literature. We incorporated it even though we had completed the manuscript. The 2nd edition contains also the ca. 30 remedies, supplementary published by Dr. Julian in his new edition of this work, now titled "Dictionnaire de Matière Médicale de 130 Nouveaux Homéothérapeutiques" by Masson, Paris (1981).

15. KÜNZLI, J.: Supplements taken from the international homoeopathic literature.

16. HAHNEMANN, S.: "Pure Materia Medica" and "Chronic diseases". Symptoms and remedies which are missing in Kent's Repertory are added according to the supplements of Künzli.

The abbreviation of the tuberculinum not otherwise defined by the authors 2, 6, 7, and 8 is tub., as for the tuberculinum Kent.

The Synthetic Repertory mentions for the first time the exact sources of symptoms or drugs added to Kent's repertory, and uses a numbering system. Symptoms and drugs from Kent's original repertory have not been numbered. Additions made by Kent in his own hand are marked[1], supplements from his "Lectures" and "New Remedies" by[1'], the figures[2-14] coincide with the enumeration of the above mentioned sources. According to Pierre Schmidt, his and Gallavardin's experiences justify classifications of certain drugs of Kent into higher grades. These drugs are marked by both figures, as[1,5] or[1,7]. Since we mention the sources of this material the reader can decide for himself the importance of the authors quoted, and test their indications in the light of his own practical experience.

The corrections of Kent which he made personally in his own Repertory, owned later on by Mr. Dr. Pierre Schmidt, were now published by Mr. Dr. D. H. Chand ("Kent's Final General Repertory", New Delhi, 1980). But we had already used them in the 1st edition of the "Synthetic Repertory", and therefore was now reason to take them into consideration anymore.

Different gradings of the drugs were found in the sources. These were adapted to the three grades of Kent with a certain amount of liberty. As the individual gradings could not be indicated for drugs added from various sources, the highest grade from among those sources has been indicated.

The grades of the drugs are clearly differentiated in print. Drugs of the first and second grades are printed in small letters, those of the second, third and fourth in bold type, those of the third and fourth in capitals, those of the fourth in underlined capitals.

The transformation of the drugs into the grading system of the Synthetic Repertory, and the transformation of varying arrangements of systems in the sources into the present system of headings, making the clearest possible differentiations, has demanded serious and difficult decisions.

The headings are indicated by printing-type, indentation and spacing. In the main heading the key word of the symptom title is printed in bold type capitals, in the sub-heading, in bold type only, whilst times of day, clock-times, and other sub-headings are printed in ordinary type. The main headings start at the beginning of a line, the first indentation indicates the first sub-heading, the second indentation indicates the next sub-heading, and so on. Each indented title refers to the key word of the main title. Under each symptom title the remedies are printed in normal spacing to show that they belong together.

The titles were partly clarified by supplements, whereas in Vol. I – delusions – and in Vol. III – dreams – they were simplified by using the indicative or the infinitive.

Headings and symptom titles are given in English, French, and German, with the exception of clock-times and Latin terms. The English titles were mostly taken from the English literature, without changing American expressions and spelling. Most of the French and German titles are translations from the English whenever they have been found in existing French and German sources.

The preference given to English titles comes from the importance of the English literature on Homeopathy, and the importance of English as a world language. French represents the languages of the Latin-American continent and South Europe.

The abbreviations agg. and am. have been used in all languages to mean the modalities of aggravation and amelioration respectively. They are to be understood as nouns or verbs, as the case may be.

For French- and German-speaking readers there is a complete and clearly arranged index at the end of each volume which uses the column numbering of the repertory to locate any required heading. Since the English listing of symptoms is already alphabetical, the English index is limited to synonyms and cross references (in vol. I, II). In addition the use of the repertory is facilitated by many references among the symptoms and in the index. The asterisk of the titles of symptoms refers to one of 138 new collected rubrics of the index of vol. I and II.

The remedy index of the Synthetic Repertory lists abbreviations of the drugs in alphabetical order, and, after each abbreviation, the remedy and its synonym. It contains 1594 drugs, whilst Kent's index contains 591. Obsolete drugs like Electricitas, Galvanism, Magnes Artificialis and the complex snake drug ophiotoxicum were not retained. Double entries, lack of clarity, and wrong nomenclature were corrected wherever possible. The traditional nomenclature of homeopathic drugs has been in use for the last 170 years, and this establishes its priority over the modern pharmacological, pharmaceutic terminology. Since homeopathic drugs have always been used in the same way, homeopathic literature remains valid regardless of its age, and can only be understood in the traditional nomenclature.

For practical reasons Kent's abbreviations have been kept, in spite of certain inconsistencies like arg-m. and nat-m. Only inconsistent abbreviations of small drugs were changed. The different abbreviations in the sources, including those of Clarke, were changed to conform to the more comprehensible, accentuated abbreviations of Kent. We tried to establish a uniform abbreviation throughout, e. g. ar. for the anion arsenicosum (compare with Kent's kali-ar. and nat-a.).

Whenever possible wrong spellings of drug abbreviations in the literature have been corrected.

In the field of general symptoms the Synthetic Repertory represents the synthesis of the homeopathic knowledge of the last 170 years. By internationalizing the nomenclature of the drugs, by using three languages for the symptoms and the indexes, we hope to have contributed to a closer understanding among homeopathic physicians in the world. The common language of homeopathic physicians can only come from commonly used terms for drugs and symptoms.

Dr. med. Horst Barthel   Dr. med. Will Klunker
Alte Römerstraße 70   Am Rosenberg 1375
D-6901 Wilhelmsfeld   CH-9410 Heiden

PRÉFACE

Au cours des années, le projet de parfaire et de parachever le Répertoire de Kent, nous a conduit à la publication de ce Répertoire Synthétique de la Matière Médicale homoeopathique en un tout, formant une synthèse de leurs symptômes à la fois concrets et abstraits.

Ce titre de synthèse, retenu puis abandonné, fut finalement repris avec un triple but: 1. Tenir compte de la littérature homoeopathique depuis son origine jusqu'aux écrits les plus contemporains, 2. Recherche circonstanciée des synonymes, 3. Enfin, synthèse de groupes de symptômes, comme, par exemple, « suites de » (traumas psychiques etc.).

Les progrès de l'homoeothérapie se manifestent d'une part par ses résultats thérapeutiques, par leur vérification grâce aux Répertoires et à la Matière Médicale homoeopatique, puis par l'adjonction de médicaments nouveaux, vérifiés et contrôlés par la clinique. C'est la raison pour laquelle les auteurs seraient enchantés d'obtenir la collaboration de leurs Confrères homoeopathes pour les vérifications et les adjonctions possibles à apporter à la Matière Médicale. Ils apprécieraient également qu'on leur signale toutes les inexactitudes ou les fautes relevées au cours de cette lecture.

Cette présentation trilingue a exigé un effort considérable de la part des auteurs et créé bien des problèmes difficultueux. La version anglaise du texte a été établie grâce aux textes anglais des Répertoires et des Matières Médicales consultés.

Le Dr. Schmidt, de Genève, avec compétence s'est chargé de la traduction, certes fort difficile, des symptômes mentaux et de la présente préface et de l'introduction. Les termes français du tome III ont également profité de son examen critique. Nous tenons ici à le remercier tout particulièrement pour ses conseils auxquels nous attachons une grande valeur, ainsi que pour son dévouement coutumier, grâce auxquels il a pu contribuer efficacement à la réalisation de cette publication. Nous tenons à remercier vivement le Docteur Roger Schmidt, ainsi que Monsieur Alain Naudé, tous deux de San Francisco, pour leur traduction en anglais de la préface et de l'introduction.

Le Dr. Jacques Baur de Lyon n'a pas seulement traduit toutes les têtes de rubriques du volume II. Il a aussi traduit les nouveaux symptômes qui ont été ajoutés. Nous remercions particulièrement de cette contribution.

Les Éditeurs remercient le Dr. Jost Künzli von Fimelsberg de St· Gallen, qui leur a permis de publier les adjonctions qu'il avait faites à son propre Répertoire d' après ses recherches dans la littérature homoeopathique classique. Ainsi se trouve maintenant rendu public et mis à la portée de tous le résultat d'un travail de longue haleine, d'un effort sans précédent de retour aux sources, et en particulier « Reine Arzneimittellehre » et à « Chronische Krankheiten » de S. Hahnemann.

Nous exprimons notre gratitude au Dr. Artur Braun et à cand. med. Klaus-Henning Gypser pour la correction du vol. III, et nous voulons aussi remercier Mr. Martin Weber de Genève, pour son aide dans la traduction française des nouvelles rubriques du vol. III.

Les auteurs sont également très reconnaissants au Dr. Herbert Schindler, de Karlsruhe, connu pour l'établissement et la vérification de la nomenclature internationale des médicaments homoeopatiques. Ils ont apprécié sa grande compétence en Matière Médicale par ses corrections, ainsi que de sa vérification finale de la liste détaillée des médicaments homoeopathiques.

Quant aux additions nombreuses enrichissant ce Répertoire synthétique, les

auteurs tiennent tout particulièrement à témoigner leur vive gratitude aux
Drs Julian, de Paris, J. Mezger ✝, de Stuttgart, P. Schmidt, de Genève et Dr.
Stephenson, de New York, pour leur autorisation de les inclure dans le texte
et d'être capables ainsi de faire pouvoir bénéficier les lecteurs de leurs précieuses
connaissances en Matière Médicale.

Nous tenons également à remercier les Maisons d'Edition Peyronnet, de Paris,
Roy et Cie, de Bombay et Ternet-Martin, de Vienne en Isère. De plus, c'est
grâce au Dr. E. Fischer, éditeur et à Monsieur le Directeur Sieber, que cet
ouvrage a pu être réalisé et mis au point, aussi leur exprimons-nous ici notre
vive reconnaissance.

INTRODUCTION

La nécessité d'un Répertoire résulte de la nature-même de l'homoeopathie. Toute l'homoeopathie repose sur la Loi de similitude d'Hahnemann (1755–1843):

SIMILIA SIMILIBUS CURENTUR.

D'après cette loi, le « tableau médicamenteux » obtenu par l'expérimentation sur l'homme sain et le tableau symptomatique caractéristique présenté par le malade, doivent coïncider et présenter une concordance aussi étroite que possible.

C'est en fait la recherche du « simillimum » du patient.

L'application de l'homoeopathie au malade comprend la connaissance de la Matière Médicale, résultant des expérimentations sur l'homme sain et leurs comparaisons avec sa symptomatologie clinique. Pour cela, une étude séméiologique rigoureuse doit être faite, dont on doit chercher la correspondance avec celle du sujet à traiter. C'est pour cette raison qu'ont été créés des Répertoires de symptômes.

S'il est vrai que la Matière Médicale nous fournit la symptomatologie médicamenteuse, les Répertoires nous indiquent les médicaments et leurs correspondances à cette symptomatologie. Ainsi, Matière Médicale d'une part et Répertoire d'autre part se complètent mutuellement et se parachèvent, ce dernier devenant absolument indispensable au practicien.

Depuis le début de l'homoeopathie, le nombre des symptômes présentés par les médicaments s'est si considérablement accru, qu'il est devenu impossible de pouvoir les mémoriser. C'est pourquoi, en 1817 déjà, Hahnemann a établi lui-même un premier Répertoire personnel, appelé « Lexique symptomatique », en deux volumes.

Dès lors, le Répertoire devient un complément vraiment indispensable de tout homoeopathe réfléchi, car c'est un recueil de symptômes – avec toutes leurs modalités – permettant au praticien de faire son choix pour arriver à déterminer le simillimum recherché – aucune mémoire, fut-elle la meilleure, ne pouvant lui être substituée.

Jusqu'à ce jour, à notre connaissance, plus de cent-dix Répertoires ont déjà été publiés : essentiellement en anglais, en français et en allemand. C'est James Tyler Kent, (1849–1916), médecin homoeopathe américain, qui, par la publication de son volumineux Répertoire – des plus de 1400 pages – a édité l'ouvrage le plus complet, le plus utile et certes le plus pratique connu jusqu'à ce jour.

Kent l'a établi par un labeur si considérable – car il y a travaillé jour et nuit pendant des mois – que cet ouvrage lui a coûté sa propre santé, et on peut le dire, abrégé sa vie. Il a compulsé en détail tous les ouvrages sérieux de Matière Médicale publiés jusqu'alors et les a complétés de sa vaste expérience personnelle. Il a laissé de côté, avec un sévère sens critique, tous les symptômes insuffisamment expérimentés ou ne méritant pas d'être retenus et en accordant à chaque médicament le degré conforme à sa vaste pratique personnelle.

Cette œuvre répertoriale exige non seulement le respect, parmi tous ceux cités dans la littérature homoeopathique jusqu'alors, des symptômes ayant fait leurs preuves, mais surtout leurs confirmations par des guérisons, en tenant compte de toutes les expérimentations – même primaires – cependant répétées par de auteurs contemporains compétents. Une des tâches de l'homoeopathe actuel consiste à sanctionner, au point de vue symptomatologique, ce qui s'est révélé, depuis Kent, par la pratique journalière, comme valable et permanent, mais en plus et surtout, de mettre à l'honneur des symptômes anciens: solt ceux confirmés par un nombre suffisant de malades guéris, soit encore ceux dont la valeur jusqu'alors inférieure, se sont révélés par la pratique plus caractéristiques.

Désirant conserver le patrimoine apporté par Kent, avec sa richesse symptomatique, les auteurs ont tenu à divulguer d'une façon complète, en tenant compte de toutes les publications existantes et à ne retenir dans leur Répertoire synthétique que la symptomatologie des cinq grandes classes des symptômes essentiels et indispensables pour toute étude de cas, à savoir, par ordre d'importance:

1. Les symptômes mentaux; 2. Les symptômes généraux; 3. Les désirs, aversions et aggravations alimentaires; 4. Les symptômes du sommeil; 5. Les symptômes sexuels.

Cette liste comprend ce que tout homoeopathe sérieux doit connaître comme indispensable pour l'étude de chaque malade à traiter, cela tout particulièrement pour les cas chroniques.

Pour les symptômes localisés aux différents organes de l'économie du corps humain, la consultation du Répertoire de Kent reste certes le meilleur ouvrage de références.

Conformément aux règles établies par Kent, pour la hiérarchisation des symptômes, le Répertoire synthétique comprend trois volumes :

Volume I : comprenant les **symptômes psychiques.**

Volume II : les **symptômes généraux,** symptômes météoropathiques, aggravations horaires, aggravations et améliorations par mouvement, position, etc.

Quant aux aggravations et améliorations concernant les aliments et les boissons, ainsi que les aversions et les désirs alimentaires contenus dans le Répertoire de Kent – répartis dans des rubriques les plus diverses – ils seront regroupés en un tout homogène.

Le **volume III :** exposera les symptômes du **sommeil,** des **rêves** et comprendra les **symptômes sexuels** concernant les deux sexes.

Références et sources du Répertoire synthétique

1. KENT, J. T., médecin américain :

Dans l'évolution des Répertoires, le « Repertory » de Kent, occupe sans conteste la place d'honneur à tous les points de vue : la richesse de son contenu, le choix et la disposition si logique des symptômes, sa retenue quant aux généralisations si fréquentes dans les autres Répertoires, sa concision, sa présentation typographique si claire et si pratique, l'extrême richesse de ses modalités, ainsi que la sécurité qu'il apporte au praticien, en font un livre unique et de valeur universelle.

Depuis plus de 70 ans, ce Répertoire a fait ses preuves dans les mains de plusieurs générations d'homoeopathes. Il a déjà atteint une sixième édition américaine et une troisième édition hindoue ! De plus, deux traductions allemandes ont paru – la deuxième en 1971 et récemment une traduction abrégée, en français.

Des erreurs typographiques ont été corrigées. On a compulsé également et tenu compte des « Lectures on homoeopthic Materia Medica » de Kent ainsi que de ses « New Remedies ».

2. KNERR, Calvin B., médecin américain, élève de C. Hering, a écrit un des Répertoires – après celui de Gentry en 10 volumes – le plus complet et le plus riche actuellement connu – en deux volumes – résumant les dix tomes de la Matière Médicale de Hering, enrichi de symptômes d'expériences cliniques. C'est véritablement le résumé des dix gros volumes de Hering, avec une symptomatologie et des modalités extrêmement fouillées. Mais, c'est un Répertoire difficile à consulter, vu sa disposition typographique trop serrée et qui exige de celui qui l'utilise beaucoup trop de temps. Ces inconvénients sont précisément évités dans le Répertoire synthétique actuel.

3. VON BOENNINGHAUSEN, C.; BOGER, C. M.: Von Boenninghausen, un Hollandais, sur les recommandations d'Hahnemann, publia le tout premier Répertoire homoeopathique connu. Il est encore utilisé de nos jours et dont C. M. Boger s'est inspiré dans sa traduction anglaise. L'auteur a tendance à généraliser, c'est-à-dire à décrire tous les médicaments avec leurs modalités dans la rubrique principale, y mélangeant malheureusement les symptômes locaux avec les symptômes généraux.

Les symptômes et remèdes qui ont été ajoutés à cette deuxième édition proviennent des ouvrages suivants de C. M. Boger:
– Additions to Kent's Repertory;
– A Synoptic Key of the Materia Medica, Répertoire.
Pour des raisons techniques nous indexons toutes ces additions par le chiffre 3.

4. JAHR, H. G. – un médecin allemand, qui a publié, en 1848 déjà, son Répertoire alphabétique et systématique de la Matière Médicale homoeopathique – qu'on ne peut plus se procurer, hélas ! Il est précieux, par sa richesse symptomatique, mais l'abondance des synonymes et sa mauvaise disposition typographique le rend malheureusement peu pratique.

5. GALLAVARDIN, Dr. J. P., un médecin français :
Les indications concernant le traitement des affections psychiques signalées par Dulac, des œuvres de Jahr, furent revues complètement et reclassées par Gallavardin dans ses excellents ouvrages : « Psychisme et homoeopathie » – œuvre posthume publiée en 1960.

6. STAUFFER, K., un médecin allemand, qui, dans sa remarquable publication « Symptomen-Verzeichnis », expose d'une façon systématique ses précieuses connaissances cliniques contrôlées par ses résultats pratiques. En plus de nombreuses vérifications de symptômes médicamenteux, son ouvrage apporte des renseignements nouveaux comportant des acquisitions de Matière Médicale plus récentes et vérifiées par sa vaste expérience.

7. SCHMIDT, Pierre, médecin suisse, qui possède quatre éditions du Répertoire de Kent, contenant de nombreuses adjonctions, fruit de ses lectures et de son expérience de 50 ans de pratique.

Nous avons inclus également dans notre Répertoire synthétique le résultat de ses nombreuses conférences comprenant les vérifications précieuses publiées dans « Les Cahiers du Groupement hahnemannien de Lyon ».

Préparé par un des disciples préférés de Kent, et par ses connaissances acquises au cours de ses 50 ans d'expérience, il a publié une liste de symptômes vérifiés tout au long de sa carrière, qu'il a cités comme méritant un q u a t r i è m e d e g r é, alors que Kent n'en indique que trois. La valeur indicatrice de ces symptômes rendra certes de grands services au praticien, puisqu'ils sont la réalisation de résultats probants, confirmés depuis un demi-siècle de pratique médicale avec des hautes dynamisations.

8. BOERICKE, O. E., médecin américain :

C'est d'après la petite Matière Médicale de William Boericke, qui a dépassé neuf éditions – une des plus utilisées par le praticien de langue anglaise – que O. E. Boericke – médecin américain – a composé un Répertoire homoeopathique de 303 pages. C'est le Répertoire présentant le plus de médicaments rares et peu utilisés dans la littérature anglo-américaine et le plus complet. Mais, il y manque une liste des abréviations des médicaments indiqués. De plus, il contient pas mal d'erreurs dans la nomenclature des remèdes. Sa disposition typographique n'est, hélas, pas toujours logique.

9. STEPHENSON, J., médecin américain, a publié une « Matière Médicale » avec des médicaments nouveaux, de provenances anglo-saxonne et allemande (de 1924 à 1959).

10. MEZGER, J., médecin allemand, a publié sa « Gesichtete homöopathische Arzneimittellehre », avec trente-cinq remèdes nouveaux ou vérifiés.

11. ALLEN, T. F., médecin américain, dont la célèbre « Encyclopaedia of pure Materia Medica » comprenant dix volumes, est considérée comme une œuvre de titan à laquelle il consacra sa vie ! Ouvrage ne contenant que des symptômes purs, c'est-à-dire expérimentés sur l'homme sain et dont l'excellent Index a été repris dans notre Répertoire synthétique. Ainsi des expérimentations anciennes sont devenues accessibles pour des vérifications futures. Il contient également toute une série de médicaments rares.

12. CLARKE, J. H., médecin anglais, dont le « Répertoire clinique » se base sur son fameux « Dictionnaire de Matière Médicale » qui, en trois gros volumes, reste encore aujourd'hui, une des Matières Médicales cliniques la plus originale.

13. Une liste d'expérimentations récentes de nouveaux médicaments, publiée dans nos revues homoeopathiques contemporaines.

14. JULIAN, O. A., médecin français, dont la Matière Médicale d'homoeothérapie, parue en 1971, contient une liste des expérimentations médicamenteuses les plus récentes signalées dans la littérature contemporaine. Pour cette 2ième édition, nous avons aussi pris en considération les nouveaux remèdes de l'édition, que Dr. Julian vient de publier, titré «Dictionnaire de Matière Médicale de 130 Nouveaux Homéothérapeutiques», chez Masson, Paris. Il s'agit donc de ca. 30 remèdes supplémentieres.

15. KÜNZLI, J.: Additions d'après la littérature homoeopathique internationale.

16. HAHNEMANN, S.: « Matière Médicale Pure » et « Maladies Chroniques ». Les symptômes et les remèdes qui manquent dans le Répertoire de Kent ont été rajoutés d'après les suppléments de Künzli.

La tuberculine pas exactement définie des auteurs 2, 6, 7 et 8 sera abrégée par tub. comme la tuberculine de Kent.

Ce Répertoire synthétique est le premier indiquant, grâce à un Index numéroté, la source exacte et précise de chacun des symptômes et de chaque médicament ajoutés au Répertoire de Kent.

Les chiffres en petites annotations après chaque reméde indiquent leurs sources bibliographiques. Par exemple « 2 » pour celles signalées par Knerr, « 4 » pour celles de Jahr, etc. « 1 » par contre, représente les annotations manuscrites de Kent lui-même, 1' les symptômes provenant de « Lectures on Homoeopathic Materia Medica » et de « New Remedies » de Kent.

Les corrections personnelles que Kent avait apportées à son propre Répertoire et que Dr. P. Schmidt a mis à notre disposition pour la 1ère édition, ont été publiées récemment par le Dr. Diwan Harish Chand dans son Kent's Final General Repertory, New Delhi, 1980. Pour cette raison, nous ne nous sommes plus référés à ce dernier.

D'après P. Schmidt et J. P. Gallavardin, certains médicaments cités par Kent méritent un degré plus élevé. Ces médicaments sont marqués par deux chiffres, 1,5 ou 1,7 ; c'est-à-dire « 1 » indique Kent et « 5 » ou « 7 » : modification apportée par Gallavardin ou Schmidt.

Cette indication des sources, signalée pour chaque remède permet, d'après les auteurs cités, d'attribuer une signification plus ou moins importante à chacun d'eux et de vérifier ces indications par la propre expérience de chaque lecteur.

La gradation symptomatique signalée dans les ouvrages originaux a été modifiée selon les trois degrés de Kent. Quand plusieurs auteurs ont signalé certains médicaments par des différents degrés, c'est le degré supérieur, qui a été adopté au Répertoire synthétique.

L'importance du degré de la valeur de chaque médicament a été rendue par des caractères d'imprimerie différenciés. Les médicaments au **premier** degré, donc moins typiques et moins vérifiés, sont indiqués en minuscules. Ceux du **deuxième** degré, en caractères gras, mais minuscules. Enfin, ceux en grands caractères gras et en majuscules, correspondent au **troisième** degré. Quant à ceux au quatrième degré signalés par P. Schmidt, ils sont également en gros caractéres, mais en plus, soulignés. On se rend compte ainsi de la complexité des problèmes qui se sont présentés aux auteurs pour la rédaction claire et précise de chaque symptôme et de leur valorisation. L'incorporation des médicaments dans le système graduel du Répertoire synthétique, selon leurs sources et leurs valeurs, a posé des questions et des difficultés véritablement considérables.

Le titre principal de chaque rubrique est imprimé en lettres grasses majuscules et dans la sous-rubrique, en grasses minuscules, alors que les indications horaires et journalières ainsi que des symptômes accessoires le sont en caractères ordinaires. Toute rubrique principale commence à la ligne, le premier retrait concerne les sous-rubriques, avec un retrait supplémentaire pour des modalités ; tout cela dépendant bien sûr de la rubrique principale. Certains titres ont été rendus plus compréhensibles par des synonymes et les rubriques concernant les illusions et les rêves rendues plus claires en utilisant l'indicatif et infinitif. Le titre des rubriques et de chaque symptôme (à part les heures et les termes latins) sont trilingues, soit en anglais, français et allemand. Les titres anglais ont été rapportés de la littérature le plus souvent anglo-saxonne, sans que certains « américanismes » aient pu être modifiés. Si les dénominations n'étaient pas déjà indiquées de sources françaises ou allemandes, la plupart d'entre elles ont dû être traduites ici de la langue « anglo-américaine ».

La primauté accordée aux titres anglais, vient de l'importance de la littérature homoeopathique et de la langue anglaise en tant que langue mondiale, le français représentant les langues de l'Amerique latine et des pays méditerranéens.

Communes à tous les idiomes, les modalités d'aggravation et d'amélioration sont indiquées par « agg. » et « am. », soit par le substantif ou par le verbe.

Pour faciliter les recherches, les pages sont divisées en deux colonnes, dont chacune possède un numéro de page.

Les Francophones et les Germanophones trouveront à la fin de chaque volume un Index dans leur langue respective avec le numéro de la colonne correspondant à la rubrique cherchée. L'astérisque ajouté aux titres des symptômes renvoie à une des 138 nouvelles rubriques collectives de l'index de vol. I et II.

Les synonymes, ainsi que des renvois facilitant les recherches, sont indiqués dans les trois langues.

Le Répertoire médicamenteux est placé en tête du volume ; il donne la liste des remèdes homoeopathiques par ordre alphabétique de leurs abréviations.

Ce Répertoire synthétique contient 1594 médicaments homoeopathiques, soit 1002 en plus que ceux signalés dans le Répertoire de Kent, qui n'en contient que 591. Certains médicaments inaccoutumés (comme Ophiotoxicon, Electricitas, Galvanismus, Magnes artificialis) et toute la série des médicaments complexes, n'ont pas été inclus dans ce Répertoire.

Il ne faut pas oublier que la nomenclature des médicaments homoeopathiques repose sur une tradition de plus de 170 ans et a été exprimée dans la terminologie latine. C'est là une nécessité pour la compréhension de la littérature homoeopathique ancienne. De ce fait, elle possède droit de priorité vis-à-vis des dénominations pharmacologiques modernes.

Pour des raisons pratiques, les abréviations indiquées par Kent, dans son grand Répertoire, ont été conservées en général, malgré quelques inconséquences comme par exemple Arg-m. et Nat-m.

Seules quelques abréviations de remèdes secondaires chez Kent ont été changées; par exemple Nat-ar. au lieu du Nat-a. de Kent, pour normaliser ces mots abrégés.

Les abréviations des remèdes que nous avons ajoutés et n'existant pas chez Kent, ont été établies selon son mode d'abréviation, en évitant ce qu'on trouve dans Clarke, qui supprime trop souvent les voyelles.

De plus, les fautes typographiques des abréviations des médicaments, signalées pour certains d'entre eux dans la littérature homoeopathique, ont été corrigées.

Ce Répertoire synthétique constitue, en fait – par l'exposition des symptômes généraux – une véritable synthèse des connaissances homoeopathiques de ces dernières 170 années.

Grâce à l'internationalisation de la nomenclature médicamenteuse et des symptômes en trois langues, ce Répertoire permettra aux médecins du monde entier de mieux se comprendre, car l'union linguistique des médecins homoeopathes ne peut être réalisée que grâce à l'adoption, pour les symptômes comme pour les médicaments, d'une nomenclature commune.

Dr. med. Horst Barthel
Alte Römerstraße 70
D-6901 Wilhelmsfeld

Dr. med. Will Klunker
Am Rosenberg 1375
CH-9410 Heiden

VORWORT

Der Plan einer Ergänzung und Weiterführung des Kentschen Repertoriums führte im Verlauf von Jahren über verschiedene Zwischenkonzeptionen zu dem jetzigen Synthetischen Repertorium. Die Wiederaufnahme des primär gewählten Titels ergab sich aus einer dreifachen Synthese: der Ergänzung aus der älteren bis neuesten homöopathischen Literatur, der Zusammenstellung von Sachgruppen sowie dreisprachigen Indizes und aus der Tatsache, daß die Homöopathie als ein apriorisches, gewisses, mathematisches Heilverfahren einen synthetischen Charakter besitzt.

Der Fortschritt der Homöopathie vollzieht sich einerseits in der Sammlung sowie praxisgerechten Zusammenstellung der Materia medica zum Repertorium und andererseits in der Hinzugewinnung neuer gesicherter Arzneimittelsymptome. Deshalb bitten die Verfasser alle Kollegen, an der zunehmenden Verifizierung von Arzneimittelsymptomen mitzuarbeiten. Gebeten wird überdies um Mithilfe bei der Beseitigung von teils aus den Quellen übernommenen, teils trotz aller Sorgfalt den Verfassern unterlaufenen Fehlern.

Die Dreisprachigkeit brachte für die deutschsprachigen Verfasser Übersetzungsprobleme mit sich. Die englischen Titel konnten meistens aus den Originalarbeiten übernommen werden. Herr Dr. Pierre Schmidt, Genf, hat mit größter Kompetenz die sehr schwierige Übersetzung der Gemütssymptome übernommen. Für diesen Band hat er außerdem Vorwort und Einleitung ins Französische übersetzt. Auch die französischen Formulierungen des III. Bandes zogen aus seiner kritischen Durchsicht Gewinn. In ihren wärmsten Dank für die Arbeit an der Übersetzung schließen die Verfasser noch den Dank für die Ratschläge und die Sympathie ein, womit Dr. P. Schmidt das Entstehen des Werkes begleitet hat. Herrn Dr. Roger Schmidt und Herrn Alain Naude in San Franzisko sind wir für die wesentliche Verbesserung der englischen Übersetzung von Vorwort und Einleitung zu Dank verpflichtet.

Herr Dr. med. Jacques Baur, Lyon, hat nicht nur die französische Übersetzung der Titel in Band II übernommen, sondern auch die neu ergänzten Symptome übersetzt. Ihm sei für seine wertvolle Hilfe ausdrücklich gedankt.

Die Verfasser danken Herrn Dr. med. Jost Künzli von Fimelsberg, St. Gallen, für die Erlaubnis, seine Nachträge aus der klassischen homöopathischen Literatur in seinem Kent für die Neuauflage übernehmen zu dürfen. Damit wird eine langjährige und entsagungsvolle Bemühung um die Quellen, vor allem um die Arzneimittellehren Hahnemanns selbst, der Öffentlichkeit zugänglich gemacht.

Herrn Dr. med. Artur Braun und Herrn cand. med. Klaus-Henning Gypser ist für Korrekturen zu Band III zu danken. Für die neuen französischen Rubriken in Band III leistete Herr Martin Weber, Genf, dankenswerte Übersetzungshilfe.

Herrn Dr. Herbert Schindler, Karlsruhe, der sich um die internationale Nomenklatur homöopathischer Arzneimittel besonders verdient gemacht hat, verdanken die Verfasser zahlreiche Auskünfte sowie Korrekturen und die Schlußkontrolle des Arzneimittelverzeichnisses.

Von den Autoren der aufgenommenen Werke können die Verfasser den Herren Dr. O. A. Julian, Paris, Dr. J. Mezger †, Stuttgart, Dr. P. Schmidt, Genf, und Dr. J. Stephenson, New York, für die freundliche Erlaubnis der Benutzung danken. Ebenso gilt unser Dank den Verlagen Peyronnet in Paris, Roy & Co. in Bombay und Ternet-Martin in Vienne (Isère).

Herr Dr. E. Fischer als Verleger und Herr Sieber als Herstellungsleiter haben, indem sie den Vorschlägen der Verfasser zur Druck- und Buchgestaltung in großzügigster Weise entsprachen, eine optimale Praktikabilität des Werkes ermöglicht. Ihnen gebührt deshalb ganz besonderer Dank.

EINLEITUNG

Die Notwendigkeit des Repertoriums ergibt sich aus dem Wesen der Homöopathie selbst. Homöopathie ist ärztliches Handeln nach dem Ä h n l i c h k e i t s - g e s e t z Hahnemanns (1755–1843): similia similibus curentur. Nach diesem Gesetz haben sich Arzneibild des Mittels und wahlanzeigendes Symptomenbild des Patienten optimal zu entsprechen. Gesucht ist also das Simillimum für den Patienten.

Für die Lehre der Homöopathie ordnet die Materia medica homoeopathica die Ergebnisse der Arzneimittelprüfungen und der klinischen Beobachtungen nach Mitteln. Die Arzneiwahl in der Praxis dagegen erfordert die Ordnung der Mittel nach den Symptomen. Diese Aufgabe wird vom Repertorium übernommen. Es ist also die für den Praxisgebrauch zweckmäßige Umkehrung der Arzneimittellehre. Bringt die M a t e r i a m e d i c a die S y m p t o m e d e r M i t t e l, so das R e p e r t o r i u m die M i t t e l d e r S y m p t o m e. Die Lehre von den Arzneimitteln und die Therapie nach den Symptomen mit Hilfe des Repertoriums ergänzen sich gegenseitig.

Die Arzneimittelsymptome waren schon in den Anfängen der Homöopathie unübersehbar angewachsen und gedächtnismäßig nicht mehr vollständig zu behalten. Deshalb hat schon Hahnemann 1817 das erste seiner beiden „Symptomen-Lexika", also das erste Repertorium, ausgearbeitet. Gegenüber der Zufälligkeit der teilweisen gedächtnismäßigen Verfügbarkeit der Materia medica ermöglicht das Repertorium jederzeit die Arzneiwahl aufgrund des umfassend dargestellten homöopathischen Wissens.

Bis jetzt sind etwa 110 Repertorien veröffentlicht worden. J. T. Kent (1849 bis 1916) hat mit dem „Repertory of the Homoeopathic Materia Medica" von allen das zweckmäßigste, vollständigste und zuverlässigste Werk verfaßt. Kent benutzte ältere Werke der Materia medica und klinische Beobachtungen, ließ aber zahlreiche noch nicht genügend bestätigte Symptome und Mittel weg. Bis zu seinem Tode ergänzte er in seinen eigenen Exemplaren handschriftlich Symptome sowie Arzneimittel und stufte Mittel nach seinen Erfahrungen in einen anderen Grad ein.

Die ständige Weiterführung des Repertoriums fordert einerseits, die im Repertorium Kents nicht angeführten Symptome und Mittel nicht nur zu bewahren, sondern auch durch Heilungen zu bestätigen. Auf der anderen Seite gilt es, die Erst- und Wiederholungsprüfungen neuerer Autoren zusätzlich verfügbar zu machen.

Die sich aus den Ergänzungen der Allgemein- und Teilsymptome ergebende Materialfülle zwingt zur Entscheidung, ob die Zahl der Autoren und Rubriken eingeschränkt oder nur die Allgemeinsymptome dargestellt werden sollen. Diese entscheiden aber in der Arzneiwahl für chronisch Erkrankte. Deshalb beschränkt sich das hier vorgelegte S y n t h e t i s c h e R e p e r t o r i u m nur auf die A l l - g e m e i n s y m p t o m e. Für die Teilsymptome bildet das Repertorium Kents weiterhin das beste Nachschlagewerk.

Entsprechend der Hierarchisierung der Allgemeinsymptome ist das Synthetische Repertorium in folgende drei Bände gegliedert: Band I enthält das Kapitel der Gemütssymptome. Band II umfaßt das Kapitel der Allgemeinsymptome im engeren Sinne. Für die Nahrungsmittel und Getränke sind die auf verschiedene Kapitel und Rubriken des Kentschen Repertoriums verteilten Symptome von Verschlimmerung, Besserung, Abneigung und Verlangen zu einem einzigen Abschnitt zusammengestellt. Band III bringt die Kapitel der Schlafsymptome und Träume sowie der männlichen und weiblichen Sexualsymptome.

Quellen für das Synthetische Repertorium

1 = KENT, J. T.: In der Evolution des Repertoriums hat Kents Repertory wegen seines Inhaltsreichtums und logischen Aufbaus, seines Maßhaltens zwischen Verallgemeinerungs- und Differenzierungstendenzen anderer Autoren, seiner Verläßlichkeit und Praktikabilität einen Gipfel erreicht. Es hat sich seit über 70 Jahren in aller Welt bewährt; es liegt englisch in der 6. amerikanischen und 3. indischen Auflage vor. Davon gibt es eine auszugsweise französische Übersetzung; eine deutsche Übersetzung erschien 1971 in 2. Auflage. Die Kapitel und Rubriken der genannten Allgemeinsymptome wurden vollständig übernommen. Bei der Bearbeitung erkannte Fehler wurden verbessert. Als weitere Quellen wurden Kents „Lectures on Homoeopathic Materia Medica" und „New Remedies" herangezogen.

2 = KNERR, C. B.: Mit den zehnbändigen „Guiding Symptoms" hat C. Hering eine klassische, durch klinische Erfahrungen bereicherte Arzneimittellehre geschrieben. Herings Schüler Knerr hat dieses Werk in ein zweibändiges Repertorium umgestaltet. Dieses nach Modalitäten und klinischen Symptomen sehr detaillierte Erfahrungsmaterial ist aber wegen seiner unübersichtlichen Anordnung schwierig zugänglich, ein Nachteil, der durch das Synthetische Repertorium wegfällt.

3 = VON BOENNINGHAUSEN, C.; BOGER, C. M.: Das im Auftrag Hahnemanns von v. Boenninghausen verfaßte Repertorium wurde zum ersten publizierten homöopathischen Repertorium überhaupt. Es ist noch heute in Gebrauch. Dem Synthetischen Repertorium wurde die englische Übersetzung und Erweiterung C. M. Bogers zugrundegelegt. Die Verallgemeinerungstendenz mit der Aufnahme aller Mittel aus den Modalitäten in die Hauptrubrik und aus den lokalen in die Allgemeinsymptome ist bei der Benutzung dieser Zitate zu berücksichtigen.

In der 2. Auflage wurden die „Additions to Kent's Repertory" und das Repertorium aus „A Synoptic Key of the Materia Medica" von C. M. Boger aufgenommen. Aus technischen Gründen wurden diese Zusätze ohne eigene Kennzeichnung durch die Ziffer 3 kenntlich gemacht.

4 = JAHR, G. H. G.: Sein 1848–49 erschienenes, nicht mehr erhältliches „Systematisch-alphabetisches Repertorium der Homöopathischen Arzneimittellehre" zeichnet sich durch Symptomenreichtum aus. Es ist aber wegen seiner Aufsplitterung in Synonyma und seiner Anordnungsweise unpraktisch.

5 = GALLAVARDIN, J. P.: Die von Dulac aus den Werken Jahrs vermittelten Indikationen für die Behandlung psychisch Kranker hat Gallavardin in seiner Sprechstunde für Gemütskranke geprüft und erweitert. Als Quellen dienten das Repertorium und die Arzneimittellehre des postum veröffentlichten Werks „Psychisme et Homoeopathie".

6 = STAUFFER, K.: Das „Symptomen-Verzeichnis" repräsentiert die große und kritisch kontrollierte Praxiserfahrung Stauffers. Es vermittelt neben Verifikationen von Arzneimittelsymptomen ebenfalls Neuzugänge der Materia medica.

7 = SCHMIDT, P.: Die Ergänzungen von 35 Autoren in seine vier Kentschen Repertorien sind vollständig übernommen. Weitere Zusätze haben sich aus den

Kursen des „Groupement Hahnmannien de Lyon" ergeben, die in den Rechen-schaftsberichten dieser Tagungen niedergelegt sind. P. Schmidts Nachfolge und indirekte Schülerschaft Kents sowie seine fünfzigjährige Praxiserfahrung berechtigen ihn zu Höherwertungen der Grade und zur Einführung des 4. Grades für Arzneimittel einzelner Symptome. Diese haben sich ihm vor allem dann bewährt, wenn sich mangels differenzierender Symptome keine andere Mittelwahl innerhalb der Rubrik ergibt.

8 = BOERICKE, O. E.: Aus der Materia Medica von W. Boericke, einer der im englischen Sprachraum häufig gebrauchten Arzneimittellehren, hat O. E. Boericke ein Repertorium angefertigt. Es bietet den Vorteil einer Vielzahl seltener und neuerer Mittel der angelsächsischen Literatur. Aber es enthält keine Liste der Mittelabkürzungen sowie Fehler in der Nomenklatur der Mittel und komplexe Symptome. Seine Gliederung ist nicht immer folgerichtig.

9 = STEPHENSON, J.: Das entsprechend dem Kentschen Repertorium übersichtlich aufgebaute Werk enthält Arzneimittelprüfungen aus den Jahren 1924–59, die vorwiegend aus dem angelsächsischen und deutschen Sprachraum stammen.

10 = MEZGER, J.: Aus dem kritischen Werk „Gesichtete Homöopathische Arzneimittellehre" werden die Symptome von 35 nachgeprüften oder neuen Mitteln verwendet. .

11 = ALLEN, T. F.: Zur zehnbändigen „Encyclopedia of Pure Materia Medica", die nur Prüfungssymptome enthält, besteht ein zweibändiger Index „A General Symptom Register of the Homoeopathic Materia Medica", der in den einschlägigen Teilen dem Synthetischen Repertorium eingefügt wurde. Damit werden ältere Prüfungssymptome für künftige Verifizierungen zugänglich gemacht. Er enthält auch zahlreiche seltene Mittel.

12 = CLARKE, J. H.: „A Clinical Repertory to the Dictionary of Materia Medica" aus seiner dreibändigen Arzneimittellehre, auch heute noch einer der besten, gibt vorwiegend klinische Indikationen und auch seltene Mittel.

13 = NEUESTE ARZNEIMITTELPRUFUNGEN, die in einzelnen Zeitschriften veröffentlicht wurden.

14 = JULIAN, O. A.: Seine 1971 erschienene große „Matière Médicale d'Homéothérapie" ist die bis heute vollständigste Zusammenfassung der Arzneiprüfungen neuester Zeit unter Berücksichtigung des internationalen Schrifttums. Sie wurde noch nach teilweisem Abschluß der Manuskripte aufgenommen. In dieser 2. Auflage wurden außerdem die ca. 30 zusätzlichen neuen Mittel berücksichtigt, die Dr. Julian in der Neuauflage unter dem Titel „Dictionnaire de Matière Médicale de 130 Nouveaux Homéothérapeutiques" (Masson, Paris) 1981 publiziert hat.

15 = KUNZLI, J.: Nachträge aus der internationalen homöopathischen Literatur.

16 = HAHNEMANN, S.: Reine Arzneimittellehre und Chronische Krankheiten. Im Kent noch fehlende Symptome und Mittel wurden entsprechend den Nachträgen von J. Künzli ergänzt.

Das nicht näher definierte Tuberkulin der Autoren 2, 6, 7, 8 wird wie das tuberculinum bovinum Kent mit tub. abgekürzt.

Das Synthetische Repertorium gibt erstmalig die exakte Quellenangabe für jedes zum Repertorium Kents zugefügte Symptom bzw. Mittel durch beigefügte K e n n z i f f e r n an. Symptome und Mittel des Kentschen Repertoriums blieben unbezeichnet. Mit [1] sind die handschriftlichen Ergänzungen Kents, mit [1'] Zufügungen aus seinen „Lectures" und „New Remedies" gekennzeichnet. Die Ziffern [2-14] sind mit der Numerierung der obigen Quellen identisch. Nach P. Schmidt berechtigen seine und Gallavardins Erfahrungen, einzelne Mittel Kents in einem höheren Grad einzustufen. Diese Mittel sind durch beide Ziffern, also [1, 5] oder [1, 7] bezeichnet. Aufgrund der Quellenangaben kann der Benutzer jedem Autor das Gewicht beimessen, das er ihm zubilligt und Mittelindikationen aus der Praxiserfahrung heraus kritisch prüfen und bestätigen.

Die eigenhändigen Korrekturen Kents in seinem, später in den Besitz von Dr. Pierre Schmidt übergegangenen Repertorium, die jetzt von D. H. Chand im „Kent's Final General Repertory" (New Delhi, 1980) publiziert worden sind, sind bereits in der 1. Auflage des Synthetischen Repertoriums enthalten, so daß dieses neue Repertorium nicht mehr berücksichtigt zu werden brauchte.

In den Quellen fanden sich für die Arzneimittel unterschiedliche G r a d e i n - t e i l u n g e n. Diese wurden mit einer gewissen Freiheit den drei Graden von Kent angeglichen. Da bei den aus mehreren Werken ergänzten Mitteln nicht auch die jeweiligen Grade genannt werden konnten, wurde das Mittel entsprechend seiner zunehmenden Bestätigung in den höchsten vorkommenden Grad gesetzt.

Im D r u c k sind die Grade der Arzneimittel augenfällig differenziert. Die Mittel des 1. und 2. Grades werden in Kleinbuchstaben, die des 2., 3. und 4. Grades fett, die des 3. und 4. Grades in Großbuchstaben gesetzt; der 4. Grad wird außerdem unterstrichen.

Sowohl die Übertragung der Mittel in das Gradsystem des Synthetischen Repertoriums als auch die Übertragung der verschiedenartigen Symptomenanordnungen aus den Quellen in ein möglichst optimal differenzierendes Rubrikensystem stellten die größten Entscheidungsschwierigkeiten für die Verfasser dar.

Die R u b r i k e n sind durch Drucktypen, Einrückungen und Zwischenabstände gegliedert. Das Stichwort des Symptomentitels ist in der Hauptrubrik durch fette Großbuchstaben und in der Unterrubrik durch bloßen Fettdruck gekennzeichnet, während die Tages- und Uhrzeiten sowie weitere Unterrubriken normal gedruckt sind. Die Hauptrubriken beginnen am Zeilenanfang; die erste Einrückung betrifft deren Unterrubriken und die zweite wieder deren Unterrubriken. Jeder eingerückte Symptomtitel übernimmt das Stichwort des übergeordneten Titels. Unter den Symptomtiteln stehen in Einrückung im normalen Zeilenabstand die Arzneimittel, so daß beide eine Einheit bilden.

Die Titel wurden zum Teil durch Ergänzungen verdeutlicht, andererseits bei Wahnideen (Band I) und Träumen (Band III) durch Gebrauch des Indikativs oder Infinitivs vereinfacht.

Die Rubriken- oder Symptomtitel sind mit Ausnahme der Uhrzeiten und lateinischer Termini in Englisch, Französisch und Deutsch, also d r e i s p r a c h i g formuliert. Die englischen Titel wurden aus der zumeist angelsächsischen Literatur übernommen, ohne daß Amerikanismen geändert werden konnten. Die französischen und deutschen Titel mußten, soweit sie nicht in den französischen und deutschen Quellen vorformuliert waren, also im überwiegenden Anteil, für das Synthetische Repertorium aus dem Englisch-Amerikanischen übersetzt werden.

Die Voranstellung des englischen Titels folgte aus dem Gewicht der englischsprachigen Literatur und der englischen Sprache als einer Weltsprache. Französisch vertritt außerdem noch die Sprachen des lateinamerikanischen Kontinents und der Mittelmeerländer.

Die für alle Sprachen gemeinsamen Abkürzungen a g g. und a m. bedeuten die Modalitäten der Verschlechterung (aggravation, Aggravation) bzw. Besserung (amelioration, amélioration, Amelioration). Sie verstehen sich je nach Zusammenhang substantivisch oder verbal.

Für die französisch- und deutschsprachigen Benutzer wurde am Schluß jedes Bandes ein umfassender und übersichtlicher I n d e x zusammengestellt, mit dessen Hilfe die gesuchte Rubrik über die Spaltennumerierung des Repertoriums mühelos gefunden werden kann. Der englische Index konnte wegen der ohnehin alphabetischen Reihenfolge der englisch formulierten Symptome auf Synonyma und Crossreferences beschränkt werden (in Band I, II). Außerdem wird der Gebrauch des Repertoriums durch zahlreiche Hinweise unter den Symptomen und im Index zusätzlich erleichtert. Der Stern an den Symptomtiteln verweist auf die 138 neuen Sammelrubriken der Indizes von Band I und II.

Das A r z n e i m i t t e l v e r z e i c h n i s des Synthetischen Repertoriums bringt hinter den alphabetisch geordneten Abkürzungen die Mittel und deren gebräuchliche Synonyma. Es ist gegenüber dem Verzeichnis Kents mit 591 Mitteln auf 1594 Mittel angewachsen. Problematische Mittel wie Electricitas, Galvanismus, Magnes artificialis und das komplexe Schlangenmittel Ophiotoxicum wurden nicht aufgenommen. Doppelführungen, Unklarheiten und Fehler in der Nomenklatur wurden nach bestem Vermögen beseitigt. Die traditionelle Nomenklatur homöopathischer Arzneimittel besitzt aufgrund ihrer 170jährigen Geschichte ein eigenes Recht gegenüber den jeweils modernen pharmakologisch-pharmazeutischen Benennungen. Da die homöopathischen Mittel stets im gleichen Gebrauch geblieben sind, bleibt auch ihre ältere Literatur gültig und ist nur durch die traditionelle Nomenklatur zu verstehen.

Aus praktischen Gründen wurden die Abkürzungen Kents im allgemeinen trotz einiger Inkonsequenzen (zum Beispiel arg-m./nat-m.) beibehalten; nur inkonsequente Abkürzungen kleiner Mittel wurden geändert. Die unterschiedlichen Abkürzungen der Quellen bis hin zu den betont konsonantischen von Clarke wurden nach dem verständlicheren, betont vokalischen Modus Kents vereinheitlicht. Im ganzen Verzeichnis wurde nach Möglichkeit einheitlich abgekürzt, zum Beispiel ar. für das Anion arcenicosum (vgl. bei Kent kali-ar. mit nat-a.). Nach Möglichkeit wurden in der Literatur vorkommende Druckfehler in der Schreibweise der Arzneimittelabkürzungen verbessert.

Das Synthetische Repertorium stellt für den Bereich der Allgemeinsymptome eine S y n t h e s e h o m ö o p a t h i s c h e n W i s s e n s aus 170 Jahren dar. Es möchte durch die Internationalisierung der Nomenklatur von Arzneimitteln, durch .die Dreisprachigkeit der Symptome und der Indizes zur Verständigung unter den homöopathischen Ärzten der ganzen Welt beitragen. Denn die Sprachgemeinschaft homöopathischer Ärzte kann erst über gemeinsame Arznei- und Symptomenbezeichnungen entstehen.

Dr. med. Horst Barthel
Alte Römerstraße 70
D-6901 Wilhelmsfeld

Dr. med. Will Klunker
Am Rosenberg 1375
CH-9410 Heiden

BIBLIOGRAPHY/BIBLIOGRAPHIE/BIBLIOGRAPHIE

1 KENT, J. T.: Repertory of the Homoepathic Materia Medica. 6th Edition, Ehrhart & Chicago (1957)

Kent's Repertorium der homöopathischen Arzneimittel. Herausgegeben von G. v. Keller und J. Künzli von Fimelsberg. 2., verb. Auflage, Karl F. Haug Verlag, Heidelberg (1971)

KENT, J. T.: Lectures on Homoeopathic Materia Medica. 1st ind. Edition, M. Bhattacharyya, Calcutta (1965)

KENT, J. T.: New Remedies. Ind. Edition, Sett Dey & Co., Calcutta (1963) pp. 1—151

2 KNERR, C. B.: A Repertory of Hering's Guiding Symptoms of our Materia Medica. M. Bhattacharyya, Calcutta (1951)

3 BOGER, C. M.: Boenninghausens's Characteristics and Repertory. 2nd Edition, Roy & Co., Bombay (1952)

BOGER, C. M.: Additions to Kent's Repertory. Jain Publishing Co., Chuna Mandi, Paharganj, New Delhi-55 (1972)

BOGER, C. M.: A Synoptic Key of the Materia Medica. Salzer & Co., Calcutta 6th Edition

4 JAHR, G. H. G.: Systematisch-alphabetisches Repertorium der Homöopathischen Arzneimittellehre. Herrmann Bethmann, Leipzig (1848)

5 GALLAVARDIN, J.-P.: Psychisme et Homoeopathie. Ed. Ternet-Martin, Vienne (Isère) (1960)

6 STAUFFER, K.: Symptomen-Verzeichnis nebst vergleichenden Zusätzen zur Homöopathischen Arzneimittellehre. Joh. Sonntag, Regensburg (1951)

7 SCHMIDT, P.: Annotations in Kent's Repertory/Annotations dans le Repertoire de Kent/Anmerkungen in Kents Repertorium

SCHMIDT, P.: passim in: Groupement Hahnemannien de Lyon, Comptes rendus des réunions

8 BOERICKE, O. E.: Repertory; in: W. Boericke, Pocket Manual of Homoeopathic Materia Medica. 9th Edition, Boericke & Runyon, New York (1927)

9 STEPHENSON, J.: A Materia Medica and Repertory, Hahnemannian Provings 1924—1959. Roy & Co., Bombay (1963)

10 MEZGER, J.: Gesichtete Homöopathische Arzneimittellehre. 3. Auflage, Karl F. Haug Verlag, Ulm (1964, 1966)

11 ALLEN, T. F.: Index ("A General Symptom Register of the Homoeopathic Materia Medica"); in: The Encyclopedia of Pure Materia Medica, vol. XI, Gregg Press Inc., Ridgewood N. J. (1964)

12 CLARKE, J. H.: A Clinical Repertory to the Dictionary of Materia Medica. The Homoeopathic Publishing Comp., London (1904)

13 KLUNKER, W.: Eine Arzneiprüfung von Espeletia grandiflora. Allg. homöop. Ztg. 217: 5—14 (1972)

KLUNKER, W.: Zu den Rubriken der Säuglings- und Stillbeschwerden im Kentschen Repertorium, Ztschrft. f. Klass. Homöop. Bd. 17/6, 269—272 (1973)

LODISPOTO, A.: Diät und Homöopathie, Ztschrft. f. Klass. Homöop. Bd IV/3, 95-141 (1960)

SÉROR, R.: Pathogénésies homéopathiques françaises. Cahiers de Biothér. (1966), 79—86

14 JULIAN, O. A.: Matière Médicale d'Homéotherapie. Peyronnet, Paris (1971). Dictionnaire de Matière Médicale de 130 Nouveaux Homéothérapeutiques. Masson, Paris (1981)

15 KÜNZLI, J.: Nachträge aus der internationalen homöopathischen Literatur

16 HAHNEMANN, S.: Reine Arzneimittellehre. 3., vermehrte Auflage. Dresden und Leipzig (1830), Nachdruck Karl F. Haug Verlag, Heidelberg (1979)

HAHNEMANN, S.: Die chronischen Krankheiten. 2., vermehrte Auflage. Dresden und
Leipzig (1835), Nachdruck Karl F. Haug Verlag, Heidelberg (1979)

REMEDIES AND THEIR ABBREVIATIONS
LES REMÈDES ET LEURS ABRÉVIATIONS
ARZNEIMITTEL UND IHRE ABKÜRZUNGEN

abel.	abelmoschus (= hibiscus abelmoschus)	agar.	agaricus muscarius (= amanita muscaria)
abies-c.	abies (pinus) canadensis	agar-cit.	agaricus citrinus
abies-n.	abies nigra	agar-cpn.	agaricus campanulatus
abr.	abrus precatorius (= **jequirity**)	agar-cps.	agaricus campestris
		agar-em.	agaricus emeticus
abrot.	abrotanum (= artemisia **abrotanum**)	agar-pa.	agaricus pantherinus
		agar-ph.	agaricus phalloides (= amanita phalloides)
absin.	absinthium (= artemisia absinthium)		
acal.	acalypha indica	agar-pr.	agaricus procerus
	acanthia lectularia = cimx.	agar-se.	agaricus semiglobatus
		agar-st.	agaricus stercorarius
	acarus = trom.	agar-v.	agaricus vernus (= amanita verna)
	acer negundo = neg.		
acet-ac.	aceticum acidum	agarin.	agaricinum
acetan.	acetanilidum (= antifebrinum)	agav-a.	agave americana
		agav-t.	agave tequilana
	achillea millefolium = mill.	agn.	agnus castus
achy.	achyranthes calea	agra.	agraphis nutans
	acokanthera schimperi = car.	agre.	agremone ochroleuca
		agri.	agrimonia eupatoria
acon.	aconitum napellus		agropyrum repens = tritic.
acon-a.	aconitum anthora		
acon-c.	aconitum cammarum	agro.	agrostema githago
acon-f.	aconitum ferox	ail.	ailanthus glandulosa
acon-l.	aconitum lycoctonum	alco.	alcoholus (= aethanolum)
acon-s.	aconitum septentrionale	ald.	aldehydum
aconin.	aconitinum	alet.	aletris farinosa
	actaea racemosa = cimic.	alf.	alfalfa (= medicago sativa)
			alkekengi = physal.
act-sp.	actaea spicata	all-c.	allium cepa (= cepa)
adel.	Adelheid aqua	all-s.	allium sativum
adeps-s.	adeps suis	allox.	alloxanum
adlu.	adlumia fungosa	aln.	alnus rubra (serrulata)
adon.	adonis vernalis	aloe	aloe socotrina
adonin.	adonidinum	alst.	alstonia constricta
adox.	adoxa moschatellina	alst-s.	alstonia scholaris
adren.	adrenalinum	alth.	althaea officinalis
	adrenocorticotropinum = cortico.	alum.	alumina (= argilla)
		alum-p.	alumina phosphorica
aesc.	aesculus hippocastanum	alum-sil.	alumina silicata (= bolus alba = kaolinum)
aesc-g.	aesculus glabra		
	aethanolum = alco.	alumin.	aluminium metallicum
aeth.	aethusa cynapium	alumin-a.	aluminium aceticum
aether	aether	alumin-m.	aluminium muriaticum
aethi-a.	aethiops antimonialis	alumn.	alumen
aethi-m.	aethiops mineralis (= mercurius sulphuratus niger = mercurius cum kali)		alumen chromicum = kali-s-chr.
			amanita muscaria = agar.
			amanita phalloides = agar-ph.
aethyl-n.	aethylium nitricum		
	aethylium nitrosum = nit-s-d.		amanita verna = agar-v.

am-a.	ammonium aceticum	anil-s.	anilinum sulphuricum
	ammonium auricum	anis.	anisum stellatum
	= aur-fu.		(= illicium stellatum)
am-be.	ammonium benzoicum		antifebrinum = acetan.
am-br.	ammonium bromatum	ant-ar.	antimonium arsenicosum
am-c.	ammonium carbonicum	ant-c.	antimonium crudum
am-caust.	ammonium causticum		(= antimonium
	(hydratum)		sulphuratum nigrum)
am-i.	ammonium iodatum	ant-i.	antimonium iodatum
am-m.	ammonium muriaticum	ant-m.	antimonium muriaticum
am-n.	ammonium nitricum	ant-o.	antimonium oxydatum
am-p.	ammonium phosphoricum	ant-s-aur.	antimonium sulphuratum
am-pic.	ammonium picricum		auratum (aureum,
am-t.	ammonium tartaricum		aurantiacum)
am-val.	ammonium valerianicum		antimonium sulphuratum
am-van.	ammonium vanadinicum		nigrum = ant-c.
ambr.	ambra grisea	ant-t.	antimonium tartaricum
ambro.	ambrosia artemisiaefolia		(= tartarus emeticus)
amgd-p.	amygdalus persica	anth.	anthemis nobilis
	(= persica amygdalus)		(= chamomilla romana)
aml-ns.	amylenum nitrosum	antho.	anthoxanthum odoratum
ammc.	ammoniacum gummi	anthraci.	anthracinum
amn-l.	amnii liquor	anthraco.	anthracokali
amor-r.	amorphophallus rivieri	antip.	antipyrinum
ampe-qu.	ampelopsis quinquefolia	ap-g.	apium graveolens
ampe-tr.	ampelopsis trifoliata	ap-v	apium virus
amph.	amphisbaena vermicularis	aphis	aphis chenopodii glauci
amyg.	amygdalae amarae aqua		(= chenopodii glauci aphis)
amylam.	amylaminum	apiol.	apiolum
	hydrochloricum	apis	apis mellifica
anac.	anacardium orientale	apisin.	apisinum (= apium virus)
anac-oc.	anacardium occidentale	apoc.	apocynum cannabinum
anag.	anagallis arvensis	apoc-a.	apocynum
anagy.	anagyris foetida		androsaemifolium
anan.	anantherum muricatum	apom.	apomorphinum
	(= cuscus)		hydrochloricum
	ancistrodon mokeson	aq-calc.	aqua calcarea
	= cench.	aq-chl.	aqua chlorata
	andira inermis = geo.		aqua glandium quercus
	andromeda arborea		= querc.
	= oxyd.	aq-mar.	aqua marina
andr.	androsace lactea	aq-pet.	aqua petra
ane-n.	anemone nemorosa		aqua regia = nit-m-ac.
	anemone pratensis = puls.	aq-sil.	aqua silicata
ane-r.	anemone ranunculoides	aqui.	aquilegia vulgaris
anemps.	anemopsis californica	arag.	aragallus lamberti
	(= yerba mansa)	aral.	aralia racemosa
ang.	angustura vera (= galipea	aral-h.	aralia hispida
	cusparia)		aralia quinquefolia = gins.
ange.	angelica atropurpurea		aranea avicularia = mygal.
ange-s.	radix angelicae sinensis	aran.	aranea diadema
ango.	angophora lanceolata		(= diadema aranea)
	angustura spuria = bruc.	aran-ix.	aranea ixobola
anh.	anhalonium lewinii	aran-sc.	aranea scinencia
	(= lophophora williamsii		araneae tela = tela
	= peyotl)	aranin.	araninum
anil.	anilinum	arb.	arbutus andrachne
		arbin.	arbutinum
			arctium lappa = lappa

arec.	areca catechu	asper.	asperula odorata
aren.	arenaria glabra		aspidium filix-mas = fil.
arg-cy.	argentum cyanatum		aspidium panna = pann.
arg-i.	argentum iodatum		aspidosperma quebracho
arg-m.	argentum metallicum		= queb.
arg-mur.	argentum muriaticum		assaku = hura
arg-n.	argentum nitricum	astac.	astacus (cancer) fluviatilis
arg-o.	argentum oxydatum	aster.	asterias rubens
arg-p.	argentum phosphoricum	astra-e.	astragalus excapus
arge.	argemone mexicana	astra-m.	astragalus menziesii
	argilla = alum.	atha.	athamanta oreoselinum
arist-cl.	aristolochia clematitis	atra-r.	atrax robustus
arist-co.	aristolochia colombiana	atri.	atriplex hortensis
arist-m.	aristolochia milhomens		atropa belladonna = bell.
	aristolochia serpentaria	atro.	atropinum purum aut
	= serp.		sulphuricum
	armoracia sativa = coch.		aurantium = cit-v.
arn.	arnica montana	aur.	aurum foliatum
ars.	arsenicum album		(metallicum) aut aurum
ars-br.	arsenicum bromatum		colloidale
ars-h.	arsenicum hydrogenisatum	aur-ar.	aurum arsenicicum
ars-i.	arsenicum iodatum	aur-br.	aurum bromatum
ars-met.	arsenicum metallicum	aur-fu.	aurum fulminans
ars-n.	arsenicum nitricum		(= ammonium auricum)
ars-s-f.	arsenicum sulphuratum	aur-i.	aurum iodatum
	flavum	aur-m.	aurum muriaticum
ars-s-r.	arsenicum sulphuratum	aur-m-k.	aurum muriaticum
	rubrum		kalinatum
	artanthe elongata = mati.	aur-m-n.	aurum muriaticum
	artemisia abrotanum		natronatum
	= abrot.	aur-s.	aurum sulphuratum
	artemisia absinthium	auran.	aurantii cortex
	= absin.	aven.	avena sativa
	artemisia maritima (cina)	aza.	azadirachta indica
	= cina		(= melia azadirachta
art-v.	artemisia vulgaris		indica)
arum-d.	arum dracontium	bac.	bacillinum Burnett
arum-dru.	arum dracunculus	bac-t.	baccillinum testium
arum-i.	arum italicum	bach	bacillus Bach-Paterson
arum-m.	arum maculatum		bacillus Calmette-Guérin
arum-t.	arum triphyllum		= v-a-b.
arund.	arundo mauritanica	bad.	badiaga
arund-d.	arundo donax	baj.	baja
asaf.	asa foetida		balsamum copaivae
	asagraea officinalis		= cop.
	= sabad.	bals-p.	balsamum peruvianum
asar.	asarum europaeum	bals-t.	balsamum tolutanum
asar-c.	asarum canadense	bapt.	baptisia tinctoria
asc-c.	asclepias cornuti (syriaca)	bapt-c.	baptisia confusa
asc-i.	asclepias incarnata	bar-a.	baryta acetica
asc-t.	asclepias tuberosa	bar-c.	baryta carbonica
	asclepias vincetoxicum	bar-i.	baryta iodata
	= vince.	bar-m.	baryta muriatica
asim.	asimina triloba	bar-p.	baryta phosphorica
	(= papaya vulgaris)	bar-s.	baryta sulphurica
ask.	askalabotes laevigatus	barb.	barbae cyprini ova
aspar.	asparagus officinalis	baros.	barosma crenulatum
			(= buchu)

bart.	Bartfelder aqua		bry.	bryonia alba aut dioica
	basaka = just.			buchu = baros.
bell.	belladonna (= atropa		bufo	bufo rana (= rana bufo)
	belladonna)		bufo-s.	bufo sahytiensis
bell-p.	bellis perennis		bung.	bungurus fasciatus
ben.	benzinum		buni-o.	bunias orientalis
ben-d.	benzinum dinitricum			bursa pastoris = thlas.
ben-n.	benzinum nitricum		but-ac.	butyricum acidum
benz-ac.	benzoicum acidum		buth-a.	buthus australis
benzo.	benzoinum oderiferum			(= prionurus australis)
benzol.	benzolum		buth-af.	buthus afer
berb.	berberis vulgaris		buth-oc.	buthus occitanus
berb-a.	berberis aquifolium		bux.	buxus sempervirens
	(= mahonia)		cac.	cacao (= theobroma
berbin.	berberinum			cacao)
beryl.	beryllium metallicum		cact.	cactus (selenicereus)
beta	beta vulgaris			grandiflorus
betin.	betainum muriaticum		cadm-br.	cadmium bromatum
beto.	betonica aquatica		cadm-i.	cadmium iodatum
betu.	betula alba		cadm-m.	cadmium muriaticum
bism.	bismuthum subnitricum		cadm-met.	cadmium metallicum
	(„oxidum" Hahnemann,		cadm-o.	cadmium oxydatum
	Kent)		cadm-s.	cadmium sulphuratum
bism-met.	bismuthum metallicum		cael.	caela zacatechichi
bism-o.	bismuthum oxydatum		caes.	caesium metallicum
bism-val.	bismuthum valerianicum			caffeinum = coffin.
bix.	bixa orellana		cain.	cainca (cahinca) racemosa
blatta	blatta orientalis			(= chiococca racemosa)
blatta-a.	blatta americana		caj.	cajuputum (= oleum
bol-la.	boletus laricis			cajuputi = oleum
	(= polyporus officinalis)			wittnebianum)
bol-lu.	boletus luridus			calabar = phys.
bol-s.	boletus satanas		cal-ren.	calculus (lapis) renalis
bold.	boldo (= peumus boldo)		calad.	caladium seguinum
	bolus alba = album-sil.		calag.	calaguala
bomb-chr.	bombyx chrysorrhea		calam.	calamus aromaticus
bomb-pr.	bombyx processionea		calc.	calcarea carbonica
bond.	Bondonneau aqua			Hahnemanni (= calcarea
bor.	borax veneta			ostrearum = conchae
bor-ac.	boricum acidum			praeparatae)
both.	bothrops lanceolatus		calc-a.	calcarea acetica
	(= lachesis lanceolatus)		calc-ar.	calcarea arsenicosa
botul.	botulinum		calc-br.	calcarea bromata
	bounafa = ferul.		calc-caust.	calcarea caustica
bov.	bovista lycoperdon		calc-chln.	calcarea chlorinata
brach.	brachyglottis repens		calc-f.	calcarea fluorica naturalis
bran.	branca ursina		calc-hp.	calcarea hypophosphorosa
brass.	brassica napus		calc-i.	calcarea iodata
	brayera anthelmintica		calc-lac.	calcarea lactica
	= kou.		calc-m.	calcarea muriatica
brom.	bromium			calcarea ostrearum = calc.
bruc.	brucea antidysenterica		calc-o-t.	calcarea ovi testae (= ovi
	(= angustura spuria)			testa = testa praeparata)
brucel.	brucella melitensis		calc-ox.	calcarea oxalica
brucin.	brucinum		calc-p.	calcarea phosphorica
	brugmansia candida		calc-pic.	calcarea picrica
	= dat-a.		calc-s.	calcarea sulphurica

calc-sil.	calcarea silicata	cast.	castoreum canadense
	calcarea silico-fluorica		aut sibiricum
	= lap-a.	cast-eq.	castor equi
calc-st-sula.	calcarea stibiato-	cast-v.	castanea vesca
	sulphurata	caste.	castella texana
	calcarea sulphurata	catal.	catalpa bignonoides
	Hahnemanni = hep.	catar.	cataria nepeta
calen.	**calendula officinalis**	caul.	caulophyllum
calli.	calliandra houstoni		thalictroides
	(= pambotano)	caust.	causticum Hahnemanni
	calomel = merc-d.	cean.	ceanothus americanus
calo.	calotropis gigantea	cean-tr.	ceanothus thrysiflorus
	(= madar)	cecr.	cecropia mexicana
calth.	caltha palustris	cedr.	cedron (= simaruba
camph.	camphora (= laurus		ferroginea)
	camphora)	celt.	celtis occidentalis
camph-ac.	camphoricum acidum	cench.	cenchris contortrix
camph-br.	camphora bromata		(= ancistrodon mokeson)
	cancer fluviatilis = astac.	cent.	centaurea tagana
canch.	canchalagua		cepa = all-c.
	(= erythraea chilensis)	ceph.	cephalanthus occidentalis
cann-i.	cannabis indica	cer-ox.	cerium oxalicum
cann-s.	cannabis sativa	cere-b.	cereus bonplandii
canna	canna angustifolia	cere-s.	cereus serpentinus
canth.	cantharis (lytta)	cerv.	cervus brasilicus
	vesicatoria		(campestris)
canthin.	cantharidinum	ceto.	cetonia aurata
capp.	capparis coriaccea	cetr.	cetraria islandica
	capsella bursa pastoris		(= lichen islandicus)
	= thlas.	cham.	chamomilla
caps.	capsicum annuum		**chamomilla romana** = anth.
	carbamidum = urea-n.	chamae.	chamaedrys (= teucrium
car.	carissa (acokanthera)		chamaedrys)
	schimperi	chap.	chaparro amargoso
carb-ac.	carbolicum acidum	chaul.	chaulmoogra
	(= phenolum)	cheir.	cheiranthus cheiri
carb-an.	carbo animalis	chel.	chelidonium majus
carb-v.	carbo vegetabilis	chel-g.	chelidonium glaucum
carbn.	carboneum	chelin.	chelidoninum
carbn-chl.	carboneum chloratum	chelo.	chelone glabra
carbn-h.	carboneum		chenopodii glauci
	hydrogenisatum		aphis = aphis
carbn-o.	carboneum oxygenisatum	chen-a.	chenopodium
carbn-s.	carboneum sulphuratum		anthelminticum
carc.	carcinosinum Burnett	chen-v.	chenopodium vulvaria
card-b.	carduus benedictus	chim.	chimaphila umbellata
card-m.	carduus marianus	chim-m.	chimaphila maculata
cardam.	cardamine pratensis	chin.	china officinalis (regia)
carl.	Carlsbad (Karlsbad) aqua		(= cinchona calisaya aut
caru.	carum carvi		cinchona succirubra)
cary.	carya alba	chin-ar.	chininum arsenicosum
cas-s.	cascara sagrada	chin-b.	china (cinchona) boliviana
	(= rhamnus purshiana)	chin-m.	chininum muriaticum
casc.	cascarilla	chin-s.	chininum sulphuricum
cass.	cassada (= manihot	chin-val.	chininum valerianicum
	utilissima)	chinid.	chinidinum
	cassia acutifolia = senn.		hydrochloricum
			chiococca racemosa = cain.

chion.	chionanthus virginica (americana)	cocc.	cocculus indicus
		cocc-s.	coccinella septempunctata
chlf.	chloroformium	coch.	cochlearia armoracia
chlol.	chloralum hydratum		(= armoracia sativa)
chlor.	chlorum	coch-o.	cochlearia officinalis
chloram.	chloramphenicolum	cod.	codeinum purum aut
chlorpr.	chlorpromazinum		phosphoricum aut
cho.	cholas terrapina		sulphuricum
chol.	cholesterinum	coff.	coffea cruda (arabica)
cholin.	cholinum	coff-t.	coffea tosta
chr-met.	chromium metallicum	coffin.	coffeinum (= caffeinum)
chr-ac.	chromicum acidum	colch.	colchicum autumnale
chr-o.	chromium oxydatum	colchin.	colchicinum
chr-s.	chromium sulphuricum	coli.	colibacillinum
chrys-ac.	chrysophanicum acidum	coll.	collinsonia canadensis
chrysan.	chrysanthemum leucanthemum	coloc.	colocynthis (= cucumis colocynthis = citrullus colocynthis)
chrysar.	chrysarobinum		
cic.	cicuta virosa	colocin.	colocynthinum
cic-m.	cicuta maculata	colos.	colostrum
cice.	cicer arietinum	com.	comocladia dentata
cich.	cichorium intybus		(= guao)
cimic.	cimicifuga racemosa (= actaea racemosa = macrotys racemosa)		condurango = cund.
		con.	conium maculatum
			conchae praeparatae = calc.
cimx.	cimex lectularius (= acanthia lectularia)	conch.	conchiolinum (= mater perlarum = perlarum mater)
cina	cina maritima (= artemisia maritima aut cina)		
		conin.	coniinum
		conin-br.	coniinum bromatum
	cinchona boliviana = chin-b.	conv.	convallaria majalis
		convo-a.	convolvulus arvensis
	cinchona calisaya = chin.	convo-d.	convolvulus duartinus
	cinchona succirubra = chin.		(= ipomoea bona-nox)
		convo-s.	convolvulus stans
cinch.	cinchoninum sulphuricum		(= ipomoea stans)
cine.	cineria maritima	cop.	copaiva (= balsamum copaivae)
cinnb.	cinnabaris (= mercurius sulphuratus ruber)		
		cor-r.	corallium rubrum
cinnm.	cinnamomum ceylanicum	corh.	corallorhiza odontorhiza
cist.	cistus canadensis	cori-m.	coriaria myrtifolia
cit-ac.	citricum acidum	cori-r.	coriaria ruscifolia
	citrullus colocynthis = coloc.	corn.	cornus circinata
		corn-a.	cornus alternifolia
cit-d.	citrus decumana	corn-f.	cornus florida
cit-l.	citrus limonum	corn-s.	cornus sericea
cit-v.	citrus vulgaris (= aurantium)	cortico.	corticotropinum (= adrenocortico- tropinum)
clem.	clematis erecta		
clem-vir.	clematis virginiana	cortiso.	cortisonum
clem-vit.	clematis vitalba	cory.	corydalis formosa
cloth.	clotho arictans		(= dicentra canadensis)
cob.	cobaltum metallicum	cot.	cotyledon umbilicus
cob-n.	cobaltum nitricum	coto	coto
coc-c.	coccus cacti	crat.	crataegus oxyacantha et monogyna
coca	coca (= erythroxylon coca)		
			cresolum = kres.
cocain.	cocainum hydrochloricum		cresylolum = kres.

croc.	crocus sativus	del.	delphinus amazonicus
crot-c.	crotalus cascavella	delphin.	delphininum
crot-chlol.	croton chloralum		delphinium staphysagria
crot-h.	crotalus horridus		= staph.
crot-t.	croton tiglium	dema.	dematium petraeum
cryp.	cryptopinum	der.	derris pinnata
cub.	cubeba officinalis		dextrum lacticum acidum
	cucumis colocynthis		= sarcol-ac.
	= coloc.		diadema aranea = aran.
cuc-c.	cucurbita citrullus		dicentra canadensis = cory.
cuc-p.	cucurbita pepo	des-ac.	desoxyribonucleinicum
culx.	culex musca		acidum
cumin.	cumarinum	dicha.	dichapetalum
cund.	cundurango	dict.	dictamnus albus
	(= condurango)	dig.	digitalis purpurea
cuph.	cuphea viscosissima	digin.	digitalinum
cupr.	cuprum metallicum	digox.	digitoxinum
cupr-a.	cuprum aceticum	dios.	dioscorea villosa
cupr-am-s.	cuprum ammoniae	diosm.	diosma lincaris
	sulphuricum	dip.	dipodium punctatum
cupr-ar.	cuprum arsenicosum	diph.	diphtherinum
cupr-c.	cuprum carbonicum	diphtox.	diphtherotoxinum
cupr-cy.	cuprum cyanatum		dipterix odorata = tong.
cupr-m.	cuprum muriaticum	dirc.	dirca palustris
cupr-n.	cuprum nitricum	ditin.	ditainum (= echitaminum)
cupr-o.	cuprum oxydatum nigrum	dol.	dolichos (mucuna) pruriens
cupr-s.	cuprum sulphuricum	dor.	doryphora decemlineata
cupre-au.	cupressus australis		dracontium foetidum
cupre-l.	cupressus lawsoniana		= ictod.
cur.	curare	dros.	drosera rotundifolia
curc.	curcuma javanensis	dub.	duboisinum
	cuscus = anan.	dubo-h.	duboisia hopwoodi
cycl.	cyclamen europaeum	dubo-m.	duboisia myoporoides
cyd.	cydonia vulgaris	dulc.	dulcamara (= solanum
cymin.	cymarinum		dulcamara)
	cynanchum = vince.		durum = scir.
cyn-d.	cynodon dactylon	dys.	bacillus dysenteriae
cyna.	cynara scolymos	eaux	Eaux bonnes aqua
cyno.	cynoglossum officinale	eberth.	eberthinum
cypr.	cypripedium pubescens		ecballium elaterium = elat.
cyt-l.	cytisus laburnum	echi.	echinacea (rudbeckia)
	(= laburnum		angustifolia
	anagyroides)	echi-p.	echinacea purpurea
cytin.	cytisinum		echitaminum = ditin.
	cytisus scoparius	echit.	echites suberecta
	= saroth.	elae.	elaeis guineensis
dam.	damiana (= turnera	elaps	elaps corallinus
	aphrodisiaca)	elat.	elaterium officinarum
daph.	daphne indica		(= ecballium elaterium
	daphne mezereum = mez.		= momordica elaterium)
dat-a.	datura arborea	elem.	elemuy gauteria
	(= brugmansia candida)	emetin.	emetinum
dat-f.	datura ferox	enteroc.	enterococcinum
dat-m.	datura metel	eos.	eosinum
dat-s.	datura sanguinea	ephe.	ephedra vulgaris
	datura stramonium = stram.	epig.	epigaea repens
datin.	daturinum	epih.	epihysterinum
datis.	datisca cannabina	epil.	epilobium palustre

epiph.	epiphegus virginiana (= orobanche)	eupi.	eupionum exogonium purga = jal.
equis.	equisetum hyemale	eys.	eysenhardtia polystachia (= orteaga)
equis-a.	equisetum arvense		
eran.	eranthis hymnalis	fab.	fabiana imbricata (= pichi-pichi)
erech.	erechthites hieracifolia		
ergot.	ergotinum	faec.	bacillus faecalis
erig.	erigeron canadensis (= leptilon canadense)	fago.	fagopyrum esculentum
		fagu.	fagus silvatica
erio.	eriodyction californicum (glutinosum) (= yerba santa)		farfara = tus-fa.
		fel	fel tauri
		ferr.	ferrum metallicum
erod.	erodium cicutarium	ferr-a.	ferrum aceticum
ery-a.	eryngium aquaticum	ferr-ar.	ferrum arsenicosum
ery-m.	eryngium maritimum	ferr-br.	ferrum bromatum
	erythraea chilensis = canch.	ferr-c.	ferrum carbonicum
		ferr-cit.	ferrum citricum
eryt-j.	erythrophlaeum judiciale	ferr-cy.	ferrum cyanatum
eryth.	erythrinus	ferr-i.	ferrum iodatum
	erythroxylon coca = coca	ferr-lac.	ferrum lacticum
esch.	eschscholtzia californica	ferr-m.	ferrum muriaticum (sesquichloratum)
	escoba amargo = parth.		
esin.	eserinum (= physostigminum)	ferr-ma.	ferrum magneticum
		ferr-o-r.	ferrum oxydatum rubrum
esp-g.	espeletia grandiflora	ferr-p.	ferrum phosphoricum
	esponjilla = luf-op.	ferr-pern.	ferrum pernitricum
eucal.	eucalyptus globulus	ferr-p-h.	ferrum phosphoricum hydricum
eucal-r.	eucalyptus rostrata		
eucal-t.	eucalyptus tereticortis	ferr-pic.	ferrum picricum
eucol.	eucalyptolum	ferr-prox.	ferrum protoxalatum
	eugenia cheken = myrt-ch.	ferr-py.	ferrum pyrophosphoricum
		ferr-r.	ferrum reductum
eug.	eugenia jambosa (= jambosa vulgaris)		ferrum sesquichloratum = ferr-m.
euon.	euonymus europaea	ferr-s.	ferrum sulphuricum
euon-a.	euonymus atropurpurea	ferr-t.	ferrum tartaricum
euonin.	euonyminum	ferul.	ferula glauca (= bounafa)
eup-a.	eupatorium aromaticum		ferula sumbul = sumb.
eup-per.	eupatorium perfoliatum		ficus indica = opun-f.
eup-pur.	eupatorium purpureum	fic.	ficus religiosa (= pakur)
euph.	euphorbium officinarum (= euphorbia resinifera)	fic-v.	ficus venosa
		fil.	filix-mas (= aspidium filix-mas)
euph-a.	euphorbia amygdaloides		
euph-c.	euphorbia corrolata	fl-ac.	fluoricum acidum
euph-cy.	euphorbia cyparissias	flav.	flavus (= neisseria flava)
euph-he.	euphorbia heterodoxa	foll.	folliculinum
euph-hy.	euphorbia hypericifolia	flor-p.	flor de piedra (= lophophytum leandri)
euph-ip.	euphorbia ipecacuanhae		
euph-l.	euphorbia lathyris	foen.	foeniculum sativum
euph-m.	euphorbia marginata	form.	formica rufa
euph-pe.	euphorbia peplus	form-ac.	formicicum acidum
euph-pi.	euphorbia pilulifera	formal.	formalinum
euph-po.	euphorbia polycarpa (= golondrina)	frag.	fragaria vesca
		fram.	framboesinum
euph-pr.	euphorbia prostata	franc.	franciscaea uniflora (= manaca)
euph-re.	euphorbia resinifera = euph.		
			frangula = rham-f.
euphr.	euphrasia officinalis	franz.	Franzensbad aqua

frax.	fraxinus americana	gunp.	gunpowder
fuc.	fucus vesiculosus	gymne.	gymnema silvestre
fuch.	fuchsinum	gymno.	gymnocladus canadensis
fuli.	fuligo ligni	haem.	haematoxylum
gad.	gadus morrhua		campechianum
gaert.	bacillus Gaertner	hall	Hall aqua
gal-ac.	gallicum acidum	halo.	haloperidolum
gala.	galanthus nivalis	ham.	hamamelis virginiana
galeg.	galega officinalis	harp.	harpagophytum
galeo.	galeopsis ochroleuca		procumbens
	galipea cusparia = ang.	hecla	Hecla (Hekla) lava
gali.	galium aparine		[= lava Heclae (Heklae)]
galin.	galinsoga parviflora	hed.	hedera helix
galph.	galphimia glauca	hedeo.	hedeoma pulegioides
gamb.	gambogia (= gummi gutti	hedy.	hedysarum ildefonsianum
	= garcinia morella)	helia.	helianthus annuus
	gardenalum = phenob.	helin.	heloninum
gast.	Gastein aqua	helio.	heliotropinum
gaul.	gaultheria procumbens		peruvianum
gels.	gelsemium sempervirens	hell.	helleborus niger
genist.	genista tinctoria	hell-f.	helleborus foetidus
gent-c.	gentiana cruciata	hell-o.	helleborus orientalis
gent-l.	gentiana lutea	hell-v.	helleborus viridis
gent-q.	gentiana quinquefolia	helm.	helminthochortos
geo.	geoffroya vermifuga	helo.	heloderma suspectum
	(= andira inermis)	helon.	helonias dioica
ger.	geranium maculatum	helx.	helix tosta
gerin.	geraninum	hep.	hepar sulphuris calcareum
get.	Gettysburg aqua		(= calcarea sulphurata
geum	geum rivale		Hahnemanni)
gink-b.	ginkgo biloba		hepar sulphuris kalinum
gins.	ginseng (= panax		= kali-sula.
	quinquefolia = aralia	hepat.	hepatica triloba
	quinquefolia	hera.	heracleum sphondylium
	glanderinum = hippoz.	heuch.	heuchera americana
	glandula thyreoidea = thyr.		hibiscus abelmoschus
glech.	glechoma hederacea		= abel.
glon.	glonoinum		hippomane mancinella
glyc.	glycerinum		= manc.
gnaph.	gnaphalium polycephalum	hip-ac.	hippuricum acidum
	golondrina = euph-po.	hipp.	hippomanes
gonotox.	gonotoxinum	hippoz.	hippozaeninum
goss.	gossypium herbaceum		(= glanderinum
gran.	granatum		= malleinum)
graph.	graphites naturalis	hir.	hirudo medicinalis
grat.	gratiola officinalis		(= sanguisuga officinalis)
grin.	grindelia robusta aut	hist.	histaminum muriaticum
	squarrosa		hoang-nan = strych-g.
gua.	guaco (= mikania guaco)	hoit.	hoitzia coccinea
guaj.	guajacum officinale		holarrhena antidysenterica
guajol.	guajacolum		= kurch.
guan.	guano australis	hom.	homarus
	guao = com.	home.	homeria collina
guar.	guarana (= paullinia	hume.	humea elegans
	sorbilis)		humulus lupulus = lup.
guare.	guarea trichiloides	hura	hura brasiliensis
guat.	guatteria gaumeri		(= assaku)
	gummi gutti = gamb.	hura-c.	hura crepitans

hydr.	hydrastis canadensis
hydr-ac.	hydrocyanicum acidum
hydrang.	hydrangea arborescens
hydrc.	hydrocotyle asiatica
hydrin-m.	hydrastinum muriaticum
hydrin-s.	hydrastinum sulphuricum
hydro-v.	hydrophyllum virginicum
hydrobr-ac.	hydrobromicum acidum
hydroph.	hydrophis cyanocinctus
	hydrophobinum = lyss.
	hydropiper = polyg-h.
hyos.	hyoscyamus niger
hyosin.	hyoscyaminum bromatum aut sulphuricum
hyper.	hypericum perforatum
hypo.	hypophyllum sanguineum
	hypophysis posterior = pitu.
hypoth.	hypothalamus
iber.	iberis amara
ichth.	ichthyolum
	ichthyotoxinum = ser-ang.
ictod.	ictodes foetida (= pothos foetidus = dracontium foetidum)
ign.	ignatia amara
	ikshugandha = trib.
ille.	illecebrum verticillatum
ilx-a.	ilex aquifolium
ilx-c.	ilex casseine
	ilex paraguariensis = maté
	illicium stellatum = anis.
imp.	imperatoria ostruthium
ind.	indium metallicum
indg.	indigo tinctoria
indol.	indolum
influ.	influenzinum
ins.	insulinum
inul.	inula helenium
iod.	iodium purum
iodof.	iodoformium
	iodothyrinum = thyr.
ip.	ipecacuanha
	ipomoea bona-nox = convo-d.
ipom.	ipomoea purpurea
	ipomoea stans = convo-s.
irid.	iridium metallicum
irid-m.	iridium muriaticum
iris	iris versicolor
iris-fa.	iris factissima
iris-fl.	iris florentina
iris-foe.	iris foetidissima
iris-g.	iris germanica
iris-ps.	iris pseudacorus
iris-t.	iris tenax (minor)
itu	itu (= resina itu)

jab.	jaborandi (= pilocarpus pennatifolius aut microphyllus)
jac.	jacaranda gualandai
jac-c.	jacaranda caroba
	jacea = viol-t.
jal.	jalapa (= exogonium purga)
	jambosa vulgaris = eug.
jasm.	jasminum officinale
jatr.	jatropha curcas
jatr-u.	jatropha urens
	jequirity = abr.
joan.	joanesia asoca (= saraca indica)
jug-c.	juglans cinerea (cathartica)
jug-r.	juglans regia (= nux juglans)
junc-e.	juncus effusus
junc-p.	juncus pilosus
	juniperus sabina = sabin.
juni.	juniperus virginiana
juni-c.	juniperus communis
just.	justicia adhatoda (= basaka)
kali-a.	kali aceticum
kali-ar.	kali arsenicosum
kali-bi.	kali bichromicum
kali-biox.	kali bioxalicum
kali-bit.	kali bitartaricum (= tartarus depuratus)
kali-br.	kali bromatum
kali-c.	kali carbonicum
kali-caust.	kali causticum
kali-chl.	kali chloricum
kali-chls.	kali chlorosum
kali-chr.	kali chromicum
kali-cit.	kali citricum
kali-cy.	kali cyanatum
kali-f.	kali fluoratum
kali-fcy.	kali ferrocyanatum
kali-hp.	kali hypophosphoricum
kali-i.	kali iodatum
kali-m.	kali muriaticum
kali-n.	kali nitricum (= nitrum)
kali-ox.	kali oxalicum
kali-p.	kali phosphoricum
kali-perm.	kali permanganicum
kali-pic.	kali picricum
kali-s.	kali sulphuricum
kali-s-chr.	kali sulphuricum chromicum (= alumen chromicum)
kali-sal.	kali salicylicum
kali-sil.	kali silicicum
kali-sula.	kali sulphuratum (= hepar sulphuris kalinum)

kali-sulo.	kali sulphurosum
kali-t.	kali tartaricum
kali-tel.	kali telluricum
kali-x.	kali xanthogenicum
kalm.	kalmia latifolia
kam.	kamala
	kaolinum = alum-sil.
kara.	karaka
karw-h.	karwinskia humboldtiana
	Karlsbad aqua = carl.
	kava-kava = pip-m.
kerose.	kerosenum
keroso.	kerosolenum
kino	kino australiensis
kiss.	Kissingen aqua
kola	kola (= nux colae)
kou.	kousso (= brayera
	anthelmintica)
kreos.	kreosotum
	krameria triandra = rat.
kres.	kresolum (= cresolum
	= cresylolum)
kurch.	kurchi (= holarrhena aut
	wrightia antidysenterica)
	laburnum anagyroides
	= cyt-l.
	lacticum acidum dextrum
	= sarcol-ac.
lac-ac.	lactis acidum
lac-c.	lac caninum
lac-d.	lac vaccinum defloratum
lac-f.	lac felinum
lac-v.	lac vaccinum
lac-v-c.	lac vaccinum coagulatum
lac-v-f.	lactis vaccini flos
lacer.	lacerta agilis
	lachesis lanceolatus
	= both.
lach.	lachesis muta
	(trigonocephalus)
lachn.	lachnanthes tinctoria
lact.	**lactuca virosa**
lact-s.	**lactuca sativa**
lactrm.	**lactucarium thridace**
lam.	**lamium** album
lap-a.	lapis albus (= calcarea
	silico-fluorica)
	lapis renails = cal-ren.
lapa.	lapathum acutum
	(= rumex obtusifolius)
lappa	lappa arctium (major)
	(= arctium lappa)
laps.	lapsana communis
	latrodectus curassavicus
	= ther.
lat-h.	latrodectus hasselti
lat-k.	latrodectus katipo
lat-m.	latrodectus mactans

lath.	lathyrus sativus aut
	cicera
laur.	laurocerasus
	laurus camphora
	= camph.
	lava Heclae (Heklae)
	= hecla
lec.	lecithinum
led.	ledum palustre
lem-m.	lemna minor
leon.	leonurus cardiaca
lepi.	lepidium bonariense
lept.	leptandra virginica
	leptilon canadense = erig.
lesp-c.	lespedeza capitata
lesp-s.	lespedeza sieboldii
lev.	Levico aqua
levist.	levisticum officinale
levo.	levomepromazinum
liat.	liatris spicata
	(= serratula)
	lichen islandicus = cetr.
lil-a.	lilium album
lil-s.	lilium superbum
lil-t.	lilium tigrinum
lim.	limulus cyclops
limx.	limex ater
lina.	linaria vulgaris
linu-c.	linum catharticum
linu-u.	linum usitatissimum
lip.	lippia mexicana
lipp.	Lippspringe aqua
lith-be.	lithium benzoicum
lith-br.	lithium bromatum
lith-c.	lithium carbonicum
lith-lac.	lithium lacticum
lith-m.	lithium muriaticum
lith-sal.	lithium salicylicum
loa.	loasa tricolor
lob.	lobelia inflata
lob-a.	lobelia acetum
lob-c.	lobelia cardinalis
	lobelia coerulea = lob-s.
lob-d.	lobelia dortmanna
lob-e.	lobelia erinus
lob-p.	lobelia purpurascens
lob-s.	lobelia syphilitica
	(coerulea)
lobin.	lobelinum
lol.	loleum temulentum
lon-c.	lonicera caprifolium
lon-p.	lonicera pericylmenum
lon-x.	lonicera xylosteum
	lophophora williamsii
	= anh.
	lophophytum leandri
	= flor-p.
	luesinum = syph.

luf-act.	luffa actangula	mati.	matico (= piper
luf-op.	luffa operculata		angustifolium = artanthe
	(= esponjilla)		elongata)
lup.	lupulus humulus	matth.	matthiola graeca
	(= humulus lupulus)	mec.	meconium
lupin.	lupulinum		medicago sativa = alf.
lyc.	lycopodium clavatum	med.	medorrhinum
lycpr.	lycopersicum esculentum	medus.	medusa
	(= solanum	mela.	melastama ackermanni
	lycopersicum)	melal.	melaleuca hypericifolia
lycps.	lycopus virginicus		melia azadirachta
lycps-eu.	lycopus europaeus		indica = aza.
lysi.	lysimachia nummularia	meli.	melilotus officinalis
lyss.	lyssinum	meli-a.	melilotus alba
	(= hydrophobinum)	melis.	melissa officinalis
	lytta vesicatoria = canth.	melit.	melitagrinum
m-arct.	magnetis polus arcticus	melo.	melolontha vulgaris
m-aust.	magnetis polus australis	meningoc.	meningococcinum
macro.	macrotinum	menis.	menispermum canadense
	macrotys racemosa = cimic.	menth.	mentha piperita
macroz.	macrozamia spiralis	menth-pu.	mentha pulegium
	madar = calo.	menth-v.	mentha viridis
mag-c.	magnesia carbonica	mentho.	mentholum
mag-bcit.	magnesia borocitrica	meny.	menyanthes trifoliata
mag-f.	magnesia fluorata	meph.	mephitis putorius
mag-i.	magnesia iodata	merc.	mercurius solubilis
mag-m.	magnesia muriatica		Hahnemanni aut
mag-p.	magnesia phosphorica		mercurius vivus
mag-s.	magnesia sulphurica	merc-a.	mercurius aceticus
mag-u.	magnesia usta	merc-aur.	mercurius auratus
magn-gl.	magnolia glauca		mercurius bi(n)iodatus
magn-gr.	magnolia grandiflora		= merc-i-r.
	mahonia = berb-a.	merc-br.	mercurius bromatus
	majeptilum = thiop.	merc-c.	mercurius corrosivus
maland.	malandrinum		(sublimatus)
malar.	malaria officinalis		mercurius cum kali
malatox.	malariatoxinum		= aethi-m.
	malleinum = hippoz.	merc-cy.	mercurius cyanatus
	manaca = franc.	merc-d.	mercurius dulcis
manc.	mancinella (= hippomane		(= calomel)
	mancinella)	merc-i-f.	mercurius iodatus flavus
mand.	mandragora officinarum		(= mercurius
mang.	manganum aceticum aut		protoiodatus)
	carbonicum	merc-i-r.	mercurius iodatus ruber
mang-coll.	manganum colloidale		(= mercurius bi(n)iodatus)
mang-m.	manganum muriaticum	merc-k-i.	mercurius biniodatus cum
mang-o.	manganum oxydatum		kali iodato
	nativum	merc-meth.	mercurius methylenus
mang-s.	manganum sulphuricum	merc-ns.	mercurius nitrosus
mangi.	mangifera indica		(= mercurius nitricus
	manihot utilissima = cass.		oxydulatus)
manz.	manzanita		mercurius oxydatus
	mapato = rat.		= merc-pr-r.
marr.	marrubium album	merc-p.	mercurius phosphoricus
	marum verum = teucr.	merc-pr-a.	mercurius praecipitatus
mate	maté (= ilex		albus
	paraguariensis)	merc-pr-f.	mercurius praecipitatus
	mater perlarum = conch.		flavus

merc-pr-r.	mercurius praecipitatus ruber (= mercurius oxydatus)	muscin.	muscarinum
		mut.	bacillus mutabilis
	mercurius protoiodatus = merc-i-f.	mygal.	mygale lasiodora (avicularia) (= aranea avicularia)
	mercurius sublimatus = merc-c.	myos-a.	myosotis arvensis
		myos-s.	myosotis symphytifolia
merc-s-cy.	mercurius sulphocyanatus	myric.	myrica cerifera
	mercurius sulphuratus niger = aethi–m.	myris.	myristica sebifera
		myrrha	myrrha
	mercurius sulphuratus ruber = cinnb.		myrtillus = vacc-m.
		myrt-c.	myrtus communis
merc-sul.	mercurius sulphuricus (= turpethum minerale)	myrt-ch.	myrtus cheken (= eugenia cheken)
merc-tn.	mercurius tannicus	myrt-p.	myrtus pimenta
	mercurius vivus = merc.	mytil.	mytilus edulis
merl.	mercurialis perennis	nabal.	nabalus serpentaria
mesp.	mespillus germanica	naja	naja tripudians
meth-ae-ae.	methylium aethylo-aethereum	napht.	naphta
		naphtin.	naphtalinum
meth-sal.	methylium salicylicum	narc-po.	narcissus poeticus
methyl.	methylenum coeruleum	narc-ps.	narcissus pseudonarcissus
methys.	methysergidum	narcin.	narceinum
mez.	mezereum (= daphne mezereum)	narcot.	narcotinum
		narz.	Narzan aqua
micr.	micromeria douglasii (= yerba buena)	nast.	nasturtium aquaticum
		nat-a.	natrum aceticum
	mikania guaco = gua.	nat-ae-s.	natrum aethylosulphuricum
mill.	millefolium (= achillea millefolium)	nat-ar.	natrum arsenicosum
	millipedes = onis.	nat-be.	natrum benzoicum
mim-h.	mimosa humilis	nat-br.	natrum bromatum
mim-p.	mimosa pudica	nat-bic.	natrum bicarbonicum
mit.	mitchella repens	nat-c.	natrum carbonicum
moly-met.	molybdaenum metallicum	nat-cac.	natrum cacodylicum
mom-b.	momordica balsamica	nat-ch.	natrum choleinicum
mom-ch.	momordica charantia	nat-f.	natrum fluoratum
	momordica elaterium = elat.	nat-hchls.	natrum hypochlorosum
		nat-hsulo.	natrum hyposulphurosum
monar.	monarda didyma	nat-i.	natrum iodatum
moni.	monilia albicans	nat-lac.	natrum lacticum
mono.	monotropa uniflora	nat-m.	natrum muriaticum
mons.	monsonia ovata	nat-n.	natrum nitricum
morb.	morbillinum	nat-ns.	natrum nitrosum
morg.	bacillus Morgan	nat-p.	natrum phosphoricum
morph.	morphinum aceticum aut muriaticum aut sulphuricum	nat-s.	natrum sulphuricum
		nat-s-c.	natrum sulphocarbolicum (sulphophenolicum)
mosch.	moschus	nat-sal.	natrum salicylicum
muc-u.	mucuna urens	nat-sel.	natrum selenicum
mucor	mucor mucedo	nat-sil.	natrum silicicum
mucot.	mucotoxinum	nat-sil-f.	natrum silicofluoricum
	mucuna pruriens = dol.	nat-suc.	natrum succinicum
mur-ac.	muriaticum acidum	nat-sula.	natrum sulphuratum
muru.	murure leite	nat-sulo.	natrum sulphurosum
murx.	murex purpureus	nat-taur.	natrum taurocholicum
musa	musa sapientum	nat-tel.	natrum telluricum

nect.	nectandra amare
nectrin.	nectrianinum
neg.	negundium americanum
	(= acer negundo)
	neisseria flava = **flav.**
nep.	nepenthes distillatoria
nepet.	nepeta cataria
	nerium oleander = olnd.
neur.	neurinum
nicc.	niccolum carbonicum aut
	metallicum
nicc-s.	niccolum sulphuricum
	nicotiana tabacum = tab.
nicot.	nicotinum
nid.	nidus edulis
nig-d.	nigella damascena
nig-s.	nigella sativa
nit-ac.	nitri acidum
nit-m-ac.	nitromuriaticum acidum
	(= aqua regia)
nit-s-d.	nitri spiritus dulcis
	(= spiritus nitrico-
	aethereus = aethylium
	nitrosum)
nitro-o.	nitrogenium oxygenatum
	nitrum = kali-n.
nuph.	nuphar luteum
	(= nymphaea lutea)
nux-a.	nux absurda
	nux colae = kola
	nux juglans = jug-r.
nux-m.	nux moschata
nux-v.	nux vomica
nyct.	nyctanthes arbor-tristis
	nymphaea lutea = nuph.
nymph.	nymphaea odorata
oci.	ocimum canum
oci-s.	ocimum sanctum
oena.	oenanthe crocata
oeno.	oenothera biennis
	oestronum = foll.
oest.	oestrus cameli
okou.	okoubaka aubrevillei
ol-an.	oleum animale aethereum
	Dippeli
	oleum cajuputi = caj.
ol-car.	oleum caryophyllatum
ol-j.	oleum jecoris aselli
ol-myr.	oleum myristicae
ol-sant.	oleum santali
ol-suc.	oleum succinum
	oleum **wittnebianum**
	= caj.
olnd.	oleander (= nerium
	oleander)
onis.	oniscus asellus
	(= millipedes)
onon.	ononis spinosa (arvensis)

onop.	onopordon acanthium
onos.	onosmodium virginianum
	oophorinum = ov.
op.	opium
oper.	operculina turpenthum
opl.	oplia farinosa
opop.	opopanax chironium
opun-f.	opuntia ficus (= ficus
	indica)
opun-v.	opuntia vulgaris
orch.	orchitinum
oreo.	oreodaphne californica
orig.	origanum majorana
orig-cr.	origanum creticum
orig-v.	origanum vulgare
orni.	ornithogalum umbellatum
	orobanche = epiph.
	orteaga = eys.
oscilloc.	oscillococcinum
osm.	osmium metallicum
ost.	ostrya virginica
ouabin.	ouabainum
ov.	ovininum (= oophorinum)
ovi-p.	ovi gallinae pellicula
	ovi testa = calc-o-t.
ox-ac.	oxalicum acidum
oxal.	oxalis acetosella
oxyd.	oxydendron arboreum
	(= andromeda arborea)
oxyg.	oxygenium (= ozonum)
oxyt.	oxytropis lamberti
	ozonum = oxyg.
paeon.	paeonia officinalis
	pakur = fic.
pall.	palladium metallicum
palo.	paloondo
	pambotano = calli.
pana.	panacea arvensis
	panax quinquefolia = gins.
pann.	panna (= aspidium panna)
papin.	papaverinum
	papaya vulgaris = asim.
par.	paris quadrifolia
paraf.	paraffinum
paraph.	paraphenylendiaminum
	parathormonum
	= parathyr.
parat.	paratyphoidinum
parathyr.	parathyreoidinum
	(= parathormonum)
pareir.	pareira brava
pariet.	parietaria officinalis
paro-i.	paronychia illecebrum
parot.	parotidinum
parth.	parthenium hysterophorus
	(= escoba amargo)
passi.	passiflora incarnata
past.	pastinaca sativa

paull.	paullinia pinnata
	paullinia sorbilis = guar.
pect.	pecten jacobaeus
ped.	pediculus capitis
pedclr.	pedicularis canadensis
pelarg.	pelargonium reniforme
	pelias berus = vip.
pellin.	pelletierinum
pen.	penthorum sedoides
penic.	penicillinum
	perlarum mater = conch.
	persica amygdalus
	= amgd-p.
perh.	perhexilinum
peri.	periploca graeca
pers.	persea americana
pert.	pertussinum
pest.	pestinum
	petasites officinalis = tus-p.
peti.	petiveria tetrandra
petr.	petroleum
petros.	petroselinum sativum
	peumus boldus = bold.
	peyotl = anh.
ph-ac.	phosphoricum acidum
phal.	phallus impudicus
phase.	phaseolus nanus
phel.	phellandrium aquaticum
phenac.	phenacetinum
phenob.	phenobarbitalum
	(= gardenalum)
	phenolum = carb-ac.
phila.	philadelphus coronarius
phle.	phleum pratense
phlor.	phlorizinum
phos.	phosphorus
phos-h.	phosphorus hydrogenatus
phos-pchl.	phosphorus pentachloratus
phys.	physostigma venenosum
	(= calabar)
	physostigminum = esin.
physal.	physalis alkekengi
	(= alkekengi = solanum
	vesicarium)
physala-p.	physalia pelagica
phyt.	phytolacca decandra
phyt-b.	phytolacca berry
	pichi-pichi = fab.
pic-ac.	picricum (picronitricum)
	acidum
	(= trinitrophenolum)
picro.	picrotoxinum
pilo.	pilocarpinum
	hydrochloricum aut
	nitricum aut purum
	pilocarpus pennatifolius
	aut microphyllus = jab.

pime.	pimenta officinalis
pimp.	pimpinella saxifraga (alba)
	pinus canadensis
	= abies-c.
pin-c.	pinus cupressus
pin-l.	pinus lambertiana
pin-s.	pinus silvestris
	piper angustifolium aut
	elongatum = mati.
pip-m.	piper methysticum
	(= kava-kava)
pip-n.	piper nigrum
pipe.	piperazinum
pisc.	piscidia erythrina
pitu.	pituitarium posterium
	(= hyophysis posterior)
pitu-gl.	pituitaria glandula
pituin.	pituitrinum
pix	pix liquida
	planifolia = vanil.
plan.	plantago major
plan-mi.	plantago minor
plat.	platinum metallicum
plat-m.	platinum muriaticum
plat-m-n.	platinum muriaticum
	natronatum
platan.	platanus occidentalis
plb.	plumbum metallicum
plb-a.	plumbum aceticum
plb-c.	plumbum carbonicum
plb-chr.	plumbum chromicum
plb-i.	plumbum iodatum
plb-n.	plumbum nitricum
plb-p.	plumbum phosphoricum
plect.	plectranthus fruticosus
plumbg.	plumbago litteralis
plume.	plumeria celinus
pneu.	pneumococcinum
	(= pneumococcus)
podo.	podophyllum peltatum
pole.	polemonium coeruleum
poll.	pollen
	polygala senega = seneg.
polyg-a.	polygonum aviculare
polyg-h.	polygonum
	hydropiperoides aut
	punctatum
	(= hydropiper)
polyg-m.	polygonum maritimum
polyg-pe.	polygonum persicaria
polyg-s.	polygonum sagittatum
polym.	polymnia uvedalia
	polyporus officinalis
	= bol-la.
polyp-p.	polyporus pinicola
polytr.	polytrichum juniperinum
pop.	populus tremuloides
pop-c.	populus candicans

pot-a.	potentilla anserina	ran-fi.	ranunculus ficaria
pot-au.	potentilla aurea	ran-fl.	ranunculus flammula
pot-e.	potentilla erecta	ran-g.	ranunculus glacialis
pot-r.	potentilla reptans	ran-r.	ranunculus repens
pot-t.	potentilla tormentilla	ran-s.	ranunculus sceleratus
pota.	potamogeton natans	raph.	raphanus sativus
	pothos foetidus = ictod.	raphani.	raphanistrum arvense
prim-f.	primula farinosa	rat.	ratanhia peruviana (= kra-
prim-o.	primula obconica		meria triandra = mapato)
prim-v.	primula veris	rauw.	rauwolfia serpentina
prin.	prinos verticillatus	rein.	Reinerz aqua
	prionurus australis =		resina itu = itu
	buth-a.	res.	resorcinum
prop.	propylaminum (= trime-	reser.	reserpinum
	thylaminum)	rham-cal.	rhamnus californica
prot.	bacillus proteus	rham-cath.	rhamnus cathartica
prun.	prunus spinosa	rham-f.	rhamnus frangula (= fran-
prun-d.	prunus domestica		gula)
prun-m.	prunus mahaleb		rhamnus purshiana = cas-s.
prun-p.	prunus padus	rheum	rheum palmatum (offi-
prun-v.	prunus virginiana		cinale)
prune.	prunella vulgaris		rhodallinum = thiosin
psil.	psilocybe caerulescens	rhod.	rhododendron chrysan-
psor.	psorinum (= psoricum)		thum (aureum)
psoral.	psoralea bituminosa	rhodi.	rhodium metallicum
ptel.	ptelea trifoliata	rhodi-o-n.	rhodium oxydatum nitricum
pulm-a.	pulmo anaphylacticus	rhus-a.	rhus aromatica
pulm-v.	pulmo vulpis	rhus-c.	rhus cotinus
pulmon.	pulmonaria vulgaris	rhus-d.	rhus diversiloba
puls.	pulsatilla pratensis (nigri-	rhus-g.	rhus glabra
	cans) (= anemone pra-	rhus-l.	rhus laurina
	tensis)	rhus-r.	rhus radicans
puls-n.	pulsatilla nuttalliana	rhus-t.	rhus toxicodendron
pulx.	pulex irritans	rhus-v.	rhus venenata
pyrar.	pyrarara	rhus-ver.	rhus vernix
pyre-o.	pyrethrum officinarum	rib-ac.	ribonucleinicum acidum
pyre-p.	pyrethrum parthenium	ric.	ricinus communis
pyre-r.	pyrethrum roseum e	rob.	robinia pseudacacia
	floribus	ros-ca.	rosa canina
pyro-ac.	pyrolignosum acidum	ros-ce.	rosa centifolia
pyrog.	pyrogenium	ros-d.	rosa damascena
pyrol.	pyrola rotundifolia	rosm.	rosmarinus officinalis
pyrus	pyrus americanus	rub-t.	rubia tinctorum
quas.	quassia amara	rubu.	rubus villosus
queb.	quebracho (= aspido–		rudbeckia angustifolia
	sperma quebracho)		= echi.
querc.	quercus e glandibus	rudb-h.	rudbeckia hirta
	(= aqua glandium	rumx.	rumex crispus
	quercus)	rumx-a.	rumex acetosa
quill.	quillaya saponaria		rumex obtusifolius = lapa.
rad.	radium metallicum	russ.	russula foetens
rad-br.	radium bromatum	ruta	ruta graveolens
	radix angelicae sinensis	sabad.	sabadilla (asagraea)
	= ange-s.		officinalis
raja-s.	rajania subsamarata	sabal	sabal serrulatum
	rana bufo = bufo	sabin.	sabina (= juniperus
ran-a.	ranunculus acris		sabina)
ran-b.	ranunculus bulbosus		saccharomyces = tor.

sacch.	saccharum officinale (album)
sacch-l.	saccharum lactis
sacchin.	saccharinum
sal-ac.	salicylicum acidum
sal-am.	salix americana
sal-n.	salix nigra
sal-p.	salix purpurea
salam.	salamandra maculata
salin.	salicinum
salol.	salolum
salv.	salvia officinalis
salv-sc.	salvia sclarea
samb.	sambucus nigra
samb-c.	sambucus canadensis
samb-e.	sambucus ebulus
sang.	sanguinaria canadensis
sang-n.	sanguinarinum nitricum
sang-t.	sanguinarinum tartaricum
sanguiso.	sanguisorba officinalis
	sanguisuga officinalis = hir.
sanic.	Sanicula aqua
sanic-eu.	sanicula europaea
santa.	santalum album
santin.	santoninum
sapin.	saponinum
sapo.	saponaria officinalis
	saraca indica = joan.
sarcol-ac.	sarcolacticum acidum (= dextrum lacticum acidum = lacticum acidum dextrum)
saroth.	sarothamnus scoparius (= cytisus scoparius = spartium scoparium)
sarr.	sarracenia purpurea
sars.	sarsaparilla (smilax) officinalis
sass.	sassafras officinalis
saur.	saururus cernuus
saxi.	saxifraga granulata
scam.	scammonium
scarl.	scarlatinum
schin.	schinus molle
	scilla maritima = squil.
scir.	scirrhinum (= durum)
scol.	scolopendra morsitans
scolo-v.	scolopendrium vulgare
scop.	scopolia carniolica
scopin.	scopolaminum bromatum
scor.	scorpio europaeus
scroph-m.	scrophularia marylandica
scroph-n.	scrophularia nodosa
scut.	scutellaria laterifolia
sec.	secale cornutum
sed-ac.	sedum acre
sed-r.	sedum repens (alpestre)

sed-t.	sedum telephium
sedi.	sedinha
	selenicereus grandiflorus = cact.
sel.	selenium
seli.	selinum carvifolium
sem-t.	semen tiglii
semp.	sempervivum tectorum
senec.	senecio aureus
senec-j.	senecio jacobaea
senecin.	senecinum
seneg.	**senega** (= **polygala** senega)
senn.	senna (= cassia acutifolia)
sep.	sepia succus
septi.	septicaeminum
	serratula = liat.
ser-ang.	serum anguillae (= ichthyotoxinum)
serp.	serpentaria aristolochia (= **aristolochia serpentaria**)
sieg.	siegesbeckia orientalis
sil.	silicea terra (= silica)
sil-mar.	silica marina
silpho.	silphion cyrenaicum
silphu.	silphium laciniatum
sima.	simaruba amara (officinalis) aut glauca
	simaruba ferroginea = cedr.
sin-a.	sinapis alba
sin-n.	sinapis nigra
sisy.	sisyrinchium galaxoides
sium	sium latifolium
skat.	skatolum
skook.	Skookum chuck aqua
slag	slag
	smilax officinalis = sars.
sol-a.	solanum arrebenta
sol-c.	solanum carolinense
	solanum dulcamara = dulc.
	solanum lycopersicum = lycpr.
sol-m.	solanum mammosum
sol-n.	solanum nigrum
sol-o.	solanum oleraceum
sol-ps.	solanum pseudocapsicum
sol-t.	solanum tuberosum
sol-t-ae.	solanum tuberosum aegrotans
	solanum vesicarium = physal.
solid.	solidago virgaurea
solin.	solanium aceticum aut purum

soph.	sophora japonica	sul-ac.	sulphuricum acidum
	spartium scoparium	sul-h.	sulphur hydrogenisatum
	= saroth.	sul-i.	sulphur iodatum
sphing.	sphingurus (spiggurus)		sulphur sublimatum
	martini		= sulph.
spig.	spigelia anthelmia	sul-ter.	sulphur terebinthinatum
	(anthelmintica)	sulfa.	sulfanilamidum
spig-m.	spigelia marylandica	sulfon.	sulfonalum
	spiggurus martini	sulfonam.	sulfonamidum
	= sphing.	sulo-ac.	sulphurosum acidum
spil.	spilanthes oleracea	sulph.	sulphur lotum
	spiritus nitrico-aethereus		(sublimatum)
	= nit-s-d.	sumb.	sumbulus moschatus
spir-sula.	spiritus sulphuratus		(= ferula sumbul)
spira.	spiranthes autumnalis	syc.	bacillus sycoccus
spirae.	spiraea ulmaria	sym-r.	symphoricarpus racemosus
spong.	spongia tosta	symph.	symphytum officinale
squil.	squilla (scilla) maritima	syph.	syphilinum (= luesinum)
stach.	stachys betonica	syr.	syringa vulgaris
stann.	stannum metallicum	syzyg.	syzygium jambolanum
stann-i.	stannum iodatum		(cumini)
stann-m.	stannum muriaticum	tab.	tabacum (= nicotiana
stann-pchl.	stannum perchloratum		tabacum)
staph.	staphysagria	tam.	tamus communis
	(= delphinium	tama.	tamarix germanica
	staphysagria)	tanac.	tanacetum vulgare
staphycoc.	staphylococcinum	tang.	tanghinia venenifera
staphytox.	staphylotoxinum	tann-ac.	tannicum acidum
stel.	stellaria media		(= tanninum)
stict.	sticta pulmonaria	tarax.	taraxacum officinale
stigm.	stigmata maydis (= zea	tarent.	tarentula (tarantula)
	maydis)		hispanica
still.	stillingia silvatica	tarent-c.	tarentula (tarantula)
stram.	stramonium (= datura		cubensis
	stramonium)	tart-ac.	tartaricum acidum
strept-ent.	bacillus		tartarus depuratus
	strepto-enterococcus		= kali-bit.
streptoc.	streptococcinum		tartarus emeticus = ant-t.
stront.	strontium metallicum	tax.	taxus baccata
stront-br.	strontium bromatum	tela	tela araneae (= araneae
stront-c.	strontium carbonicum		tela)
stront-i.	strontium iodatum	tell.	tellurium metallicum
stront-n.	strontium nitricum	tell-ac.	telluricum acidum
stroph-h.	strophantus hispidus	tep.	Teplitz aqua
stroph-s.	strophantus sarmentosus	ter.	terebinthiniae oleum
stry.	strychninum purum	tere-ch.	terebinthina chios
stry-ar.	strychninum arsenicosum	terebe.	terebenum
stry-n.	strychninum nitricum		testa praeparata
stry-p.	strychninum phosphoricum		= calc-o-t.
stry-s.	strychninum sulphuricum	tet.	tetradymitum
stry-val.	strychninum valerianicum	tetox.	tetanotoxinum
strych-g.	strychnos gaultheriana		teucrium chamaedrys
	(= hoang-nan)		= chamae.
	strychnos tieuté = upa.	teucr.	teucrium marum verum
stryph.	stryphnodendron		(= marum verum)
	barbatimam	teucr-s.	teucrium scorodonia
succ.	succinum	thal.	thallium metallicum aut
succ-ac.	succinicum acidum		aceticum

thal-s.	thallium sulphuricum	tub-d.	tuberculinum Denys
thala.	thalamus	tub-k.	tuberculinum Koch
	thaspium aureum = ziz.	tub-m.	tuberculinum Marmoreck
thea	thea chinensis	tub-r.	tuberculinum residuum
thebin.	thebainum		Koch
	theobroma cacao = cac.	tub-sp.	tuberculinum Spengler
ther.	theridion curassavicum		turnera aphrodisiaca
	(= latrodectus		= dam.
	curassavicus)		turpethum minerale
thev.	thevetia nerifolia		= merc-sul.
thiop.	thioproperazinum	tus-fa.	tussilago farfara
thiosin.	thiosinaminum		(= farfara)
	(= rhodallinum)	tus-fr.	tussilago fragans
thlas.	thlaspi bursa pastoris	tus-p.	tussilago petasites
	(= bursa pastoris		(= petasites officinalis)
	= capsella bursa pastoris)	typh.	thypha latifolia
thuj.	thuja occidentalis	ulm.	ulmus campestris (fulva)
thuj-l.	thuja lobii	upa.	upas tieuté (= strychnos
thym-gl.	thymi glandulae extractum		tieuté)
thymol.	thymolum	upa-a.	upas antiaris
thymu.	thymus serpyllum	ur-ac.	uricum acidum
thyr.	thyreoidinum (= glandula	uran.	uranium metallicum
	thyreoidea = thyroidi-	uran-n.	uranium nitricum
	num = iodothyrinum)	uranoth.	uranothorium
thyreotr.	thyreotropinum	urea	urea pura
	(= thyreostimulinum)	urea-n.	urea nitrica
til.	tilia europaea		(= carbamidum)
tinas.	tinaspora cordifolia	urt-c.	urtica crenulata
titan.	titanium metallicum	urt-g.	urtica gigas
tol.	toluidinum	urt-u.	urtica urens
tong.	tongo (= dipterix odorata	usn.	usnea barbata
	= tonca)	ust.	ustilago maydis
tor.	torula cerevisiae	uva	uva ursi
	(= saccharomyces)	uvar.	uvaria triloba
torm.	tormentilla erecta	uza.	uzara
tox-th.	toxicophloea thunbergi	v-a-b.	vaccin atténué bilié
toxi.	toxicophis pugnax		(= bacillus Calmette-
trach.	trachinus draco		Guérin)
trad.	tradescantia diuretica	vac.	vaccininum
trib.	tribulus terrestris		(= vaccinotoxinum)
	(= ikshugandha)	vacc-m.	vaccinium myrtillus
trich.	trichosanthes amara		(= myrtillus)
trif-p.	trifolium pratense	valer.	valeriana officinalis
trif-r.	trifolium repens	vanad.	vanadium metallicum
tril.	trillium pendulum	vanil.	vanilla aromatica
tril-c.	trillium cernuum		(= planifolia)
	trimethylaminum = prop.	vario.	variolinum
	trinitrophenolum = pic-ac.	ven-m.	venus mercenaria
trinit.	trinitrotoluenum	verat.	veratrum album
trios.	triosteum perfoliatum	verat-n.	veratrum nigrum
tritic.	triticum (agropyrum)	verat-v.	veratrum viride
	repens	verb.	verbascum thapsus aut
trito	trito		thapsiforme
trom.	trombidium muscae	verb-n.	verbascum nigrum
	domesticae (= acarus)	verbe-h.	verbena hastata
trop.	tropaeolum majus	verbe-u.	verbena urticaefolia
tub.	tuberculinum bovinum Kent	verin.	veratrinum
tub-a.	tuberculinum avis	vero-b.	veronica beccabunga

vero-o.	veronica officinalis	wye.	wyethia helenoides
vesi.	vesicaria communis	x-ray	x-ray
vesp.	vespa crabro	xan.	xanthoxylum fraxineum
vib.	viburnum opulus		(americanum)
vib-od.	viburnum oderatissinum	xanrhi.	xanthorrhiza apifolia
vib-p.	viburnum prunifolium	xanrhoe.	xanthorrhoea arborea
vib-t.	viburnum tinus	xanth.	xanthium spinosum
vichy-g.	Vichy aqua, grande grille	xero.	xerophyllum
vichy-h.	Vichy aqua, hôpital	xiph.	xiphosura americana
vinc.	vinca minor		yerba buena = micr.
vince.	vincetoxicum officinale		yerba mansa = anemps.
	(= asclepias vincetoxi-		yerba santa = erio.
	cum = cynanchum)	yohim.	yohimbinum
viol-o.	viola odorata	yuc.	yucca filamentosa
viol-t.	viola tricolor (= jacea)	zea-i.	zea italica
vip.	vipera berus (torva)		zea maydis = stigm.
	(= pelias berus)	zinc.	zincum metallicum
vip-a.	vipera aspis	zinc-a.	zincum aceticum
vip-l-f.	vipera lachesis fel	zinc-ar.	zincum arsenicosum
vip-r.	vipera redi	zinc-br.	zincum bromatum
	vipera torva = vip.	zinc-c.	zincum carbonicum
visc.	viscum album	zinc-cy.	zincum cyanatum
visc-q.	viscum quercinum	zinc-fcy.	zincum ferrocyanatum
vit.	vitex trifolia	zinc-i.	zincum iodatum
vitr.	vitrum antimonii	zinc-m.	zincum muriaticum
voes.	Voeslau aqua	zinc-o.	zincum oxydatum
	vulpis pulmo =	zinc-p.	zincum phosphoricum
	pulm-v.	zinc-pic.	zincum picricum
wies.	Wiesbaden aqua	zinc-s.	zincum sulphuricum
wildb.	Wildbad aqua	zinc-val.	zincum valerianicum
wildu.	Wildungen aqua	zing.	zingiber officinale
	wrightia antidysenterica	ziz.	zizia aurea (= thaspium
	= kurch.		aureum)

DAYTIME
JOURNÉE, pendant la
TAGSÜBER
   agar.[3], **alum.,** am-c.[3], am-m.,
   arg-m.[3], arg-n.[3], calc.[3], caust.[3],
   cimic., **euphr.**[3], **ferr.,** guaj., lac-d.[1'],
   lach.[3], **med., nat-ar.,** nat-c., **nat-m.,**
   nit-ac., nux-v.[6], phos.[3], **puls.,**
   rhust-t., sang., SEP., STANN.,
   SULPH.

   sunrise till sunset[7]
   du lever au coucher du soleil
   von Sonnen-Aufgang bis -Unter-
      gang
      med.

   am.[3, 6]
   acon.[6], **agar.,** arn., bry., cham.,
   cob-n.[9], **cycl.,** helon., **jal.,** kali-c.[8],
   mag-p., merc.[1'], nat-p.[1'], nat-s.[1'],
   petr., sep., syph.[8]

MORNING (5–9 h)
MATIN
MORGENS
   abies-n., abrot., absin., **acal.**[8],
   acon., aesc., **AGAR.,** agn., all-c.[3],
   aloe, alum., ALUM-P.[1'], alumn.[2],
   am-c., **AM-M., ambr., anac.,**
   ang.[2, 3, 6], **ant-c.,** ant-t.[2, 3], **apis,**
   aran.[3], aran-ix.[10], **ARG-M., arg-n.,**
   arist-cl.[10], **arn., ars., ARS-I.,**
   ars-s-f.[1'], asaf., asar., **AUR.,**
   aur-ar.[1'], aur-i.[1'], **AUR-S.**[1'], **bapt.,**
   bar-c., bar-i.[1'], **bar-m., bar-s.**[1'], bell.,
   benz-ac., **berb.,** bism., **bor., bov.,**
   BRY., bufo, cadm-met.[9, 14], calad.,
   CALC., calc-i.[1'], **CALC-P.,** calc-sil.[1'],
   cann-i.[8], cann-s., **canth., caps.,**
   CARB-AN., CARB-V., CARBN-S.,
   cast.[3, 6], **caust., CHAM., CHEL.,**
   chin., **chr-ac.,** cic., cimic., **CINA,**
   cinnb., cist., clem., cob.[3],
   cob-n.[9, 10, 14], coc-c., **coca, cocc.,**
   cod., **coff.,** colch., coloc., **con.,**
   convo-s.[9, 14], corn., cortico.[9, 14],
   cortiso.[9, 14], **CROC.,** crot-h., crot-t.,
   cupr., cycl., **dig., dios., dros., dulc.,**
   echi.[3], elaps[3], erig.[10], **eup-per.,**

   euph., **euphr., ferr., ferr-ar.,** ferr-i.,
   ferr-p., fl-ac.[3, 8], form., **gamb., gels.,**
   gran., **graph.,** grat., **guaj.,** harp.[14],
   hed.[9, 10, 14], hell., **hep., hydr.,**
   hydroph.[14], hyos., **ign.,** iod., ip.,
   iris[3], **kali-ar., KALI-BI., kali-c.,**
   kali-i., kali-m.[1'], **KALI-N., kali-p.,**
   kali-sil.[1'], **kalm., kreos.,** lac-c.[8],
   LACH., laur., led., lept.[3], lil-t.[3, 8],
   lith-c.[8], lob.[3], lyc., **mag-c.,**
   mag-f.[10, 14], **mag-m.,** mag-s.[9, 10, 14],
   magn-gr.[8], mang., med.[7, 8], meny.,
   meph.[4], **merc.,** merc-c., **merc-i-f.,**
   mez., mosch., mur-ac., **naja**[3, 6],
   NAT-AR., nat-c., **NAT-M.,**
   nat-n.[3, 6], **nat-p., NAT-S.,** nat-sil.[1'],
   nicc., **NIT-AC.,** nuph.[8], **nux-m.,**
   NUX-V., oci-s.[9, 14], olnd.[2, 3], **ONOS.,**
   op., ox-ac., par., pareir., perh.[14],
   PETR., PH-AC., PHOS., phyt.,
   pic-ac., **plan., plat.,** plb., **PODO.,**
   psor., ptel., **PULS., ran-b.,** ran-s.,
   rheum, RHOD., RHUS-T., RUMX.,
   ruta, sabad., **sabin., sal-ac.,** samb.,
   sang., sars., sec., **sel., senec.,**
   seneg., **SEP., sil., SPIG.,** spong.,
   SQUIL., stann., staph., stell.[8],
   stram., stront-c., stry.[8], **SUL-AC.**[1],
   sul-i.[1'], **SULPH.,** tab., **tarax.,** tell.[14],
   teucr., **thuj., TUB.**[7], **VALER.,**
   ven-m.[14], **verat., verat-v.,** verb.,
   viol-o., viol-t., visc.[9, 14], **zinc.,**
   zinc-p.[1']

5 h
   aloe[3], apis[3, 6], bov., **chin.**[3], cob.,
   dros.[3], helon., **kali-c.**[1', 3], kali-i.,
   nat-m.[3], nat-p.[3], ph-ac.[3], **podo.,**
   rumx.[3], sep.[3], sil.[3], sulph.[3]

6 h
   aloe, **alum.**[3], arn.[3], bov.[3], calc-p.,
   ferr.[3], **hep.**[3], lyc.[3], **nux-v.**[3], ox-ac.,
   sep., sil., sulph., verat.

7 h
   eup-per., **hep.**[3], nat-c.[3], **nux-v.**[3],
   podo., sep.[3]

8 h[3]
   eup-per., nux-v.

   breakfast/petit déjeuner/Frühstück

and afternoon[3]
et l'après-midi
und nachmittags
  sars.

and evening[3]
et le soir
und abends
  alum., bov., **calc.**, caust., coc-c.,
  graph., guaj., **kali-c.**, lach., **lyc.**,
  phos., psor., **rhus-t.**, sang., **SEP.**,
  stram., **stront-c.**, **thuj.**, verat.,
  zinc.

and night[3]
et la nuit
und nachts
  iod., nat-c.

morning of one day and the afternoon of the next[3]
un jour **le matin** et l'après-midi le
  lendemain
am **Morgen** des einen und am Nach-
  mittag des nächsten Tages
  lac-c.

am.[3, 6]
  acon., am-m., ambr.[4], apis[8],
  cench.[1'], jugl-c.[8], merc.[3, 4, 6],
  phos.[2, 3, 6], sang., still.[8], xero.[8],
  zinc.[4]

bed, in[3]
lit, au
Bett, im
  aloe, **am-m.**, ambr., bry., con.,
  kali-c., **lyc.**, **nux-v.**, phos., sep.,
  sulph.

daybreak am.[3]
pointe du jour am.
Tagesanbruch am.
  colch., syph.

sunrise, agg. before[3]
lever du soleil, agg. avant le
Sonnenaufgang, agg. vor
  lyc.

sunrise, after
lever du soleil, après le
Sonnenaufgang, nach
  cham., **nux-v.**, puls., syph.[7]

waking see sleep–after–morning

FORENOON (9–12 h.)
MATINÉE
VORMITTAGS
  aloe, alum., alum-p.[1'], **alumn.**[2],
  am-c., am-m., ambr., anac.[3], ang.[2, 3],
  ant-c., ant-t., aran., **arg-m.**,
  arg-n.[3, 6], ars., ars-s-f.[1'], asaf.,
  aur., aur-ar.[1'], aur-s.[1'], bar-c.,
  bar-m., **bar-s.**[1'], bell., bor., bov.,
  bry., cact., calc., calc-sil.[1'],
  CANN-I.[2], **CANN-S.**, canth.,
  carb-an., **carb-v.**, carbn-s., caust.,
  cedr., cham., chel., chin., cocc.,
  coloc., con.[2, 3], cupr., cycl., dros.,
  dulc., euph., euphr., ferr., **fl-ac.**[3],
  graph.[2, 3], **guaj.**, halo.[14], hell.,
  hep.[2, 3], ign., ip., kali-ar., kali-c.,
  kali-m.[1'], kali-n., kali-p., kali-sil.[1'],
  kreos., lach., **laur.**, lyc.[2, 3], mag-c.,
  mag-m., **mang.**, merc., mez., mosch.,
  mur-ac., **nat-ar.**, **NAT-C.**, **NAT-M.**,
  nat-p., **nat-sil.**[1'], nit-ac., **nux-m.**,
  nux-v., par., **pareir.**[2], petr., ph-ac.,
  phos., plat.[2, 3], plb., **PODO.**, puls.,
  ran-b., rhod., rhus-t., rumx.,
  SABAD., **sars.**, **sec.**, sel.[2], sil.,
  seneg., **SEP.**, **sil.**, **spig.**, spong.[2, 3],
  STANN., staph.[2, 3], stram.[3],
  stront-c., **SUL-AC.**, **SULPH.**, tarax.,
  teucr., valer., verat.[2, 3], verb.,
  viol-t., zinc., zinc-p.[1']

9 h
  bry.[3], **cham.**, **eup-per.**[3], kali-bi.[3],
  kali-c., lac-c.[3], nat-m.[3], nux-v.[3],
  podo., sep.[3], sumb., **verb.**[3]

9–11 h[6]
  stann.

9–14 h[6]
  nat-m.

10 h
ars.³, bor.³, chin.³, chin-s.³, cimic.,
eup-per.³, gels., iod.³, meli.³,
NAT-M., nux-v., petr.³, phos.³,
rhus-t.³, sep.³, sil.³, stann.³, sulph.³,
thuj.³

10–11 h agg.⁸
gels., nat-m.⁶, ⁸, sep., sulph.

10–15 h agg.⁷
tub.

11 h
arg-m., arg-n.⁶, ⁷, ars., arum-t.,
asaf.³, asar., bapt.³, berb., cact.,
chin-s.³, cimic., cob., cocc.³, gels.³,
hydr., hyos., ind.⁶, ip., lach.³, ⁶,
mag-p.³, nat-c.³, NAT-M.³, nat-p.³,
nux-v.³, phos.³, phyt., puls.³,
rhus-t.³, sep.³, stann.³, SULPH.,
zinc.³

am.
alum., lil-t.⁸, LYC., nat-sil.¹'

NOON (12 h)
MIDI
MITTAGS
alum., ant-c.³, apis, ARG-M.,
arg-n.³, ars., bol-la.³, bruc.⁴, carb-v.,
cham.³, chel.³, chin.³, cic., coloc.³,
elaps³, eup-per.³, gels.³, kali-bi.,
kali-c.³, lach.³, mag-c.³, nat-m.³,
nux-m., nux-v.³, paeon., phos.,
sang.³, sel.³, sep., sil.³, spig.³,
stram., sulph., valer., verb.³, zinc.

12–24 h⁶
lach.

eating, after⁶
mangé, après avoir
Essen, nach dem
grat.³, halo.¹⁴, mag-m., nat-c.,
nux-m., valer.

am.
CHEL., nat-s.⁶

symptoms increasing till noon,
then decreasing³, ⁶
les symptômes augmentent jusqu'à
midi, puis déclinent
Symptome nehmen bis mittags zu,
dann ab
acon.³, arg-n., bry.³, echi., gels.,
glon., kali-bi.³, kalm.¹', ³, ⁶, nat-m.³,
nux-v.³, sang.³, ⁷, sanic.⁷, spig.⁷,
stann., stram.³, stront-c., sulph.³

AFTERNOON (13–18 h)
APRÈS-MIDI
NACHMITTAGS
acon., aesc.⁸, aeth., agar., all-c.,
aloe, alum., ALUM-P.¹', alum-sil.¹',
am-c., am-m., ambr., anac., ang.², ³,
ant-c., ant-t., apis, arg-m., arg-n.,
arn., ars., ars-i., ars-s-f.¹', asaf.,
asar., aur., aur-ar.¹', aur-i.¹', aur-s.¹',
aur-sil.¹', aza.¹⁴, bar-c., bar-i.¹',
bar-m., bar-s.¹', BELL., bism., bor.,
bov., bry., buth-a.⁹, ¹⁴, cact., calad.,
calc., calc-i.¹', calc-p., calc-sil.¹',
camph., cann-s., canth., caps.,
carb-an., carb-v., carbn-s., caust.,
cedr., cench.⁷, ⁸, cham., chel., chin.,
cic., cimic., cina, coc-c., cocc., coff.,
colch., coloc., con., croc., cycl.,
cyn-d.¹⁴, cyt-l.¹⁰, ¹⁴, dig., dios., dros.,
dulc., euphr., eys.⁹, fago.⁸, ferr.,
ferr-ar., ferr-i., ferr-m.², ferr-p.,
fl-ac.³, gels., graph.², ³, grat.⁴,
guaj.³, hell., hep.², ³, hip-ac.⁹, ¹⁴,
hyos., ign., iod., ip., kali-ar.,
kali-bi., kali-c., kali-cy.⁸, kali-m.¹',
KALI-N., kali-p., kali-sil.¹', kreos.,
lach., laur., led., lil-t.⁸, lob.⁸, LYC.,
mag-c., mag-m., mang., meli.,
meny., merc., mez., mosch.,
mur-ac., naja¹⁴, nat-ar., nat-c.², ³, ⁶,
nat-m., nicc., nit-ac., nux-m.,
nux-v., ol-an., op., par., petr.,
ph-ac., phos., phyt., plan., plat.², ³,
plb., ptel., PULS., ran-b., ran-s.,
rheum, rhod., RHUS-T., rumx.,
ruta, sabad., sabin., sal-ac., sang.,
sars., sel., seneg., SEP., SIL.,
SIN-N., spig., spong.², ³, squil.,
stann., staph.², ³, still., sul-ac.,

sul-i.[1]', **sulph.**, tarax., **teucr.**,
thiop.[14], **THUJ., valer., ven-m.**[14],
verat.[2, 3], verb., **viol-t.**, wye.[1]',
x-ray[8], xero.[8], **ZINC., ZINC-P.**[1]'

13 h
arg-m., **ars.**[3], cact.[3], chel.[3], cina[3],
grat.[3], kali-c.[3], **lach.**[3], mag-c., phos.[3],
puls.[3]

13–14 h[1]'
ars.

13–21 h[6]
chel.

14 h
ars.[3], calc., chel.[3], cur.[7], **eup-per.**[3],
ferr.[3], gels.[3], lach., lob., mag-p.[3],
nit-ac., ol-an., puls., sang.

14, 15, 16 h till towards morning[6]
14, 15, 16 h jusque vers le matin
14, 15, 16 h bis gegen Morgen
syph.

14.30 h
hell.

15 h
ang.[3], ant-t.[3], **apis**, ars., asaf.[3], asar.,
BELL., bry.[1', 7], cedr.[3], cench., chel.[3],
chin-s.[3], clem., con.[3], nat-m.[3],
samb.[3], sang.[3], sil., staph., sulph.,
thuj.

15–17 h
sep.

15–18 h[6]
apis

15–3 h[1]'
bell.

16 h
aesc.[3], alum., anac., **apis**[3], ars.[3],
arum-t., cact.[3], calc-p., carb-v.,
caust., cedr.[3], chel., **chin-s.**[3], cob.,
coloc., gels., **hell.**, hep.[3], ip.[3],
kali-c., lachn., **LYC.**, mag-m.,
mang.[3], mur-ac., nat-m.[3], nat-s.,
nit-ac.[3], **nux-v.**[3], puls., rhus-t.[3],
stront-c., sulph.[3], verb.[3]

16–17 h[14]
allox.

16–18 h
alum.[16], eys.[9, 14], gels.[6], **sep.**[1]

16–19 h[6]
coloc., **lyc.**

16–20 h
alum., bov., buth-a.[9, 10], coloc.[3],
hell., LYC., mag-m., nux-m.,
sabad.[3, 8], sulph., zinc.[3]

16–22 h
alum., chel., plat.

16–4 h[6]
thuj.

17 h
alum.[3], bov.[3], caust.[3], cedr.[3], **chin.**[3],
cimic., **coloc.**, con., **gels.**[3], **hep.**,
hyper.[3], kali-c., **lyc.**[3], nat-m.[3],
nux-v.[3], **PULS.**[1, 7], **rhus-t.**[3], sulph.[3],
THUJ.[3], tub.[3], valer.[3]

17–18 h[14]
ange-s., methys.

17–20 h
lil-t.

and evening[3]
et le soir
und abends
kali-c.

am.
cinnb., cob-n.[14], cortico.[9, 14], hecla[14],
hed.[14], kali-c.[14], **nat-s.**[3], phyt.[3],
rhus-t.[3], **sep.**[3, 6]

EVENING (18–21 h)
SOIR
ABENDS
abrot., **acon.**, agar., agn., alf.[8],
all-c., aloe, **ALUM.**, alum-sil.[1]',
alumn.[2], am-br.[8], **AM-C., am-m.,**
AMBR., anac., ang.[2, 3], **ANT-C.,**

ANT-T., apis, **arg-m., arg-n., ARN.,
ars., ars-i.,** ars-s-f.[1'], **asaf., asar.,**
aur., aur-ar.[1'], aur-i.[1'], **aur-s.**[1'],
bapt., bar-c., bar-i.[1'], bar-m., bar-s.[1'],
BELL., berb., berb-a.[14], bism., **bor.,
bov., brom., BRY.,** bufo[3], buth-a.[9],
caj.[8], **calad., CALC.,** calc-ar.[1'],
calc-i.[1'], calc-p., **calc-s., CALC-SIL.**[1'],
camph., cann-s., canth., **CAPS.,
CARB-AN., CARB-V., CARBN-S.,**
carc.[9], **CAUST.,** cedr., **cench.**[1', 7],
CHAM., chel., chin., chlorpr.[14], cic.,
cimic., cina, clem., **cocc.,** coff.,
COLCH., coloc., com., **con., croc.,**
crot-h., cupr., **cupr-s.**[2], **CYCL.,**
cyn-d.[14], cyt-l.[9, 10, 14], dig., dios.[8],
dirc., dros., **dulc.,** euon-a.[8],
EUPHR., eys.[9, 14], **ferr., ferr-ar.,
ferr-i., ferr-p., fl-ac.,** flor-p.[14],
form.[6], **gamb., graph., guaj.,** hecla[14],
HELL., hep., HYOS., ign., iod., ip.,
jatr., **kali-ar., kali-bi., kali-c.,
kali-i.,** kali-m.[1'], **KALI-N., kali-p.,
kali-s.,** kali-sil.[1'], **kalm.,** kreos.,
LACH., laur., led., lil-t., **LYC.,
MAG-C., mag-m., mang., MENY.,**
meph.[4], **MERC.,** merc-c.[8], **merc-i-r.,
MEZ.,** mosch., mur-ac., **nat-ar.,
nat-c., nat-m., NAT-P.,** nat-sil.[1'],
nep.[10, 13, 14], nicc., **NIT-AC., nux-m.,
nux-v.,** olnd.[2, 3], op., osm., **ox-ac.,**
palo.[14], **par.**[2, 3], penic.[13], **petr.,
PHOS-AC., PHOS.,** phyt., pic-ac.,
pitu.[14], plan., **PLAT., PLB.,** psor.,
ptel., PULS., ran-b., RAN-S., rheum,
rhod., rhus-t., RUMX., RUTA,
sabad., **sabin.,** sal-ac., **samb., sang.,
sars.,** sel., **seneg., SEP., SIL.,
SIN-N.,** spig., **spong.,** squil.,
STANN., staph., stict., **STRONT-C.,
SUL-AC.,** sul-i.[1'], **SULPH., sumb.,**
syph.[3, 8], **tab.,** tarax., tarent.[2], teucr.,
thiop.[14], **thuj.,** trios.[14], v-a-b.[14],
VALER., verat., verb., vib., viol-o.,
viol-t., x-ray[9], **ZINC., ZINC-P.**[1']

18 h
ant-t.[3], bapt., calc.[7], calc-p., caust.,
cedr.[3], dig., hep., hyper., **kali-c.**[3],
kali-i., lachn., nat-m.[3], **NUX-V.**[3],
penic.[13], petr.[3], **puls.**[3], **rhus-t.**[3],
sep.[3], **sil.**[3], **sumb.**

18–19 h
carc.[9], culx.[1'], **hep.**

18–20 h[14]
rauw.

18–22 h[14]
kali-c.

18–4 h[7]
guaj.

18–6 h
kreos., lil-t.[6], **syph.**

19 h
alum.[3], ant-c., bov., cedr.[3], chin-s.[3],
culx.[1'], ferr.[3], gamb.[3], gels.[3], **hep.**[3],
ip.[3], **lyc.,** nat-m.[3], **nat-s.**[3], **nux-v.**[3],
petr., puls.[3], pyrog.[3], rhus-t., **sep.**[3],
sulph.[3], tarent.[3]

20 h
alum.[3], **bov.**[3], caust.[3], coff.[3], elaps[3],
hep.[3], mag-c.[3], merc.[3], merc-i-r.,
phos.[3], **rhus-t.**[3], **SULPH.**[3], tarax.

20–3 h[6]
syph.

21 h
ars.[3], **bov.**[3], **BRY.,** calc.[7], **gels.**[3],
merc.[3], mur-ac., sulph.

**and night
et nuit
und nachts**
cenchr.[1'], lil-t.[6], mag-c.[3]

air agg., in open
air agg., en plein
Freien agg., im
   am-c., carb-an., carb-v., **merc.,**
   nit-ac., sulph.

am.
   agar.[6], **alum.**, aran-ix.[10], arn.,
   arg-m., asaf., **AUR.**, bor.[8], bruc.[4],
   cast.[6], chel., cob-n.[9], cortiso.[14],
   halo.[14], hed.[10, 14], kali-n.[4],
   lob.[8], lyc., mag-c.[10], **med.**, nat-m.[6],
   nicc.[8], nux-v.[8], podo.[6], **puls.**[3, 4, 6],
   sep., stel.[8], thyr.[14], visc.[9, 14]

16 h till going to bed am.
à 16 h jusqu'au coucher am.
16 h bis zum Zubettgehen am.
   alum.

eating, after
mangé, après avoir
Essen, nach dem
   indg.

   am.
      sep.

every other evening
tous les 2 soirs
jeden 2. Abend
   puls.

lying down agg., after
mis au lit agg., après s'être
Hinlegen agg., nach dem
   ars., graph.[6], hep.[6], **ign., led.,**
   merc.[6], **phos.**, puls.[6], sel.[6],
   stront-c., **sulph.**, thuj.

   am.
      kali-n.

sleep, before going to
s'endormir, avant de
Einschlafen, vor dem
   plat.

sunset, after
coucher du soleil, après le
Sonnenuntergang, nach
   ang.[3], bry., ign., lycps.[3], merc.[3],
   phyt.[3], **puls.**, rhus-t., syph.[3]

   am.[3]
      coca, lil-t., med., sel.

till sunrise
jusqu'à son lever
bis Sonnenaufgang, von S.
   aur., cimic., colch., **merc.**[3, 8],
   phyt.[8], **SYPH.**[1, 7]

twilight agg.
crépuscule agg.
Abenddämmerung agg.
   am-m., ang.[3], arg-n.[3], **ars.,**
   ars-s-f.[1'], berb.[3], **calc., caust.,**
   cham.[3], dig., graph.[3], mang.[3],
   nat-m., nat-s.[3], **phos.**, plat.[3], plb.,
   PULS., rhus-t., staph., sul-ac.,
   valer.

   am.
      alum., bry., meny.[3], **phos.**, tab.[3]

NIGHT (21–5 h)
NUIT
NACHTS
   abel.[14], abrot., acet-ac., **ACON.,**
   agar., agn., agre.[14], aloe, alum.,
   ALUM-P.[1'], alum-sil.[1'], alumn.[2],
   am-br., am-c., **am-m.**, ambr., **ammc.,**
   anac., **ang.**[2, 3], **ant-c., ant-t.,**
   apis[3, 6, 8], apoc., **aral.**, aran.[3],
   arg-m., **ARG-N.**, arist-cl.[9], **ARN.,**
   ARS., ARS-I., ARS-S-F.[1'], asaf.,
   asar., aster.[8], **aur.**, aur-ar.[1'], aur-i.[1'],
   aur-m.[1'], **AUR-S.**[1'], bac.[8], **bar-c.,**
   bar-i.[1'], **bar-m., bar-s.**[1'], **bell.,**
   benz-ac., berb-a.[14], bism., bor.,
   bov., brom., bry., bufo[3], buni-o.[14],
   but-ac.[8], cact., caj.[8], calad., **CALC.,**
   calc-ar.[1'], **CALC-I., CALC-P.,**
   CALC-S., CALC-SIL.[1'], camph.,
   cann-i., cann-s., canth., caps.,
   carb-ac., **CARB-AN., carb-v.,**
   CARBN-S., caust., cedr., **cench.**[1',7,8],
   CHAM., chel.[1], **CHIN.**, chin-ar.,
   chion.[8], cic., cimic.[3], **cina**[1], **CINNB.,**
   clem., coc-c., **cocc., cod., COFF.,**
   COLCH., coloc., com.[8], **CON.,**
   convo-s.[14], **croc.**, crot-c.[8], **crot-h.,**
   crot-t.[4], **cupr., CYCL.**, cyt-l.[9], **dig.,**
   dios., **dol., dros., DULC.**, elaps,
   erig.[10], eucal., **euphr., equis.,**
   FERR., FERR-AR., FERR-I., ferr-p.,

fl-ac., flaw.[14], **gamb.**, **GRAPH.**,
grat.[4], guaj., hed.[9], **hell.**, **HEP.**,
hip-ac.[14], **HYOS.**, ign., **IOD.**, **IP.**,
iris[8], jal.[3, 6], **KALI-AR.**, **KALI-BI.**,
kali-br., **KALI-C.**, **KALI-I.**, kali-m.,
kali-n., **kali-p.**, **kali-sil.**[1'] kalm.[1'],
kreos., **LACH.**, laur., **led.**, **LIL-T.**,
lob.[3], **lyc.**, **MAG-C.**, **MAG-M.**,
mag-p.[3, 8], mand.[9], **MANG.**, meny.,
meph.[3, 14], **MERC.**, **merc-c.**,
merc-i-f., **mez.**, moly-met.[14], mosch.,
mur-ac., **nat-ar.**, **nat-c.**, **nat-m.**,
nat-p., **nat-s.**, **nat-sil.**[1'], nep.[10, 13, 14],
NIT-AC., **nux-m.**, **nux-v.**, olnd.,
op., **ox-ac.**, par., pareir.[2], **petr.**,
ph-ac., phenob.[13], **PHOS.**, **phyt.**,
pic-ac., plat., **PLB.**, **PSOR.**, **PULS.**,
pyrog.[3], ran-b., ran-s., rat.[3], **rheum,**
rhod., **RHUS-T.**, **RUMX.**, ruta[3, 6],
sabad., sabin., sal-ac., **samb.**, sang.,
sarcol-ac.[14], **sars.**, **sec.**, **sel.**, senec.,
seneg., **SEP.**, sieg.[10], **SIL.**, sin-n.,
spig., **spong.**, squil., **stann.**, **staph.**,
stict., still.[3], stram., **STRONT-C.**,
sul-ac., **SUL-I.**[1'], **SULPH.**,
SYPH.[1'-3, 6-8], tarax., tarent.,
TELL., ter.[3], teucr., thal.[14], thea[8],
thuj., trios.[14], valer., verat., vib.[8],
viol-t., vip.[3], visc.[14], x-ray[8], **ZINC.**,
ZINC-P.[1']

22 h
ars.[3], bov.[3], cham., **CHIN-S.**[3],
graph.[3], ign.[3], lach.[3], petr.[3], podo.,
puls.

23 h
aral.[3], ars.[3], bell., **cact.**, calc.[3],
carb-an.[3], lach., rumx., sil., sulph.[3]

night-air agg.[3]
air de la nuit **agg.**
Nachtluft agg.
am-c., carb-v., merc., nat-s., nit-ac.,
sulph.

am.[3, 6]
alum.[3, 4], ang., arg-m.[3], caust.,
cupr-a.[8], laur.[3, 4], mand.[9], med.[7],
petr.[3]

every other night
une nuit sur deux
jede zweite Nacht
    puls.

midnight[3]
minuit
Mitternacht
    ACON.[3, 7], aran.[8], arg-n.[3, 6],
    ars.[3, 7, 8], ars-i.[6], brom.[6], calc.,
    calad., canth., **caust.**, chin.[1', 3],
    dig., **dros.**, **ferr.**, hed.[14], kali-ar.[1'],
    kali-c., lach.[3, 4], lyc., **mag-m.**,
    mez.[8], **mur-ac.**, nat-m., nux-m.,
    nux-v.[3, 6], op.[3, 6], phos., puls.[3, 6],
    rhus-t., **samb.**, spong., stram.,
    sulph.[3, 7], verat., zinc.[5]

before/avant/vor
    alum., alum-p.[1'], am-m., ambr.,
    anac., **ang.**[2, 3], **ant-t.**, apis,
    ARG-N., arn., **ARS.**, ars-s-f.[1'],
    asar., **bell.**, brom., **bry.**,
    calad.[2, 3], cann-s., caps.[3],
    CARB-V., carbn-s., **caust.**,
    CHAM., chel., chin., **COFF.**,
    colch., **cupr.**, cycl., dulc., ferr.,
    ferr-ar., **fl-ac.**[3], graph., **hep.**,
    ign., **KALI-AR.**, kali-c.,
    kali-m.[1'], **lach.**, **LED.**, **LYC.**,
    mag-c.[3], **mang.**, merc., **mez.**,
    mosch., **mur-ac.**, nat-m.,
    nat-p.[1'], nat-s.[1'], **nit-ac.**, nux-v.,
    osm., petr., **PHOS.**, phyt., plat.,
    psor., **PULS.**, ran-b., **RAN-S.**,
    rhod., **rhus-t.**, **RUMX.**, **ruta,**
    SABAD., samb., **sep.**, **spig.**,
    spong., **STANN.**, **staph.**,
    stront-c., sulph., teucr., thuj.,
    valer., verat.[3], viol-t.

after/après/nach
    acon., alum., alum-p.[1'],
    alum-sil.[1'], am-m., ambr.,
    ang.[2, 3], ant-c., apis[8], arist-cl.[9],
    ARS., **ars-i.**, asaf., aur.,
    aur-ar.[1'], bar-c., bar-i.[1'], bar-m.,
    bar-s.[1'], bell., bor., **bry.**,
    calad.[2, 3], **calc.**, **calc-i.**[1'],
    calc-sil.[1'], **cann-s.**, canth.,
    caps., **carb-an.**[2, 3, 8], carb-v.,

caust., cham., **chel.**, chin.,
coc-c., cocc., coff., con., croc.,
cupr., DROS., dulc., euph.[2],
euphr., **ferr., ferr-ar.**, ferr-i.,
ferr-p., **gels.**, graph., hed.[9],
hell., hep., **ign.**, iod., **KALI-C.**,
kali-m.[1]', **KALI-N.**, kali-p.,
kali-sil.[1]', lyc.[2, 3], **mag-c.**,
mand.[9, 10], **mang., merc., mez.**,
mur-ac., **NAT-AR.**, nat-c.,
nat-m., nat-p., nat-s., nat-sil.[1]',
nit-ac., **NUX-V.**, par., **ph-ac.**,
PHOS., phyt., plat., **PODO.**,
puls., ran-b., **ran-s.**, rhod.,
RHUS-T., rumx., sabad., sabin.,
samb., sars., seneg., sep., **SIL.**,
spig., **spong.**, squil., staph.,
stram., sul-ac., sul-i.[3], **sulph.**,
tarax., **THUJ.**, viol-o.

0–4 h[6]: thuj.

1 h
ARS., carb-v.[3], caul., cocc.,
lachn., mag-m., mur-ac., psor.,
puls.[3]

1–2 h[1]'
ars.

1–3 h
kali-ar.

2 h
all-c. (non[1]: ars.), aur-m.,
benz-ac., **caust.**[3], com.[3], cur.[7],
dros., ferr., graph.[3], **hep.**, iris[3],
(non[1]: kali-ar.), **kali-bi., kali-br.**,
KALI-C., kali-p.[3], lach.[3], lachn.,
lyc.[3], mag-c., mez.[3], nat-m.[3],
nat-s.[3], **nit-ac.**[3], ptel.[3], **puls.**[3],
rumx., sars.[3], **sil.**[3], spig.[3], sulph.[3]

2–3 h
gink-b.[14], kali-bi.[6]

2–4 h
arist-cl.[9, 10], **KALI-C.**

2–5 h[8]
aesc., aeth., **aloe**, am-c., bac.,
bell., bell-p.[10], chel., cina, coc-c.,
cur., hed.[10], **kali-bi., kali-c.**,
kali-cy., kali-p., nat-s., **nux-v.**,
ox-ac., **podo.**, ptel., rhod.,
rumx., sulph., thuj., tub.

3 h
adlu.[14], **am-c., am-m.**[3], ant-c.,
ant-t., **ars.**[1], bapt., bor., **bry.**[3],
calc., canth.[3], **cedr.**[3], chin., con.,
euphr., dulc., ferr.[3], hed.[9, 10, 14],
iris, **kali-ar.**[1], kali-bi.[1]', **KALI-C.**,
kali-n., kali-p.[7], **mag-c.**[3, 10],
mag-f.[10, 14], mag-m., **nat-m.**[3],
nux-v., podo., **rhus-t.**[3], sec., **sel.**[3],
sep., sil.[3], staph., **sulph.**[3], thuj.,
zinc.

3–4 h[6]
am-m., arist-cl.[10], caust., kali-bi.,
kali-c., med.[7], nux-v.[6]

3–5 h[10]
bor.[6], calc-f., mag-c., mand.,
syph.[6]

4 h
alum.[3], alumn., **am-m.**[3], anac.[3],
apis[3], **arn.**[3], **bor.**[3], **caust.**[3],
CEDR.[3], chel., coloc.[3], **con.**[3],
cycl.[6], ferr.[3], **ign.**[3], kali-c.[3], **lyc.**[3],
mag-c.[10], **mur-ac.**[3], **nat-s.**[3],
nit-ac.[3], **NUX-V.**[3], penic.[13, 14],
podo., **puls.**[3], rad-br.[3], sep.[3], sil.[3],
stann.[3], **sulph.**[3], verat.[3]

4–16 h
kali-cy.[7], **MED.**[7], nux-v.

am.
LYC., mand.[9], nat-p.[1]', nat-s.[1]'

until noon[8]
jusqu'à midi
bis mittags
puls.

until noon
jusqu'à midi
bis mittags
ars., cist.

ABSCESSES, suppurations
ABCÈS, suppurations
ABSZESSE, Eiterungen
  acon.[8, 11], all-c.[2], **anan.,** ant-c.,
  ant-t., **ANTHRACI.**[1, 7], **apis**[2, 8, 12],
  ARN.[2, 3, 6, 8, 12], ars., **ars-i.,** ars-s-f.[1'],
  asaf., bar-c., bar-m.[11], **bell.**[2, 6, 8, 12],
  bell-p.[7], both.[11], **bry.,** bufo[3, 12],
  calc., calc-f.[1', 10], **calc-hp.**[3, 6, 8],
  CALC-I., CALC-S., calc-sil.[1'],
  CALEN.[2, 3, 7, 8, 12], **canth.**[2], caps.,
  carb-ac.[8], carb-an.[6], **carb-v.,**
  caust.[2], **cench.**[1'], **cham.**[2, 4], **chin.**[8, 12],
  chin-ar.[10], chin-s.[8, 11], cic., **cist.**[2, 6],
  cocc., con., conch.[11], **croc.,** crot-h.,
  cupr.[6,] digox.[12], **dulc., echi.**[3, 6, 7],
  elat.[12], **fl-ac.**[2, 6-8, 12], **guaj., gunp.**[7],
  HEP., hippoz.[2, 8, 12], kali-c., kali-chl.,
  kali-s.[3], **kreos.**[2, 6], **LACH., lap-a.**[2, 8],
  led.[2, 8], **lyc.**[1'-3, 6, 8], mag-c., **mang.**[1', 2],
  matth.[12], **MERC.,** merc-d.[3], methyl.[12],
  mez., **myris.**[6-8, 10, 12], nat-c., nat-m.,
  nat-sal.[12], nat-sil.[1'], **nit-ac.,** nux-v.,
  ol-j.[1] (non: olnd.), paeon., petr.,
  ph-ac.[1', 6, 8], **PHOS.**[1'-4, 6, 8],
  phyt.[2, 6], plb.[11], psor.[6], ptel.[11], puls.,
  pyrog., raja-s.[14],
  rhus-t.[1'-3, 4, 6, 8], **sec.,** sep., sieg.[7, 10],
  SIL., sil-mar.[8], staph., **stram.,**
  sul-ac.[2], sul-i.[3, 6], **sulph.,** symph.[12],
  syph.[1', 7, 8, 12], tarent.[2, 3], **tarent-c.,**
  thyr.[12], tub.[6], vesp.[8, 11, 12], **vip.**[4],
  wies.[11]

fistulae/fistules/Fisteln
reaction, lack/réaction, manque/
  Reaktionsmangel
wounds–supparating/plaies–
  suppurantes/Wunden–eiternde

abort, remedies to[8]
arrêter l'évolution d'un, remèdes
  pour
kupieren; Mittel, um A. zu
  apis, arn.[7], bell., bry., calc.[1'],
  calc-s.[2], **hep., merc.**

absorption of pus[3]
absorption de pus
Absorption von Eiter
  iod., **LACH., phos.,** sil.

bones, of[6]
os, des
Knochen, der
  ang., arg-m., arg-n., aur., calc-f.,
  calc-hp., merc-aur., phos., puls.[3],
  sil., staph., sulph.[3]

burning
brûlure, avec
Brennen, mit
  ANTHRACI., ARS., merc.[1'], **pyrog.,**
  TARENT-C.

chronic[2, 8]
chroniques
chronische
  arg-m.[14], arn.[8], **asaf.**[2], aur.[2], calc.,
  calc-f.[8], calc-i.[8], calc-p.[8], calc-s.[6],
  carb-v., cham.[8], chin.[8], con.[2],
  fl-ac.[6, 8], graph.[8], **hep., iod.,** iodof.[8],
  kali-i.[8], laur.[2], lyc.[2], mag-f.[14],
  mang.[2], **merc.,** merc-c.[2], merc-i-r.[8],
  nit-ac.[2], ol-j.[8, 12], phos.[2, 6, 8], sars.[2],
  sep.[2], **SIL.**[2, 7, 8], **sulph.**

effects from[6]
troubles à la suite d'
Folgen von Abszessen
  abrot., **chin.,** chin-ar., ferr., kali-c.,
  nat-m., ph-ac., **phos.**

fever, continued[7]
fièvre, continue
Fieber, anhaltendes
  ph-ac.

foreign bodies, elimination of
corps étrangers, élimination des
Fremdkörpern, zur Ausscheidung von
  arn.[7], hep.[1', 2], lob.[7, 12], SIL.[2, 7, 12]

gangrenous[2]
gangreneux
brandige
  ars., asaf., carb-v., chin., chin-s.,
  hep., kreos., LACH., merc., nit-ac.,
  phos., **sil., sul-ac.**

glands, of
glandes, ganglions des
Drüsenabszeß
  aur.[4], **aur-m-n.**[2], bad.[3, 6], **bar-c.**[2, 3, 6],
  bar-m., **bell.**, brom., **CALC.**,
  calc-f.[10], **calc-hp.**[3, 6, 10], calc-i.[8],
  calc-p.[10], **CALC-S.**, canth.,
  carb-an.[3, 6, 10], carb-v., cinnb.[1'],
  cist., clem.[3, 6], coloc., crot-h., **dulc.**,
  echi.[6], fl-ac.[3, 6, 10], **form.**[3, 6], **guaj.**,
  guare.[2], **HEP.**, hyos., ign., jug-r.[12],
  KALI-I., kreos., **lach.**, lap-a.[8], **lyc.**,
  MERC., myris.[10], **nit-ac.**, petr.,
  phos., **phyt.**[3], **pyrog.**, **rhus-t.**, sars.,
  sec.[12], **sep.**, **SIL.**, sil-mar.[12], spig.[3],
  squil., sul-ac.[3], **SULPH.**, **stram.**,
  syph., teucr-s.[6, 10], **tub.**, zinc.[3]

hasten suppuration remedies to[1'-3, 8]
hâter la suppuration, remèdes pour
beschleunigen; Mittel, um die
  Eiterung zu
  ars.[3], **bell.**[3], guaj.[8], **hep.**, lach.[3, 8],
  merc., nat-sil.[1'], oper.[8], phos.[8],
  phyt.[8], puls.[3], **sil.**[1-3, 7, 8], sulph.[1']

incipient[6]
commençant
Beginn, im
  apis, **arn.**[2, 6], ars., **bar-c.**[2], **bell.**,
  carb-an., euph., guaj., **hep.**, **lach.**,
  merc.[2, 6], rhus-t.

internal organs, of[2]
internes, des organes
innerer Organe
  canth., **LACH.**

joints, of[6]
articulations, des
Gelenkabszeß
  ang.[2], ars-i., bac., calc., calc-f.,
  calc-hp.[6, 8], **calc-p.**[2, 3], calc-s.,
  conch.[11], fl-ac., guaj.[1'], kali-c.,
  kali-i., **merc.**[1'-3, 6], myris.[12], nit-ac.,
  ol-j.[12], ph-ac., **phos.**[3, 6], **psor.**[3, 6],
  puls., **sil.**[2, 3, 6, 8], ter., **teucr.**, thuj.,
  tub.

muscles, of [1', 8]
muscles, des
Muskeln, der
  calc.

pus, acrid[4]
pus âcre
Eiter, scharfer
  ail.[3], **ARS.**[3, 4], **asaf.**[6], bell-p.[3],
  brom.[3], **carb-v.**, **CAUST.**[2, 4, 6],
  cham., **clem.**, echi.[3], euphr.[3],
  fl-ac.[1'], gels.[3], **hep.**, **kali-ox.**[3],
  lach., **lyc.**, **merc.**[2, 4, 6], mez., **nat-c.**,
  nat-m., **NIT-AC.**[3, 4], nux-v.,
  petr.[2], phos., plb., puls., **ran-b.**[3, 4],
  ran-s., **rhus-t.**[2, 4, 6], ruta, sabad.[3],
  sanic.[3], sars.[3], **sep.**, **sil.**[2, 4, 6],
  spig., squil., **staph.**, **sulph.**[2-4, 6],
  zinc.

excoriating[4]
excoriant
wundmachender
  am-c., anac., bell., calc., chel.,
  con., cupr., graph., ign., iod.,
  kreos.

black[4]
noir
schwarzer
  bry., chin., lyc., **sulph.**[2, 4]

bland[2]
doux
milder
  bell., **calc.**, **hep.**, **lach.**, mang.,
  merc., phos., **PULS.**, rhus-t., **sil.**,
  staph., **sulph.**

bloody[4]
sanglant
blutiger
  arg-n., arn., **ars.**[2, 4, 6], **ASAF.**[2, 4, 6],
  bell., calc-s.[1'], **carb-v.**[2, 4],
  caust.[2, 4], con., croc., dros.,
  HEP.[2, 4, 6], iod., kali-c., kreos.,
  lach., **lyc.**[2, 4], **MERC.**[2, 3, 4, 6], mez.,
  nat-m., **nit-ac.**[2, 4, 6], ph-ac., phos.,
  phyt.[2], **puls.**[2, 4], **rhus-t.**[2, 4], ruta,
  sabin., sec., **sep.**, **sil.**[2, 4, 6], sul-ac.,
  sulph., zinc.

brown[2, 4]
brun
brauner
    anac.[4], **ars.**, bry., calc.[4], **carb-v.**,
    con.[4], puls.[4], **rhus-t., sil.**

fetid[4]
fétide
stinkender
    am-c., ant-t., **anthraci.**[2], arn.[7],
    ars.[2-4, 6], **ASAF.**[2, 4, 6], aur., bapt.[3],
    bar-m., **bell.**, bov., bry., **calc.**[2, 4, 6],
    carb-an.[2], **CARB-V.**[2, 4, 6],
    caust.[2, 4], chel., **chin.**[2, 4],
    chin-s.[2, 4, 12], cic., clem., con.[2, 3, 4],
    cycl., dros., fl-ac.[6], **graph.**[2, 4],
    HEP.[2, 4, 6], kali-c., **kali-p.**[2],
    KREOS.[2, 4], **lach.**[2, 4, 6], led.[3],
    lyc.[2, 4], mang., **merc.**[2, 4], mez.,
    mur-ac., nat-c., **nit-ac.**[2, 4, 6],
    nux-m., **nux-v.**[2, 4], paeon.[6], petr.[6],
    ph-ac.[2, 4, 6], phos.[2, 4, 6], **phyt.**[2],
    plb., **psor.**[3, 6], **puls.**, pyrog.[3],
    ran-b., **ran-s., rhus-t.**[2, 4], ruta,
    sabin., sec., **sep.**[2-4], **SIL.**[2-4, 6],
    squil., stann., **staph.**, sul-ac.[4, 6],
    SULPH.[2-4, 6], syph.[3], thuj., vip.[4, 6],
    vip-r.

gelatinous[2, 4]
gélatineux
gallertiger
    arg-m.[4], arn.[4], bar-c.[4], cham.,
    ferr.[4], merc., sep.[4], **sil.**

gray[2, 4]
gris
grauer
    ambr.[4], **ars.**, carb-an.[4], **caust.**,
    chin.[4], lyc.[4], merc., sep.[4], **sil.**,
    thuj.[4]

greenish[2, 4]
verdâtre
grünlicher
    ars.[4], **asaf., aur.**, carb-v.[4], **caust.**,
    kreos.[4], **MERC.**, nat-c.[4], nux-v.[4],
    phos.[4], **puls.**, rhus-t.[4], sec.[1', 3],
    sep., sil., staph.[4], syph.[3], tub.[3]

sour, smelling[2, 4]
acide, odeur
sauer riechender
    calc., graph.[4], **hep.**, kalm., **merc.**,
    nat-c.[4], sep.[4], sulph.

suppressed[3]
supprimé
unterdrückter
    bry., calc.[2], cham.[2], dulc., **HEP.**[2],
    lach.[2, 3], **merc.**[2], puls., **sil.**[2, 3],
    stram., **sulph.**

tenacious[2, 4]
collant, adhérent
zäher
    ars.[4], asaf., bor.[3], bov., cham.[4],
    coc-c.[3], **con.**[2-4], hydr.[3], kali-bi.[3],
    merc., mez.[4], ph-ac.[4], phos.[2],
    sep., sil.[4], sulph.[4]

thick[3]
épais
dicker
    arg-n., **calc-sil.**[1'], euphr., hep.,
    kali-bi., kali-s., **puls.**, sanic.

thin[3, 4]
fluide
dünner
    ars.[3], **asaf.**[3, 4, 6], carb-v.[4],
    caust.[3, 4, 6], dros.[4], fl-ac.[3], iod.[4],
    kali-c.[4], **lyc.**[4], **merc.**[3, 4, 6], nit-ac.,
    phos.[3], plb.[4], puls.[4], ran-b.[4],
    ran-s.[4], rhus-t.[3, 4, 6], ruta[4],
    sil.[3, 4, 6], staph.[4], **sulph.**[3, 4, 6],
    thuj.[4]

watery[2, 4, 6]
aqueux
wäßriger
    agar-cps.[11], **ars., ASAF.**, calc.[2, 3, 4],
    carb-v.[2, 4], **caust.**, cench.[1'],
    cham.[2], clem.[4], con.[4], dros.[4],
    fl-ac.[3], **graph.**[4], **iod.**[4], kali-c.[4],
    lach.[4], **lyc.**[2, 4], **merc., nit-ac.**[2, 3, 4],
    nux-v.[4], **phyt.**[2], plb.[4], puls.[4],
    ran-b.[2, 4], **ran-s.**[4], rhus-t.[6], **sil.**[3, 6]

whitish[4]
blanchâtre
weißlicher
   am-c., ars., **calc.**[2, 4], carb-v., hell.,
   lyc.[2, 4], nat-m., puls., sep., sil.,
   sulph.

yellow[4]
jaune
gelber
   acon., am-c., ambr., anac., ang.,
   arg-m., ars.[2, 4], aur., bov., **bry.**,
   calc.[2, 4, 6], calc-s.[1'], caps.,
   carb-v.[2, 4, 6], **caust.**[2, 4, 6], cench.[1'],
   cic., **clem.**, con., croc., dulc.,
   euphr.[3], graph., **HEP.**[2, 4], iod.,
   kali-n., kreos., lyc., mag-c., mang.,
   merc.[2, 4, 6], **mez.**[3, 6], **nat-c.**[2, 4],
   nat-m., **nit-ac.**[4, 6], **nux-v.**,
   phos.[1', 2, 4], **PULS.**[2, 4, 6],
   rhus-t.[2, 4], ruta, sec., sel.,
   sep.[2, 4, 6], **sil.**[2, 4, 6], spig., **staph.**[2, 4],
   sul-ac., **sulph.**[2], thuj., viol-t.

yellow-green[3]
jaune-verdâtre
gelb-grüner
   ars-i., **calc-sil.**[1'], kali-bi., kali-s.,
   merc.[1'], **puls.**[2, 3]

recurrent
récidivants
rezidivierende
   pyrog., syph.

wounds–reopening/plaies–
* réouverture/Wunden–Wieder-*
* aufbrechen*

ACETONEMIA of the child[14]
ACÉTONÉMIE de l'enfant
ACETONÄMIE des Kindes
phenob.

ACTIVITY am.[3]
ACTIVITÉ am.
AKTIVITÄT am.
   cycl., helon., iod., kali-bi., lil-t.,
   mur-ac., sep.

Vol. I: occupation/Beschäftigung
Vol. I: exertion/travail/Anstrengung

desire for[2]
désir d'
Verlangen nach
   acon., ars., aur., eucal.

increased[2]
augmentée
gesteigerte
   acon., **agar.**, ant-c., ant-t., camph.,
   cic.[14], eucal., **hyos.**, lyss., nep.[13, 14],
   op., **ox-ac.**, plat., **stram.**

outer a. ceases[9]
extérieure, cessation de l'
äußere A. hört auf
   anh.

physical[11]
corporelle
körperliche
   ars., coca[7, 11], fl-ac.[7], lycps.,
   nat-s., nep.[13, 14], **op.**, phos.

   exertion/exercice/Anstrengung

   afternoon[11]
   après-midi
   nachmittags
     rhus-t.

   evening[11]
   soir
   abends
     lycps.

   midnight, until[11]
   minuit, jusqu'à
   Mitternacht, bis
     COFF.

ADHAESION of inner parts,
   sensation of[3, 7]
ADHÈRENCE des parties internes,
   sensation d'
VERWACHSUNGEN, Gefühl von
inneren
   arn., bry., coloc., **dig.**[7], euph., hep.,
   kali-c.[3], kali-n., merc.[7], **mez.**, nux-v.,
   par., petr., phos., **plb.**, puls., **ran-b.**[3],
   RHUS-T., seneg., sep., **sulph.**, thuj.,
   verb.

AGILITY[3]
AGILITÉ
BEHENDIGKEIT
apis, calc-p., coca[11], coff., form.[11, 12], lach., mang., nux-v., op., rhus-t., stram., tarent., valer.

AGRANULOCYTOSIS[9]
AGRANULOCYTOSE
cortico., lach.[10], sulfa.

AIR, draft agg.
AIR, courant d'air agg.
LUFT, Zugluft agg.
acon., alum.[1'], anac., **ars.**, ars-s-f.[1'], **bapt.[2]**, **BELL.**, benz-ac., bov., brom.[1'], **bry.[1, 7]**, cadm-s., **CALC.**, calc-f.[1', 7, 10] **CALC-P.**, **calc-s.**, calc-sil.[1'], camph., **canth.[3]**, **caps.**, carb-an., **carbn-s.[1, 7]**, **caust.**, cench.[1'], **cham.**, **chin.**, cist., cocc., colch.[3, 6], coloc., crot-h.[3], dulc.[1'], **ferr.**, gels., **graph.**, hep., ign., kali-ar., kali-bi.[3], **KALI-C.**, kali-m.[1'], kali-n., kali-p., kali-s., kali-sil.[1'], lac-c., **lach.**, led., **LYC.[1, 7]**, **lyss.**, **mag-c.[1, 7]**, **mag-p.**, med., **merc.**, mim-p.[14], mur-ac., **nat-c.**, **nat-m.[1, 7]**, nat-p., nat-sil.[1'], **nit-ac.**, **nux-m.**, **nux-v.**, ol-j., onop.[14], **petr.**, **ph-ac.**, **phos.**, psil.[14], **psor.**, **PULS.[1, 7]**, **ran-b.**, **RHUS-T.**, rumx., sang.[3, 6], **sanic.**, sars., **SEL.**, senec.[1'], **sep.**, **SIL.**, spig.[1, 7], **stann.[1']**, **stram.[1, 7]**, stront-c., **SULPH.**, **sumb.**, tep.[11], tub.[1', 3, 7], valer., verb., vichy[11], x-ray[9], **zinc.**, zinc-p.[1']

ailments from[12]
troubles à la suite de
Beschwerden infolge von
cadm-s., lach.

cold draft, when perspiring
froid pendant la transpiration
kalter Zugluft beim Schwitzen
dulc.[1'], merc-i-f.[12]

am.[3]
lycps.

sensation of, as if fanned
sensation d'un, comme éventé
angeweht, als ob von einem Luftzug
camph., canth., caust.[6], **chel.**, coloc.[6], cor-r., croc., fl-ac., graph., **lac-d.**, **laur.**, **mez.[6]**, **mosch.**, **nux-v.**, olnd., puls., rhus-t., sabin., samb., spig., squil., stram., **zinc.**

fanned/éventé/angefächelt
wind-sensation/vent-sensation/
  Wind-Gefühl

indoor air agg.[2]
chambre, agg. à l'air d'une
Zimmerluft agg.
acon., **ALUMN.**, am-c., am-m., **ambr.**, anac., **ang.**, **ant-c.**, **arg-m.**, arn., ars., **asaf.**, **asar.**, **aur.**, **bar-c.**, bell., **bor.**, **bov.**, bry., calc., camph., cann-s., canth., caps., carb-an., carb-v., **caust.**, chel., **cic.**, cina, coff., **colch.**, con., **CROC.**, dig., dulc., graph., **hell.**, hep., hyos., ign., **iod.**, ip., kali-c., kali-n., **laur.**, **lyc.**, **MAG-C.**, mag-m., mang. **meny.**, merc., **mez.**, mosch., mur-ac., nat-c., **nat-m.**, nit-ac., nux-v., **op.**, **ph-ac.**, **phos.**, **plat.**, **plb.**, **PULS.**, **ran-b.**, **ran-s.**, **rhod.**, rhus-t., ruta, **SABIN.**, **sars.**, sel., **seneg.**, sep., spig., **spong.**, **stann.**, staph., **stront-c.**, sul-ac., **sulph.**, **tarax.**, thuj., **verat.**, **verb.**, viol-t., **zinc.**

am.[2]
agar., alumn., **am-c.**, **am-m.**, ambr., anac., ang., **ant-c.**, arn., ars., bar-c., **bell.**, bor., bov., bry., **calad.**, calc., **camph.**, **cann-s.**, **canth.**, caps., carb-an., **carb-v.**, caust., **CHAM.**, **chel.**, **chin.**, cic., **Cina**, cit-v., **COCC.**, coff., **coloc.**, con., dig., **dros.**, dulc., **euph.**, **ferr.**, graph., **GUAJ.**, hell., hep., hyos., **ign.**, iod., **ip.**, kali-c., **kali-n.**, **kreos.**, lach., laur., **led.**, lyc., mag-c., mag-m., mang., meny., **merc.**, mez., **mosch.**,

mur-ac., **nat-c.**, nat-m., **nit-ac.,
NUX-M., NUX-V.**, oci-s.[9], **olnd.**,
op., **petr.**, ph-ac., phos., plat.,
plb., puls., ran-b., **rheum**, rhod.,
rhus-t., ruta, sabad., sabin., sars.,
sel., seneg., sep., **SIL., spig.**,
stann., **staph., stram.**, stront-c.,
sul-ac., sulph., tarent., **teucr.,
thuj., valer.**, verat., verb., **viol-t.,**
zinc.

night-air see night-air

open a. agg., in
plein a., agg. en
Freien agg., im
  acon., **agar.**, agn., agre.[14], alco.[11],
  all-c.[3], alum., alumn.[2], **am-c.,**
  am-m., ambr., anac., ang.[3], ant-c.,
  ant-t., arg-m.[3], arn., **ars., ars-s-f.**[1'],
  asar.[3], aur., aur-ar.[1'], aur-s.[1'],
  aza.[14], **bar-c.**, bar-m., **bell.**,
  benz-ac.[8], berb.[4], bor., bov.,
  bruc.[4], **bry.**, bufo, cact., cadm-s.[8],
  calad., **calc.**, calc-i.[1'], **calc-p.**,
  camph.[3], cann-s.[3], canth., **caps.**,
  carb-an., carb-v., carbn-o.[11],
  carbn-s.[8], **caust.**, cedr., **cham.**,
  chel., CHIN., chin-ar., cic.,
  cimic.[3], cina, cist.[3], **clem., COCC.**,
  coff., coff-t.[7], colch.[3], **coloc., con.**,
  cor-r.[3, 8], crot-h.[8], crot-t., **cycl.**[8],
  dig., dros.[8], **dulc.**, epiph.[8], euph.,
  euphr.[8], **ferr.**, ferr-ar., ferr-p.,
  fl-ac.[3], form., **graph., GUAJ.**,
  ham., hell., **helon., HEP.**, hyos.,
  ign., iod., ip., **kali-ar., kali-bi.**,
  KALI-C., kali-m.[1'], **kali-n.**,
  kali-p., kali-sil.[1'], kalm., **kreos.**,
  lach., laur., led.[3], lina.[8], **lyc.**,
  lycpr.[8], **lyss.**, mag-c., mag-m.[2],
  mag-p.[3], **mang.**, meny., **MERC.**,
  merc-c., mez.[3, 11], mosch.[3, 8],
  mur-ac., nat-ar., **nat-c.**, nat-m.,
  nat-p., nat-sil.[1'], **NIT-AC.,
  NUX-M., NUX-V.**, olnd., op.,
  par., **petr., ph-ac., phos.**, phyt.,
  plat.[3], plb., **psor.**, puls., ran-b.,
  rheum, rhod., **rhus-t., RUMX.**,
  ruta, sabad.[3], sabin.[3], sang.[3],
  sars.[3], **sel.**, senec., **seneg.**[1], **sep.**,
  SIL., spig., spong.[3], **stann.**,

staph.[3], **stram., stront-c., sul-ac.,
SULPH.**, tarax.[3], **teucr.**, thea[8],
thuj., **valer.**, verat., verb., viol-t.,
voes.[11], x-ray[8], **zinc.**

am.
  abrot., **acon.**, aesc.[3], agar., **agn.**,
  all-c., aloe, **ALUM.**, alum-p.[1'],
  alum-sil.[1'], **ALUMN.**[2], am-c.[2, 3],
  am-m., ambr., **aml-ns., anac.**[2, 3],
  ang.[2, 3], ange-s.[14], **ant-c., apis**,
  aran.[3], aran-ix.[10], **arg-m., ARG-N.**,
  arist-cl.[10], arn., **ARS.**, ars-i.,
  ars-s-f.[1'], **asaf., asar., atro., aur.**,
  aur-i.[1'], aur-m.[1'], bapt.[3],
  bar-c.[2, 3, 16], bar-i.[1'], bar-s.[1'],
  bell.[2, 3, 16], bism.[2], bor.[2, 3], **bov.,
  bry.**, buni-o.[14], **cact.**, caj., **calad.**,
  calc.[2, 3], calc-i.[1'], **calc-s., camph.,
  CANN-I.**, cann-s., canth.,
  caps.[2, 3], carb-ac., carb-an.,
  carb-v., carbn-s., carc.[9], caust.[2, 3],
  chel., chlor., cic., **cimic.**, cina[2, 3],
  cinnb., coc-c., coca, **coff.**,
  colch.[3], coloc., com., **con., CROC.,
  crot-c.**, culx.[1'], dicha.[14], dig.,
  dios., dulc.[2, 3], erig.[10], euphr.,
  ferr-i., **fl-ac.**, flor-p.[14], **gamb.**,
  gels., glon.[3], **graph.**, grat.[1'],
  hed.[10], **hell.**, hep.[2, 3], hip-ac.[9, 14],
  hydr-ac., hyos., iber.[3], ign.[2, 3],
  ind., **IOD., ip., kali-bi.**,
  kali-c.[2, 3, 14, 16], **KALI-I.**, kali-n.,
  kali-s., lac-c.[7], **lach.**, lact.,
  laur., **lil-t., lyc. MAG-C.,
  MAG-M.**, mag-p.[3], mag-s.,
  mang., **med.**[7, 15], **meli.**, meny.,
  merc.[2, 3], merc-i-f.[1'], merc-i-r.,
  mez., mosch., mur-ac., myrt.,
  naphtin., nat-c., **nat-m., NAT-S.**,
  nep.[10], nicc., nit-ac.[2, 3], nux-v.[3],
  op., **osm.**, ph-ac., **phos., phyt.**,
  pic-ac., pip-n.[3], pitu.[14], **plat.**,
  plb., pneu.[14], **PSOR.**[3, 7, 15],
  ptel., PULS., ran-b., **ran-s.**, rat.,
  rauw.[9, 14], **rhod.**[2, 3], **RHUS-T.**,
  ruta[2, 3], **SABAD., SABIN.**, sal-ac.,
  sang., sanic., saroth.[9], sars.[2, 3, 16],
  sec., sel.[2, 3], **seneg., sep.**, spig.,
  spong., stann.[2, 3], staph.[2, 3],
  stront-c.[2, 3], sul-ac.[2, 3], **sul-i.**[1'],
  sulph., tab., tarax., **tarent.**[1', 7],

tell., thiop.[14], thlas.[3], thuj., tril.,
TUB.[7, 15], valer.[3], verat.[2, 3], verb.[1],
vib., viol-t., visc.[9], **zinc.,** zinc-p.[1']

aversion to
aversion pour
Abneigung gegen frische Luft
  agar., alum., **AM-C., am-m.,**
  ambr., anac., ang.[3], aran.[3], arn.[3],
  ars.[3], ars-s-f.[1'], aur.[3], **BAPT., bell.,**
  bry., CALC., calc-ar.[1'], **CALC-P.,**
  calc-sil.[1'], camph., cann-s.[3],
  canth., **caps.,** carb-an., carb-v.,
  caust., CHAM., chel., **chin.,** cic.[3],
  cina, **cist., COCC., COFF.,** coloc.,
  con., cycl., dig., dros.[3], **ferr.,**
  ferr-ar., graph., guaj., helon.,
  hep., IGN., ip., kali-ar., **KALI-C.,**
  kali-m.[1'], kali-n., kali-p.,
  kali-sil.[1'], kreos., **lach.,** laur.,
  led.[3], **lyc., lyss.,** mag-m.[3, 11],
  mang., meny., **merc.,** merc-c.,
  mosch., mur-ac.[3], **NAT-C., nat-m.,**
  nat-p., NAT-SIL.[1'], nit-ac.,
  nux-m., NUX-V., op., **PETR.,**
  ph-ac., phos., plat.[3], **plb., psor.,**
  puls.[3], rhod., **rhust-t., RUMX.,**
  ruta[3], sabin.[3], sars.[3], sel., seneg.,
  sep., SIL., spig., staph.[3], stram.[3],
  stront-c., **sul-ac., SULPH.,** teucr.,
  thuj., tub.[3], valer., verb., **viol-t.,**
  zinc.[3]

alternating with desire for [1']
alternant avec désir de
abwechselnd mit Verlangen nach
  frischer Luft
  ars-s-f.

desire for
désir de
Verlangen nach frischer Luft
  acon., **agn.,** aloe[3], **alum.,**
  alum-p.[1'], alum-sil.[1'], am-c.[3],
  am-m., ambr., aml-ns.[11], anac.,
  ang.[3], ange-s.[14], **ant-c.,** ant-t., **apis,**
  aran-ix.[10], arg-m., **ARG-N.**[1, 7],
  arn., ars., ars-i., asaf., **asar.,**
  aster., **AUR.,** aur-ar.[1'], **aur-i.**[1'],
  AUR-M., AUR-S.[1'], **bapt.**[6], **bar-c.,**
  bar-i.[1'], bar-m., bar-s.[1'], bell.[3],

bor., bov., **brom., bry.,** bufo, calc.[3],
CALC-I., calc-s., cann-s.[3], caps.[3],
carb-an., **CARB-V.,** carbn-h.,
carbn-s., caust., chel.[11], cic.[3],
cimic.[14], cina[3], cit-v.[11], coca[11],
CROC., dig., **elaps, fl-ac.,** gels.,
graph., hell., hep.[3], hyos.[11], **IOD.,**
ip.[6], kali-bi.[3], kali-c., **KALI-I.,**
kali-n., **KALI-S., lach.,** lact.[11],
laur., **lil-t., LYC., mag-c., mag-m.,**
mang., med.[1', 7], meny., **mez.,**
mosch.[3], mur-ac., nat-c., **nat-m.,**
nat-s., op., ph-ac., phos., **plat.,**
plb.[3], **ptel., PULS.,** rhod.[3], rhus-t.,
ruta[3], sabin., **sanic.,** sars., **sec.,**
sel.[3], seneg., sep., **spig.,** spong.,
stann., staph.[3], **stram.,** stront-c.[3],
sul-ac.[3], sul-i.[1'], **SULPH., tab.,**
tarax., tarent., tell., teucr., thuj.,
tub.[1', 3, 7], tub-r.[13], verat.[3], **viol-t.,**
zinc., zinc-p.[1']

cold air see cold–air–desire

but draft agg.[7]
mais les courants d'air agg.
aber Luftzug agg.
  acon., anac., **ars.,** bor., **bry.,**
  calc-s., carb-an., **carbn-s., caust.,**
  graph., KALI-C., lach., LYC.,
  mag-c., mur-ac., **nat-c., nat-m.,**
  ph-ac., phos., PULS., RHUS-T.,
  sars., **sep., spig., stram., SULPH.,**
  zinc.

passing through glands, sensation of
traversant les glandes, sensation d'a.
geht, als ob Luft durch die Drüsen
  spong.

through him[3]
qui le traverse
durch ihn
  calc., coloc.

seashore agg., air on the
bord de la mer, agg. au
Seeküste, Seeluft agg.
  aq-mar.[8], **ars.,** brom.[3, 8, 10],
  carc.[7, 9, 10], iod.[10], kali-i., **mag-m.,**
  mag-s.[10], med.[3, 7], **nat-m.**[1, 7],
  nat-s., rhus-t.[3], **sep., tub.**[7]

bathing–sea/se baigner–mer/
Baden–See

ailments from[12]
troubles à la suite de
Beschwerden infolge von
aq-mar., brom.

am.
   brom.[1', 3, 7, 8], **carc.**[7, 9, 10], lyc.[3],
   med.[1, 7], **nat-m.**[7], **tub.**[7]

alcohol see food–alcohol agg.–
brandy agg.

ALIVE sensation, internally[3]
VIVANT intérieurement,
   sensation de qc.
LEBENDIGEM, Gefühl von etwas
   innerlich
   anac., asar., bell., berb.[3, 6], calc.,
   cann-s., chel., cocc., **CROC.**[3, 6], cycl.,
   hyos., **ign.,** kali-i., lach., led., mag-m.,
   meny., merc., nat-m., op., petr., phos.,
   plb., puls., rhod., sabad., sabin., sang.,
   sec., sil., spong., sulph., tarax.,
   THUJ.[3, 6], viol-t.

ALTERNATING states[3] ✱
ALTERNANTS, états
ABWECHSELNDE Zustände
   acon., **ars.**[1'], dulc., ign., **KALI-BI.,**
   lyc., onop.[14], prot.[14], puls.

change–symptoms/changement–
*   symptômes/Wechsel–Symptom-*
*   wechsel*
contradictory/contradictoires/
*   widerspruchsvolle*
metastasis/metastases/
*   Metastasierung*

ALUMINIUM poisoning[2, 3]
ALUMINIUM, empoisonnement par
ALUMINIUM-Vergiftung
   alum.[10], **bry.,** cadm-o.[7], camph., cham.,
   ip., puls.

ANAEMIA
ANÉMIE
ANÄMIE
   abel.[14], **acet-ac.,** acon., agar., agn.[1'],
   alet.[6, 8, 12], aloe[6], alum., alum-p.[1'],
   alum-sil.[1'], am-c.[6], ambr., anil.[11, 12],
   ant-c., **ant-t.**[2, 3], **apis**[2], apoc.[1'],
   aq-mar.[6], **arg-m., arg-n., arg-o.**[8],
   arn., **ARS., ars-i., ARS-S-F.**[1'],
   aur-ar.[8, 12], **bell.,** ben-d.[12], berb.[1'],
   beryl.[9, 14], bism.[2, 8], bol-la.[2], **BOR.,**
   bov., **bry.,** cadm-met.[9, 14], **CALC.,**
   calc-ar.[8], calc-i.[1'], calc-lac.[8],
   CALC-P., calen.[6], calo.[8], carb-an.[1'],
   carb-v., carbn-s.[2, 12], casc.[2, 12],
   caust., cedr., cham., **CHIN.,** chin-ar.,
   chin-s.[8], chlol.[12], chloram.[14],
   chlorpr.[14], cic.[8], cina, cob-n.[9, 14],
   cocc., coff., colch.[11], coloc., **con.,**
   cortico.[9], cortiso.[9], crat.[8], **crot-h.,**
   cupr., cupr-ar.[8], cupr-s.[11], **cycl.,**
   dig., eucal.[6], **FERR., FERR-AR.,**
   ferr-c.[8], ferr-cit.[8], **ferr-i., ferr-m.**[8, 12],
   ferr-o-r.[8], **ferr-p.,** ferr-pic.[6], **ferr-r.**[8],
   goss.[8], **GRAPH., ham.**[2], **HELL.,**
   helon., hep.[3], **hydr.**[2, 6, 8], **ign.,** iod.,
   ip.[6, 12], **irid.**[8, 12], **KALI-AR., kali-bi.,**
   kali-br.[2], **KALI-C.,** kali-n.[6],
   KALI-P., kalm.[2], kres.[10, 13, 14],
   lac-ac.[12], lac-d.[1', 3, 6, 12], **lach.,** lec.[8],
   lyc., mag-c., mag-m., **MANG.,**
   MED., MERC., merc-c., mez.,
   MOSCH.[3], nat-ar., **nat-c., NAT-M.,**
   nat-n.[6, 12], **nat-p., nat-s., NIT-AC.,**
   nux-m., **nux-v.,** ol-j., **olnd.,** oxyg.[12],
   petr., **ph-ac., PHOS., phyt.**[8], **pic-ac.,**
   PLAT.[3, 6, 8], **PLB., plb-a.**[8], psor.,
   PULS, rhod., **rhus-t.,** ric.[11],
   rub-t.[6, 8, 12], ruta, sabin., sacch.[8],
   sec., senec., sep., sil., spig., **SQUIL.,**
   stann., STAPH., stroph-h.[12],
   SUL-AC., sulfa.[9, 14], sulfonam.[14],
   SULPH., tab.[11, 12], ther., **thyr.**[8, 12],
   tub.[1'], urt-u.[12], valer., vanad.[7, 8],
   verat., **x-ray**[9, 14], **zinc.,** zinc-ar.[8],
   zinc-m.[8], zinc-s.[11]

faintness–anaemia/évanouisse-
*   ment–anémie/Ohnmacht–*
*   Anaemie*
weakness/faiblesse/Schwäche

exhausting disease, from[8]
épuisante, par maladie
erschöpfende Erkrankung, durch
  acet-ac., alst., **calc-p., chin.,** chin-s.,
  ferr., helon., kali-c., **nat-m., ph-ac.,**
  phos.[2, 8], sec.[2]

haemorrhage, after
hémorrhagie, après une
Blutung, nach einer
  arg-o.[8], **ars.**[8], **calc., carb-v., CHIN.,**
  crot-h.[8], **FERR.,** helon.[2], hydr.[2],
  ign.[8], **lach.,** nat-br.[8], **nat-m., nux-v.,**
  ph-ac., phos., sabin.[1'], staph.[2],
  sulph.

menorrhagia, from[8]
ménorrhagie, par
Menorrhagie, durch
  arg-o., ars., **calc.,** calc-p., **cann-i.**[2],
  crat., **cycl., ferr., graph., hydr.**[2],
  kali-c., mang., **nat-m., puls.,** sep.[7, 8]

nutritional disturbance, from[8]
alimentaires, par troubles
Ernährungsstörungen, durch
  alet., alum., **calc-p.,** ferr., helon.,
  nux-v.

pernicious[8, 12]
pernicieuse
perniziöse
  ars.[8], calc.[1'], **crot-h.**[2], mang.[1'],
  nat-m.[1'], **phos.,** pic-ac.[2, 8, 12], **thyr.,**
  trinit.[8]

ANAESTHESIA
ANESTHÉSIE
ANÄSTHESIE
  abrot., absin.[11], **acon.**[6, 11], alco.[11],
  ambr.[4, 6], **anac.**[2, 6], ant-t.[4], arg-n.[6],
  ars.[4, 6], ars-i.[1'], atro.[11], bar-m.[4, 6],
  bell.[4, 11], berb.[6], cadm-s.[1'], **camph.**[2],
  cann-i.[1', 2, 11], **caps.**[2], carb-ac.[6, 11],
  carbn-chl.[11], carbn-h.[11], carbn-o.[11],
  carbn-s.[1', 2, 11], caul.[2], **caust.**[6], cham.[6],
  chlf.[2, 11], chlol.[2, 11], **cic.**[2], cocc.[6],
  crot-chlol.[12], cupr-a.[4], cycl.[11],
  eucal.[2], **HYDR-AC.**[4-6], hyos.[6]
  hyper.[6], ign.[6], kali-br.[6, 12], **kali-i.**[2],

keroso.[11, 12], laur.[4], lyc.[4, 6], m-arct.[4],
mand.[10, 14], merc.[11], meth-ae-ae.[11],
methyl.[11], nitro-o.[11], **nux-m.**[6],
nux-v.[4], **olnd.**[2, 4, 6], **op.**[4, 6, 11],
ox-ac.[6], ph-ac.[6], **PLB.**[1', 2, 4, 6, 11, 12],
puls.[11], ran-a.[4], rhod.[4, 6], **sec.**[4, 6, 10],
spig.[6], stram.[6, 11], stront-c.[6], tab.[11],
ter.[2], verat.[4], **verat-v.**[2], vip.[4, 6],
zinc.[2, 4]

right side, of[11]
droit, du côté
rechten Seite, der
  plb.

affected parts, of[11]
affectées, des parties
leidender Teile
  plb.

ANALGESIA
ANALGÉSIE
ANALGESIE
  anh.[10], ant-c.[6], bell., chel., **cic.,**
  COCC., con., hell., **hyos.,** ign.,
  kali-br., laur., **LYC.,** mand.[10], merc.,
  mosch., **OLND., OP., PH-AC.,**
  phos., pic-ac., **PLB.**[1, 7], puls.,
  rhus-t.[1], **sec., STRAM., sulph.**

  irritability–lack/irritabilité–
    manque d'/Reizbarkeit–
    Unempfindlichkeit
  painlessness/insensibilité/
    Schmerzlosigkeit

inner parts
internes, des parties
innerer Organe
  ars., bell., bov., hyos., **OP., PLAT.,**
  spig.

parts affected
affectées, des parties
leidender Teile
  anac., asaf., **cocc.,** con., **lyc., olnd.,**
  PLAT., puls., rhus-t.

ANXIETY, general physical
ANXIÉTÉ physique générale,
  sensation d'
ANGSTGEFÜHL, körperliches
  acon., agar., alum.[4], am-m., ambr.[4],
  aml-ns., ant-t., ARG-N., arn.[4],
  ARS., ars-i., **ARS-S-F.**[1]', bar-c.,
  bar-m., bar-s.[1]', bell.[4], bor.[4], **brom.,**
  bry., calc., calc-ar.[1]', calc-i.[1]',
  CAMPH., cann-s., **canth.,** carb-v.,
  caust.[4], cench.[1]', **CHAM., chel.,**
  chin., chlor.[11], cic., cocc., **coff.,**
  colch., con., cupr., **DIG.,** euph.,
  ferr., ferr-ar., ferr-i., ferr-p.[1], guaj.,
  ign., **iod., IP.,** kreos.[4], laur., lob.,
  lyc., mag-c.[4], meph.[4], merc., mez.,
  mosch., mur-ac., nat-c.[4], nat-m.,
  nat-s.[1]', nux-m.[4], **NUX-V.,** op.[4],
  petr.[4], **PH-AC., PHOS.,** plat., plb.,
  prun.[4], **PULS.,** ran-b.[4], rhod.[4],
  rhus-t., ruta[4], sabad., sabin., sars.[4],
  sec., seneg., **sep.,** sil.[4], spig.[4],
  squil.[4], **stann., staph.,** stram.,
  sul-ac., **sul-i.**[1]', **SULPH.,** tarent.[1]',
  teucr., ther.[1]', thuj., **verat., zinc.,**
  zinc-p.[1]'

APOPLEXY *
APOPLEXIE
  ACON.[10], agar.[10], **alco.**[11],
  ANAC.[2, 3, 12], ant-c.[3, 11, 16], ant-t.[3],
  apis[12], **arn., ars.**[2, 3], ars-s-f.[12],
  asar.[3, 6], **aster.**[2, 12], **aur.,** bapt.[12],
  bar-c., **BELL.,** brom.[12], **BRY.**[2, 3, 12],
  cact.[7, 12], cadm-br.[12],
  cadm-s.[2, 3, 11, 12], calc.[3, 6], **camph.,**
  carb-v., carbn-h.[12], carbn-s.[12],
  caust.[12], chen-a.[10, 12], **chin.,** chlol.[12],
  COCC., coff., con., croc.[3], **crot-h.,**
  cupr., cupr-a.[12], dig.[3, 6, 11], erig.[10],
  ferr., fl-ac.[12], **form.**[2, 12], gast.[12],
  GELS., GLON.[2, 3, 6, 10, 12], guare.[12],
  hell.[12], hep.[3], hydr-ac.[3, 10, 11], **hyos.,**
  ign.[3], iod.[2], **IP.,** juni.[11, 12], kali-br.[12],
  kali-cy.[12], kali-m.[3], kali-n.[10], kreos.[3],
  LACH., laur., lim.[12], lith-br.[12], lol.[11],
  lyc., merc., **mill.**[1', 2, 11], morph.[11],
  nat-m., nat-n.[10], nat-ns.[12], nit-ac.,
  nux-m., nux-v., oena.[2, 12], olnd.[3, 6, 10],
  OP., ox-ac.[11], ph-ac.[3], **phos.,** plb.,

puls., ran-g.[12], rhus-t., sabad.[3],
  samb.[3], sars.[3], sec., sep., **sil.,**
  sin-n.[2, 7, 12], sol-a.[12], **stram.,**
  stront-c.[12], sulph.[3], tab.[2, 11, 12],
  thuj.[3], verat.[3, 6, 11, 12, 16],
  verat-v.[2, 6, 12], viol-o.[3], vip.[3, 6]

convulsions–apoplectic/
  convulsions–apoplexie/
  Konvulsionen–Apoplexie
paralysis-one-sided/paralysie-d'un
  côté/Paralysis-einseitige
weakness–apoplexy/faiblesse–
  apoplexie/Schwäche–Apoplexie

threatening[2]
menaçante
drohende
  aster., bell., COFF., fl-ac., **glon.**[2, 10],
  ign., kali-n.[10], **laur.**[2, 12], prim-v.[12],
  stront-c.[2, 8]

ARMS holding away from body am.[3]
BRAS en position écartée am., les
ARME vom Körper entfernt halten am.
  psor., spig., sulph.

ARSENICAL poisoning
ARSENIC, empoisonnement par
ARSENVERGIFTUNG
  camph., **carb-v.**[2, 3, 8, 12], chin.,
  chin-s.[2, 12], dig.[2], euph.[12], **ferr.,** graph.,
  HEP.[2, 3, 8, 12], iod., **ip.,** lach.[2, 3, 12],
  merc., nux-m.[12], nux-v.,
  ol-j.[3], **phos.**[2], plb.[2], samb., sulph.[12],
  tab.[2, 12], thuj.[7], **verat.**

paralysis-poisoning/
paralysie-empoisonnement/
Paralysis-Vergiftung

ARTERIOSCLEROSIS[8]
ARTÉRIOSCLÉROSE
ARTERIOSKLEROSE
adren., **am-i.**[6, 8], am-van., aml-ns.[6],
ant-ar., arg-n.[10], **arn.**[3, 6, 8, 10], ars.[6, 8],
ars-i.[6, 8], aster.[14], **aur.**[3, 6, 8, 10], aur-br.[6],
aur-i.[6, 8], aur-m-n.[6, 8], **bar-c.**[6, 8, 10],
bar-i.[6, 10], bar-m., bell-p.[10, 14], benz-ac.[6],
cact., cal-ren.[6], **calc.**[3, 6], calc-ar.[3],
calc-f.[6, 8, 14], card-m.[8], chin-s., chlol.[7],
con.[6, 8], crat.[6, 8], **cupr.**[6, 8], ergot.,
fl-ac.[3, 6], form.[3], form-ac.[6], fuc.[10],
glon.[6, 8], hed.[10, 14], hyper.[10],
iod.[3, 6, 10], **kali-i.**[6, 10], kali-sal.,
kres.[10, 14], lach.[8, 10], lith-c., mag-f.[10],
mand.[14], naja[10], **nat-i.**, nit-ac.[6], phos.,
plb.[3, 6, 8, 10], **plb-i.**[6, 8, 10, 12], **polyg-a.**,
rad-br.[10], rauw.[10], **sec.**[3, 6, 8, 10], sil.[10],
solid.[6], **stront-c.**[3, 6, 8], **stront-i.**[6, 8],
stroph-h., sumb., **tab.**[3, 6], thlas.[6], thyr.,
vanad.[6-8], **visc.**[3, 6, 14], zinc-p.[6]

hypertension/Hypertonie

ASCENDING agg.
MONTER agg.
STEIGEN agg.
acet-ac., acon., agar.[3, 6], aloe,
alum., alum-sil.[1'], **alumn.**[2], **am-c.**,
anac., **ang.**[2, 3], ant-c., arg-m., arg-n.,
arn., **ARS.**, ars-s-f.[1'], asar., aur.,
aur-ar.[1'], aur-i.[1'], aur-s.[1'], **bar-c.**,
bar-m., **bar-s.**[1'], bell., **bor.**, **BRY.**,
but-ac.[8], **cact.**[2, 8], cadm-s., **CALC.**,
calc-ar.[1'], **calc-p.**, calc-sil.[1'], cann-i.,
cann-s., canth., **carb-v.**, **carbn-s.**,
caust., chin., **COCA**, coff., **con.**[2, 3],
conv., **cupr.**, dig., dios., dros.,
euph., **ferr.**[2, 3], gels., gins.[11], **glon.**,
graph., hell., hep., hyos., ign.,
iod.[3, 6, 11], kali-ar., kali-c., **kali-i.**,
kali-n.[1], kali-p., **kalm.**, kreos., lach.,
led., lyc., mag-c., mag-m., meny.,
merc., mosch., mur-ac., nat-ar.,
nat-c., **nat-m.**, nat-n.[3, 6], nat-p.,
nit-ac., nux-m., **nux-v.**, olnd.[3, 6],
ox-ac., par., petr., ph-ac., **phos.**,
plat., plb., prot.[14], **puls.**[3], ran-b.,
rhod.[2], rhus-t., **ruta**, sabad., **sabin.**[2],
seneg., **sep.**, sil., **spig.**, **SPONG.**,

squil., **stann.**, staph., sul-ac., **sulph.**,
tab., **tarax.**, thuj., **valer.**[2], verb.,
vip-a.[14], **zinc.**, zinc-p.[1']

ailments from[12]
troubles à la suite de
Beschwerden infolge von
calc-p.

am[3]
allox.[14], am-m., arg-m., bar-c., bell.,
bry., canth., coff., **con.**, ferr., lyc.,
meny., nit-ac., plb., **rhod.**, rhus-t.,
ruta, sabin., stann., sulph., **valer.**,
verb.

high agg.
haut agg.
Hochsteigen agg.
acon., agar.[3], bell.[3], bry., **CALC.**[1, 7],
carb-v.[3], **COCA**[1, 7], conv., merc.[3],
nat-m.[3], **olnd.**, onos.[3], rhus-t.[3], **spig.**,
sulph.

mountain/mal de montagne/
Höhenkrankheit

ATROPHY[3]
ATROPHIE
ars., bar-c., chin., cupr., hep., kali-c.,
nux-v., phos., plb., sec., stann.

paralysis–atrophy/paralysie–
atrophie/Lähmung–Atrophie

glands, of
glandes, ganglions, des
Drüsen, der
anan., ars., **aur.**, bar-c., carb-an.,
cham., chim.[2], chin., **CON.**, **IOD.**,
kali-ar., kali-c., **KALI-I.**, kali-p.,
kreos., lac-d., **nit-ac.**, nux-m.,
ph-ac., plb., sars., **sec.**, sil., **staph.**,
sul-i.[1'], verat.

myatrophy/amyotrophie/
Muskelatrophie

autumn see seasons

AVIATOR'S DISEASE[7]
MAL DES AVIATEURS
FLUGKRANKHEIT
  ars.[8], bell., bor., **coca**[7, 8], psor.

BALL internally
BOULE, intérieurement sensation d'une
KUGEL, Gefühl einer inneren
  acon., **arg-n.**, arn.[3], asaf., atri[6], **bell.**,
  brom., bry., calc., **cann-i.**, caust.,
  cham.[3], chin.[3], cob.[3], coc-c., coloc.,
  con., crot-t., cupr., gels.[3], graph.,
  HEP.[7], **IGN.**, kali-ar.[3], kali-c., kali-m.[3],
  lac-c.[3], **lach.**, **lil-t.**[3, 6], mag-m.,
  merc-d.[3], merc-i-r.[3], mosch.[3], nat-m.,
  nat-s.[3], nit-ac.[3], nux-m., par., phos.[3],
  phyt., plan.[3], plat., **plb.**, **puls.**[3], raph.,
  rhus-t., ruta, **sabad.**[3], senec., **SEP.**,
  sil., spig., staph., stram., sulph., tab.,
  teucr.[3], ust.[3], valer.

knotted/nœud/Knoten
plug/cheville/Pflock
shot/grenaille/Schrotkugeln

hot[3]
chaude
heißen
  carb-ac., phyt.

BASEDOW'S disease[8, 10]
BASEDOW, maladie de
BASEDOW' Krankheit
  adren.[7], aml-ns.[8], anh.[14], antip.[8],
  aq-mar.[14], aran-ix.[14], ars., ars-i.,
  atra-r.[14], aur., bad., bar-c.[8], **bell.**,
  brom., **cact.**[8], **calc.**[8], calc-f.[10, 14],
  cann-i.[8], chin.[10], chin-ar.[10], chr-s.[8],
  cimic.[14], colch.[8], con., cupr.[10],
  cupr-a.[10], cyt-l.[14], echi.[8], ephe.[8],
  elaps[10], **ferr.**[8], ferr-i.[8], ferr-p.[8],
  ferr-s[10], **fl-ac.**, flor-p.[10], fuc.[8], **glon.**[8],
  hed[10, 14], **iod.**, jab[8], kali-c.[6], lach.[10],
  lycps., mag-c.[10], mag-f.[10], nat-m.[6, 8, 10],
  nux-v.[7], op.[10], phos.[10], **pilo.**[8], **rauw.**[14],
  saroth.[8, 14], scut.[8], sec.[10], sel.[14], spong.,
  stram.[8], thal.[14], thala.[14], **thyr.**[8, 14],
  thyreotr.[14], tub.[10]

BATHING, washing agg.
SE BAIGNER, se laver agg.
BADEN, Sichwaschen agg.
  aesc., aeth., **AM-C.**, am-m.,
  ANT-C., ant-t., **apis**[6], **aran.**, ars.[2, 3],
  ars-i., ars-s-f.[1'], **bar-c.**, bar-s.[1'], **bell.**,
  bell-p.[8], bor., bov., bry., **CALC.**,
  CALC-S., calc-sil.[1'], **canth.**, caps.[1'],
  carb-v., **carbn-s.**, **caust.**, **cham.**,
  CLEM., con., crot-c[8], **dulc.**, ferr.[8],
  form.[3, 6, 8], **graph.**, **hep.**[2], **ign.**[2, 3],
  kali-c., kali-m[1'], **kali-n.**, kali-s.,
  kali-sil.[1'], kreos.[8], **lac-d.**, lach.[8], laur.,
  lil-t.[8], **lyc.**, mag-c., **mag-p.**, **mang.**,
  merc., merc-c., **mez.**, mur-ac.,
  nat-c., nat-m., **nat-s.**[8], **nit-ac.**,
  nux-m., nux-v., **op.**[3, 6], petr., **phos.**,
  phys.[3, 8, 12], puls., rat.[3], **RHUS-T.**,
  rumx., **sars.**, **SEP.**, sil., **spig.**, stann.,
  staph., **stront-c.**, sul-ac., **SULPH.**,
  thuj.[3], urt-u.[8], zinc., zinc-p.[1']

ailments from[12]
troubles à la suite de
Beschwerden infolge von
  nux-m., phys., rhus-t.

am.
  acon., agar., **alum.**, alumn.[2],
  am-m., ant-t., **apis**, arg-n[3, 6], ars.,
  ASAR., aur., **bor.**, bry., bufo[1'],
  calc.[2], cann-i., **caust.**, cham.,
  chel., **euphr.**, **fl-ac.**, form., hell.[2],
  hyper.[3, 6], kali-chl., **lac-c.**, laur.,
  LED., mag-c., **mez.**, mur-ac.,
  nat-m.[3, 6], nux-v., phos.[3], phyt.,
  pic-ac., **psor.**, **PULS.**, rhod.,
  sabad., sep., **spig.**, staph., thlas.[3],
  thuj.[3], zinc.

affected part, of; and moistening[15]
parties affectées, baigner et
  humecter des
leidender Teile, und Befeuchten
  alum., **am-m.**, ant-t., ars., **ASAR.**,
  bor., bry., **caust.**, cham., **chel.**,
  euphr., laur., mag-c., mez.,
  mur-ac., nux-v., **PULS.**, rhod.,
  sabad., sep., **spig.**, staph., zinc.

aversion to, dread of
aversion pour
Abneigung gegen
    AM-C., am-m., **ANT-C.**, aq-mar.[14],
    bar-c., bar-m., **bell.**, bell-p.[7], **bor.**,
    bov., **bry.**, **calc.**, calc-sil.[1'], **canth.**,
    carb-v., caust.[3], **cham.**, **CLEM.**,
    coloc.[3], **con.**, dulc., **hep.**[2], kali-c.,
    kali-m.[1'], **kali-n.**, kali-sil.[1'], **laur.**,
    lyc., mag-c., mag-p.[3], mang.[3], merc.,
    mez., mur-ac., nat-c., nat-p., nit-ac.,
    nux-m., nux-v., ol-an.[3], phos.,
    phys.[2, 11], **PSOR.**, **puls.**, **RHUS-T.**,
    sars., **SEP.**, sil., **SPIG.**, stann.,
    staph., **stront-c.**, sul-ac., **SULPH.**,
    thuj.[3], **zinc.**

cold bathing agg.
froids agg., bains
kaltes Baden agg.
    acon.[1'], **AM-C**[2, 6], am-m.[2],
    ANT-C., **ANT-T.**[1', 7], apoc.[7], ars.[3],
    ars-i.[6], **bar-c.**, **bell.**, bell-p.[7, 9],
    bor.[2], bov.[2], **bry.**[2], bufo[2],
    CALC.[2], calc-sil.[1], **canth.**[2], caps.,
    carb-v.[2], carbn-s., **caust.**, **cham.**[2],
    chim.[7], cimic.[7], **CLEM.**[2, 3], **colch.**,
    con.[2], **dulc.**[2, 3, 6], elaps, **form.**,
    glon[3], **IGN.**[2, 3], **kali-c.**[2], **kali-m.**[3],
    kali-n.[2, 6], **kreos.**, **lac-d.**, lach.[7],
    laur.[2], **lyc.**[2, 6], mag-c.[2], **MAG-P.**,
    merc.[2, 6], mez.[2, 3], mosch.[3],
    mur-ac., nat-c.[2], **nit-ac.**, **nux-m.**[2],
    nux-v.[2, 5-7], phos., psor.[1'], puls.[2],
    RHUS-T., ruta[7], sars., **sep.**, **sil.**[3, 6],
    spig.[2], stann.[2], **staph.**[2], **stront-c.**[2],
    sul-ac.[2], **SULPH.**[2, 5, 7], thyr.[14],
    TUB., zinc.[2]

ailments from[12]
troubles à la suite de
Beschwerden infolge von
    mag-p., **phys.**

am.
    agar[8], aloe[8], alum[6], ambr.[8],
    apis[3, 6, 8], **arg-n.**, **arn.**, asar.,
    aster.[14], aur.[1', 3, 6], **aur-m.**, bell-p.[3],
    berb-a.[14], bism., **bry.**[3, 6, 8], bufo[8],
    calc-f.[14], **cals-s.**, camph[8], cann-i.[8],
    cann-s.[3], caust.[3], cupr.[8], fago.[8],
    fl-ac., hed.[10, 14], hyper.[3, 6], ind.,

iod., **led.**[3, 6, 8], mag-s.[9, 14],
meph., **nat-m.**, phos.[8], phyt.[3],
pic-ac.[1', 6, 8], **psor.**[6], **puls.**[3, 8],
sec.[3], sep.[8], spig.[6], sulph.[3],
syph.[7]

desire for
désir de
Verlangen nach kaltem B.
    aloe[6], **apis**[6], asar.[6], aster., caust.[6],
    chel.[6], fl-ac.[11], **hyper.**[6], iod.[6],
    led.[6], meph., nat-m., phyt.,
    puls.[6], sep.[6]

desire for[11]
désir de
Verlangen nach
    tarent.

face bathing agg.
face agg., se laver la
Gesichtes agg., Waschen des
    fl-ac.[1'], plan.[3]

am.
    asar., calc-s, lac-d.[3], mez., nat-m[2],
    phos.[3], sabad.

hot bathing agg.[3]
très chauds agg., bains
heißes Baden agg.
    APIS, arg-n., bell., bry., carb-v.,
    GELS., **IOD.**, **LACH.**, **NAT-M.**,
    op., **puls.**, sec., sulph.

am.[3]
    anac., **ARS.**, hep., rhus-t., sil.,
    thuj.

lukewarm bathing agg.[3]
tièdes agg., bains
lauwarmes Baden agg.
    acon, **ang.**[2, 3], phos.

sea agg., bathing in the
mer agg., bains de
See agg., Baden in der
    ars., lim.[8, 12], **mag-m.**, med.[7],
    nat-m.[3], **rhus-t.**, sep., zinc.[2, 3, 7]

ailments from[12]
troubles à la suite de
Beschwerden infolge von
    ars., mag-m., rhus-t.

am.[7]
    med.

warm bathing agg.[1', 3, 6]
chauds agg., bains
warmes Baden agg.
    acon.[5], ant-c.[1'], **apis,** ars-i.[6], bell.[5],
    caust.[1'], iod.[6], **lach.,** op.[3, 6],
    phos.[3, 6], sulph.[3]

am.[8]
    ant-c., bufo, flav.[14], lat-m.[9, 14],
    mim-p[14], rad-br., sec.[6],
    stront-c., thea

feet, of[14]
pieds, de
Fußbäder, warme
    pneu.

bed see hard bed

BENDING, turning **agg.**[3]
PLIER, tourner **agg.**
SICHKRUMMEN, Sichbeugen **agg.**
    am-m., anac.[14], ang., ant-t., arn.,
    bell., bov., **bry.,** calc., camph., caps.,
    carb-an., carb-v., cham., **chin., cic.,**
    cocc., coloc., **con.**[3, 8], cycl., dros.,
    dulc., euph., guaj., **hep., ign.,** iod.,
    ip., lach., laur., mag-c., merc. mez.,
    mur-ac. **nat-m.,** nit-ac., nux-v.[3, 8],
    petr., ph-ac., plat., plb., puls.[3, 8],
    ran-b., rhod., **rhus-t.,** sabad., sabin.,
    samb., **sel.,** spig., **spong., stann.,**
    staph., thuj., verat., visc.[14], zinc.

affected part agg.[3]
affectées agg., les parties
leidender Teile agg., Beugen
    acon., am-c., **am-m.,** anac., ang.,
    ant-c., ant-t., arg-m., **arn.,** asaf.,
    aur., bar-c., **bell.,** bor., bov., **bry.,**
    CALC., camph., caps., carb-an.,
    carb-v., caust., cham., **chel., chin.,**

cic., cina., cocc., **coff.,** con., croc.,
cupr., cycl., dig., dros., dulc.,
graph., hep., hyos., **IGN.,** iod.,
ip., **kali-c.,** lach., laur., led.,
lyc., mag-c., merc., mez., mur-ac.,
nat-m., nit-ac., **nux-v.,** olnd.,
par., petr., ph-ac., plat., plb.,
puls., ran-b., rhod., **rhus-t.,** ruta,
sabad., sabin., samb., **sel., sep.,**
spig., spong., stann., staph.,
sulph., tarax., teucr., thuj., valer.,
verat., zinc.

drawing up/remonté/Anziehen

am.[3]
    acon., am-m., anac., arg-m.,
    arg-n., **BELL.,** bov., calc., cann-s.,
    caust., **cham., chin.,** colch., **coloc.,**
    guaj., hep., kali-c., lach., mag-c.,
    mag-p., mang., meny., **merc.,**
    merc-c., mur-ac., nux-v., petr.,
    plb., puls., rheum, rhus-t., sabad.,
    sabin., **squil.,** teucr., **thuj.,**
    verat.

backward agg.[3]
en arrière agg.
Rückwärtsbiegen agg.
    am-c., **anac.,** ant-c., aran-ix.[14],
    asaf., atra-r.[14], aur., **bar-c.,**
    calc., caps., carb-v., caust.,
    chel., cina., coff., **con.**[3, 4], cupr.,
    dig., dros.[3, 4], dulc.[3, 4], **ign.,**
    kali-c., kali-i.[4], kreos.[4], lac-c.,
    lach.[4], lith-c.[3], mag-c[4], mang.[4],
    nat-m., nat-s.[4], **nit-ac.,** nux-v.,
    ph-ac.[4], **plat.**[3, 4, 6], plb., **puls.** [3, 4],
    rhod.[3, 4], rhus-t.[3, 4], ruta[4],
    samb.[4], **SEP.**[3, 4], stann., **sulph.,**
    teucr., thuj., tong.[4], valer.[3, 4],
    zinc.[4]

and forward agg.[3]
et en avant agg.
und Vorwärtsbeugen agg.
    asaf., **chel.,** coff., nux-v., thuj.

am.[3]
  acon., ant-c.[4], **bell.**[3, 6, 10],
  bism.[3, 6, 7, 10], bry.[4],
  calen.[4], cann-s., **cham.**, chin.,
  cimic.[3, 6], dios.[6, 10], **DROS.**,
  fl-ac.[3, 6], hep.[3], iod.[44], kali-c.,
  kreos.[3], lac-c., **lach.**, mag-m.[14],
  mand.[10, 14], med.[3], merc.[4], nux-v.,
  puls., rhus-t.[3], sabad.[3, 4], sabin.,
  sep.[4], spong.[4], squil.[4], **thuj.**,
  verat., zinc.[3], zinc-o.[4]

  stretching am./s'étirer am./
  Sichstrecken am.

bed agg., turning in[2]
lit agg., se tourner au
Bett agg., Sichumdrehen im
  acon., agar., am-m., anac., **ars.**,
  asar., **bor.**, **BRY.**, calc., **cann-s.**,
  caps., **carb-v.**, **caust.**, chin., cina,
  cocc., **con.**[2, 8], cupr., dros., **euph.**,
  ferr., graph., **hep.**, kali-c., lach.,
  led., **lyc.**, mag-c., merc., **nat-m.**,
  nit-ac., **nux-v.**[2, 8], petr., **phos.**, plat.,
  plb., **PULS.**[2, 8], ran-b., **rhod.**,
  rhus-t., ruta, **sabad.**, sabin., **samb.**,
  sais., **sil.**, **staph.**, **sulph.**, thuj.,
  valer.

double agg.[8]
en deux agg., se plier
Sichzusammenkrümmen agg.
  dios.

  am.[6, 8]
  aloe[8], arg-n.[6, 7], bov.[6], caust.[6],
  chin., colch.[6], **coloc.**[6, 8, 10],
  mag-c.[6, 10], **mag-p.**, mand.[14],
  plb.[6]

  bent holding/parties pliées/
  Beugehaltung
  doubling up/corps plié en deux/
  Zusammenkrümmen

forward agg.[3]
en avant agg.
Vorwärtsbeugen agg.
  aesc.[7], asaf., **bell.**[8], chel., **coff.**,
  kalm.[8], mag-m.[14], mang.[4],
  nux-v.[3, 8], thiop.[14], thuj.

---

am.
  apis[1'], **aur.**, coloc.[7], gels.[8],
  kali-c.[8, 14], **teucr.**

inward agg.[3]
intérieurement agg.
Einwärtsbeugen agg.
  am-m., **ign.**, staph., verat.

  am.[3]
  am-m., **bell.**

right agg., to[3]
à droite agg.
rechts agg., nach
  spig.

sideways agg.[3]
de côté agg.
Seitwärtsbeugen agg.
  bell., bor., **calc.**, canth., chel.,
  chin., cocc., **kali-c.**, lyc., **nat-m.**,
  plb., stann., staph.

  am.[3]
  meny., **puls.**

BENT HOLDING the part **agg.**[3]
PARTIES PLIÉES agg., maintenir les
BEUGEHALTUNG der Körperteile **agg.**
  hyos., lyc., **spong.**, teucr., valer.

  am.[3]
  bov., bry., **coloc.**, nat-m., puls.,
  rhus-t., squil., sulph., verat.

  bending-double/plier-en deux/
  Sichbiegen-Sichkrümmen
  doubling up/corps plié en deux/
  Zusammenkrümmen

BESNIER–BOEK–SCHAUMANN,
  morbus[14]
  aq-m., aran-ix., asar., beryl.,
  hip-ac., hist., kres., mand.,
  parathyr., thiop., v-a-b.

BINDING UP, bandaging am.[3, 6]
LIER, appliquer des bandages am.
FESTES BINDEN, Bandagieren am.
  apis, arg-n.[3], bry., chin.[3], gels.,
  mag-m.[3], mang.[3], mim-p.[14], puls.,
  rhod., sil., tril.[3]

BLACKNESS of external parts
NOIRCEUR des parties externes
SHWARZE VERFÄRBUNG äußerer
  Körperteile
  acon., agar., all-c.[12], alum., am-c.,
  ang.[3], **ant-c.,** ant-t.[3, 4], **anthraci.,** apis,
  arg-n., arn., **ARS.,** ars-i., asaf., asar.,
  aur., bapt.[3], bar-c., bell., bism.,
  both.[7, 11, 12], brass.[11, 12], brom.[3], bry.,
  calc., **calc-ar.**[2], camph., canth.,
  caps.[2, 4], carb-ac.[3, 12], **carb-an.,**
  carb-v., carbn-o.[11], caust., cham.,
  chin., chin-ar., chr-ac.[2], chr-o.[12], cic.,
  cina, cocc., com.[6], **con., crot-h.,**
  CUPR., cycl., **dig.,** dros., **echi.,** elaps[3],
  ergot.[12], euph., euph-c.[6], gels.[3], **ham.,**
  hell.[4], hep.[3], hyos., ign.[2, 3], iod., ip.,
  kali-p.[1', 2, 12], **kreos.,** kres.[13], **lach.,**
  lyc., mag-c., mag-m.[3], **MERC.,**
  merc-c.[3], **merc-cy.**[6], mur-ac.[4], nat-m.,
  nit-ac., **nux-v., OP., ph-ac., phos.,**
  phyt., plb., puls., ran-a.[12], ran-b.[3, 4],
  ran-s.[11], **rhus-t.,** ric.[12], ruta sabad.,
  sabin.[4], **samb.,** sars., **SEC.,** sep., sil.,
  solid.[3], spig., spong., squil., stann.,
  staph.[3], stram., sul-ac.[3, 4, 12], sulph.[3, 4],
  tarent.[2, 3, 11], ter.[2], thuj., **VERAT.,**
  vip.[4, 6], **vip-r.**[4]

inflammation-internally-gangrenous/
  inflammation-interne-gangreneuse/
  Entzündungs-innere-gangränöse

cold
froide
kalter Haut, mit
  ant-t., **ARS.,** asaf., bell., **canth.,**
  caps., **carb-v.,** chin.[2], con., crot-h.,
  euph., lach., merc., **PLB.,** ran-b.,
  SEC., sil., squil., sul-ac., sulph.,
  tarent-c., **ter.**[2]

diabetic[3]
diabétique
diabetische
  ars.[6, 10], con., **kreos.**[6, 10], kres.[10, 14],
  lach., **sec.**[2, 6, 10], solid.

hot
chaude
heißer Haut, mit
  acon., ars., bell., mur-ac., op.[3],
  sabin., sec.

moist
moite
feuchte
  brom.[3], **carb-v., CHIN., hell.,** lach.[6],
  ph-ac., phos.[3], tarent., **vip.**[3, 6]

senile
sénile
senile
  adren.[6], all-c.[2, 7, 8, 12], am-c.[2, 8],
  ars.[2, 6, 8, 12], **carb-v.,** chin.[2], con.[2],
  crot-h.[6], cupr.[7], echi.[6], ergot.[6],
  euph.[2], **kreos.**[6], **LACH.**[2, 6], **ph-ac.**[2],
  plb.[2, 6], **SEC.,** sul-ac.[8], vip.[6]

traumatic[2, 3, 8]
traumatique
traumatische
  am-m.[2], **arn., calen.**[2], **hyper.**[2],
  LACH., sul-ac.[2, 8]

BLOOD too **quick,** sensation of
  circulation of[16]
SANG trop **rapide,** sensation de la
  circulation du
BLUT zirkuliert zu **schnell;** Gefühl, das
  ars.

thin, sensation as if[7, 11]
fluide, comme si le s. est
verdünnt sei; Gefühl als ob das
  hell.

BREAKFAST agg., **before**
PETIT DÉJEUNER agg., **avant** le
FRÜHSTÜCK agg., **vor** dem
  alumn.[2], croc.[8]

after b. agg.
après, agg.
nach, agg.
   agar., am-m., ambr., anac., ars.,
   bell., bor., **bry., calc.,** calc-sil.[1'],
   carb-an., carb-v., carbn-s., **caust.,**
   CHAM., chin., **con.,** cycl., **dig.,**
   euph., form., **graph.,** grat.[3], **guaj.[3],**
   hell., ign., iris.[3], **kali-c., kali-n.,**
   laur., lyc., mag-c., mang., **nat-c.,**
   nat-m., nat-s.[3], nit-ac., nux-m.,
   NUX-V., par., petr., ph-ac., **PHOS.,**
   plb., puls., rhod., rhus-t., sars.,
   sep., sil., stront-c., **sulph.,**
   thuj., valer., verat., **ZINC.,** zinc-p.[1']

after b. am.
après, am.
nach, am.
   acon.[3], alum.[3], am-c.[3], **am-m.[2, 3],**
   ambr.[3], anac.[3], ars.[3], **bar-c.[2, 3],**
   bov.[2, 3], bry.[3], **calc., cann-s.[2, 3],**
   canth.[3], **carb-an.[2, 3],** carb-v.[3], caust.[3],
   chel.[2, 3], chin.[3], cina[3], **croc.,** ferr.,
   graph.[3], hell.[3], **hep.[2, 3], ign.[2, 3],**
   iod., kali-c.[3], **lach.[2, 3, 6], laur.[2, 3],**
   lyc.[2, 3], mag-c.[3], mag-m.[3], merc.[3],
   mez.[2, 3], nat-c.[3], nat-m., nat-p.[1'],
   nat-s.[1', 3, 8], nit-ac.[3], **nux-v.** [2, 3, 6],
   petr.[2, 3], phos.[3], **plat.[2, 3], plb.[2, 3],**
   puls.[3], **ran-b.[2, 3],** ran-s.[3], rhod.[3],
   rhus-t.[2, 3], sabad.[2, 3], sep.[2, 3],
   squil.[2, 3], staph., stront-c.[2, 3],
   sulph.[2, 3], tarax.[2, 3], teucr.[3], valer.,
   verat.[3], **verb.[2, 3],** zinc-p.[1']

BREATHING agg.[3]
RESPIRER agg.
ATMEN agg.
   acon., agar., alum., am-c., **am-m.,**
   anac., ant-c., arg-m., arn., ars.,
   asaf., asar., aur., **bell.,** bism., bor.,
   bov., **BRY., calc., cann-s., caps.,**
   cham., chin., **cina,** clem., cocc.,
   COLCH., coloc., con., croc., cupr.,
   dig., dros., dulc., euphr., graph.,
   hep., hyos., **kali-c.,** kali-n., led.,
   lyc., **mag-c.,** merc., mez., **mur-ac.,**
   nat-c., **nat-m., nit-ac.,** nux-v.,

ph-ac., plat., **puls.,** ran-b., rhod.,
rhus-t., sabad., sars., **sel.,** seneg.,
SEP., sil., **SPIG.,** squil., stann.,
sul-ac., **sulph.,** thuj., verat.

Cheyne-Stokes' respiration
Cheyne-Stokes, respiration de
Cheyne-Stokes' Atmen
   acon., **acon-f.[7, 8, 12],** am-c.[6],
   ang.[6], antip.[7, 8, 12], atro[7, 8, 12], bell.,
   camph[6], cann-i.[6], carb-v.[7, 8], chlol.[7],
   coca [7], cocain.[7, 8], crot-h.[6], **cupr.[6],**
   cupr-ar.[6], **dig.[6], grin.[7, 8, 12],**
   hydr-ac.[6, 10], ign., iod.[6], ip.[6],
   kali-cy.[7, 8, 12], lach.[6], **laur[6],** led.[6,]
   lob.[6], nux-v., olnd.[6], **op.[1, 7],**
   morph.[7, 8], parth.[7, 8, 12], **saroth.[7, 8],**
   spong., sul-ac.[3], sulph.[3], vanad.[7],
   verat.[6]

deep b. agg.[3]
profonde agg., respiration
Tiefatmen agg.
   ACON., agn., am-m.[2, 3], arg-m.,
   arn., asaf., **bell., bor.,** brom., **BRY.,**
   calad., calc., **canth.,** caps., carb-an.,
   caust., cina, dros., dulc., fl-ac.,
   graph., hell., hep., hist.[14], hyos.,
   ign., ip., **kali-c., kali-n.,** kreos.,
   lach., **lyc.,** mag-m., mang., **merc.,**
   merc-c., mosch., nat-c., nat-m.,
   nux-m., nux-v., **olnd., phos.,** plb.,
   puls., ran-b.[3], **ran-s.,** rheum,
   RHUS-T., rumx.[3], sabad., **SABIN.,**
   sang.[3], seneg., sep., **sil.,** spig.,
   spong., **squil.,** stram., sulph.[3],
   thuj., valer., verb.

am.
   acon., agar.[3], asaf., bar-c., **cann-i.,**
   chin., **colch., cupr.,** dig., dros.,
   ign., iod., **lach.,** meny., mygal.[3],
   nat-m.[3], olnd., osm., puls., **seneg.,**
   sep., **spig., STANN.,** staph.,
   sulph.[3], ter., verb.[3], viol-t.

desire to
désir de
Verlangen nach
acet-ac., achy.[14], acon., agar.[3],
alum., alumn., am-br., aml-ns.[3, 6],
ant-c.[6], apis[3], **aur.**, bapt., **bor.**,
brom., **BRY., CACT., CALC.,**
calc-p., camph.[6], cann-i.[6], **caps.,**
carb-ac., carb-v., card-m., caust.,
cedr., **chin.**, cimx., coca, croc.,
CROT-T.[1, 7], **cupr.**[3, 6], **dig.**, euon.,
eup-per., **glon.**, hell.[3], hydr.,
IGN., ind., **ip.**[3, 6], kali-bi.[3], **kali-c.,**
kali-n.[3, 6], **kreos., LACH., lact.,**
laur[3], lil-t., **lob.**[3, 6], **lyc.**, mag-p.[3],
med.[2], **merc.**, mez., mosch.,
NAT-S., nux-m., **op.**[3, 6], **par.,**
phos., plat.[3], podo., poth., prun.,
ran-b., rhus-t.[3], sabin.[3], samb.,
sang., SEL., seneg., sep., sil.[3, 6],
squil.[3,] stann., stram., **SULPH.,**
tab.[3,] ther., tub[1'], verb., xan.

expiration agg.[3]
Ausatmen agg.
agn., ambr., anac., ang., ant-c.,
ant-t., **arg-m.**[2, 3], ars.[2, 3], asaf.,
aur., bry., cann-s., carb-v., caust.,
cham., chel., chin., **chlor.**[2], cic.,
cina, clem., coff., **COLCH., dig.,**
dros., dulc., euphr., **fl-ac., ign.,**
iod., ip.[2,] kreos., laur., led.,
mang., mur-ac., nat-c., nux-v.,
olnd., ph-ac., **PULS.**, rhus-t., ruta,
sabad., **sep., SPIG.**, spong., squil.,
stann., **staph.**, tarax., verat.,
viol-o., viol-t., zinc.

am.[3]
ACON.[2, 3], agar., am-m., anac.,
ang., arg-m., arn.[2, 3], asaf., asar.,
bar-c., **bor., BRY.**[2, 3], calc.,
cann-s., canth., caps., carb-an.,
caust., cham., chel., chin., cina,
clem., croc., cycl., euphr., guaj.,
hell., hep., ip., kali-c., kali-n.,
kreos., lyc., **meny.**, merc.,
mosch., nux-m., olnd., op., plat.,
plb., ran-b., ran-s., **RHUS-T.,**
sabad., **SABIN.**, sars., sel.,
seneg., sep., spig., spong., **squil.,**
stann., sul-ac., sulph., tarax.
valer., verat.

inspiration agg.[3]
Einatmen agg.
ACON.[2, 3, 8], **agar.**, agn., alum.,
am-c., am-m., **anac.**, ang., **ANT-C.,**
arg-m., arg-n.[7], **arn.**[2, 3], ars., asaf.,
asar., aur., bar-c., **bell., bor.,**
bov., **BRY.**[3, 8], **calc.**, camph.,
cann-s., canth., **caps.**, carb-an.,
carb-v., caust., **cham., chel.,**
chin., cic., cina, clem., coloc.,
con., croc, **crot-h.**, cupr., cycl.,
dulc., euphr., **guaj.**, hell., hist.[10],
hyos., ign., iod., **ip., kali-c.,**
kali-n., kreos., laur., led., lob.,
lyc., mag-c., mag-m., **meny.,**
merc., mez., mosch., mur-ac.,
nat-c., nat-m., nit-ac., nux-m.,
nux-v., olnd., op., par., petr.,
ph-ac., phos.[3, 8], plat., plb., **puls.,**
ran-b.[3, 8], ran-s., rhod., **RHUS-T.,**
ruta, **sabad., SABIN.**, sars.,
sel., seneg., sep., sil., spig.[3, 8],
spong., SQUIL., stann., **staph.,**
stront., sul-ac., sulph., tarax.,
teucr., thuj., **valer.**, verat., verb.,
viol-t., zinc.

am.[3]
ant-t., asaf., bar-c., bry., cann-s.,
caust., **chin.**, cina, **COLCH.**[3 ,8],
cupr., dig., dros., dulc., **IGN.**[3, 8],
iod., **lach.**, mang., meny., nux-v.,
olnd., ph-ac., **puls.**, ruta., sabad.,
sep., **SPIG.**[3, 8], squil., **stann.,**
staph., tarax., verat., verb.,
viol-o., viol-t.

hot air, ailments from i. of[12]
air chaud, troubles à la suite d'i. d'
heißer Luft, Beschwerden infolge
von E.
carb-v.

BRITTLE BONES
OS FRAGILES
BRÜCHIGE KNOCHEN
asaf.[3], bufo[3], **calc.**, calc-p.[3], cupr.[3],
fl-ac.[3], lyc.[3], **merc.**[3], par.[3], ph-ac.[3],
ruta[3], **SIL.**[3], **sulph.**[3], **symph.**, thuj.[3]

caries-bone/carie osseuse/
Knochenkaries

BROMIDES, abuse of[3, 6]
BROMURES, abus de
BROM, Mißbrauch von
am-c.[2], camph.[2], cham., lach., mag-c.[2],
op.[2], phos., zinc-p.

BUBBLING
BULLES, sensation de
BLASENAUFSTEIGEN, Sprudeln,
Gefühl von
ambr., ant-c., asaf., bell., berb.,
caps.[3, 11], colch., coloc.[3], ip., junc-e.[7],
laur.[3], lyc., mang.[16], nux-v., **puls.,**
rheum, spig., squil., sulph.[3], tarax.

BURNS
BRÛLURES
VERBRENNUNGEN
acet-ac.[2, 7, 8, 12], **acon.**[2, 3, 4, 7, 8], agar.,
aloe[10], alum., alumn.[2], ant-c.,
arist-cl.[10, 14], arn.[2, 7, 8], **ARS., bar-c.**[4],
bell.[4,] **bry.**[4], calc., calc-p.[7],
calc-s.[2, 8, 12], **calen.**[2, 7, 8, 12],
camph.[7, 8], **CANTH.,** carb-ac.,
carb-v., carbn-s.[2, 12], **caust.,** chin.[4],
cic.[2], crot-h.[2], cycl., des-ac.[14], echi.[6],
euph., ferr.[4], gaul.[7, 8], grin.[7, 8, 10],
ham.[2, 7, 8, 12], **hep.**[2, 7, 8, 12], hoit.[14],
hyos[4, 10], **hyper**[2], **ign.**[4], jab.[7, 8, 12],
kali-bi.[7, 8, 12], kali-c.[4], kali-m.[2, 12],
kreos., lach., mag-c., **mag-m.**[4],
merc.[2, 4], **nat-c.**[4, 12], **nux-v.**[4], op.[4],
par.[4], passi.[12], petr.[2, 7, 8, 12], phos.[4],
pic-ac.[8, 12], **plan.**[2, 12], plat.[4], plb.,
puls.[2, 4], ran-b.[7], **rhus-t.,** ruta,
sabad[4], **sec.,** sep.[4], **sil.**[12], spira.[12],
stram., sul-ac.[4], **ter.**[2, 7, 8], thuj.[4],
urt-u.[2-4, 6-8, 10, 12], verat.[4]

ailments from[12]
troubles à la suite de
Beschwerden infolge von
caust., kali-m., plan., rad-br., urt-u.

x-ray, from[3, 7]
rayons X, par les
Röntgenstrahlen, durch
calc-f.

CACHEXIA
CACHEXIE
KACHEXIE
acet-ac.[6], arg-m.[14], arg-n.[7, 11, 12],
arn.[12], **ARS.,** ars-i.[6], bad.[2], bond.[11],
calc.[12], caps.[2], carb-ac.[11], chim.,
chin.[1', 4, 11, 12], clem., **coc-c.**[2],cund.[2, 6],
fl-ac.[6, 7], **form.**[2], hydr.[6], iod., **kali-bi.,**
mang.[6], merc.[11, 12], merc-ns.[11],
morph.[11], mur-ac.[11], nat-m.,
NIT-AC., phos.[12], phyt.[6], pic-ac.[12],
plb.[11], sec.[6, 12], seneg.[2], thal.[14], thuj.[1'],
vip.[11], y-ray[14]

cancerous–cachexia/cancéreuses–
cachexie/kanzeröse–Kachexie
emaciation/amaigrissement/
Abmagerung

CAGED in wires, twisted tighter and
tighter
ENSERRÉ dans des fils de fer qui se
tendent et enserrent toujours plus
fortement, sensation d'être
UMSCHLOSSEN von Drähten, die sich
immer fester zusammenziehen,
Gefühl wie
CACT.

CANCEROUS affections
CANCÉREUSES, affections
KANZERÖSE Erkrankungen
acet-ac., alum., alumn., anan.[8, 12],
anil.[12], **ant-m.**[8], **apis,** apoc.[7], **ambr.,**
arg-m.[1'], arg-n.[10], **ARS.,** ars-br.[8],
ars-i., aster., aur., aur-ar.[1', 8, 12],
aur-i.[1', 14], **aur-m.,** aur-m-n.[7, 8],
aur-s.[1'], **bapt.**[7, 8, 12], bar-c.[1', 3],
bar-i.[7, 12], bell.[2], bism., **BROM.,**
bry.[7, 12], **bufo, cadm-s., calc.,**
calc-i.[7, 8, 12], calc-ox.[8, 12], **calc-s.,**
calen.[2, 8], calth.[12], **carb-ac.,**
CARB-AN., carb-v., carbn-s.,
carc.[8, 9], caust., chel.[12], cholin.[8],
cic.[8, 12], cinnm.[8, 12], **cist.,**
cit-ac.[2], cit-l.[12], clem., **CON.,**
cory.[7], crot-h.[12], **cund.**[2, 3, 7, 8, 12],
cupr., cupr-a.[8], cur.[12], dulc.,
elaps[12], eos.[8], epiph.[12], eucal.[7],
euph.[8, 12], euph-he.[12], ferr-i.[12],

ferr-p.[2], ferr-pic.[7], form.[8], form-ac.[8],
fuli.[8], **gali.**[7, 8, 12], gent-l.[7], **graph.,**
gua.[7, 8], **ham.**[8, 12], hep., **hippoz.**[2, 12],
hydr., hydrin-m.[12], **iod.**[3, 7, 8, 12],
kali-ar., kali-bi., kali-chl.[3],
kali-cy.[2, 7, 8, 12], **kali-i.**[3, 8, 12], **kali-p.**[7],
kali-s., kreos., kres.[10], **lach., lap-a.,**
lob-e.[12], **LYC.,** maland.[8], matth.[12],
med.[7, 8], **merc., merc-i-f.,** methyl.[12],
mill.[2, 12], **morph.**[2], nat-m., nectrin.[12],
NIT-AC., ol-an.[12], **op.**[12], orni[12],
oxyg.[12], ph-ac., **PHOS., PHYT.,**
pic-ac.[12], psor.[12,] rad-br.[3, 8],
rumx-a.[8], **sang.**[7, 8, 12], sarcol-ac.[10],
scir.[8, 12], sed-r.[8], **semp.**[7, 8], sep.,
sieg.[10], sec.[3], **SIL.,** silphu.[12], squil.[4],
strych-g.[8], sul-ac., **sulph.,** symph.[3, 8],
tax.[8], tarax.[7, 14], **ter.**[2], **thuj.,**
trif-p.[7, 12], viol-o.[12], visc.[10, 14],
x-ray[9, 14], zinc.

Hodgkin's disease/lymphogranulo-
matose/Hodgkin' Syndrom
leukaemia/leucémie/Leukämie

sarcoma/sarcome/sarkom
tumors/tumeurs/Tumoren

bones, of[8, 12]
os, des
Knochen, der
   aur-i.[8], con.[2], hecla[12], **phos.,** symph.

cachexia, emaciation, with
cachexie, amaigrissement, avec
Kachexie, Abmagerung, mit
   acon.[7], **hydr.**[2], pic-ac.[12], thuj.[1']

cicatrices, in old[1', 7]
cicatrices vieilles, des
Narben, in alten
   graph.

colloid cancer[2]
colloïde, cancer
Gallertkrebs
   lach., phos.

contusions, after[2]
contusions, après
Quetschungen, nach
   con.

encephaloma see tumors

epithelioma
épithélioma
Epitheliom
   abr.[8, 12], acet-ac., alum.[1', 6],
   alumn.[1', 2, 8], arg-m., arg-n., **ars.,**
   ARS-I., ars-s-f.[1'], aur., aur-ar.[1'],
   bell., brom., calc., calc-p., calc-sil[1'],
   carb-ac.[6], carb-an.[2], chr-ac.[8],
   cic.[6, 8, 12], clem., **CON., cund.**[2, 6, 8, 12],
   euph.[8], fuli.[8], **hydr., hydrc.**[6],
   kali-ar.[6, 8, 12], kali-chl.[12], kali-m.[6],
   kali-s., kreos., lap-a.[2, 3, 6, 8, 12],
   lob-e.[8], **LYC.,** mag-m.[14], mag-s.[12],
   merc., merc-c.[2], methyl.[12], nat-cac.[8],
   nat-m.[2], nectrin.[12], nit-ac.[2], phos.,
   phyt., puls.[2], rad-br.[8], raja-s.[14],
   ran-b., scroph-n.[8], sep., **sil.,**
   strych-g.[8], sulph., thuj., uran-n.[2]

fungus haematodes see tumors–
angioma

glands, of
glandes, des
Drüsen, der
   aur-m., buni-o.[14], **CARB-AN., CON.,**
   sieg.[10], strych-g.[8], sul-i.[1'], syph.[7]

lupus, carcinomatous
lupus carcinomateux
Lupus carcinomatosus
   agar., alum., alumn., ant-c.,
   arg-n., **ARS., ars-i.,** aur-m., **bar-c.,**
   calc., **carb-ac., carb-v., carbn-s.,**
   caust., **cist.,** graph., hep., **hydrc.,**
   kali-ar., **kali-bi.,** kali-c., **kali-chl.,**
   kali-s., **kreos.,** lach., **LYC.,**
   nit-ac., phyt., psor., sep., **sil.,**
   spong., staph., sulph., **THUJ.**

   in rings/annulaire/ringförmig
   sep.

melanoma
mélanome
Melanomkarzinom, -sarkom
  arg-n., card-m., **lach.,** ph-ac.

pains see pain–cancerous affections

sarcoma/sarcome/Sarkom

scirrhus
squirrhe
Scirrhus
  alumn., **anac.**[2], arg-m., arn.[2], **ars.,**
  ars-s-f.[1'], **aster.,** bell-p.[3], **calc-s.,**
  calen.[2], **CARB-AN., carb-v.,**
  carbn-s., clem.[1'], **CON.,** cund.[2],
  graph., hydr., lap-a., nux-v.[2], petr.[3],
  phos., phyt., sep., **SIL.,** squil.[16],
  staph., **sulph.**

ulcers of glands
ulcères cancéreux des glandes
Drüsengeschwüre
  arn., **ARS.,** ars-i.[1], aur., **bell.,**
  BUFO, calc., carb-an., carb-v.,
  caust., clem., **CON.,** cupr., dulc.,
  hep., kali-ar.[1'], **kali-c., kreos.,** lyc.,
  merc., merc-i-f., nit-ac., ph-ac.,
  phos., rhus-t., **sep., sil.,** squil.[1],
  sul-ac., **SULPH.,** zinc.

of skin
de la peau
Hautgeschwüre
  ambr., ant-c., **anthraci.,** apis,
  ARS., ars-i., ARS-S-F.[1'], **aster.**[8],
  aur., aur-ar.[1'], aur-i.[1'], **AUR-S.**[1'],
  bell., **BUFO,** calc., **calc-s.,**
  carb-ac., carb-an., carb-v.,
  carbn-s., caust., chel., chim.[8, 12],
  chin-s.[2, 4, 11], clem., **con., crot-c.,**
  cund., dor.[11], dulc., **ferr.**[3], fl-ac.[6],
  fuli.[8], **gali.**[8], **graph., HEP.,**
  hippoz., hydr., kali-ar., kali-bi.[1'],
  kali-c., **kali-i., kreos., lach., LYC.,**
  lyss., mang., **merc., mill.**[2],
  mur-ac., **nit-ac., petr., ph-ac.,**
  phos., phyt., rhus-t., rumx., sars.,
  sep., SIL., spong., squil., **staph.,**
  sul-i.[1'], **SULPH.,** tarent-c.[8], **thuj.**

CARIES of bone
CARIE osseuse
KNOCHENKARIES
  ANG., anthraco.[2], arg-m.[2], arn.[2],
  ars., ASAF., Aur., aur-ar.[1'], aur-i.[1'],
  aur-m., aur-m-n., bell., both.[11], bry.,
  calc., **calc-f.,** calc-hp.[8], **calc-p.,**
  calc-s., caps., carb-ac., caust.[2],
  chin., cinnm.[2], **cist.,** clem., con.,
  cupr., dulc., euph., ferr., **FL-AC.,**
  graph., **guaj., guare.,** hecla[6], **hep.,**
  iod., kali-bi., **KALI-I.,** kreos., lach.,
  LYC., mang.[1', 8], **MERC., mez.,**
  nat-m., **nit-ac., ol-j.**[2], op., petr.,
  ph-ac., phos., psor.[2], **puls.,** rhod.,
  rhus-t., ruta, sabin., sal-ac.[2, 12], sec.,
  sep., SIL., spong., **staph.,** stront-c.[10],
  sulph., symph.[8], syph.[1', 7], tarent.[2],
  tell.[3], ter.[2], **THER.,** thuj., tub-k.[12]

brittle bones/os fragiles/brüchige
  Knochen
necrosis bone/nécrose–os/
  Knochennekrose
softening bones/ostéomalacie/
  Knochenerweichung

periosteum, of
périoste, du
Periost, des (chron. entzündl.
  Granulationen)
  ant-c., **ASAF.,** aur., bell., **chin.,**
  cycl., hell., **merc.,** mez., **PH-AC.,**
  puls., rhod., rhus-t., ruta, sabin.,
  sil., staph.

CARRYING, ailments from[7]
PORTER, troubles à la suite de
TRAGEN, Beschwerden infolge von
  carb-ac., caust., ruta[12]

am.[3]
  ant-c., ant-t.[8], ars., **cham.**[8], coloc.,
  ferr., ip., kali-c., nat-c., nat-m.,
  ph-ac., sep.

back agg., on the
dos, agg. en portant sur le
Rücken agg., auf dem
  alum.

head agg., on the
tête, agg. en portant sur la
Kopf agg., auf dem
  calc.

CARTILAGES, affection of[6] ✱
CARTILAGES, affections des
KNORPEL, Erkrankungen der
  ARG-M.[1, 2, 6, 7, 12], cimic., guaj.,
  led., merc., nat-m.[2], olnd., plb., ruta,
  sil.[1, 6]

enchondroma/enchondrome/Knorpel-
  geschwulst
inflammation–c./Entzündungen–K.
swelling–c./tuméfaction–c./
  Schwellung–K.

ulcers of
ulcères des
Ulcera der
  merc-c.

CATALEPSY
CATALEPSIE
KATALEPSIE
  abies-c.[12], acon., aether[11, 12], **agar.**,
  aran., **art-v.**, asaf.[6] bell.,
  camph-br.[8], cann-i., canth.[11],
  caust.[6], cham., chlol., **cic., cocc.,**
  coff., con., crot-c.[8], crot-h.[6], **cupr.**[6],
  cur., ferr., gels., GRAPH.,
  hydr-ac.[2, 4, 6, 8], hyos., ign., indg.[12],
  iod.[11], **ip.**, lach., laur.[4], **mag-m.**[6],
  merc.[4, 8], **morph.**[8], **mosch.**[4, 6, 12],
  nat-m., nux-m., ol-an.[6], **op., petr.,**
  ph-ac., pip-m.[6, 12], **plat.**, plb.[11],
  raph.[12], reser.[14], sabad.[8], spong.[12],
  staph., stram., stry.[11], sulph., tab.[12],
  tanac.[11] thuj., **valer.**[6], verat., **zinc.**[6]

Vol. I: *automatisms/automatismes/*
  unwillkürliche Handlungen
  gestures/gesticule/Gebärden
  sits/assis/sitzt
  unconsciousness–conduct/
  inconscience–conduite/
  Bewußtlosigkeit–Verhalten

afternoon[11]
après-midi
nachmittags
  grat.

evening in bed
soir au lit
abends im Bett
  cur.

anger, from[2]
colère, par
Zorn, durch
  bry., **cham.**

fright, after
frayeur, par
Schreck, nach
  acon., bell., **gels.**, ign., **OP.**

grief, after
chagrin, par
Kummer, nach
  ign., **ph-ac.**, staph.

jealousy, from
jalousie, par
Eifersucht, durch
  hyos., **LACH.**

joy, from
joie, par
Freude, durch
  COFF.

love, from unrequited
amour désappointé, par
Liebe, durch unerwiderte
  hyos., **ign.**, lach., **ph-ac.**

menses, before[8]
menstruation, avant la
Menses, vor den
  mosch.

  during
  pendant la
  während der
    plat.

religious excitement, from
religieuse, par excitation
religiöse Erregung, durch
  stram., sulph., verat.

sexual excess, from[2]
sexuels, par excès
sexuelle Ausschweifungen, durch
chin., nux.

excitement, from
excitation sexuelle, par
Erregung, durch
con., plat., stram.

worm affections, in[1']
vermineuses, au cours d'affections
Wurmbefall, bei
sabad.

CATHETERISM, ailments from[6]
CATHÉTERISME, troubles à la suite de
KATHETERISIERUNG, Beschwerden
infolge von
arn., mag-p.[6, 12], nux-v.

CAUTERY (with arg-n.), antidote to[12]
CAUTÉRISATION (par le nitrate
d'argent) antidote
KAUTERISATION (mit arg-n.),
Antidot bei
nat-m.

CHANGE of **position** agg.
CHANGEMENT de **position** agg.
WECHSEL, Lagewechsel agg.
acon., **bry., CAPS., carb-v.,**
caust., **chel., con., EUPH., FERR.,**
lach., lyc., petr., ph-ac., **phos.,**
plat., plb., **PULS.,** ran-b., rhod.,
rhus-t., sabad., **samb.,** sil.,
SYPH.[3], thuj.

am.
agar., apis[8], arn.[3, 6], ars., buni-o.[14],
caust.[8, 15], cench.[1'], **cham., dulc.**[3],
IGN., meli., nat-s., ph-ac., plb.[3],
puls., **RHUS-T.,** sep.[3], staph.[3],
syph.[3], tab.[3], teucr., valer., zinc.

desire for change of position[3, 6]
désir de changement de position
Verlangen nach Lagewechsel
acon., alum.[3, 4, 6], **arn.**[4, 6], **ars.**[2, 3, 6],
bapt., bell.[3, 4, 6], **bry.**[3, 4, 6], caust.,
cham., **eup-per.,** ign., lyc.[3, 4, 6],
nat-s., **rhus-t.**[3, 6], sil.[3, 4, 6], tarax.[3, 4, 6],
zinc., **zinc-val.**

symptoms, constant ch. of[8]
symptômes, continuel des
Symptomwechsel, ständiger
apis, berb., carc.[10], cimic.[1', 7],
crot-t.[1'], **ign.**[3, 8], **kali-bi.**[1', 7, 8],
kali-c.[1'], **kali-s., lac-c.**[7, 8], lil-s.[1'],
lil-t., **mang.,** paraf., **phyt.,** podo.[1'],
puls.[7, 8], sabin.[1'], sanic.[7, 8],
tub.[1', 7, 8], valer.[1']

alternating/alternants/
abwechselnde
contradictory/contradictoires/
widerspruchsvolle
metastasis/métastases/Metasta-
sierung

rapid[3, 6]
rapide
schneller
ambr., ant-c.[1'], arn., benz-ac.,
berb., caul., caust., cimic., kalm.,
led., meph.[11], plat.[3], plb.[3], puls.,
sal-ac.[6], sul-ac.[6], tub., **valer.**

temperature agg., off
température agg., de
Temperaturwechsel agg.
acon., act-sp.[2, 7], aesc.[1'], alum.,
alumn.[2], ant-c.[8], **ant-t.**[2, 7], **ARS.,**
bar-c.[3, 6], bufo[3], calc.[6], **calc-p.**[3, 6],
carb-v., caust., dulc.[3, 6],
FL-AC.[2, 7], graph., ip.[3, 7, 8],
kali-i.[3], **lach.**[2, 3, 7, 8], lyc., **mag-c.,**
meli.[3], merc-c.[3], nit-ac.[6],
nux-v.[1, 7], **phos.**[1, 7], phys.[11], **puls.,**
RAN-B., ran-s., rhod.[3, 6],
rhus-t.[1, 7], rumx.[3, 6], sabad.[3],
sabin., sang.[3, 6], sep.[3], sil.[1', 3, 6],
spong.[1, 7], sul-i.[3], sulph., verat.,
VERB.

ailments from[12]
troubles à la suite de
Beschwerden infolge von
nat-c., ran-b.

weather see weather–change

CHILDBED, ailments from (1897) ✳
COUCHES, troubles à la suite des
WOCHENBETT, Beschwerden infolge
von
cimic., sep., stram.

convulsions–puerperal/convulsions–
puérpérales/Konvulsionen–
Kindbett
faintness–puerperal/évanouisse-
ment–puerpéral/Ohnmacht–
Kindbett

CHILDREN, affections in
(Kent's Rep. 1897) ✳
ENFANTS, affections chez les
KINDERN, Erkrankungen bei
abrot.[6], acet-ac.[12], **ACON.,** aeth.,
agar., **all-c.,** alum.[3, 6], ambr.,
ang.[2, 3], ant-c., ANT-T., apis[6], arn.,
ars., asaf., **aur., bar-c., BELL., BOR.,**
bry., CALC., calc-f.[14], **calc-p.,**
camph., canth., **CAPS.,** caust.[3],
CHAM., chel.[2], chin., chlol.[2],
chlorpr.[14], **cic.,** cic-m.[12], **cina,**
clem., coc-c.[6], **cocc., cocc-s.[2],** coff.,
con., **croc.,** cupr., dig., dros., euph.,
ferr., ferr-p.[3, 6, 7], **gels.,** graph., hell:,
hep.[3], **HYOS.,** ign., iod., **IP.,**
kali-br.[2, 12], kali-c., **kali-m.[2],**
kali-p.[2], kreos., lach., laur., **lyc.,**
mag-c., mag-p.[2], meph.[14], **MERC.,**
mill.[2], mosch.[2], mur-ac., nat-c.,
nat-m.[2, 6], nux-m., nux-v., OP.,
ped.[12], phos.[6], phyt.[3], plb., **podo.,**
psor., PULS., rheum, rhod.[3], rhus-t.,
rib-ac.[14], ruta, sabad., sabin.,
samb.[3, 6], sec., seneg., senn.[4], sep.,
SIL., spig., **spong., squil.,** stann.,

staph., stram.[6, 12], sul-ac., **SULPH.,**
ter.[2], **teucr.,** thuj., thyr.[14], verat.,
viol-o., viol-t., zinc.

dentition/Dentitio
development, arrested/
développement arrêté/
Entwicklungshemmung
emaciation-children/
amaigrissement-enfants/
Abmagerung-Kindern
growth/croissance/Längen-
wachstum
Vol. I: *feces-urinating/défèque-*
urinant/Stuhl-urinieren

biting nails[3, 7]
ronger les ongles, se
Nägelkauen
acon., am-br.[7], arn.[7], ars., **ARUM-T.,**
bar-c., calc.[3, 15], cina, hura[3],
hyos.[5, 7], lyc., lyss.[3], med.[3],
nat-m.[7, 15], nit-ac.[3], phos.[3], plb.[3],
sanic.[7], senec., **sil.[5, 7],** stram.,
sulph.[5, 7]

delicate, puny, sickly[3, 6]
maladifs, délicats, chétifs
zarte, schwächliche, kränkelnde
brom., calc-p., **caust.[2],** irid.[12],
lyc.[2, 3, 6, 12], mag-c.[12], phos., psor.[2, 12]

emaciation–pining boys/
amaigrissement–jeunes garçons/
Abmagerung–Jugendlicher

fingers in the mouth, put
doigts dans la bouche, fourrent
Finger in den Mund, stecken die
calc., **cham., IP.,** kali-p.[15], lyc.[5],
nat-m.[15], sil.[15], tarent.[7]

growing too fast[8, 12]
croissance trop rapide
wachsen zu schnell
calc.[7, 8], **calc-p.[8],** ferr.[3], ferr-a.[6, 8],
iod.[3, 6], irid., kreos.,
PH-AC.[2, 3, 4, 6-8, 12], phos.[1'-3, 6-8, 12]

growth/croissance/Längen-
wachstum

CHILL, feels better before
FRISSON, se sent mieux avant le
FIEBERFROST besser,
  fühlt sich vor dem
  psor.

CHINA (without quinine cachexia)
QUINQUINA (sans cachexie), suite
  d'intoxication
CHINARINDE (ohne Chininkachexie),
  Folgen von
    ant-t.[6], aran.[2], arn.[2, 6], **ars.[2, 4, 6]**,
    bell.[2, 4], **calc.[2, 4, 6]**, **carb-v.[2, 4, 6]**, cham.[2],
    coff.[2], eup-per.[2], ferr.[2, 6], **hell.[2]**, **HEP.[2]**,
    iod.[2, 6], **ip.[2, 4, 6]**, lach.[2, 4, 6], led.,
    meny.[2, 4], merc.[2, 4, 6], nat-c.[2], **nat-m.[2, 6]**,
    nux-v.[2, 6], ph-ac.[6], **puls.[2, 6]**, rhus-t.[2],
    salv.[3], **sel.**, sep.[2, 6], **sulph.[2, 6]**, thea[3],
    verat.[2, 4, 6]

CHLOROSIS
CHLOROSE
    abrot.[2, 6], absin.[2, 12], **acet-ac., alet.,**
    alum., alum-p.[1'], **alumn., am-c.,**
    ambr.[2], ant-c., ant-t.[2], aq-mar.[6],
    arg-m., arg-n., **ARS.,** ars-i.,
    ars-s-f.[1'], aur-ar.[12], bar-c., **BELL.,**
    bry.[12], cadm-met.[14], **CALC.,**
    calc-ar.[1'], **CALC-P., carb-an.,**
    carb-v., CARBN-S., caust., cham.[12],
    chin., chin-ar., chlor.[12], cina[2],
    cob-n.[14], **COCC.,** coch.[2], **con., cupr.,**
    cycl., dig., **FERR., FERR-AR., ferr-i.,**
    FERR-M., ferr-p., **ferr-s.[2],** franz.[12],
    GRAPH., guar.[2], hell., helon., hep.,
    ign., **ip.[2], kali-ar.,** kali-bi.[6], **kali-c.,**
    kali-fcy., kali-p., kali-perm.[6],
    kali-s., lac-c.[6], lach.[12], **LYC., lyss.,**
    MANG., med.[7], merc., **mill.[2, 12],**
    nat-c. nat-hchls.[12], **NAT-M.,** nat-p.,
    NIT-AC., nux-v., olnd., **petr.,**
    ph-ac., **PHOS.,** phyt.[2], pic-ac.,

PLAT., plb., PULS., sabin.,
    sacch.[11, 12], **SENEC., SEP., sin-n.[2, 12],**
    spig., staph., sul-ac., **SULPH.,** thuj.,
    ust., valer., vanad.[7], **xan.[2],** zinc.

symptoms agg. alternate days
symptômes agg. tous les 2 jours
Symptome agg. jeden zweiten Tag
  alum.

winter, in
hiver, en
Winter, im
  ferr.

CHOREA
CHORÉE
CHOREA
    abrot.[2], absin.[8], acon., **AGAR.,**
    agar-ph.[12], agarin.[8], agre.[14], **ambr.[2],**
    aml-ns.[2, 12], ant-c.[12], **ant-t.,** apis,
    arg-n., arn.[12], **ars.,** ars-i., ars-s-f.[1'],
    ART-V., asaf., aster., **atro.[2],** aven.[8],
    bell., bufo, cact., CALC., calc-i.[1'],
    calc-p.[8, 12], cast.[2, 12], caul., **CAUST.,**
    cedr., **cham., chel.,** chin.[1], chlol.,
    CIC., CIMIC., CINA, cocain.[8],
    cocc., coch.[2], **cod.[2, 12],** coff., **con.,**
    croc., crot-c., crot-h., **CUPR.,**
    cupr-a.[8, 10, 12], cupr-ar., cypr., **dios.,**
    dulc., eup-a.[8], **ferr.,** ferr-ar.,
    ferr-cit.[6], ferr-cy.[8], **ferr-i., ferr-r.[8],**
    ferr-s.[2, 12], form., **gels.[2], guar.[2],**
    hipp., hyos., IGN., iod., ip., kali-ar.,
    kali-br., kali-c., kali-i., kali-p.,
    kali-s.[2, 12], lach., lat-k.[8, 12], laur.,
    levo.[14], **lil-t.,** lyss.[10], **mag-p.,**
    mand.[14], mang.[7], merc., mez., **mill.[2],**
    morph.[2, 12], mur-ac.[12], **MYGAL.,**
    nat-m., nit-ac., nux-m., nux-v.,
    ol-an.[6], **op.,** passi.[6], ph-ac., **phos.,**
    phys.[2, 6, 8, 10, 12], phyt.[2], picro.[8], **plat.,**
    plb., psor., **puls.,** rhod., **rhus-t.,**
    russ.[12], sabin., **santin.[8],** scut.[8, 12],
    sec., sep., sil., sin-n.[2, 12], sol-n.[8, 12],
    spig.[8], stann., stict.[2], **STRAM.,**

stry.[8], stry-p.[6, 8], sul-ter.[12], sulfon.[8],
sulph., sumb., tanac.[8, 12], **TARENT.,**
tarent-c.[12], **ter.**[2, 12], thal.[11, 14],
thiop.[14], thuj., **tub.**[7], valer.[6],
verat-v., visc., **zinc.,** zinc-ar.[8],
zinc-br.[8, 12], zinc-cy.[6, 8, 12], zinc-p.[1'],
zinc-val.[6, 8], ziz.[2, 6, 8]

side, crosswise left arm and right leg[8]
côté, croisé bras gauche et jambe
  droite
Seite, kreuzweise linker Arm und
  rechtes Bein
      agar., cimic., **stram.**[2]

    right arm and left leg[8]
    bras droit et jambe gauche
    rechter Arm und linkes Bein
      tarent.

  left
  gauche
  linke
    cimic., cupr., rhod.

  one sided
  unilatéral
  einseitige
    calc., cocc., cupr., nat-s., phys.,
      tarent.[7]

  right
  droit
  rechte
    ars., caust., **nat-s.,** phys., **tarent.,**
    zinc.[15]

  side lain on
  côté où il se couche, sur le
  Seite, auf der man liegt
    cimic.

daytime
journée, pendant la
tagsüber
  art-v., tarent.

morning
matin
morgens
  arg-n.[15], mygal.

afternoon
après-midi
nachmittags
  nat-s.

noon[15]/midi/mittags
  arg-n.

evening agg.
soir agg.
abends agg.
  zinc.

night
nuit
nachts
  arg-n., CAUST.[1, 7], cupr.[1']

  am.[2]
    art-v., tarent.

anxiety, from[6]
anxiété, par
Angst, durch
  stram.

begins see face

children who have grown too fast
enfants avec croissance trop rapide
Kinder, die zu schnell gewachsen sind
  phos.

  ch.-puberty/e.-puberté/
    K.-Pubertät

climacteric period, during[6]
ménopause, pendant la
Klimakterium, während des
  cimic.

coition (woman), after
coït (chez une femme), après le
Koitus (bei einer Frau), nach dem
  agar., cedr.

cold bath, after
bain froid, après un
kaltem Bad, nach
  rhus-t.

dentition, in second
dentition permanente, au cours de
Zahnen, beim zweiten
    bell.[8], **calc.**[2]

dinner, after
déjeuner, après le
Mittagessen, nach dem
    zinc., ziz.[2]

dry weather
sec, quand il fait
trockenem Wetter, bei
    caust.

eating, after
mangé, après avoir
Essen, nach dem
    ign.

emotional
émotionelle, par excitation
Gemütsbewegung, durch
    agar., arg-n.[6], cimic.[1'], **ign., laur.,**
    nat-m.[6], **op., phos., tarent.**[2]

exercise am.
exercises, am. par
Körperübungen am.
    zinc.

face, agg. in[8]
face, agg. à la
Gesicht, agg. im
    caust., cic., **cupr.**[2, 8]**,** hyos.,
    mygal., nat-m., zinc.

    begins in f. and spreads to body
    débute à la f. et de là s'étend au
      corps
    beginnt im G. und breitet sich über
    den Körper aus
      sec.

falling, with[2]
chutes, avec
Fallen, mit
    calc.

fear, from[7]
peur, par
Furcht, durch
    calc.

fright, from
frayeur, par
Schreck, durch
    acon., agar., arg-n.[6], **calc., CAUST.,**
    cimic.[8], cupr., **cupr-a.**[2]**,** cupr-ar.[6],
    gels., ign., kali-br., laur., nat-m.,
    op., phos., **stram.,** tarent.[8]**, zinc.**

grief, after
chagrin, par
Kummer, nach
    cimic.[8], **cupr-a.**[2]**,** ign., tarent.[8]

hyperaesthesia, with excessive[2]
hyperesthésie excessive, avec
Hyperästhesie, mit excessiver
    tarent.

imitation, from
imitation, par
Imitation, durch
    caust., cupr., mygal., **tarent.**

light agg.
lumière agg.
Licht agg.
    ign.[8], ziz.[2]

loss of animal fluids, from
perte de fluide vital, par
Verlust von Körperflüssigkeit, durch
    chin.

lying on back am.
couché sur le dos am., en étant
Liegen auf dem Rücken am.
    cupr., cupr-a.[2]**, ign.**

masturbation, from
masturbation, par
Masturbation, durch
    agar.[8], **calc.,** chin., cina[2]

menses, before[6]
menstruation, avant la
Menses, vor den
    caul.

    during
    pendant la
    während der
      caul.[6], caust.[1', 7]**, ZINC.**

after, am.[2]
après la, am.
nach den, am.
   sep.

moon, at full[15]
lune, à la pleine
Vollmond, bei
   nat-m.

at new[6]
à la nouvelle
bei Neumond
   cupr.

motions agg.[2]
mouvements agg.
Bewegungen agg.
   cupr-a., ziz.

backward, with[2]
en arrière
Rückwärtsbeugen, mit
   bell.

gyratory, with[7]
giratoires, avec
drehenden, mit
   stram.

rhythmical, with[8]
rythmiques, avec
rhythmischen, mit
   agar., caust., cham., cimic., lyc.,
   tarent.

music am.[7, 8]
musique am.
Musik am.
   tarent.

noise agg.
bruits agg.
Geräusche agg.
   ign.[8], ziz.[2]

numbness of affected parts, with[15]
engourdissement des parties
   souffrantes, avec
Taubheit leidender Teile, mit
   nux-v.

nymphomania, with[2]
nymphomanie, avec
Nymphomanie, mit
   tarent.

periodic
périodique
periodische
   cupr., cupr-a.[2], nat-s.

every seven days[2, 7]
tous les 7 jours
jeden 7. Tag
   croc.

pollutions, with[2]
pollutions, avec
Pollutionen, mit
   dios.

pregnancy, during
grossesse, pendant la
Schwangerschaft, in der
   bell.[8], **caust., chlol.**[2], **cupr.**

puberty, in[6, 8]
puberté, dans la
Pubertät, in der
   agar.[6], asaf.[8], caul.[1', 2, 8], **cimic.,**
   ign.[8], puls.

punishment, from[2]
châtiments, par
Bestrafung, durch
   ign.

rest, during
repos, pendant le
Ruhe, in der
   zinc.

rheumatic
rhumatismal
rheumatische
   CAUST., cimic., kali-i., **rhus-t.,**
   spig.[8], stict.

run or jump, cannot walk must
courir ou sauter, ne peut marcher
   doit
laufen oder springen, kann nicht
   gehen, muß
   bufo, kali-br., nat-m., **stram.**[2]

sight of bright colors am.[8]
vue de couleurs vives am., par la
Anblick heller, leuchtender Farben
   am.
   tarent.

sleep, during
dormant, en
Schlaf, im
   cupr.[6], tarent.[8], **ziz.**[2, 6, 8, 12]

   am.
      AGAR., cupr.[8], hell., ziz.

spinal
spinale
   asaf., cic., cocc., **cupr.,** mygal.,
   nux-v.

strabism, with[2]
strabisme, avec
Strabismus, mit
   stram.

suppressed eruptions, from
supprimées, par éruptions
unterdrückte Hautausschläge, durch
   caust., cupr.[6, 8], **SULPH.,** zinc.

thinking of it, when
pensant, en y
Darandenken, beim
   caust.

thunderstorm, before
orage, avant un
Gewitter, vor
   agar., rhod., sep.

   during
   pendant un
   beim
      phos.

touch agg.[2]
touche, agg. quand on le
Berührung agg.
   ziz.

uterine[2]
utérine
Uterus-Erkrankungen, bei
   caul., **CIMIC.,** croc., **ign., lil-t.,**
   nat-m., puls., sec., **sep.**

waking, on[2]
s'éveillant, en
Erwachen, beim
   chlol.

wet, after getting
humidité, après exposition à l'
Naßwerden, nach
   rhus-t.

wine agg.
vin agg., le
Wein agg.
   zinc.

worms, from
vermineuses, au cours d'affections
Würmer, durch
   asaf.[8], **calc., cina,** santin.[8], **spig.**[8]

clear weather see weather–clear

CHRONIC DISEASES,
   to begin treatment[8]
MALADIES CHRONIQUES,
   pour commencer le traitement des
CHRONISCHER KRANKHEITEN,
   zum Behandlungsbeginn
   calc., calc-p., **nux-v.,** puls., **sulph.**

CHRONICITY[3]
CHRONICITÉ
CHRONISCHER Krankheitsverlauf
   alum., **arg-n., ars., calc., caust., con.,**
   kali-bi., kali-i., **lyc.,** mang., phos.,
   plb., psor., **sep., sulph.,** syph., tub.

CLOTHING, intolerance of
VÊTEMENTS, intolérance à la pression des
KLEIDUNG wird **nicht ertragen**
agar.[3], **am-c.**, aml-ns.[3], **apis,
ARG-N.**, arn., asaf., asar., **bov.,
bry., CALC., caps., carb-v.,
carbn-s., caust.**, cench.[1, 7], chel.[3],
chin., clem.[3], coc-c.[1, 3], coff., con.,
CROT-C., crot-h., dios.[6], euph.[11],
glon.[3], **graph., hep.**, ign., kali-bi.,
kali-c., kali-i.[3], kali-m.[2], kali-n.,
kreos., **lac-c.[7], LACH.**, lil-t.[3, 6],
LYC., merc.[3, 4, 6, 11], merc-c.[3],
nat-m.[3], nat-s., nit-ac.[3], nux-m.[3],
NUX-V., olnd., **ONOS.**, op., phos.[3],
polyg-h.[2, 7], psor.[3], **puls., ran-b.,
sanic., sars.**, sec.[3], **sep., spig.,
SPONG., stann.**, sulph., **tarent.**,
tub.[3], verat-v.[3], vip.[3]

*covers–agg./couvertures–agg./
Hüllen–agg.
warm–desire/chaleur–désir/
Wärme–Verlangen*

woolen
de laine
wollene
phos., psor., puls., **sulph.**

loosing, am.
dégrafant, am. en se
Lösen der K. am.
am-c., arn., asar., ars.[2], **bry., CALC.,
cann-i., caps., carb-v., caust.**, chel.,
chin., coff., **hep., LACH., LYC.**,
mag-m.[16], **NIT-AC., NUX-V.**, olnd.,
op., **puls.**, ran-b., **sanic., sars., sep.,
spig.**, spong., stann., sulph.

pressure of, am.[3]
pression par les, am.
Kleiderdruck am.
fl-ac., nat-m.

cloudy weather see weather–cloudy

COAL GAS, from
GAZ d'éclairage, intoxication par le
GASVERGIFTUNG
acet-ac.[7, 8], am-c.[8], arn., bell.[2, 8],
bor.[7, 8], bov., **carbn-s.**, carb-v., coff.[8],
ip.[2], lach.[7], **op.[2, 7, 8, 12]**, phos.[12], sec.[3]

*death–carbon/mort–carbone/
Scheintod–Kohlenmonoxyd
sewer–gas poisoning/gaz
méphitiques/Faulschlammgas-
vergiftung*

COAT of skin drawn over inner parts,
sensation of
PEAU tirée sur les parties internes,
sensation de la
HAUTÜBERZUGS über die inneren
Organe, Gefühl eines
ant-t.[3], ars.[3], bar-c.[3], brom.[3], bry.[3],
calc.[3], caust., cina[3], cocc., dig.[3], dros.,
hep.[3], merc., nat-m.[3], nux-m., ph-ac.[3],
phos., pip-n.[3], **puls.**, sulph.[3]

COBWEB, sensation of a[2, 3]
TOILE D'ARAIGNÉE, sensation d'une
SPINNGEWEBES, Gefühl eines
alum.[3], alumn.[2], **bar-c., bor.**, brom.[3],
calc., chin.[3], **graph.**, mag-c., ph-ac.,
phos.[3], plb., **ran-s.**, sul-ac., sumb.[3, 11]

COITION, during*
COÏT, troubles **pendant le**
KOITUS, Beschwerden **beim**
alum.[3, 4], anac., asaf., bar-c.,
berb.[4], bor.[4], **bufo**[3], calad., calc.[4],
canth., carb-v.[4], caust.[4], clem.[4],
ferr., **graph., kali-c.**, kreos., lyc.,
nit-ac.[4], **nux-v.**[4], petr.[4], plat.,
plb.[4], **sel.**, sep., tax.[4], thuj.

after
après le
nach dem
AGAR., agn., alum.[4], am-c.,
ambr.[6], anac., anan., **apis**, arg-n.,
asaf., bar-c., berb.[4], bor., **bov.**,

bufo³, **calad., CALC.,** calc-i.¹′,
calc-s.⁸, calc-sil.¹′, canth.,
carb-an.⁴, carb-v.³, **cedr., chin.,**
con., daph.⁴, dig.⁴, eug.⁴, **graph.,**
kali-bi.³, **KALI-C., KALI-P.,**
kreos.³, ⁴, led.⁴, lyc., mag-m.,
merc.³, ⁴, mez.⁴, mosch., **nat-c.,**
nat-m., **nat-p.,** nat-sil.,¹′, **nit-ac.,**
nux-v., petr., ph-ac., phos., plb.,
puls.³, rhod., **sel., SEP., SIL.,**
staph., sul-ac.⁴, tab.⁴, tarent.,
ther.

am.³, ⁶
    CON., merc.³, **staph.**

interrputed agg.³
réservé agg.
interruptus agg.
    bell.

COLD in general **agg.**
FROID agg. en général, le
KÄLTE im allgemeinen **agg.**
    abrot.¹⁵, acet-ac.¹′, achy.¹⁴, **acon.,**
act-sp.³, adon.⁶, aesc., **agar., agn.**⁷,
alum., alum-p.¹, **alum-sil.**⁷, alumn.,
am-c., am-m.¹′, anac.², ³, ¹⁶, **ant-c.,**
ant-t.³, **apoc., aran.,** aran-ix.¹⁰, ¹⁴,
arg-m., arg-n., arist-cl.⁹, ¹⁰, arn.,
ARS., ars-i.¹′, ³, asar., **aur.,** aur-ar.¹⁵,
aur-s.¹′, **bad., BAR-C., bar-m.**¹, ⁷,
bar-s.¹′, **bell.,** bell-p.⁹, ¹⁰, ¹⁴,
benz-ac.¹⁵, **bor., bov., brom.**³, ⁷, ¹¹,
bry., cadm-s., **CALC., CALC-AR.,**
CALC-F., CALC-P., calc-s.,
CALC-SIL., CAMPH.¹′⁻⁴, ⁵, ⁸, ¹¹,
canth.¹, ⁷, **CAPS., carb-an., carb-v.,**
carbn-s., **card-m.**¹′, **carl.**¹¹, cast.³,
caul.¹′, ⁷, **CAUST., cham.,** chel.,
CHIN., chin-ar., chin-s.³, **cic.,**
cimic., cinnb., cist., clem.,
coc-c.¹′, **cocc.,** coch.¹², **coff.**¹, ⁷,
colch., coll.⁸, **coloc., con.,** cop.¹¹,
crot-c.⁸, **cycl.,** cyt-l.⁹, ¹⁰, ¹⁴,
dig., DULC., elaps, **eup-per.**³, ⁷,
euphr.⁷, **FERR.**¹, ⁷, **ferr-ar.,** ferr-p.¹¹,
flav.¹⁴, **form.**⁷, ⁸, ¹¹, franz.¹¹, gins.¹¹,
GRAPH., guaj., gymno., ham.¹′,
hed.¹⁰, **hell., helon., HEP.,** hydr.,

hyos., **HYPER.,** hypoth.¹⁴, **ign.,**
iod.¹¹, **ip., KALI-AR., kali-bi.,**
KALI-C., kali-i.⁶, ¹¹, kali-m.¹′,
KALI-P., kali-sil.⁷, **kalm., kreos.,**
lac-ac.¹¹, **lac-d.,** lach., laur., **led.,**
lob.⁸, **LYC.,** lycps., **MAG-C.**¹, ⁷,
mag-m.¹, ⁷, **MAG-P.,** mand.¹⁴,
mang., med.¹′, meny., **merc., mez.,**
mit.¹¹, moly-met.¹⁴, **MOSCH.,**
mur-ac.¹, **NAT-AR., nat-c.**¹, ⁷,
nat-m., nat-p., nat-s.¹′, nat-sil.¹′,
NIT-AC., nux-m., NUX-V.,
oci-s.⁹, ¹⁴, **onop.**¹⁴, **ox-ac., petr.,**
ph-ac., PHOS., phys.¹¹, **phyt.,**
pimp.¹¹, **plb.**¹, ⁷, **podo.**⁷, polyg-h.¹¹,
polyg-pe.¹², psil.¹⁴, **PSOR.,** ptel.¹¹,
puls., pyre-p.¹¹, **PYROG.,** raja-s.¹⁴,
RAN-B., rheum, **rhod., RHUS-T.,**
rib-ac.¹⁴, **RUMX., ruta, SABAD.,**
samb., saroth.¹⁰, **sars.**¹, ⁷, sec.¹¹, sel.⁸,
senec., seneg., **SEP.,** sieg.¹⁰, **SIL.,**
sol-n.¹¹, sol-t-ae.³, **SPIG.,** spong.,
squil., **stann.,** staph., stram.,
STRONT-C., stry.¹¹, **sul-ac., sulph.,**
sumb., tab.⁸, **tarent.,** teucr., thala.¹¹,
ther., thuj., tub., valer.¹⁵, verat.², ³, ⁸,
verb., vichy¹¹, **viol-t.**¹, ⁷, x-ray¹⁴,
xero.⁸, **zinc.**

am.²
    acon.², ³, aesc.¹′, ⁶, all-c.⁸, aloe¹′, ³, ⁶,
alumn., am-m.⁶, **ambr., anac., ant-c.,**
ant-t.², ³, **apis**¹′, ³, ⁶, **arg-n.**³, ⁶, arn.,
asar., aur.², aur-i.¹′, bar-c., bell.,
bell-p.⁸, beryl.¹⁴, bor.², ⁸, **bry.**¹′, ², ³, ⁶, ⁸,
calad., calc., **cann-i.,** carb-v., caust.,
cham., chin., **cina,** coc-c.¹′, cocc.,
colch., coloc., **croc.,** cycl.³, **dros.,**
dulc., **euph.,** fago.⁸, ferr.,
FL-AC.², ³, ⁷, **glon.**³, graph.,
guaj.³, ⁷, hell., hep., hist.⁹, **HYOS.,**
iber.¹⁴, ign., **IOD.**², ³, ⁶⁻⁸, **ip.**², kali-c.,
kali-i.³, kali-m.³, **lac-c.**¹′, lach.,
laur., **led.**², ³, ⁶⁻⁸, ¹², lil-t.³, ⁶,
lyc.², ³, ⁶⁻⁸, mag-m.⁶, mag-s.⁹,
med.³, ⁷, merc., mez., moly-met.¹⁴,
mur-ac., nat-c., **nat-m.**², ³, ⁶, **nat-s.**³,
nit-ac.², ⁴, nux-m., nux-v., onos.⁸,
op.², ³, ⁸, ph-ac., **phos.**², ⁸, **plat.,**
PULS.¹′⁻³, ⁶, ⁷, rhus-t., sabad., **sabin.,**
sang.³, sec.¹′⁻³, ⁸, **sel., seneg.,** sep.,
sil., spig., spong., staph., **sulph.**², ³, ⁶,
teucr.², ⁸, **thuj.**², ⁴, trios.¹⁴, verat.

air agg.
air, agg.
Luft agg., kalte
   abrot., acon., aesc., AGAR.,
   ALL-C., alum., alum-p.[1'],
   alum-sil.[1'], **alumn.,** am-br.[2],
   am-c., ammc., anac.[2, 3], ant-c.,
   apis[3], apoc.[1'], **aran.,** arn., **ARS.,**
   ars-s-f.[1'], asar., astac.[2], **AUR.,**
   aur-ar.[1'], aur-s.[1'], bac.[8], **BAD.,**
   bapt.[2], **BAR-C., bar-m.,** bar-s.[1'],
   bell., bor., bov., brom.[11], **bry.,**
   bufo[2, 3], cadm-s., **CALC.,**
   CALC-P., calc-sil.[1'], calen.[2],
   CAMPH., canth., caps., **carb-ac.,**
   carb-an., carb-v., carbn-s., carl.[11],
   CAUST., cham., chin., chin-ar.,
   cic., **CIMIC.,** cina, **CIST.,** clem.[6],
   coc-c.[2], **coca, cocc.,** coff., **colch.,**
   coloc., con., cupr.[7, 8], cur.[8],
   cycl.[2, 3], **dig., DULC., elaps,**
   euph.[8], **ferr.,** ferr-ar., ferr-p., fl-ac.,
   graph., guaj.[3], ham.[1'], **HELL.,**
   HEP., hyos., HYPER., ign., ind.[2],
   ip., KALI-AR., kali-bi., **KALI-C.,**
   kali-m.[1'], kali-p., **kreos.,** lac-c.[11],
   lac-d., lach., lappa[3], laur., **LYC.,**
   lycps., lyss.[2], **mag-c.,** mag-m.,
   MAG-P., mang., med.[2], meny.,
   merc., merc-i-r.[2], mez., **MOSCH.,**
   mur-ac., **nat-ar.,** nat-c., nat-m.,
   nat-p., nat-s.[3, 7], nat-sil.[1'], nit-ac.,
   nit-s-d.[2], **NUX-M., NUX-V.,**
   osm., ox-ac.[1'], par., **petr., ph-ac.,**
   phos., phys.[3], physal.[3], **plan.,**
   plat.[3], plb.[3, 8], psil.[14], **PSOR.,**
   ptel.[11], **puls., RAN-B., RHOD.,**
   RHUS-T., RUMX., ruta, **SABAD.,**
   samb., sars., sel.[6, 8], senec.[11],
   seneg., **SEP., SIL.,** sol-n., spig.,
   spong., squil., staph., stram.,
   STRONT-C., sul-ac., sulph.,
   sumb., tarent., thuj., tub.[8],
   urt-u.[3, 8], **verat., verat-v.**[2], verb.,
   viol-o.[3, 8], viol-t., visc.[8], **zinc.,**
   zinc-p.[1'], **zing.**[2]

am.[8]
   acon.[7, 8], aesc.[6, 8], aeth.,
   all-c.[1', 8], aloe[6, 8], **alum.**[6, 8],
   am-m.[6, 8], ambr.[2, 6, 8], **aml-ns.,**
   anac.[2], anan.[2], ang.[6], **ant-c.**[2, 6, 8],

ant-t.[2, 8], **apis**[6, 8], aran.[6],
aran-ix.[14], **arg-n.**[6-8], arist-cl.[14],
asaf.[6, 8], **asar.**[2], aur-i.[1'], bapt.[1', 3],
bar-c., bar-i.[1'], bell-p.[14],
beryl.[14,] **bry.**[1', 2, 6, 8], **bufo**[1', 8],
cact., calad.[1', 2], calc.[2, 8],
calc-f.[14], cann-i.[2, 8], **carb-v.**[2],
cham.[2], **chin.,** cina[2], cit-v.[2],
clem., **coc-c.**[2, 6], coca,
colch.[2], com., conv., crat.,
croc.[2, 8], dig., dios., **dros.**[2, 8],
dulc.[8], euon-a., euph.[2],
euphr., foll.[14], gels., **glon.**[1', 6, 8],
graph., hed.[14], iber.[14], ign.[2],
IOD.[2, 6, 8], ip.[2], kali-bi.[6],
kali-i.[1', 2, 6, 8], **kali-s.**[1', 6, 8],
lach.[2, 6, 8], **led.**[2, 3], **lil-t.**[6, 8],
luf-op.[14], **LYC.**[2, 6, 8], **mag-c.,**
mag-m.[1', 6, 8], med.[1'], meph.[14],
merc.[2], merc-i-r., mez.,
mosch.[6, 8], naja, **nat-m.**[2, 6, 8],
nat-s., nep.[13, 14], **nit-ac.**[2, 3],
nux-v.[2], ol-an., **op.**[2, 6], phos.[2, 8],
pic-ac.[1', 8], pitu[14], plat.[2, 3, 8],
psil.[14], **PULS.**[2, 6, 8], rad-br.[3, 8],
rauw.[14], rhus-t.[2, 8], **sabad.,**
sabin.[2, 8], **sec.**[1', 2, 6, 8], **sel.**[2],
seneg.[2], **sep.**[2, 6, 8], stel.,
stront-c.[6], stry-p., **sulph.**[2, 6, 8],
syph.[1'], **tab.**[6, 8], **tarent.,**
tere-ch.[14], teucr.[2], thala.[14],
thuj.[2], tub.[7], tub-r.[14], vib.,
visc.[14]

windows open, must have[1']
fenêtres ouvertes, exige les
Fenster offen haben, muß
   aml-ns.[8], apis[6], **arg-n.**[6-8],
   bapt.[6, 8], **bry.**[1'], calc.[8], camph.,
   carb-v.[7], **carbn-s.,** glon., graph.,
   iod.[6], **ip.**[6], **lach.**[1', 8], lyc.[6], med.[8],
   puls.[1', 8], sabin., sec.,
   sulph.[1', 6, 8], tub.

aversion to[6]
aversion pour
Abneigung gegen
   am-c., **aran., ars.,** bart.[11], bell.,
   bry., **calc.,** caps.[6, 11], caust.,
   cham., chin., graph., grat., **hep.,**
   kali-c., nat-c., nat-m., nux-m.,
   nux-v., petr., sel., **sil.,** sulph.,
   tub.

desire for
désir d'
Verlangen nach
achy.[14], aloe, **apis**, arg-n.[1', 6],
asaf., asar., **aur.**, camph.[1'],
carb-v., cic.[11], **croc.**, gran.[11],
iod., kali-s.[1'], lil-t., **puls.**[1', 6], **sec.**,
sul-i.[1'], sulph.

open air see air–open–desire

inspiring of, agg.[3]
inspirer de l', agg.
Einatmen kalter Luft agg.
aesc., alum., **am-c.**, ant-c., **ars.**,
aur., bell., bry., calc., camph.,
CAUST., cham., **cimic.**, cina, cist.,
dulc., hep., hydr., **HYOS., ign.**,
kali-bi., **kali-c., MERC.**, mosch.,
nat-m., **nux-m., NUX-V.**, par.,
petr., phos., psor., puls., **rhod.**,
rhus-t., RUMX., SABAD., sars.,
sel.[14], seneg., **sep.**, sil., spig.,
staph., **stront-c.**, sulph., syph.,
thuj., verat.

becoming cold
refroidir, se
Abkühlung, bei
acon., aesc., **agar., alumn., am-c.**,
ant-c., arg.-n., **arn., ARS.**, ars-i.,
asar., **AUR.**, aur-s.[1'], **bad.**,
BAR-C., bar-m., bar-s.[1'], **bell.**,
bor., bov., **bry., calc., calc-p.**,
calc-sil.[1'], **camph.**, canth., **caps.**,
carb-an., carb-v., carbn-s., caust.,
cham., chin., chin-ar., cic., **cimic.**,
clem., cocc., con., dig., dulc.,
elaps, **ferr.**, ferr-ar., ferr-p.,
graph., hell., **HEP., hyos., hyper.**,
ign., ip.[3], **KALI-AR., KALI-BI.**,
KALI-C., kali-p., kali-s., **kreos.**,
lach., **LYC., mag-c.**, mag-m.,
mag-p., mang., **med.**, meny.,
merc., merc-i-r., mez., **MOSCH.**,
mur-ac., **nat-ar.**, nat-c., nat-m.,
nat-p., nicc., nit-ac., nux-m.,
NUX-V., petr., PH-AC., phos.,
psor., puls.[3], **PYROG., RAN-B.**,
rhod., **RHUS-T., rumx.**, ruta,
SABAD., samb., sars., **SEP.**,
SIL., spig., spong., squil., staph.,

stram., **stront-c., SUL-AC.**,
sulph., sumb., tarent., thuj.,
verat.[2, 3], verb., viol-t., **zinc.**

ailments from[12]
troubles à la suite d'
Beschwerden infolge von
kalm., phyt.

when heated[12]
en ayant chaud
wenn erhitzt
kali-s.

am.
acon., aesc.[3], agn., all-c.[3], aloe[3],
alum., alumn.[2], am-c.[3], am-m.[3],
ambr., anac.[2, 3], ang.[3], ant-c.,
ant-t., **apis**[3], **arg-n.**, arn., asaf.[3],
asar.[2, 3], aur., bapt.[3], bar-c., bell.,
bov., brom.[3], **bry.**, calad.,
calc.[2, 3], calc-i[1'], cann-i.[2], cann-s.,
carb-v., caust.[2, 3], **cham.**, chin.[2, 3],
cina[2, 3], clem., coc-c.[3], cocc.,
coff., colch., coloc., croc., **dros.**,
dulc., euph., **fl-ac.**[3], **glon.**,
graph.[2, 3], guaj.[3], hell., ign.[2, 3],
IOD., ip., kali-bi.[2], kali-c.[3], kali-i.[3],
kali-s.[3], kalm.[3], **lac-c., lach.**,
led., lil-t.[3], **LYC.**, mang., **merc.**,
mez., mur-ac., nat-c., **nat-m.**,
nit-ac., **nux-m.**[2, 3], nux-v.[2, 3], olnd.,
op., **petr.**, ph-ac., phos., plat.,
PULS., rhus-t.[2, 3], sabad., **sabin.**,
sars., **sec.**, sel., seneg., sep.[2, 3],
sil.[2, 3], spig., spong., staph.,
sulph., teucr., thuj., verat.

after, agg.
après s'être refroidi, agg.
nach, agg.
acon., agar., **alum.**, alum-p.[1'],
alum-sil[1'], **alumn., am-c.**,
anac.[2, 3], **ant-c.**[2, 3], ant-t., **arg-n.**,
arn., **ARS.**, ars-s-f.[1'], aur.
aur-s.[1'], **BAR-C.**, bar-s.[1', 3], **BELL.**,
bor., **BRY., CALC., CALC-P.**,
calc-s., calc-sil.[1'], camph.,
carb-v., carbn-s., caust.[2, 3],
CHAM., CHIN., cimic.[3], **coc-c.**[2],
cocc., **coff.**, colch.[1', 3], **coloc., con.**,
croc., cupr., cupr-s.[2], **cycl.**, dig.,

dros., **DULC.**, ferr., ferr-ar[1]',
FL-AC.[3], **GRAPH.**, guaj.[3], **HEP.**,
hydr.[3], **HYOS.**, hyper., ign., **ip.**,
kali-ar.[1]', **kali-bi., kali-c.**,
kali-m[1]', kali-p., **kali-sil.**[1]', kalm.,
led., **lyc.**, mag-c., **mang., med.**,
MERC., nat-c., **nat-m.**, nat-p.,
nat-sil.[1]', **nit-ac., nux-m.**,
NUX-V., op., **petr., ph-ac.**,
PHOS., phyt.[1]', plat., polyg-h.[3],
psor., PULS., PYROG., RAN-B.,
RHUS-T., ruta, sabin., **samb.**,
sang.[1]', sars., sel., **SEP., SIL.**,
SPIG., stann., staph., stront-c.,
SUL-AC., sul-i.[1]', **sulph., tarent.**,
thuj., tub.[1]', valer., **verat., xan.**[2],
zinc-p.[1]'

uncovering/découvrir/entblößen

a part of body agg.
une partie du corps agg.
eines Körperteils agg.
 agar.[3], am-c.[3], **bar-c., bell.**,
 calc.[3], cham., **hell., HEP.**, ip.[2],
 led.[1], **nux-v.**[3], ph-ac., **phos.**[3],
 psor.[3], puls., **RHUS-T., sep.**,
 SIL., tarent.[3], thuj.[3], zinc.[3]

uncovering-single part/
* decouvrir-seule partie/*
* entblößen - einzelner Teile*

back[7]
dos, le
Rücken
 pilo.

extremities
membres, ses
Extremitäten
 aur., bry., con., **HEP., nat-m.**,
 RHUS-T., SIL., squil., stront-c.,
 THUJ.

feet
pieds, ses
Füße
 alum[3], am-c.[3], ars.[3], **bar-c.**,
 bufo[3], cham., clem.[3], **con.**,
 cupr.[1], kali-ar.[3], kali-c.[3],
 lach.[3], lyc.[3], mag-p.[3], nit-ac.[3],

nux-m.[3], **NUX-V.**[3], phos.[3],
phys.[3], **puls.**[1], sep.[3], **SIL.**,
stann.[16], zinc.[3]

hand out of bed
mains du lit, en sortant ses
Hand aus dem Bett
 acon.[3], **BAR-C.**, canth., **con.**,
 HEP., merc.[3], phos., **RHUS-T.**,
 sil.

head
tête, la
Kopf
 am-c.[16], arg-n.[3], **BELL., hep.**[3],
 hyos.[3], led., nux-v.[3], puls.,
 rhus-t.[3], **SEP., SIL.**

heated, when[1]'
chaud, en ayant
erhitzt, wenn
 acon.[3], **bell-p.**[7], bry.[3], kali-ar.,
 ran-b.

perspiration, during[3, 7]
transpiration, pendant la
Schwitzen, beim
 ACON., ars-s-f.[1]', calc-sil.[1]',
 dulc.[7], sul-i.[1]'

sitting on cold steps[3, 8]
s'asseoir sur des escaliers froids
Sitzen auf kalten Stufen
 chim., **nux-v.**, rhod.[3]

dry weather see weather–cold dry

feeling in blood vessels
impression de f. dans les vaisseaux
sanguins
Kältegefühl in den Blutgefäßen
 abies-c.[3], **ACON.**, ant-c., ant-t.,
 ARS., bell.[6], lyc., op.[3], plb.[3],
 RHUS-T., sulph.[6], **verat.**

bones
os, dans les
Knochen, in den
 aran., ars., berb.[1], **calc.**, elaps,
 eup-per.[3], kali-i.[3], lyc., merc.,
 pyrog.[3], sep., sulph., **verat.**, zinc.

inner parts
organes internes, dans les
inneren Organen, in
    anh.[10], ars., **calc., hura**[7]**, laur.,**
    lyc., meny., nux-v., par., sep.,
    sulph.

single parts[10]
certaines parties, dans les
einzelnen Teilen, in
    agar., aran., aran-ix., buth-a.,
    elaps, helo.

heat and cold
chaud et par le froid, par le
Wärme und Kälte
    alum., alum-p.[1]', ang.[3], **ant-c.,**
    ant-t.[7], arn.[7, 8], **ars-i.,** asar.[3],
    aur-s.[1]', bar-s.[1]', calc.[3], calc-s.[1]',
    caps.[3], **carbn-s., caust.,** cina[3],
    cinnb., **cocc.,** cor-r.[3], ferr.[3, 6],
    flav.[14], **FL-AC.,** glon.[3], **graph.,**
    ip., kali-c., **lach.,** lyc., mag-c.[3],
    mag-m., **merc.,** nat-c., **nat-m.,**
    nux-v.[7, 16], **ph-ac.,** phys.[3], **psor.,**
    puls., ran-b., rob.[7], sanic.[3], **sep.,**
    sil., sul-ac.[3], **sulph., syph.**[1'-3, 7],
    tab.[3], thala.[14], **tub.**[7, 15]

hot days with cold nights[3]
jours chauds et nuits fraîches
heiße Tage mit kalten Nächten
    acon., dulc., merc-c., rumx.

one part cold, with heat of another[3]
une partie est froide, une autre est
    chaude
ein Körperteil kalt, ein anderer heiß
    apis, bry., cham.

place agg., entering a
local f., agg. en entrant dans un
Raumes agg., Betreten eines kalten
    ARS., bell.[3], calc-p., **camph.**[2, 3],
    carb-v., caust., con., **dulc., ferr.,**
    ferr-ar., graph., hep., ip.[3],
    KALI-AR., kali-c., kali-p.,
    kali-sil.[1]', mosch., nux-m., **nux-v.,**
    petr., phos., psor., puls., **RAN-B.,**
    rhus-t., sabad., **SEP.,** sil., spong.,
    stront-c., **tub., verb.**

take c., tendency to ✱
refroidissements, tendance aux
Erkältungen, Neigung zu
    ACON., aesc.[6], agar.[6], all-c.[6],
    ALUM., alum-p.[1]', alum-sil.[1]',
    alumn.[1]', am-c., am-m., anac.,
    ant-c., ant-t., aral.[6], aran.[6], **arg-n.,**
    arn., ars., ars-i., ars-s-f.[1]', **bac.**[7],
    BAR-C., bar-i.[1]', bar-m.[6], bar-s.[1]',
    bell., benz-ac.[3], bor., **BRY.,**
    calad.[6], **calc.,** calc-i.[1]', **CALC-P.,**
    calc-s., calc-sil.[1]', **calen.**[7], camph.,
    caps.[10], carb-an.[6], **carb-v.,**
    carbn-s., caust., **CHAM.,** chin.,
    chin-ar., cimic.[1', 6], cinnb.[6], cist.[6],
    clem.[6], coc-c., cocc., coff.,
    colch.[1]', coloc., **con.,** croc.,
    crot-h.[4], cupr., cycl.[6], dig., dros.,
    DULC., elaps[6], eup-per.[1]',
    euphr.[6], **ferr.,** ferr-ar., ferr-i.,
    ferr-p., **form.,** gast.[11, 12], **gels.,**
    goss., **graph.,** ham., hed.[10, 14],
    HEP., hyos., hyper.[6], ign., iod.,
    ip., kali-ar., **kali-bi., KALI-C.,**
    KALI-I.[1], kali-p.[1], kali-s.,
    kali-sil.[1]', **lac-d.,** lach.[4, 6], led.,
    LYC., m-arct.[3], m-aust.[3], mag-c.[10],
    mag-m., **MED.**[7]**, MERC.,** mez.,
    naja[3], **NAT-AR., nat-c., NAT-M.,**
    nat-p., nat-sil.[1]', **NIT-AC.,**
    nux-m., NUX-V., ol-j.[3, 6], op.,
    osm.[12], **petr., ph-ac., phos.,** plat.,
    PSOR., puls., rhod.[6, 12], **rhus-t.,**
    RUMX., ruta, sabad., sabin.,
    samb., sang., sars., sel.,
    senec.[1', 6], **SEP., SIL.,** solid.[3],
    spig., stach.[11], stann., staph.,
    sul-ac., sul-i.[1]', **sulph., thuj.**[2, 6],
    TUB., valer., verat., verb.[6],
    zinc.[6]

faintness–cold/évanouisse-
    ment–r./Ohnmacht–E.
paralysis–cold/paralysie–r./
    Lähmung–E.

ailments from[12]
troubles à la suite des
Beschwerden infolge von
    coloc., kali-c., rhod.

spring, in[12]
printemps, au
Frühling, im
   all-c.

feet, from c.[7]
pieds froids, par
Füße, durch kalte
   con., **sil.**

becoming cold–a part–feet/
se refroidir–partie–pieds/
Abkühlung–Körperteils–Füße

menses, during[3]
menstruation, pendant la
Menses, während der
   bar-c., graph., mag-c., senec.

wet weather see weather–cold wet

COLDNESS of affected parts[3]
REFROIDISSEMENT des parties
   atteintes
KÄLTE erkrankter Teile
   alum-sil.[1]', **ang.,** ars., bry., calc.,
   caust., cocc., colch., crot-h., dulc.,
   graph., lach., **led.,** meny., merc.,
   mez., petr., plat., plb., rhod., **rhus-t.,**
   sec., sil., thuj.

lain side morning in bed, on[16]
couché, le matin au lit r. du côté
   sur lequel on est
unten liegenden Seite morgens
   im Bett, der
   arn.

one side of body in septic fever[16]
seul côté du corps dans les fièvres
   septiques, d'un
einer Körperseite bei septischem
   Fieber
   meny., **puls.,** rhus-t.

COLLAPSE
COLLAPSUS
KOLLAPS
   acet-ac., acetan.[8], acon.[3, 8, 10, 11],
   aconin.[11], adren.[7], aeth.[3], **AM-C.,**

ampe-qu.[11], amyg., **ant-t.**[3, 8], apis,
aran-ix.[10], arn.[3, 8], **ARS., ars-h.,**
bar-c., **CAMPH.,** cann-i., canth.,
carb-ac., carb-an.[2, 10], **CARB-V.,**
CARBN-S., cench.[11], **CHIN.**[2], cina,
cit-l.[2, 11], colch.[3, 8], colchin.[11], con.[3],
crat.[8], **crot-h.,** crot-t., **cupr.,**
cupr-a.[8, 11], **cupr-ar.,** cupr-s.,
cyt-l.[2, 9-11], **dig.**[8], diph.[8], dor., euon.,
hell., home.[11, 12], **hydr-ac.**[3, 6-8],
hyos.[2], iod., ip.[3], jab., kali-br.[6],
kali-chl.[11], kali-chr.[11], kali-cy.[11],
kali-n., **lach.**[6, 11], lat-m.[9], **laur.,**
lob.[8], lob-p.[8], lol.[11], lyc.[6], **med.,**
merc., merc-c., merc-cy.[3, 8],
merc-ns.[11], merc-pr-a.[11], morph.,
mosch.[2], mur-ac.[8], naja, nicot.[8, 12],
nit-s-d.[11], olnd., op., ox-ac., **phos.,**
phys., pitu.[9], plb., sabad.[10], santin.[11],
scam.[11], **sec., seneg.**[2], sep.[3], stram.,
sul-ac., **sulph.**[3], tab.[3], tarent.[10],
tarent-c.[6], tax., **verat.,** verat-v.[3],
vip., **zinc.**[6, 8]

faintess/évanouissement/
   Ohnmacht
weakness–sudden/faiblesse–
   subite/Schwäche–plötzliche

diarrhoea, after
diarrhée, après
Diarrhoe, nach
   ant-c.[2], **ARS., CAMPH., CARB-V.,**
   ric.[11], **VERAT.**

fainting-diarrhoea/
   évanouissement-diarrhée/
   Ohnmacht-Diarrhoe

needle, prick of a[16]
aiguille, piqûre d'
Nadelstich, durch
   calc.

paralysis, at beginning of general
paralysie générale, au début d'une
Lähmung, am Anfang einer
   con.

sudden
subit
plötzlicher
    ARS., colch.[2], phos.

weakness-rapid, sudden/faiblesse-
rapide, subite/Schwäche – schnell
zunehmende, plötzliche

vomiting, during
vomissement, pendant le
Erbrechen, beim
    ars., ric.[11], **verat.**[2]

after
après le
nach dem
    ARS., lob., phys., ric.[11], **verat.**

COMPLEXION (color of eyes, face,
    hair), **dark,** brunette (Kent 1897)
TEINTE des yeux, du visage et des
    cheveux, **foncée**
AUSSEHEN (Augen-, Gesichts-, Haar-
    farbe) **dunkel,** dunkelbraun
    acon.[1, 7], alum., anac., arn., ars.,
    aur.[2, 6, 12], brom.[12], **bry., calc.,**
    calc-i.[6], caps.[6], **CAUST.,** cham.[12],
    chin.[2, 12], cina[3, 6, 7, 15], coff.[2, 12],
    con.[12], graph.[12], **IGN.,** iod.[6, 12],
    KALI-C., kreos., lac-c.[2], lach.[3],
    lyc.[12], lycpr.[12], mag-p.[6], mur-ac.[12],
    nat-m., **NIT-AC., nux-v.,**
    PHOS.[1, 7], pic-ac.[12], **PLAT.,**
    PULS.[1, 7], **RHUS-T.**[7], sang.[12],
    sec.[6], sep., staph.[7], sulph.,
    thuj.[12], viol-o.[12]

eyes[12]
yeux
Augen
    aur., graph., iod., lach., lycpr.,
    mur-ac., nit-ac.

rigid fibre, with[2]
rigide, avec tissu conjonctif
straffer Faser, mit
    acon., anac., arn., **ars., bry.,**
    caust., kalm., nat-m., **nit-ac.,**
    NUX-V., plat., puls., **sep.,** staph.,
    sulph.

blue eyes and **dark** hairs[15]
yeux **bleus,** et cheveux **foncés**
blaue Augen und **dunkle** Haare
    lyc., nat-m., sep.

fair, blonde, light (Kent 1897)
claire, blonde
hell, blond
    agar., **apis,** aur.[12], bell.[4, 6, 12], bor.,
    brom., bry., **CALC., caps.,**
    cham.[12], chel.[12], clem.[12], cocc.[6, 12],
    coloc.[12], con.[12], cupr.[12], cycl.[12],
    dig.[12], **graph., hep.,** hyos., ip.[4, 12],
    kali-bi., kreos.[12], lob., lycps.[12],
    merc., mez.[12], nat-c.[6, 12], op.[12],
    PETR., PHOS., PULS., rhus-t.,
    sabad., sel.[12], sep.[4, 12], **sil.,** spig.[12],
    SPONG., stann-i.[3, 6, 12], sul-ac.[12],
    sulph., thuj.[12], vario.[12], viol-o.[12]

eyes[12]
yeux
Augen
    bell., brom., caps., lob., puls.,
    spong.

lax fibre, with[2]
lâche, avec tissu conjonctif
schlaffer Faser, mit
    agar.[7], **bell., BROM., CALC.,**
    caps., cham., clem., cocc., con.,
    dig., **GRAPH.,** hyos., **kali-bi.,**
    lach., **lyc.,** merc., **rhus-t.,** sil.,
    SULPH.

relaxation/relâchement/
    Erschlaffung

red hair[2, 12]
cheveux roux
rote Haare
    calc-p.[15], lach., phos., sep.,
    sulph.[7, 12]

CONGESTION of blood
CONGESTION du sang
BLUTANDRANG, Kongestion
    ACON., act-sp.[2], **AESC.,** agar.[3],
    agn.[3], **aloe, alum.,** alum-p.[1'],
    alum-sil.[1'], am-c., am-m., ambr.,
    aml-ns.[3], ang.[3], anis.[2], ant-c., ant-t.[3],
    anthraci.[2], **apis,** aq-mar.[14], arist-cl.[9],
    arn., ars.[1', 3], asaf., aster.[14], **aur.,**

aur-ar.[1'], aur-i.[1'], aur-s.[1'], bar-c.,
bar-i.[1'], **BELL., bor.,** bov., brom.[3],
bry., CACT., calad.[3], **calc.,**
calc-hp.[12], calc-sil.[1'], camph.,
cann-s., canth., carb-an., **carb-v.,**
carbn-s., caust., cham., chel.,
CHIN., chin-s.[4], cinnb.[7], clem.,
cocc., **coff.,** colch., coloc., con.,
conv., croc., cupr., cycl., dig., dulc.,
erig.[6], eucal.[6], euphr.[3], **FERR.,**
ferr-i., ferr-p., **ferr-s.**[2, 6], fl-ac.[3, 6],
gels.[1', 3], **GLON., graph.,** guaj., **ham.,**
hell., hep., hir.[14], hydr.[6], hydr-ac.[11],
hyos., hypoth.[14], ign., iod., ip.[3],
jab.[12], kali-c., kali-i.[6], kali-n.,
kreos.[6], **lach.,** laur., led., **lyc.,**
mag-c., mag-m., mand.[10], mang.,
MELI., merc., merc-c.[3], mez., **mill.**[2-4],
mosch., nat-c., **nat-m.,** nat-s.[3],
nit-ac., nux-m., **NUX-V.,** op., petr.,
ph-ac., **PHOS.,** plat., plb., podo.[6],
psor., PULS., raja-s.[14], **ran-b.,** rhod.,
rhus-t., sabin., samb., **sang.**[3, 6],
sars.[3], sec., sel.[3], **seneg., sep., sil.,**
spig., **spong.,** squil., staph.,
stram., stront-c.[6], **stront-i.**[6], sul-ac.,
SULPH., tarax., ter.[3], thuj., valer.,
verat., verat-v., **VIOL-O.,** zinc.[3]

heat, flushes of/bouffées de
  chaleur/Hitzewallungen
orgasm of blood/afflux de sang/
  Blutwallungen
plethora/pléthore/Plethora

coldness of legs, with[15]
refroidissement des jambes, avec
Kälte der Beine, mit
  bell., nat-m., stram.

haemorrhage, after[1']
hémorrhagie, après une
Blutung, nach einer
  mill.

internally
interne
innerlicher
  aloe, apis, ars., aur-i.[1'], bar-i.[1'],
  CACT., camph., canth., **colch.,**
  conv., cupr., **glon., hell., MELI.,**
  phos., sars.[1'], sep., **verat.,** verat-v.

sudden[3]
soudaine
plötzlicher
  acon., bell., glon., verat-v.

CONSTIPATION am.
VERSTOPFUNG am.
  calc., carb-v.[3], merc., **psor.**

CONSTRICTION, sensation of **external**
CONSTRICTION externe, sensation de
ZUSAMMENSCHNÜREN, Gefühl von
  äußerlichem
  abrot., **acon., aesc.,** aeth.,
  aether[11], **agar., all-c.,** all-s.[11],
  alum., alum-sil.[1', 8], **alumn.**[2],
  am-c., am-m., **ammc., aml-ns.,**
  anac., ang.[3], ant-c., **ant-t., apis,**
  aral., arg-m., arg-n., arn., **ars.,**
  ars-i., arum-t., asaf., **asar.,** atro.[11],
  aur., **bar-c.,** bar-s.[1'], bell., berb.,
  bism., bor., bov., brom.[3], **bry.,**
  cact., cadm-s.[3], calc., **calc-p.,**
  cann-i., cann-s., canth., **caps.,**
  carb-ac., carb-an., carb-v.,
  carbn-o.[11], **carbn-s.,** caust., cham.,
  chel., chin., CIMIC., cina, coc-c.[3],
  COCC., coff., colch., **coloc.,** con.,
  croc.[2, 3], crot-h.[3], **cupr.,** dig.,
  dios., **dros.,** dulc., euphr., **ferr.,**
  gels., **glon., GRAPH.,** guaj., **hell.,**
  hep., hist.[9, 10], hydr-ac., **HYOS.,**
  IGN.[2], **iod., ip.,** kali-c., kali-n.,
  kreos., **lach.,** laur., led., lil-t.,
  lob., lyc., mag-c., mag-m., **mag-p.,**
  manc.[3], mang., meny., **MERC.,**
  merc-c., merc-i-r., mez., mosch.,
  mur-ac., naja, nat-c., nat-m.,
  nat-n.[3], **NIT-AC.,** nitro-o.[11],
  nux-m., **NUX-V.,** oena.[3], olnd.,
  op., ox-ac., par., petr., **ph-ac.**[2],
  phos., phys.[3], pic-ac.[1'], **plat.,**
  PLB., puls., ran-b., ran-s., rheum,
  rhod., **RHUS-T.,** ric.[11], russ.[11],
  ruta, sabad., sabin., sars., sec.,
  sel., **sep.,** sil., sin-n.[11], spig.,
  spong., squil., **STANN.,** staph.,
  STRAM., stront-c., sul-ac.,
  sulph., tab., thuj., **verat.,**
  verat-v.[11], verb., viol-o.[3], viol-t.,
  visc.[9], zinc.

as if caged with wires twisted
tighter and tighter
par des fils qui serrent progressive-
ment toujours davantage
wie mit immer fester zusammen-
ziehenden Drähten
CACT.

small areas, of[9]
petits endroits, localisés, de
kleiner Flächen
hist.

internal
interne
innerlichem
acon., aesc., agar., agn., **alum.,**
am-c., ambr., aml-ns., anac., ang.[3],
ant-c., ant-t., arg-m., **arn.,** ars.,
ars-i., asaf., **asar.,** aur., **bapt.,** bar-c.,
BELL., benz-ac., bism., bor., bov.,
brom., bry., bufo[3], **CACT., calad.,**
calc., camph., cann-i., cann-s.,
canth., caps., carb-an., carb-v.,
carbn-s., caust., **cham., chel.,**
CHIN., chlol., cic., cina, **clem.,**
cocc., coff., colch., **COLOC., con.,**
croc., crot-h., crot-t., cub., **cupr.,**
dig., dios., **dros.,** dulc., euph., ferr.,
glon., graph., guaj., hell., hep.,
hyos., **IGN., iod., ip.,** kali-c., kali-n.,
kreos., **lach., laur., led.,** lyc.,
mag-c., mag-m., **MAG-P.,** mang.,
meny., merc., merc-c., mez., **mosch.,**
mur-ac., **naja,** nat-ar., nat-c.,
NAT-M., NIT-AC., nux-m.,
NUX-V., olnd., op., ox-ac., par.,
petr., **ph-ac., phos., PLAT., PLB.,**
PULS., ran-s., rheum, rhod., rhus-t.,
ruta, sabad., **sabin.,** samb., **sars.,**
sec., sel., seneg., **sep.,** sil., **spig.,**
spong., **squil.,** stann., staph., still.,
STRAM., stront-c., **sul-ac., SULPH.,**
sumb., tab.[3], tarax., teucr., **thuj.,**
valer., **verat., verat-v.,** verb.,
viol-t., zinc.

bones, of
os, des
Knochen, der
am-m., anac., aur., chin., cocc.,
coloc., con., graph., kreos., lyc.,

merc., nat-m., **NIT-AC.,** nux-v.,
petr., phos., **PULS.,** rhod., **rhus-t.,**
ruta, sabad., sep., sil., stront-c.,
SULPH., zinc.

glands, in[3]
glandes, ganglions, des
Drüsen, der
ign., iod.

joints, of[3]
articulations, des
Gelenke, der
acon., am-m., **ANAC.,** apis[6], **AUR.,**
calc., carb-an., chin., coloc., ferr.,
GRAPH., kreos., lyc., meny.,
NAT-M., NIT-AC., nux-m., nux-v.,
petr., ruta, sil., spig., squil., stann.,
stront-c., sulph., zinc.

orifices, of; sphincter spasm
orifices, des; spasme des sphincters
Körperöffnungen, der; Sphinkter-
spasmus
acon., alum., alum-sil.[1]', ars., ars-i.,
bar-c., **BELL., brom., CACT.,** calc.,
calc-sil.[1]', carb-v., **chel.,** cic., cocc.,
colch., con., crot-h., dig., dulc., ferr.,
form., graph., hep., **hyos.,** ign., iod.,
ip., **LACH., lyc., MERC., merc-c.,**
mez., **nat-m., NIT-AC.,** nux-v., op.,
phos., plat., **plb.,** rat., rhod.,
RHUS-T., sabad., sars., sep., **SIL.,**
staph., STRAM., sulph., sumb.,
tarax., **thuj., verat., verat-v.**

band, sensation of a
bande, sensation d'une
Bandes, Gefühl eines
acon., **alum.,** alum-p.[1]', alumn.,
am-br., **ambr., ANAC.,** ant-c., ant-t.,
arg-n., arn., ars., ars-i.[1]', ars-s-f.[1]',
asaf., **asar.,** aur., aur-ar.[1]', aur-i.[1]',
aur-s.[1]', **bell.,** benz-ac., brom., bry.,
CACT., calc., cann-i., **CARB-AC.,**
carb-v., **carbn-s.,** caust., **CHEL.,**
chin., coc-c., **cocc.,** colch., coloc.,
CON., croc., dig., dios.[3], gels.,
graph., hell., hyos., iod., kreos.,
lach.[3], laur., lyc., mag-m., **mag-p.,**
manc., mang.[16], **merc., merc-i-r.,**
mosch., **nat-m., nat-n.**[3]**, NIT-AC.,**

nux-m., nux-v., olnd., op., ox-ac.[3], petr., **phos.**, pic-ac.[1'], **PLAT., PULS.,** rhus-t.[3], sabad., sabin., sang., sars., **sec.**[3], sep.[3], **SIL., spig.,** stann., **stram.**[3], sul-ac., sul-i.[1'], **SULPH.,** tarent., til., zinc., zinc-p.[1']

belt, sensation of a[6]
ceinture, sensation d'une
Gürtels, Gefühl eines
  cact., chin., phos., rhus-t., visc.[9]

CONTRACTIONS, strictures, stenoses, after inflammation
CONTRACTIONS, strictures, sténoses après inflammation
ZUSAMMENZIEHUNGEN, Strikturen, Stenosen nach Entzündung
acon.[2, 3], **agar.**, alum., **alumn.**[2], ant-c., arg-m., **arn.**[2, 3], **ars.**[2, 3], asaf., **bell., bry.**, calc., **camph.**, canth., caust., chel., **chin., CIC., clem., cocc.,** con., dig., dros., dulc., euph., guaj.[3], hyos.[2, 3], **ign.**[2, 3], lach., led., meny.[3], **MERC., mez.,** nat-m., nit-ac., **NUX-V.,** op.[2, 3], petr., **phos.,** plb., **psor., puls.,** ran-b., **RHUS-T.,** ruta, sabad., sep., **spong.,** squil., staph., stram., sulph., teucr., thuj., **verat.**[2, 3], zinc.

CONTRADICTORY
and alternating states
CONTRADICTOIRES
et alternants, états
WIDERSPRUCHSVOLLE
und abwechselnde Zustände
abrot.[7], **aloe**[7], ambr.[3], **carc.**[7], cimic.[3, 7], croc., **IGN.,** kali-c.[1'], **nat-m., plat.**[1], plb.[3], **PULS.,** sanic.[7], **sep.**[7], **staph.**[7], **thuj.**[1], **TUB.**[7]

alternating states/alternants/ abwechselnde change-symptoms/changement- symptômes/Wechsel-Symptom- wechsel metastasis/métastases/Metasta- sierung

CONVALESCENCE, ailments during[3, 6]
CONVALESCENCE, troubles pendant la
REKONVALESZENZ, Beschwerden in der
  ail.[7], **alet.**[2, 7], am-c.[1'], apoc.[1'], aur.[7], **aven.,** bac.[7], cadm-met.[14], **CALC.**[2, 7], **calc-p.,** caps.[1'], **cast.**[3, 6, 7, 10], **CHIN.**[3, 6, 7, 10], **chin-ar.**[3, 6, 7], coca[6, 7], cocc.[7], cupr.[7, 11], **cur.**[7], cypr.[7], **ferr.**[3, 6, 10], ferr-a.[6], gels.[3], guar.[7], **kali-c.,** kali-m.[1'], kali-p.[3, 7], laur.[1'], lob.[7], mang.[1'], med.[7], meph., **nat-m.,** nat-p.[7], okou.[14], op., ph-ac., phos.[3], prot.[14], psor.[1', 3, 6, 7], **scut.**[7], **sel.**[1', 3, 6], **sil.**[2, 7], sul-ac., sul-i.[10], **sulph.**[1', 3, 6, 10], syph.[1'], **TUB.**[7], tub-a.[7], zinc.[3, 6, 7]

reaction, lack-convalescence/ réaction, manque-convalescence/ Reaktionsmangel-Rekon- valeszenz weakness–fever/faiblesse–fièvre/ Schwäche–Fieber

fever, ailments from[12]
fièvre, troubles à la suite de
Fieber, Beschwerden infolge von lyc.

infectious diseases, ailments from[6]
infectieuses, troubles à la suite des maladies
Infektionskrankheiten, Beschwerden infolge von
  form-ac., gels.[3], psor., puls., sulph., thuj., tub., vario.

metapneumonic[7]
postpneumonique
Pneumonie, nach
  calc., carb-v., **kali-c.,** lyc., phos., sang., sil., sulph.

never well since pneumonia[7]
jamais bien été depuis une pneumonie
schlechtes Befinden seit einer **kali-c.**

meningitis, after[7]
méningite, après
Meningitis, nach
  calc., sil.

parturition, after[2]
accouchement, après
Entbindung, nach
  graph.

postdiphtheric[7]
postdiphtérique
Diphtherie, nach
  alet., cocain., cocc., fl-ac., helon.[2],
  lac-c.[2]

postinfluenzal[7]
postgrippal
Grippe, nach
  abrot., cadm-met.[14], okou.[14],
  scut.[7, 12], sulfonam.[14], tub.

rheumatism after tonsillitis[3]
rhumatisme après amygdalite
Rheuma nach Tonsillitis
  echi., guaj., lach., phyt.

typhoid, ailments from[1']
typhoïde, troubles à la suite de
Typhoid, nach
  carb-v., pyrog.[12], sulph.

CONVULSIONS
CONVULSIONS
KONVULSIONEN
  absin., acet-ac., **acon.**, aconin.[12],
  aesc., aesc-g.[11], aeth., aether[11, 12],
  agar., agar-pa.[11], agar-se.[11], agre.[14],
  alco.[11], **alet.**[2, 12], alum., alum-p.[1'],
  alum-sil.[8], am-c., am-caust.[11],
  am-m.[6], ambr., **aml-ns.**[2, 6], amyg.[11],
  ang.[3, 4, 6], anis.[8], **ant-c., ant-t.**,
  anthraci.[2], antip.[8], **apis, aran.**,
  arg-m.[6], **arg-n.**, arist-cl.[9], **arn., ars.**[1],
  ars-s-f.[1', 2], **ART-V.**, arum-m.[2],
  asaf., aster., **ATRO.**, aur., aur-ar.[1'],
  aur-fu.[4], bar-c., **bar-m.**, bar-s.[1'],
  bart.[11], **BELL.**, ben-n.[2, 11, 12], bism.[4],
  both.[11], bov.[3], brom.[6], bruc.[4], **bry.**,
  BUFO, buth-a.[9], cact., **CALC.**,

calc-i.[1'], **camph.**, cann-i., cann-s.,
canth., carb-ac., carb-an.[4], carbn.[12],
carbn-h.[11], **carbn-s.**, cast.[3, 8, 12],
caul.[3], **CAUST., CHAM.**, chen-a.,
chin., **chlf.**[2, 8, 12], chlor.[12], **CIC.**,
cic-m.[8, 11], **cimic.**[6], **CINA**, cit-ac.[4],
clem., coca, coc-c., **cocc.**, cod.[11, 12],
coff., colch., colchin.[12], coloc., **con.**,
convo-s.[9], cop., cortico.[9, 10],
cortiso.[9, 10], croc., **crot-c., crot-h.**,
cryp.[11], cub., **CUPR., cupr-a.**[8, 11],
cupr-ar., cupr-s.[11], cur., **cypr.**[6, 12],
cyt-l.[8, 9, 11, 12], dat-m.[11, 12], dat-s.[11],
dig., dios.[3, 6], dor.[2], dulc., euon.[8, 12],
eupi., fagu.[11], ferr., ferr-ar.,
ferr-m.[4, 11], ferr-s.[12], form., frag.[12],
gels., glon., gran.[11], **graph.**, grat.[1'],
guare.[11], **hell., hydr-ac., HYOS.**,
hyper.[8], **ign.**, indg.[6], iod., **ip.**,
iris-fl.[8, 12], jasm.[11, 12], jatr.[4],
juni.[11, 12], **kali-br., kali-c., kali-chl.**,
kali-cy.[11], kali-i., kali-m.[1'],
kali-ox.[11, 12], kali-p.[6], kalm.,
keroso.[11, 12], lach., lact.[4, 11],
lat-m.[9], laur., linu-c.[11], linu-u.[12],
LOB., lol.[11], lon-x.[8, 11, 12], **lyc., lyss.**,
mag-c., mag-m., **mag-p.**, mag-s.[9],
manc., mand.[9], med.[3, 12], meli.,
meph., **merc., merc-c.**, merc-d.[11],
merc-ns.[11], merc-p-r.[11], methyl.[12],
mez.[6], mill.[3], morph.[8, 11, 12], **mosch.**,
mur-ac., nat-f.[9], **nat-m.**, nat-s.,
nicot.[8, 12], nit-ac., nitro-o.[11],
NUX-M., NUX-V., oena.,
ol-an.[3, 4, 6], ol-j.[6], olnd., **OP.**,
ox-ac., passi.[8, 12], petr., **phos., phyt.**,
pic-ac.[6], pitu.[9], plat., **PLB.**,
plb-chr.[8, 12], **podo.**[3, 6], **psor., puls.**,
pyre-p.[12], ran-b.[6], ran-s., **rat.**[6],
rauw.[9], rhus-t., ric.[11], rob.,
rumx-a.[11, 12], russ.[11, 12], ruta,
sabad., sal-ac.[6], samb., **santin.**[8, 11, 12],
scol.[12], **sec.**, sep., **sil.**, sin-n., sium[12],
sol-c.[8, 12], **sol-n.**, spig., spirae.[12],
squil., stann., staph., **STRAM.**,
stront-c., stroph-h.[3], **STRY., stry-s.**[6],
sul-ac.[6], sul-h.[12], sul-i.[1'], **sulph.**,
tab., tanac.[4, 11], tax., **ter.**, thal.[14],
thea, thuj.[6], thymol.[9, 14], **tub.**[7],
upa.[8, 12], upa-a.[8], valer., **vario.**[2],
verat., verat-v., verb.[6], verbe.[8],

vesp.[1'], vib.[3], vip., zinc., zinc-cy.[12],
zinc-m.[11, 12], zinc-o.[8], zinc-p.[1'],
zinc-s.[8, 12], zinc-val.[3, 6], zing.[2], ziz.

Vol. I: *anger, anxiety, cheerful,
clinging, cursing, delirium, impa-
tience, insanity, irritability,
lamenting, laughing, moaning,
morose, prostration, rage, restlessness, shrieking, striking, stupe-
faction, stupor, unconsciousness,
weeping, wildness.*

*agitation, s'agrippe, anxiété,
colère, criant, délire, férocité, folie,
frapper, gai, gémissements, impa-
tience, inconscience, irritabilité,
jurer, se lamente, morose, pleurer,
prostration, rage, rire, stupéfac-
tion, stupeur.*

*Angst, Betäubung, Bewußtlosig-
keit, Delirium, Erschöpfung,
Fluchen, froh, Geisteskrankheit,
Jammern, klammert sich, Lachen,
mürrisch, Raserei, Reizbarkeit,
Ruhelosigkeit, Schlagen, Schreien,
Stöhnen, Stupor, Ungeduld,
Weinen, Wildheit, Zorn.*

Vol. III: *Menses-copious, painful,
scanty. Metrorrhagia. Pollutions.
Sleep-comatose, convulsions,
disturbed, sleepiness, sleeplessness, yawning.*

*Menstruations-douloureuses,
copieuses, insuffisantes.
Métrorrhagies. Pollutions.
Sommeil comateux, convulsions,
insomnie, somnolence, troublé.*

*Menses-reichliche, schmerzhafte,
spärliche. Metrorrhagie. Pollutionen. Schlaf-Gähnen, gestörter,
komatöser, Konvulsionen,
Schläfrigkeit, Schlaflosigkeit.*

**one-sided
côté, d'un
einseitige**
apoc., **art-v.,** bell., brom.[6],
calc-p., caust., chin-s.[4], cina[8],
dulc., elaps, gels., graph., hell.,
ip., plb.

left side of body
côté gauche, du
linken Körperseite, der
bell.[4], **calc-p.,** chin-s.[4], colch.[11],
cupr., elaps, graph., **ip.,**
nat-m., nit-ac.[4], plb., sabad.[4],
stram.[4], **sulph.**

to right[2, 16]
de gauche à droite
von der linken zur rechten
sulph.

paralyzed side
paralysé, du côté
gelähmten Seite, der
phos., sec.

paralysis of the other
paralysie, du côté opposé à la
Lähmung auf der anderen Seite
apis, **art-v.,** bell., hell.[1], lach.[6],
phos.[6], **stram.**

right side of body
côté droit, du
rechten Körperseite, der
bell., caust., chen-a.[1], **LYC.,**
nux-v., sep.[4, 16], tarent.[6]

left paralyzed
côté gauche paralysé
linke Seite gelähmt
art-v.

to left
de droite à gauche
von der rechten zur linken
visc.

daytime[2]
journée, pendant la
tagsüber
art-v., kali-br.

morning
matin
morgens
    arg-n., art-v., **calc.**, **caust.**, cocc.,
    crot-h., kalm., **lyc.**, **mag-p.**,
    nux-v., plat., sec., sep., sulph.,
    tab.

4–16 h
    calc.

5 h[11]
    plb.

9–10 h
    nat-m.[2], plb.[11]

afternoon
après-midi
nachmittags
    arg-m., stann.

evening
soir
abends
    alum., **alumn.**[2], **CALC.**, **caust.**,
    croc., gels. graph.[4], kali-c.[4], laur.,
    merc-ns., nit-ac.[4], **op.**, plb-chr.[11],
    stann., stram., sulph.

air, in open
air, en plein
Freien, im
    caust.

20 h
    ars.

21 h
    lyss.

night
nuit
nachts
    arg-n., ars., **art-v.**, aur., bufo,
    calc., calc-ar., **caust.**, cic., cina,
    cupr., dig., **hyos.**, kali-c., kalm.,
    lach.[4], lyc., **merc.**, nit-ac., nux-v.,
    oena., **OP.**, **plb.**, sec., **SIL.**, **stram.**,
    sulph., zinc.

midnight
minuit
Mitternacht
    bufo, cina, **cocc.**, santin., zinc.

after/après/nach
    nit-ac.

3 h[2]
    stram.

absences see Vol. I unconsciousness–
frequent

Addison's disease, in
maladie bronzée, pendant la
Addisonscher Krankheit, bei
    calc., iod.[2]

alternating with excitement of mind
alternant avec excitation
abwechselnd mit Erregung
    STRAM.

    rage
    rage
    Raserei
        STRAM.

    relaxation of muscular system[11]
    relaxation du système musculaire
    Muskelentspannung
        acet-ac.

    rigidity[11]
    rigidité
    Starre
        stry.

    unconsciousness
    inconscience
    Bewußtlosigkeit
        agar., aur.

anger, after
colère, à la suite de
Zorn, infolge von
    bufo, **CHAM.**, cina, **CUPR.**[2],
    kali-br., lyss., **NUX-V.**, op., plat.,
    sulph.

epilepsy from[2]
épilepsie à la suite de
Epilepsie infolge von
    art-v., **CALC.**

vexation/contrariété/Ärger

amenorrhoe, in[2]
aménorrhée, pendant l'
Amenorrhoe, bei
    art-v.

anxiety, from[6]
anxiété, par
Angst, durch
    stram.

apoplectic
apoplexie, après
Apoplexie, nach
    bell., crot-h., cupr., lach., nux-v.,
    stram., **verat-v.**[2]

begin in the abdomen
commençant dans le ventre
beginnen im Abdomen
    aran., **bufo**

    arm
    bras, dans le
    Arm
        arum-t.[2], **bell.**

        left[7]
        gauche, dans le
        linken
            sil.

    back
    dos, dans le
    Rücken
        ars.[4], sulph.

    calf muscles[16]
    mollet, dans les muscles du
    Wadenmuskeln, in den
        lyc.

    face
    face, dans la
    Gesicht
        absin., **bufo,** cina, dulc., **hyos.,**
        ign., lach., santin., sec.

    left side
    gauche, à l'hémiface
    linke Seite
        lach.

fingers[2]
doigts, dans les
Fingern, in den
    cupr-a.

    and toes
    et orteils
    und Zehen
        cupr., cupr-a.[2]

head
tête, dans la
Kopf
    cic.

legs[2]
jambes, dans les
Beinen, in den
    cupr-a.

toes[2]
orteils, dans les
Zehen, in den
    cupr-a., hydr-ac.

bending elbow am.
flexion du coude am., la
Beugen des Ellbogens am.
    nux-v.

    head backwards, from
    tête en arrière, en mettant la
    des Kopfes nach hinten, durch
    NUX-V.

biting, with
mordre, avec tendance à
beißen, mit Tendenz zu
    croc.[4], **cupr.**[2], lyss., **tarent.**[2]

bone in the throat, from
os dans la gorge, par un
Knochen im Hals, durch einen
    cic.

bright light, from
lumière vive, par
helles Licht, durch
   bell., **canth.**[2], lyss., nux-v., op.,
   STRAM.

light agg./lumière agg./Licht agg.

cerebral softening
cérébral, du cours du ramollissement
Gehirnerweichung, bei
   bufo[2], **caust.**

changing in character
à caractère variable
wechseln den Charakter
   bell., ign., **puls., STRAM.**

children, in
enfants, chez les
Kindern, bei
   absin.[8], acon., **aeth.,** agar.,
   agre.[14], **ambr., aml-ns.**[2], ant-t.[2, 4],
   apis, arn.[1, 2], ars.[2], **ART-V.,**
   asaf.[4], **BELL.,** bry., bufo[8],
   calc., calc-p.[1, 3, 6], **camph.,**
   camph-br.[6, 8], canth.[4], caust.,
   cham., chlol.[2, 8], **cic.,** cimic.[2],
   CINA, cocc., **coff.,** colch.[2],
   crot-c., cupr., **cupr-a.**[2], **cypr.**[3, 6, 8],
   dol., **gels.,** glon.[8], **guare.**[2], **HELL.,**
   hep., **hydr-ac., hyos.,** ign., **ip.,**
   kali-br.[2, 7, 8], kali-c., kali-p.[3, 6],
   kreos.[2, 8], **lach.,** laur., **lyc., mag-p.,**
   meli.[2, 8], merc.[1, 2], mosch.[8], nux-m.[4],
   nux-v., oena.[3, 6, 8], **OP.,** passi.[12],
   ph-ac.[6], phos.[6], plat., **santin.**[8],
   scut.[8], sec., **sil., stann.**[2, 3, 4, 6, 8],
   STRAM., sulph., ter.[2], **VERAT.,**
   verat-v.[2], **ZINC., zinc-cy.**[6],
   zinc-s.[8], **zinc-val.**[3, 6]

infants, in[2]
petits enfants, chez les
Kleinkindern, bei
   art-v., bell., bufo, **cham., cupr.,**
   HELL.[1, 2], **hydr-ac., mag-p., meli.**

newborns, in[2]
nouveaux-nés, chez les
Neugeborenen, bei
   art-v., bell.[2, 4], **cupr.,** nux-v.[4]

strangers, from approach of
étrangers, à l'approche d'
Fremde sich nähern, wenn
   lyss., op., tarent.[6]

chill, during
frissons, pendant les
Fieberfrost, während
   ars., camph.[2], **lach.,** merc., nux-v.

climacteric period, during
ménopause, pendant la
Klimakterium, während des
   glon.[6], **lach.**[2, 7]

clonic
cloniques
klonische
   acon., **AGAR.,** alum-p.[1], am-c.,
   am-m., ambr., anac., ang.[3], ant-c.,
   ant-t., **anthraci.**[2], **arg-m.,** arg-n.[3],
   arn., **ars., art-v.,** asar.[1] (non: asaf.),
   aster., aur., **bar-c.,** bar-m., bar-s.[1],
   BELL., bor., bov.[3], brom.[6], **bry.,**
   BUFO, calc., calc-i.[1], **calc-p.,**
   camph., cann-s., canth., carb-v.,
   carbn-o., **carbn-s.,** caul.[3], **caust.,**
   CHAM., chin., **chin-s., chlf.**[2], **CIC.,**
   cimic., **cina, clem.,** cocc., coff.,
   coloc., **con.,** croc., **CUPR.,** dig.,
   dulc., graph., guaj., hell., hep.,
   HYOS., ign., iod., **ip.,** kali-ar.,
   kali-bi.[3], **kali-c.,** kali-m.[1], **kalm.,**
   kreos., lach., lat-m.[9], laur., **lyc.,**
   LYSS., mag-c., mag-m., **mag-p.,**
   mang., med.[12], meny., **merc., mez.,**
   mosch., mur-ac., mygal., nat-c.,
   nat-f.[9], **nat-m.,** nit-ac., **nux-m.,**
   nux-v., **oena.,** ol-an.[3], olnd.[1], **OP.,**
   petr., ph-ac., phos., phys., **plat.,**
   PLB., podo.[3], puls., ran-b., ran-s.,
   rheum., rhod., rhus-t., russ.[11], ruta,
   sabad., samb., sars., **sec.,** sel.,
   seneg., **SEP., sil.,** spig., spong.,
   squil., **stann.,** staph., **STRAM.,**
   stront-c., stry.[3], **stry-s.**[6], sul-ac.,
   sulph., tab.[3], tarent., tarax., teucr.,
   thuj., thymol.[9], valer.[3], verat.,
   verat-v., visc., **zinc.,** zinc-p.[1],
   zinc-val.[3, 6]

alternating with tonic
alternant avec c. toniques
abwechselnd mit tonischen
  bell.[1',3,6], **cimic.**[2], con.[3,6], **ign.**[3,6],
  mosch.[3,6], nux-v.[6], plat.[3,6],
  sep.[3,6], stram., **tab.**[2], verat-v.[3,6]

closing a door, on
fermant une porte, en
Schließen einer Tür, beim
  stry.

noise/bruits/Geräusche

coition, during
coït, pendant le
Koitus, während des
  bufo

  after/après le/nach
  agar.

cold air, from
froid, par l'air
kalte Luft, durch
  ars., bell., **cic., indg.**[2], merc.,
  nux-v.

  drinks, from
  boissons froides, par l'ingestion de
  Getränke, durch
  caust.[4], cupr., lyc.[4]

  water am.
  eau froide am.
  Wasser am., kaltes
  caust., lyc.[4]

cold, becoming
refroidissement
Abkühlung, durch
  bell., **caust.,** cic., **mosch.**[1], **nux-v.**

coldness of the body
froideur du corps, avec
Kälte des Körpers, mit
  anan.[1], bell.[8], **camph.,** caust., cic.,
  hell., hydr-ac.[6,8], hyos., mosch.,
  nicot.[8], **OENA.,** op., stram., **verat.**

feet, of
pieds, des
Füße, der
  bell.[8], **cupr.**[2]

hands, of[2]
mains, des
Hände, der
  cupr.

head hot, feet cold[8]
tête très chaude et pieds froids,
  avec
heißem Kopf und kalten Füßen, mit
  bell.

of one side of body
d'un seul côté du corps
einer Seite des Körpers
  sil.

colic, during
coliques, pendant les
Koliken, bei
  CIC.[2], **cupr.**[2], plb., sec.[2]

commotion of the brain, from[2]
commotion cérébrale, par
Commotio cerebri, durch
  ARN., CIC., hyper., nat-s.

compression on spinal column
compression sur la colonne vertébrale, par
Druck auf die Wirbelsäule, durch
  tarent.

congenital[2]
congénitales
angeborene
  hell., **kali-br.,** verat.

consciousness, with
conscience, avec
Bewußtsein, mit
  ang.[3], ars., aur-ar.[1'], bar-m.[1'],
  bell., calc., camph., **canth.,** caust.,
  CINA, grat., **hell.,** hyos., **ign.**[3],
  ip., kali-ar., **kali-c.,** lyc., **mag-c.,**
  merc., mur-ac., **nat-m.,** nit-ac.,
  nux-m., nux-v., phos., plat., plb.,
  sec., **sep.,** sil., **STRAM.,** stry.,
  sulph.

without
inconscience, avec
ohne
    absin., acet-ac., acon., **aeth.,**
    agar.[2], agre.[14], aml-ns.[2], ant-t.,
    ARG-N., ars., aster., aur., **bell.,**
    BUFO, CALC., calc-ar., calc-p.[2],
    calc-s., camph., CANTH.,
    carb-ac., **caust.,** cham., chin.,
    CIC., cina, **cocc.,** crot-h., **cupr.,**
    cupr-a.[8], cupr-ar.[8], cur.[2], dig.,
    ferr., glon., hydr-ac., **HYOS.,**
    ign.[1',2,4], **ip., kali-c.,** lach.,
    laur., led., lyc., merc., **mosch.,**
    nat-m., nit-ac., nux-v., **OENA.,**
    op., phos., **plat., PLB.,** sec., **sep.,**
    sil., **stann.[2,4],** staph., **stram.,**
    sulph., tanac., **tarent.,** verat.,
    vesp.[1'], **VISC.**

contradiction, from
contradiction, par
Widerspruch, durch
    aster.

cough, during[2]
toux, pendant la
Husten, beim
    bell., **calc.,** ign., meph., stram.[2,11],
    sulph.

    after/après la/nach
    cupr., ip., verat.[2]

    whooping cough, in[2]
    coqueluche, au cours de
    Keuchhusten, beim
        brom., **calc., cupr.[2,8], hydr-ac.,**
        ip.[1',2], KALI-BR.[2,8]

croup, in[2]
croup, pendant l'accès de
Krupp, bei
    lach.

cyanosis, with[2]
cyanose, avec
Zyanose, mit
    cupr., cupr-a.[8], **hydr-ac.[2,6,8],** verat.

delirium tremens, in[2]/par/bei
    hyos.

dentition, during
dentition, pendant la
Zahnen, beim
    acon., aeth., art-v., arum-t.[2], **bell.,**
    CALC., calc-p.[2], caust.[2], CHAM.,
    cic., cina, coff.[3,6], **colch.[2], cupr.,**
    cupr-a.[2], cypr.[2,6], gels.[3,6], hyos.,
    ign., ip.[2], KALI-BR.[2,3,6], kreos.,
    lach.[2], mag-p.[1'-3,6,7], meli.[2], merc.,
    mill.[2], nux-m.[3,6], passi.[6], **podo.,**
    rheum[3,6], sin-n.[2], **stann., stram.,**
    sulph.[4], thyr.[14], **verat-v.[2,3,6],**
    zinc.[2,3,6]

diarrhoea am.
diarrhée am.
Diarrhoe am.
    lob.

downwards, spread
bas, s'étendent vers le
nach unten, erstrecken sich
    cic., sec.

draft agg.
courant d'air agg.
Zugluft agg.
    ars., cic.[1'], **lyss., NUX-V., STRY.**

drawing-up of legs, alternately[9]
remonte les jambes alternativement
Anziehen eines Beines,
    abwechselndes
    cyt-l.

drinking, after
bu, après avoir
Trinken, nach dem
    ars., art-v.[2], **bell.,** hyos., **stram.[3]**

    water[15]
    de l'eau
    von Wasser
        calc., canth.

drugs, after[2]
drogues, après
Medikamenten, nach
    acon., **ARN.**

drunkards, in
ivrognes, chez les
Trinkern, bei
   anthraci.[2], glon., **hyos.**[2], **nux-v.,**
   ran-b.

eating, while
mangeant, en
Essen, beim
   plb.

   after
   après avoir mangé
   nach dem
      aster.[2], **calc-p.**[2], cina, grat., hyos.,
      nux-v.[6]

emission of semen, during
éjaculation, pendant l'
Ejakulation, bei der
   art-v., grat., **nat-p.**

   from[2]/par/durch
   lach.

epileptic
épilepsie
Epilepsie
   absin., acet-ac., acon.[3], **aeth.,**
   agar., agre.[14], alco.[11], all-c.[11],
   alum., alum-p.[1'], alum-sil.[1'],
   alumn.[2], **am-br.**[2, 8, 12], am-c.,
   ambr.[2], ambro.[12], **aml-ns.**[2, 6, 8, 12],
   amyg.[12], **anac., anag.**[2, 12], ang.[3],
   anil.[11], anis.[8], ant-c.[3], ant-t.[3],
   antip.[12], apis[3], aran-ix.[10], **ARG-M.,**
   ARG-N., arn.[3], **ars., art-v.,** asaf.[3],
   aster., atro.[2, 8, 12], aur.[3],
   aur-br.[8, 12], aven.[8], **bar-c.,**
   BAR-M., bar-s.[1'], **bell.,** ben-n.[12],
   bism.[6], bor.[8], bry.[3], **BUFO,** caj.[2, 12],
   calc., CALC-AR., calc-p., **calc-s.,**
   calc-sil.[1'], camph., cann-i., **canth.,**
   carb-an., carb-v., carbn-s., **cast.**[2],
   cast-eq.[2, 12], caste.[14], caul.[6],
   CAUST., cedr., cham.[3, 4], chen-a.[12],
   chin., chin-ar.[2, 12], chin-s., **chlol.**[2],
   chlorpr.[14], **cic.,** cic-m.[8, 11, 12],
   cimic.[2, 8, 12], **cic.,** cina, cinnm.[2], **cocc.,**
   coloc.[3], **con.,** convo-s.[9, 14],
   cori-r.[11], **crot-c., crot-h., CUPR.,**

cupr-a.[2, 8, 11], **cupr-ar., cur.,**
cypr.[2, 12], dat-m.[12], des-ac.[14], dig.,
dros.[2, 3, 4, 12], dulc.[3], fago.[11],
fagu.[12], ferr.[3], **ferr-cy.**[8], ferr-p.[8],
form., gels., glon., graph.[1'], **hell.,**
hell-v.[12], hep.[8], hydr-ac., **HYOS.,**
hyper.[2], **ictod.**[2], **ign., indg.,** iod.,
ip.[3], irid.[8], kali-ar.[1'], kali-bi.[1', 2, 12],
kali-br., kali-c., **kali-chl.,**
kali-cy.[8, 11, 12], kali-m.[1', 8, 12],
kali-p.[2, 8], kali-s., kres.[10, 14], **lach.,**
laur., led.[3], levo.[14], lith-br.[12], lol.[6],
lyc., lyss., mag-c., mag-p., mand.[14],
med., meli.[8, 12], merc., methyl.[8],
mill.[12], mosch., mur-ac.[3], naja,
nat-m., nat-s., nicot.[12], nit-ac.,
nitro-o.[12], nux-m., **nux-v., OENA.,**
oest.[8], onis.[12], onon.[12], **op.,**
paeon.[10], passi.[6, 8, 12], perh.[14],
petr.[2, 3], **ph-ac., phos.,** phys.[10, 12],
picro.[8], **plat., PLB.,** polyg-pe.[12],
psor., puls., ran-b., ran-s.[3, 4],
rauw.[14], rhus-t.[3], rib-ac.[14], ruta[3],
salam.[6, 8], santin.[8, 12], **sec.,** sep.,
SIL., sin-n.[2], **sol-c.**[8, 12], sol-n.[4],
spirae.[8, 12], **stann.,** staph., **stram.,**
stry., sulfon.[12], **SULPH.,**
sumb.[8, 10, 12], **syph.,** tab.,
tanac.[12], tarax.[3], **tarent., ter.**[2, 12],
thea[11], thiop.[14], thuj.[3, 12],
tub.[8], valer.[3, 8], verat., verat-v.[6],
verb.[7, 8], verbe-h.[12], vip., **VISC.,**
zinc.[3, 6, 10], zinc-cy.[8, 12], zinc-o.[10],
zinc-p.[6], **zinc-val.**[6, 8, 12],
ziz.[2, 8, 11, 12]

Vol. I: *anxiety, delusions,*
dementia, fear, indifference,
laughing-spasmodic, prostration,
rage, unconsciousness.

anxiété, démence, imaginations,
inconscience, indifférence, peur,
prostration, rage, rire-spasmo-
dique.

Angst, Bewußtlosigkeit, Demenz,
Erschöpfung, Furcht, Gleich-
gültigkeit, Lachen-krampfhaftes,
Raserei, Wahnideen.

Vol. III: *Masturbation-m.*
Menses-pale, scanty. Sleep-
restless.

Masturbation-m. Menstruations-
insuffisantes, pâles. Sommeil-
agité.

Masturbation-m. Menses –
blasse, spärliche. Schlaf –
unruhiger.

aura/Aura
   Vol. I: *absent–minded, anger,*
   anxiety, confusion, delusions–
   small, dullness, eccentricity,
   excitement, foolish, forgetfull,
   imbecility, irritability, lascivious,
   laughing–spasmodic, sadness,
   sighing, speech–unintelligible

   anxiété, colère, confusion,
   distrait, esprit gourd, excen-
   tricité, excitation, imaginations–
   petits, imbécillité, irritabilité,
   lascif, langage–unintelligible,
   oublieux, ridicule, rire–
   spasmodique, soupire, tristesse

   albernes, Angst, Erregung,
   Exzentrizität, Imbezillität,
   Lachen–krampfhaftes, lasziv,
   Reizbarkeit, Seufzen, Sprechen–
   unverständliches, Stumpfheit,
   Traurigkeit, vergeßlich, Ver-
   wirrung, Wahnideen–klein,
   zerstreut, Zorn

   Vol. II: *shock electric-like,*
   epilepsy/choc–électrique–
   épileptique/Schock–elektrischer–
   epileptischen
   shuddering/frisonnement/
   Schaudern

abdomen to head
abdomen irradiant à la tête,
   partant de l'
Abdomen zum Kopf, vom
   indg.

absent[3]
absente
fehlende
   ars., art-v.[3, 6], atro., bell., camph.,
   canth., cham., cic., cupr., cupr-ar.,
   dios., hydr-ac.[3, 6], lach.[3, 6], nat-s.,
   oena.[3, 6], plb., podo., tarent.,
   valer., zinc.[3, 6], zinc-val.[6, 8]

arms, in
bras, dans les
Armen, in den
   calc., **calc-ar.**[1], bell.[6], **lach.**,
   sulph.

left arm, in
gauche, dans le bras
linken Arm, im
   calc-ar.[2, 7], cupr.[2, 6], **sil.**[2, 6, 8],
   sulph.[6, 7]

forearms, in[7]
avant-bras, dans les
Unterarmen, in den
   bell., calc., sulph.

auditory disturbances[3, 6, 8]
auditifs, troubles
Gehörstörungen
   bell., calc.[8], cic.[3, 6], hyos.[3, 6],
   sulph.

back, in[4]
dos, dans le
Rücken, im
   ars., sulph.

   and left arm[7]
   et dans le bras gauche
   und im linken Arm
      calc-ar., sulph.

creeping down spine[2]
rampe en bas de la colonne
   vertébrale
kriecht die Wirbelsäule herunter
   lach.

blind
aveugle
blind
   cupr.

cold air over spine and body
air froid sur le corps et le long
   de la colonne vertébrale
kalte Luft über Wirbelsäule und
   Körper
      agar.

cold feet, with
pieds froids, avec
kalten Füßen, mit
      cina[6], **lach.**[2]

coldness, with[3]
froid, avec
Kälte, mit
      cina, sil., sep.[16]

between scapulae[16]
entre les omoplates
zwischen den Schulterblättern
      sep.

running down spine
descendant l'épine dorsale
läuft die Wirbelsäule herunter
      ars.

   on left side
   du côté gauche
   auf der linken Seite
      sil.

confusion[2, 3, 6]
confusion
Verwirrung
      lach.

congestion of blood to head[6]
congestion du sang à la tête
Blutandrang zum Kopf
      calc-ar., op., sulph.

descending[8]
descendante
erstreckt sich nach unten
      calc.

drawing in limbs
tiraillement dans les membres
Ziehen in den Gliedern
      ars.

in left chest[16]
dans le thorax à gauche
in der linken Brust
      nit-ac.

ear noises[7]
bruits de l'oreille
Ohrgeräusche
      hyos.

epigastrium to uterus, legs[2, 7]
épigastre jusqu'à l'utérus,
   aux jambes, partant de l'
Epigastrium zum Uterus,
   zu den Beinen, vom
      CALC.

eructations[2, 6]
renvois
Aufstoßen
      lach.

expansion of body, sensation of
expansion du corps, sensation d'
Ausdehnung des Körpers,
   Gefühl der
      arg-n.

eyes, sparks before
yeux, éclairs devant les
Augen, Funken vor den
      hyos.

   turned upwards to left
   tournés en haut et à gauche
   verdreht nach links oben
      bufo

face, chewing motion
face, mouvement de mâchonnement
Gesicht, Kaubewegungen
      calc.

formication in[6]
formication dans la
Ameisenlaufen im
      nux-v.

twitching[3]
contraction
Zucken
      laur.

fear[2]
peur
Furcht
    aml-ns., arg-n., cupr., nat-m.

fingers and toes, in[2]
doigts et dans les orteils, dans les
Fingern und Zehen, in
    cupr.

formication[3]
Ameisenlaufen
    bell., calc., nit-ac., **nux-v.**

general nervous feeling
nervosité générale, sensation de
allgemeines nervöses Gefühl
    arg-n., **nat-m.**

hand, in right[2]
main droite, dans la
Hand, in rechter
    cupr.

hands to head, from[2]
mains jusqu'à la tête, dans les
Händen bis zum Kopf, von den
    sulph.

head, from[3]
tête, partant de la
Kopf, ausgehend vom
    caust., lach., stram., sulph.

    trembling sensation
    tremblement de la, sensation de
    Zittern des Kopfes, Gefühl von
        caust.

headache[2]
maux de tête
Kopfschmerzen
    bell., calc., **calc-ar.**, cann-i.,
    caust.[2, 6], cina[2, 16], **lach.**[2, 6], staph.,
    zinc.

heart, from
cœur, partant du
Herzen ausgehend, vom
    CALC-AR., lach., naja, nat-m.[3],
    op.[3], sulph.[3]

heat, flushes of
bouffées de chaleur
Hitzewallungen
    calc-ar.[7], indg.[8]

heel to occiput, right
talon droit à l'occiput, du
Ferse zum Hinterkopf,
    von der rechten
    stram.[1]

jerk in nape
secousse dans la nuque
Ruck im Nacken
    bry.[2], bufo

knees, in
genoux, dans les
Knien, in den
    cupr., cupr-a.[7]

    ascending[6, 8]
    ascendante
    aufsteigende
    cupr.

legs, in[6]
jambes, dans les
Beinen, in den
    lyc., plb.

    right leg to abdomen, from[6]
    jambe droite irradiant
        à l'abdomen, partant de la
    rechten Bein zum Abdomen, vom
        lyc.

limbs, in[3]
membres, dans les
Gliedern, in den
    bell.[3, 7], calc.[3, 7], cina, cupr.,
    lyc.[3, 8], plb., sil., sulph.

    left[3]
    gauches
    linken
    cupr., sil., sulph.

morose[6]
morose
mürrisch
    zinc., zinc-val.

mouse, running like a
souris qui court, comme une
Maus läuft, als ob eine
    ars.[6], aur.[6], **BELL., CALC.**, ign.,
    nit-ac., sep.[6], **sil.**, stram.[6], **sulph.**

mouth wide open
bouche grande ouverte, avec la
Mund weit offen
    bufo

nausea[2]
nausée
Übelkeit
    cupr., **sulph.**

numbness of brain
engourdissement du cerveau
Betäubung
    bufo, indg.[8]

palpitation
Herzklopfen
    absin.[3, 6], ars., **calc., calc-ar.**,
    cupr., ferr.[3], **lach.**, nat-m.[6]

pupils dilated
pupilles dilatées
Pupillen, weite
    ARG-N., bufo

ravenous appetite
faim canine
Heißhunger
    calc., HYOS.

perspiration scalp
transpiration du cuir chevelu
Kopfschweiß
    caust., hell-v.[12]

restlessness
agitation
Ruhelosigkeit
    arg-n.[1'], bufo[2], caust.[3, 6]

sadness
tristesse
Traurigkeit
    art-v.[2], zinc.[6], zinc-val.[3]

shocks
chocs
Schock, Schläge
    ars., **laur.**

shoulders, pain between[3, 6, 8]
épaules, douleur entre les
Schultern, Schmerz zwischen den
    indg.

shrieking
cris
Schreien
    CIC.[2, 3, 6], **cupr.**[2, 3, 6, 8],
    hydr-ac.[6, 8], stram.[3, 6]

solar plexus, from
plexus solaire, du
Solarplexus aus, vom
    art-v., bell., **bufo**[1, 7], **calc.**[1, 7],
    caust., CIC., cupr., **indg.**,
    NUX-V., sil., SULPH.

to head
jusqu'à la tête
jusqu'à la tête
bis zum Kopf
    calc.[7], **sil.**[2]

speech, unintelligible[6]
language, inintelligible
Sprechen, unverständliches
    bufo

stomach, in
estomac, dans l'
Magen, im
    art-v., bell., bism.[3, 6], bufo,
    calc., calc-ar.[3], **caust.**[7], **CIC.**,
    cupr., **HYOS., indg., NUX-V.**,
    sil., SULPH.

to head
jusqu'à la tête
bis zum Kopf
    CALC.

teeth, grinding of[2]
grincement de dent, avec
Zähneknirschen, mit
    sulph.

throat, narrow sensation[3, 6]
gorge étroite, sensation de
Halsenge, Gefühl von
  lach.

tongue swelling[3, 6]
gonflement de la langue, avec
Zunge schwillt an
  plb.

trembling
tremblement, avec
Zittern
  absin.[3, 6-8], arg-n.[7], aster.[8]

urging stool[7]
envie d'aller à la selle
Stuhldrang
  calc-ar.

uterus, in
utérus, dans l'
Uterus, im
  bufo

  to stomach
  jusqu'à l'estomac
  bis zum Magen
    bufo

  to throat
  jusqu'à la gorge
  bis zum Hals
    lach.

vertigo
vertige, avec
Schwindel, mit
  ars., **calc-ar.**, **caust.**, **HYOS.**,
  indg.[3, 6], **lach.**, **plb.**, sil.[3, 6], **sulph.**,
  tarent., visc.[3, 6]

visual disturbance
visuels, troubles
Sehstörungen
  bell.[3, 6, 8], calc.[8], hyos.[3, 6], lach.[3],
  sulph.[6, 8]

voice, loss of
aphonie
Stimmverlust
  calc-ar.

vomiting
vomissement
Erbrechen
  cupr., op.

warm air streaming up spine
air chaud qui souffle sur la colonne
    vertébrale de bas en haut, de l'
warme Luft strömt die Wirbelsäule
    hoch
  ars.

waving sensation in brain
vague dans le cerveau,
    avec sensation de
wogendes Gefühl im Gehirn
  cimic.

ailments during e. attack
troubles au cours des crises d'é.
Beschwerden während epileptischer
  Anfälle

Vol. I: *delirium/délire/Delirium*
laughing-spasmodic/rire-spasmodi-
que/Lachen – krampfhaftes
shrieking/criant/Schreien
weeping-c./pleurer-c./Weinen-K.
Weinen-K.

biting tongue
morsure de la langue
Zungenbiß
  art-v., **bufo**, camph., **caust.**, cocc.,
  cupr., **oena.**, **op.**, sec., stram.[1'],
  tarent., valer.

eyes turned upwards to right[2]
yeux tournés en haut et à droite,
    avec
Augen nach rechts oben verdreht
  hydr-ac.

  downwards[4]
  en bas
  nach unten
    aeth.

face, bluish
face cyanosée, avec
Gesicht, bläuliches
    absin.[2], agar.[2], atro.[2], **bell.**[2],
    cic., cina[2, 4], **CUPR., hyos.**,
    ign.[4], **ip.**, nux-v.[2], **oena., OP.**[2],
    phys., plb.[2], stry., **verat.**[2]

pale[2]
pâle
blasses
    am-c., ars.[2, 4], bell., calc.,
    caust., chin., cic.[2, 4], cina, **cupr.**,
    ip., lach.[2, 4], mosch.[4], nat-m.,
    plb., puls., sil., stann.[2, 4], sulph.,
    verat.

red
rouge
rotes
    aeth.[2, 4, 8], **bell.**[2, 4], bufo,
    camph.[2, 4], caust.[2], **CIC.**[2, 4],
    cina[2], cit-ac.[4], cocc.[4], **cupr.**[2],
    GLON., ign.[2, 4], ip.[2, 4], lyc.[2, 4],
    nux-v.[2], **oena., OP.**, stram.[2, 4]

yellow
jaune
gelbes
    cic.[2, 4], plb.[2]

froth, foam from mouth
écume à la bouche, avec de l'
Schaum vor dem Mund
    aeth.[4, 8], agar., ars., **art-v.,**
    aster.[2], bell., **bufo**, camph.,
    canth., **caust., cham., cic.**[2, 6], **cina,**
    cocc., colch., **cupr.**, gels., **glon.,**
    hydr-ac.[6], **hyos.**, ign.[2], **ind.**[2],
    lach.[2], laur.[2, 4], lyc.[2], lyss., med.[2],
    oena., op., plb.[2], **sil.**[2, 4], staph.,
    stry., sulph., tax., vip.[6]

involuntary discharges[2]
involontaires, avec écoulements
unwillkürliche Absonderungen
    cocc.

urination[2]
énurésie
Urinabgang, unwillkürlicher
    art-v., **BUFO, caust.**, cocc.,
    cupr., **HYOS.**, lach.[2], nat-m.[2],
    nux-v., **oena., plb.**, stry., **zinc.**

pupils contracted[2]
pupilles contractées
Pupillen, enge
    cic., **op.**, phyt.

dilated[2]
dilatées
weite
    aeth.[4, 8], **bell.**, carb-ac., cic.,
    cina, cocc., oena., plb., verat-v.

shrieking[2]
criant
Schreien
    bufo, cedr., **CIC.**[2, 3, 6, 8], crot-h.,
    cupr.[2, 3, 6, 8], hydr-ac.[6, 8], **HYOS.**,
    ign., **ip., kali-bi.**, lach., **lyc.**,
    nit-ac., **nux-v., oena.**, op., **sil.**,
    stann., stram.[2, 3, 6], sulph.,
    verat-v.

teeth, grinding of
grincement de dents, avec
Zähneknirschen, mit
    bufo, HYOS., sulph. tarent.

throwing backwards[2]
se jette en arrière
wirft sich zurück
    camph.

forwards[2]
en avant
nach vorn
    cupr.

winking of eyes
clignotement des yeux, avec
Blinzeln der Augen, mit
    kali-bi.

ailments after e. attack
troubles après les crises d'é.
Beschwerden nach epileptischen
Anfällen

Vol. I: *delirium, laughing–spasmodic, memory–loss, mildness, rage, speech–incoherent, unconsciousness.*

délire, douceur, inconscience, langage incohérent, mémoire–perte, rage, rire–spasmodique.

Bewußtlosigkeit, Delirium, Gedächtnisverlust, Lachen–krampfhaftes, Milde, Raserei, Sprechen–unzusammenhängendes.

weakness-c./faiblesse-c./
Schwäche-K.

blind
aveugle
blind
   sec.

ear noises
bruits d'oreille
Ohrgeräusche
   caust.

headache
maux de tête
Kopfschmerzen
   calc.[2], **caust.**, cina, cupr., kali-br.[15]

hiccough[8]
'hoquet
Schluckauf
   cic.

prostration[8]
Erschöpfung
   aeth., **chin-ar.**[2,8], **cic.**, hydr-ac., sec., sil., **stry.**, sulph.

ravenous appetite[16]
faim canine
Heißhunger
   calc.

restlessness[8]
agitation
Ruhelosigkeit
   cupr.

urine, copious
miction abondante, avec
Urinmenge, vermehrte
   caust.[4], **cupr.**, lach.[4]

vomiting
vomissement
Erbrechen
   acon., **ars.**, bell.[8], **calc.**[2], colch., **cupr.**, glon.

epileptiform
épileptiformes
epileptiforme
   absin.[2,3,6], acon., aeth., **AGAR.**, alum., alum-sil.[1'], am-c., aml-ns.[2,3,6], **anac.**, ant-c., ant-t., arg-m.[1], **ARG-N.**, arn., **ars.**, art-v.[6], asaf., aur., aur-ar.[1'], **BELL.**, bism.[3,6], bry., **bufo, CALC.**, calc-i.[1'], calc-p.[3,6], calc-s., **camph.**, canth., carbn-s., caul.[3,6], **CAUST.**, cedr., **cham.**, chin., **chin-ar.**[2], chlorpr.[14], **CIC., CINA, cocc.**, coloc., con., **convo-s.**[9,14], cortico.[9], **CUPR., cur.**, dig., dros., dulc., ferr., ferr-ar., gal-ac.[7], **gels., GLON.**, graph.[1'], hell., hydr-ac.[6], **HYOS., hyper.**, hypoth.[14], ign., indg.[3], iod., **ip.**, kali-br., **kali-c.**, kali-i.[2], kali-m.[1',3,6], kali-s., **lach.**, laur., led., lob.[3,6], lol.[6], **lyc.**, mag-c., mag-p.[3], **med.**, merc., mosch., mur-ac., **nat-m., nit-ac., nux-m., nux-v.**, oena., op., passi.[6], petr., ph-ac., phos., **phys.**[2], **plat., PLB.**, prot.[14], **psor., puls., ran-b.**, ran-s., rauw.[14], rhus-t., ruta, salam.[6], **sec., sep., sil.**, stann., staph., **STRAM., stry.**, sul-i.[1'], **SULPH.**, tarax., **tarent.**, teucr., thuj., valer., verat., verat-v., verb.[3], verbe-h.[6], vip.[3,6], **VISC.**, zinc., zinc-cy.[12], zinc-p.[1',3,6], **zinc-val.**[3,6]

errors in diet
erreurs diététiques, par
Diätfehler, durch
   cic.

eructations am.
renvois am.
Aufstoßen am.
   kali-c.

eruptions fail to break out, when
éruptions qui ne « sortent » pas,
   à l'occasion d'
Hautausschläge nicht herauskommen,
wenn
   ant-t., CUPR., ZINC.

exanthemata repelled or do not
   appear, when
exanthèmes supprimés ou qui ne
   sortent pas, par
Exantheme, durch nicht heraus-
   gekommene oder unterdrückte
   ant-t., apis[1, 8], ars.[8], **bry., camph.,**
   cupr., cupr-a.[2], **gels., hep.**[2]**, ip.,** op.[8],
   stram., sulph., ZINC., zinc-s.[8]

excitement, from
excitation, par
Erregung, durch
   acon., **agar.,** art-v.[6]**, aster., bell.,**
   cann-i.[11]**, cham.,** cic., cimic., **coff.,**
   cupr., gels., HYOS., ign., kali-br.,
   nux-v., OP., plat., **puls.,** sec.,
   tarent., **zinc.**[2]

   nervousness/nervosité/
     Nervosität

   religious[2]
   religieuse
   religiöse
     verat.

exertion, after
exercices physiques, après
Anstrengungen, nach körperlichen
   alum., alumn.[2]**, calc., glon.,** kalm.,
   lach., lyss., nat-m., petr., sulph.

extension of body am., forcible
extension forcée du corps am.
Ausstrecken des Körpers am.,
   forciertes
   nux-v., stry.

extensor muscles
extenseurs, des **muscles**
Streckermuskeln, der
   CINA

eyelids, while touching
paupières, en touchant les
Augenlider, beim Berühren der
   coc-c.

falling, with
chute, avec
Fallen, mit
   agar., alum., alum-p.[1']**, am-c.,**
   ars., aster., BELL., bufo[1']**, calc.,**
   calc-i.[1']**, calc-p.,** camph.[4]**, canth.,**
   caust., cedr., CHAM., chin-ar.[2]**,**
   cic., cina, cocc., **con., CUPR.,**
   dig., dulc., **HYOS.,** ign., **iod.**[1]**,** ip.,
   lach.[4], laur., lyc., lyss.[2]**,** merc.,
   nit-ac., **OENA.,** op., petr., ph-ac.,
   phos., plb., sec., sep., sil., **stann.,**
   staph., **stram.,** sulph., verat., zinc.

   backwards
   en arrière
   nach rückwärts
     ang.[2]**, bell.,** camph.[2]**,** canth., chin.,
     cic., cic-m.[11]**, ign., ip.,** kalm.[2]**,**
     nux-v., **oena., OP.,** rhus-t., spig.,
     stram.

   forward
   en avant
   nach vorwärts
     arn., **aster.,** calc-p., canth., cic.,
     cupr., ferr., rhus-t., sil., sulph.,
     sumb.

   left side
   à gauche
   nach links
     bell., caust., lach., sabad., sulph.[7]

   right side
   à droite
   nach rechts
     bell.

runs in a circle to
tourne en rond vers la droite
läuft im Kreis und fällt nach
   rechts
   caust.

sideways[2]
sur le côté
auf die Seite
   bell., **calc.,** con., nux-v., sulph.

fear, from[6]
peur, par
Furcht, durch
   acon., arg-n.[7], **CALC.**[2, 7], **caust.,**
   cupr.[6, 7], glon., kali-p., **op.,** sil.

fingers, spread[7]
doigts étendus, des
Finger, der gespreizten
   sec.

fluids, from
eau ou des liquides, provoquées par l'
Wasser oder Gewässer, durch
   bell., canth., hyos., **LYSS., STRAM.**

forcible aroused from a trance, when
brusquement d'un état de transe,
   quand on le réveille
gewaltsam aus einem Trancezustand
   geweckt, wenn
   nux-m.

fright, from
frayeur, par
Schreck, durch
   acon., agar., apis, **arg-n., art-v.,**
   bell.[6, 7], **bufo, CALC., caust.,** cic.,
   cina[6], **cupr., gels.**[2, 7], glon.[6],
   HYOS., IGN., INDG., kali-br.,
   kali-p.[2], laur.[7], lyss., nat-m.[7], **OP.,**
   plat., sec., sil.[7], **stram.,** sulph.,
   tarent., verat., **zinc.**

of the mother (infant)
de la mère (chez les petits enfants)
der Mutter (beim Kleinkind)
   bufo[2], **OP.**

grief, after
chagrin, par
Kummer, durch
   ars.[2, 7], art-v., **hyos.,** ign., indg.[7],
   nat-m., nux-v.[5], **op.,**

haemorrhage, with
hémorrhagies, avec
Blutungen, bei
   chin., hyos., ip.[15], **plat., sec.**

after[3]/après/nach
   ars., bell., calc., cina, con., ign.,
   lyc., nux-v., puls., sulph., verat.

heat, during the
chaleur fébrile, pendant la
Fieberhitze, bei
   ars.[3], **bell.**[2, 3], camph.[3], carb-v.[3],
   caust.[2], **cic., cina,** cur., **ferr-p.**[2],
   hyos., ign.[2], **nat-m.**[2], **NUX-V.,** op.,
   sep.[3], **STRAM.,** verat.[3]

hydrocephaly with[2]
hydrocéphalie avec
Hydrozephalie mit
   arg-n., art-v., calc., kali-i., merc.,
   nat-m., stram., sulph., zinc.

hydrophobia with[2]
hydrophobie avec
Tollwut mit
   bell., canth., cur., gels., **stram.**

hypochondriasis with[8]
hypocondrie avec
Hypochondrie mit
   mosch., stann.

hysterical
hystériques
hysterische
   absin., acet-ac.[2], acon.[4, 11], **alum.,**
   alum-p.[1'], ambr.[3, 6], **apis,** ars.,
   ASAF., asar.[2, 3, 6, 8], **aur.,** aur-ar.[1'],
   aur-s.[1'], **bell., bry., calc.,** calc-s.,
   cann-i.[2], cann-s., cast.[8], caul.[2, 6, 8],
   caust., cedr., cham., chlf.[2], **cic.,**
   cimic., cocc., coff., **coll., CON.,**
   croc., cupr.[1', 7, 8], dig.[3], **gels.,**
   graph.[1'], hydr-ac.[2, 8], hyos., **IGN.,**
   iod., ip., kali-ar.[1'], kali-p.[3, 6, 8],

lach., lact.[4], **lil-t.**[3, 6], lyc.,
mag-c.[3, 6], **mag-m.**, meph.[3, 6],
merc., **mill.**[2], **MOSCH.**, **nat-m.**,
nit-ac., **nux-m.**, nux-v., oena.[6, 8],
op., petr., phos., **plat.**, plb., puls.,
ruta[3], sec., **sep.**, **sol-c.**[8],
stann.[3, 4, 8], staph., **stram.**, sul-i.[1'],
sulph., sumb., tarent., thyr.[12],
valer., **verat.**, **verat-v.**, visc.[3],
zinc., zinc-p.[1'], **zinc-val.**[3, 6, 8, 12]

before menses[6]
avant les menstruations
vor den Menses
   hyos., ign., lach.

indigestion, from
indigestions, par
Verdauungsstörungen, durch
  IP.

indignation, from
indignation, par
Entrüstung, durch
  staph.

injuries, from
traumatismes, par
Verletzungen, durch
  ang.[2], arn., art-v., **cic.**, con.[8],
  cupr.[8, 10], cupr-a.[10], **HYPER.**,
  meli.[8], **nat-s.**, op., oena., puls.[2],
  rhus-t., sil.[10], sulph., **valer.**

head, of the[2]
tête, de la
Kopfverletzungen
  ARN., CIC., cupr., hyper., led.,
  meli.[7], **nat-s.**

commotion/Commotio

intermittent
intermittentes
intermittierende
  absin.

internal
internes
innerliche
  acon., agar., alum.[3], am-c., ambr.,
  anac., ang.[3], ant-c.[3], ant-t.[3], arg-m.,

arn., ars., **asaf.**, asar.[3], bar-c.[3], **bell.**,
bism., bor.[3], bov., **bry.**, calad., **calc.**,
camph., canth., caps., carb-an.[3],
carb-v., CAUST., cham., cina,
COCC., coff., colch., coloc., con.,
cupr., dig., dulc.[3], euph.[3], **ferr.**,
graph., hep.[3], **HYOS., IGN.**, iod.,
ip., kali-c., kali-m.[1'], kali-n.[3], kreos.,
lach.,laur., led., **lyc.**, mag-c.,
mag-m., merc.[3], **mosch.**, mur-ac.,
nat-c., nat-m., nit-ac., nux-m.,
NUX-V., op., petr., ph-ac., **phos.**,
plat., plb., **PULS.**, rhod., rhus-t.[3],
sabad., sars.[3], **sec.**, seneg., **sep.**, sil.,
spong., **STANN., staph.**, stram.,
stront-c., sul-ac., sulph., teucr.,
thuj., valer., verat., **zinc.**, zinc-p.[1']

interrupted by painful shocks
interrompues par des chocs
  douloureux
unterbrochen durch schmerzhafte
  Schläge
  stry.

isolated groups of muscles, of[8]
groupes isolés des muscles, de
isolierter Muskelgruppen
  acon., **cic.**, cina, cupr., ign., nux-v.,
  stram., stry.

jealousy, from[2, 8]
jalousie, par
Eifersucht, durch
  lach.

labor see parturition

laughing, from[2]
rire, par
Lachen, durch
  coff., cupr.

with/avec/mit
  coff., graph.

leucorrhoea, with[2]
leucorrhées, avec
Fluor, mit
  caust., lach.

light agg.
lumière agg.
Licht agg.
    bell., **LYSS.**, op., nux-v., **STRAM.**

    bright light/lumière vive/helles
      Licht

love, from disappointed
chagrin d'amour, par
Liebe, durch enttäuschte
    hyos., ign.[1']

lying on side, on
couché sur le côté, étant
Liegen auf der Seite, beim
    puls.

    convulsively turned on the back
    se tourne convulsivement
      sur le dos
    dreht sich in Konvulsionen auf den
      Rücken
      cic.

    on abdomen with spasmodic
      jerking of pelvis upward[16]
    sur l'abdomen, avec tressaillements
      spamodiques du pelvis vers le
      haut
    auf dem Bauch mit krampfhaften
      Rucken vom Becken nach oben
      cupr.

masturbation, from
masturbation, par
Masturbation, durch
    bufo, calad., **calc.**, dig., elaps,
    kali-br., **lach.**, naja, nux-v., **PLAT.**,
    plb., sep., sil., stram., **sulph.**

meningitis, in cerebrospinal[2]
méningite cérébrospinale dans la
Meningitis cerebrospinalis, bei
    ant-t., apis, arg-n., crot-h., glon.,
    hell., tarent., verat.

menses, before
menstruations, avant les
Menses, vor den
    bell.[2], brom.[2], **bufo,** carb-v.,
    caul.[6], **caust.**, cimic.[2], **cupr.**,
    hyos., kali-br., mag-c.[6], mag-m.[6],
    oena., plat.[2], **puls.**, sulph.[2]

during
pendant les
während der
    apis, **arg-n., art-v.**[2], **bell.**, bufo[1, 7],
    caul., caust., **cedr., cimic., cocc.,**
    coll., cupr.,** gels., glon.[3, 6], **hyos.,**
    ign., kali-br., kali-m.[6], **lach.**[1, 7],
    mosch.[6], **nat-m.,** nux-m., **nux-v.,**
    OENA., phys., **plat.,** plb., puls.,
    sec., stram., **sulph.,** tarent., **zinc.**

after
après les
nach den
    kali-br.[7], syph.

instead of
au lieu des
an Stelle der
    oena.

suppressed, from
supprimées, par les
unterdrückte, durch
    bufo, calc-p., cocc., cupr., **gels.,**
    mill.[2, 8, 15], **puls.**

mental exertion, after
intellectuel, après travail
geistiger Anstrengung, nach
    bell., cann-i.[11], **glon.**

mercurial vapors, from
mercurielles, par vapeurs
Quecksilberdämpfe, durch
    stram.

metastasis
métastatiques
„Metastase" eines anderen
    Symptoms, als
    cupr.

mirror, from a[10]
miroir, par une
Spiegel, durch einen
    lyss.

miscarriage, after
avortement, après
Abort, nach
    ruta

moon, at full[2, 6-8]
lune, par pleine
Vollmond, bei
    CALC., caust.[6], **nat-m.**[2]

new m., at[2, 7, 8]
nouvelle l., par
Neumond, bei
    bufo[2, 7], **caust.**[2, 6, 8], **cupr., kali-br.,**
    sil.[2, 4, 6, 8, 11]

mortification, from
mortification, par
Kränkung, durch
    calc., cham.[1'], **staph.**[2]

motion agg.
mouvement agg.
Bewegung agg.
    ars., bell., **cocc.,** graph., **nux-v.,**
    stry.

nervousness, from
nervosité, par
Nervosität, durch
    arg-n.

excitement/excitation/Erregung

newborns see children

noise, from
bruits, par
Geräusche, durch
    ang.[4], ant-c., arn., **cic.,** ign., **lyss.,**
    mag-p.[2], nux-v., stry.

arrests the paroxysm
bruit arrête les paroxysmes, un
Geräusch unterbindet den Anfall
    hell.

odors, from strong
odeurs fortes, par
Gerüche, durch starke
    bruc.[4], **lyss.** (non[1]: sil., stram.,
    sulph.)

old age, in[10]
personnes âgées, chez les
Alter, im
    plb.

douleurs, pendant les
Schmerzen, während der
    ars.[11], **bell.,** coloc., ign., kali-c.,
    lyc., nux-v., plb-chr.[11]

renewed at every[2]
recrudescence de la douleur,
    à chaque
erneuert durch jeden Schmerz
    bell.

palpitation, after
palpitations, après
Herzklopfen, nach
    glon.

paralysis, with
paralysie, avec
Lähmung, mit
    arg-n., bell., **CAUST.,** cic., cocc.,
    cupr., **hyos.,** lach., laur., **nux-m.,**
    nux-v., phos., plat., **plb., rhus-t.,**
    sec., **stann., tab.,** vib., zinc.

*followed by see paralysis–
    convulsions*

paresis, followed by[8]
parésie, suivies par
Parese, gefolgt von
    acon., **elaps,** lon-x., plb.

parturition, during[8]
accouchement, pendant l'
Entbindung, während der
    acon.[4, 8], aeth., aml-ns., arn.,
    bell.[3, 4, 8], **canth.,** cham.[3, 4, 8], **chin.**[1'],
    chin-s.[3, 15], chlf.[2], **chlol., CIC.**[2, 3, 8],
    cimic.[3, 8, 15], cinnm.[2], cocc.[3],
    coff.[2, 4, 8], **cupr.**[2, 7, 8], **cupr-ar.,**
    gels., glon., **hydr-ac.**[8, 12],
    HYOS.[2, 3, 7, 8, 15], **IGN.**[3, 4, 8],
    ip.[3, 4, 8], **KALI-BR.**[2, 8], merc.,
    merc-d., mosch.[3], **oena.,** op.,
    pilo., **plat.**[2, 3, 4, 8], **sec.**[1', 6], sol-n.,
    spirae., stram.[3, 8], **VERAT-V.**[3, 8],
    zinc., ziz.[2, 8]

after[2]
après l'
nach der
   cupr.[7], **mill., plat.**

periodic
périodiques
periodische
   agar., ars., bar-m., calc., **cedr.,**
   chin.[2], chin-s., cupr., ign., indg.,
   lach.[2], lyc., nat-m., nux-v.[2], plb.[2],
   sec., stram., vip[3]

every 5 or 6 days[2]
tous les 5 ou 6 jours
alle 5 oder 6 Tage
   lyc.

   7 days/jours/Tage
      agar., chin-s., **indg., kali-br.[2],**
      nat-m.

   10 days[2]/jours/Tage
      kali-br.

   14 days/jours/Tage
      cupr., **kali-br.[2],** oena.

   15 or 20 days[2]/jours/Tage
      tarent.

   21 days[2]/jours/Tage
      camph.[1'], **cupr.[2], ferr.,** stram.,
      cupr., op.

perspiration during
transpiration pendant la
Schwitzen bei
   ars., **bell., BUFO,** camph.,
   nux-v., op., sep.

   cold
   froide
   kalter Schweiß
      camph.[1'], **cupr.[2], ferr.,** stram.,
      verat.[2]

   after/après la/nach
      acon., ars., **bry.[2],** cedr., cupr.,
      sec., stry.

pregnancy, during
grossesse, dans la
Schwangerschaft, in der
   acon.[8,] aeth.[8], aml-ns.[8], arn.[8],
   bell.[2, 3, 4, 8], canth.[3, 8], cast.[12], **cedr.,**
   cham., chlol.[3, 8], cic., cimic.[3, 8],
   cina[4, 11], coff.[8], croc.[3], **cupr.,**
   cupr-ar.[3, 8], gels.[2, 3, 8], glon[6, 8],
   hell.[3], **hydr-ac.[8], hyos.,** ign.[3, 8,]
   ip.[1', 2, 8], kali-br.[8], lyc., lyss.[8, 12],
   mag-c.[6], mag-m.[6], merc-c.[8], merc-d.[8],
   mill., mosch.[4], nux-m.[4], **oena.[2, 3, 8],**
   op.[3, 8], pilo.[8], pitu.[9], plat.[3, 4, 8,]
   rhus-t.[2], sec.[3], sol-n.[8], spirae.[8],
   stram.[3 4, 8], stry.[3], **verat-v.[2, 3, 8],**
   zinc.[3, 8]

pressure on a part, from
pression sur une partie du corps, par
Druck auf einen Körperteil, durch
   cic.

   on spine
   sur la colonne vertébrale
   auf die Wirbelsäule
      tarent.

   on stomach
   gastrique
   auf den Magen
      canth., cupr., cupr-a.[11], nux-v.

puberty, at
puberté, dans la
Pubertät, in der
   caul.[2, 6], caust., cupr.[1', 6], hypoth.[14],
   lach.[3], puls.[3, 6], zinc.[6], zinc-val.[3, 6]

puerperal
puerpérales
Kindbett, im
   acon.[2], ambr., **ant-c.[2],** ant-t.[2, 15],
   apis, **arg-n.,** arn.[2], ars., art-v.,
   atro.[2], BELL., benz-ac.[2], **CALC.[3]**
   canth., **carb-v.,** caul.[2], caust.,
   cham., chin.[3], chin-s.[2, 12], chlf.[2, 12],
   chlol.[2, 12], **CIC.,** cimic., cinnm.[2],
   cocc., coff., crot-c., **crot-h.[2], cupr.,**
   gels., glon., hell., helon.[2],
   hydr-ac., **HYOS., ign., ip., jab.[2],**
   KALI-BR.[2], KALI-C.[2, 3], kali-p.[2],
   lach., laur., lyc., lyss., mag-p.,

merc.², merc-c., mill.², ¹², mosch.,
nat-m.², nux-m., nux-v., oena.,
op., ph-ac.², ³, ¹², phos.¹, pilo.¹²,
plat., puls., sec., sol-n.¹²,
STRAM., sulph.³, ter., thyr.¹²,
verat., verat-v., zinc.

blindness, with
aveuglement, avec
Blindheit, mit
   aur-m., cocc., cupr.

haemorrhage, with
hémorrhagies, avec
Blutungen, mit
   chin., hyos., plat., sec.,

perspiration and fear, with⁷
transpiration et peur, avec
Schwitzen und Furcht, mit
   stram.

shrieking, with
cris, avec
Schreien, mit
   hyos., iod., lach.²

punishment, after
châtiments, après
Bestrafung, nach
   agar.¹', ⁷, cham., cina, cupr.⁷, IGN.

reproaches, from
reproches, par
Tadel, durch
   agar.¹' ⁶, ign.⁶

riding in a carriage am.
en voiture am.
Fahren am.
   nit-ac.

rubbing am.
massage am.
Reiben am.
   phos., sec., stry.⁷

running, after
courir, par
Laufen, durch
   sulph.

sexual excesses, from²
sexuels, par excès
sexuelle Exzesse, durch
   bufo², kali-br., phos.

excitement
excitation sexuelle
Erregung
   art-v.⁸, bar-c.³, bufo, calc.³, ⁸,
   KALI-BR.², lach., plat., stann.⁸,
   sulph.⁸, visc.³

shining objects, from
brillants, par les objets
glänzende Gegenstände, durch
   bell., LYSS., STRAM.

*bright light/lumière vive/helles
   Licht*

shock, after
choc, par un
Schock, durch einen
   aesc.¹', op.

shrieking, with²
cris, avec
Schreien, mit
   acon.⁴, aml-ns., ant-t.⁴, apis, art-v.,
   bell.⁴, calc.⁴, ⁶, camph., canth.⁴,
   caust.², ⁴, cedr., cic.², ⁴, ⁶, cina², ⁴,
   crot-h.², ⁴, cupr., HYOS.¹', ², ⁴, ign.,
   ip.², ⁴, lach.², ⁴, lyc.⁴, merc.², ⁴,
   nux-v.², ⁴, nit-ac., oena.⁶, OP.², ⁴, ⁶, ¹¹,
   stann., stram., sulph.², ⁴, verat-v.,
   vip.⁴, zinc.

sleep, during
sommeil, pendant le
Schlaf, im
   arg-n.⁶, bell.², ⁶, bufo, calc.⁴,
   caust., cham.⁶, cic., cina⁴, cocc.⁶,
   cupr., cupr-ar.⁶, gels.², hyos.,
   ign., kali-c., lach., mag-c.⁴, ⁶,
   merc.⁴, oena., op., puls.⁴, ⁶,
   rheum², rhus-t.⁴, ⁶, sec., sil.,
   stram., tarent.³, ⁶

loss of, after
manque de, par
Schlafmangel, durch
   COCC.¹

on going to[6]
avant de s'endormir
vor dem Einschlafen
   arg-m., sulph.

sleeplessness, with or after[3]
insomnie, avec ou après
Schlaflosigkeit, mit oder nach
   alum., art-v.[2], bell., bry., calc.,
   carb.-an., carb-v., cic.[2], cupr.,
   cypr.[2], hep., hyos.[3, 4], ign., ip.,
   KALI-BR.[2], kali-c., merc., mosch.,
   nux-v., passi.[6], ph-ac., phos., puls.,
   rheum, rhus-t., sel., sep., sil.,
   stront-c., thuj., verbe-h.[6], zinc.[6],
   zinc-val.[6]

small pox fails to break out, when
petites véroles qui ne « sortent » pas,
   à l'occasion de
Pocken nicht herauskommen, wenn
   ANT-T.

speak, on attempting to
parler, en essayant de
sprechen, beim Versuch zu
   lyss.

strange person, sight of
étrange, à la vue d'une personne
Fremden, beim Anblick eines
   lyss., op., tarent.[6]

stretching out parts am.
s'étirer am.
Ausstrecken der befallenen Teile am.
   sec.

   of limbs before c.
   des membres avant les c.
   der Glieder vor den K.
      calc.

      during c.[16]
      pendant les c.
      während der K.
         bell.

sudden
subites
plötzliche
   ars.[6], bell.[2, 8], hydr-ac.[6], mez.[6],
   oena.[6], stry., verat-v.[2]

suppressed discharges, from
supprimés, par écoulements
Unterdrückung von Absonderungen,
   durch
      asaf., cupr., stram.

eruption
éruptions
Hautausschlägen
   agar., ant-c.[2], bry., calc., camph.[2],
   caust., cupr., cupr-a.[2], hyos.[2],
   ip.[2], kali-m.[2], psor.[8], stram.,
   sulph., urt-u.[2], zinc.

footsweat, after
transpiration des pieds, par
   suppression de la
Fußschweiß, durch U. von
   SIL.

mother milk
lactation supprimée
Muttermilch, der
   agar.

perspiration[6]
transpiration supprimée, par
Schweiß, durch U. von
   sil.

secretions and excretions
sécrétions et excretions
Sekretionen und Exkretionen, von
   stram.

suppuration, during
suppuration, au cours de la
Eiterung, bei
   ars., bufo, canth., lach., tarent.

swallow, during attempt to
avaler, en essayant d'
schlucken, beim Versuch zu
   LYSS., mur-ac., nux-m., nux-v.[11],
   stram.

swing, letting legs, exites c.
balancement des jambes excite les c.,
   le
Pendeln der Beine erregt K.
   calc.

syphilitic
syphilis, au cours de
Syphilis, bei
    aur.[2], iod.[2], **kali-br.**[2, 8], **KALI-I.**[2],
    merc-c[2], mez.[2], **nit-ac.**

tetanic rigidity
tétanique, rigidité
tetanische Starre, Starrkrampf
    abel.[14], absin., acet-ac.[11], **acon.**,
    aconin.[12], aesc., agar-ph.[11], agre.[14],
    alum., **am-c., am-m.**[3], **aml-ns.**[2],
    amyg.[2, 11, 12], **anac., ang.**[2, 3, 4, 6, 12],
    ant-t.[2], aran-ix.[14], **arn., ars.,** asaf.,
    atro.[2, 12], **bell.,** ben-n.[11, 12], both.[11],
    bruc.[4], bry.[3, 4], **calc.**[3, 6, 7, 10],
    calc-f.[14], calc-p.[3, 6], **calen.**[6, 12],
    camph., cann-i., cann-s., **canth.,**
    carbn.[12], carbn-h.[12], carbn-o.,
    carbn-s.[12], **cast.**[2, 12], caust., **cham.,**
    chin-s., chlf.[12], **chlol., CIC.,**
    cic-m.[12], cimic.[3], cina[3], **cocc.,**
    con., cori-m.[11], cortico.[9],
    crot-h.[2, 12], **cupr.,** cupr-a.[10]
    cupr-ar., **cur.,** dig.[3, 6], dros.,
    dulc.[11], **gels.,** grat.[4, 12], **hell.,**
    hep., **hydr-ac., hyos., HYPER.,**
    ign., ip., jasm.[11, 12], juni.[12],
    kali-bi.[11], **kali-br.**[2, 12], kali-c.[3],
    kali-cy.[11], kali-n.[11], kreos.,
    kres.[10], **lach., laur., led.,** linu-c.[11],
    lob., lyc., lyss., mag-c.[3, 10],
    mag-m.[14], **mag-p.,** meph.[14],
    merc., methys.[14], **mill.**[2, 12],
    morph.[11, 12], **mosch.,** mur-ac.,
    nat-f.[14], nicot.[12], nux-m.[3],
    NUX-V., oena., ol-an.[3], **OP.,**
    ox-ac.[12], passi.[8, 12], **PETR.,** phos.,
    phys., phyt., PLAT., plb., puls.,
    pyre-p.[7], rhod., **rhus-t**[1], santin[12],
    scor.[11, 12], **sec.,** seneg.,**SEP.,**
    sium[12], sol-c.[12], **sol-n.,** solin[12],
    stann.[3, 6], **stram., stry.,** stry-p.[6],
    sul-ac.[11], sul-h.[12], sulph., tab.[12],
    tanac.[11], **ter.**[2, 12], teucr., **ther.,**
    thyr.[12], upa.[7, 8, 12], valer.[3], verat.,
    verat-v., verin.[12], vib-p.[12], zinc.

dashing cold water on face am.
asperger de l'eau froide sur la
    figure am.
Bespritzen des Gesichtes mit
    kaltem Wasser am.
    ben-n.

injured parts become cold as ice
    and spasms begin in the wound
les parties traumatisées deviennent
    froides comme la glace et les
    spasmes débutent dans la plaie
verletzte Teile werden eiskalt und
    die Krämpfe beginnen in der
    Wunde
    LED.

traumatic[2]
traumatiques
traumatische
    acon., **arn.**[2, 7], **chlol., cic., cur.,**
    hell., hydr-ac., HYPER., nux-v.,
    stram.[7], tetox.[7], teucr.[12]

trismus, with[2]
trismus, avec
Trismus, mit
    ant-t., bell., cupr-a., oena., stram.,
    verat-v.

wiping perspiration from face agg.
essuyer la transpiration du visage
    agg.
Abwischen des Gesichtsschweißes
    agg.
    nux-v.

wounds in the soles, finger or
    palm
plaies plantaires, palmaires ou des
    doigts
Wunden an Sohlen, Fingern oder
    Handtellern, durch
    bell., HYPER., led.

thunderstorm
orage, pendant l'
Gewitter, bei
    agar., **gels.**

tight grasp am.
maintien serré am., un
fester Griff am.
  nux-v.

tightly binding the body am.
bandage serré du corps am., un
festes Binden des Körpers am.
  mez.

tonic
toniques
tonische
  acon., agar., alum., alum-p.[1'],
  alum-sil.[1'], am-c., am-m., ambr.[3, 6],
  anac., **ANG.**[3, 6], ant-t., apis, arg-m.,
  arn., ars.[3], asaf., asar., **BELL.**, bor.,
  bry., **BUFO, calc.**, camph., cann-s.,
  canth., caps., carbn-o., **caust.**,
  cham., chin., chlf.[2], **CIC.**, cina, clem.,
  cocc., coloc., con., cupr., **cur.**[3, 6],
  cycl., dig., **dros.**[3], dulc., euph., **ferr.**,
  ferr-ar., graph., guaj., hell.[3],
  hep., hydr-ac.[2], hyos., **hyper.**[3, 6],
  ign., ip., kali-c., lath.[6], laur., led.,
  lyc., mag-p., mang., med.[2], meny.,
  merc., mez., **mosch.**, nat-c., nat-m.,
  nit-ac., nux-v., olnd., op., **PETR.**,
  ph-ac., **phos., phys.**[3, 6], phyt.[3, 6],
  PLAT., plb., puls., rhod., rhus-t.,
  sabad., sars., **sec.**, seneg., **SEP.**, sil.,
  spig., spong., stann., **stram.**, stry.[3],
  stry-s.[6], sumb., **sulph.**, tab.[3, 6], thuj.,
  verat., verat-v.[6], visc.[9], zinc.,
  zinc-p.[1']

tooth extraction, after[7]
extraction dentaire, après
Zahnextraktion, nach
  bufo

touched, when
touche, quand on le
Berührung, bei
  acon., **bell.**, carbn-o., **CIC.**, cocc.,
  lyss., mag-p.[2], nux-v., stram., stry.

turning the head
tournant la tête, en
Drehen des Kopfes, beim
  cic.

in bed[11]
au lit
im Bett
  chen-a.

unjustly accused, after being
injustes, après des accusations
Unrecht beschuldigt, wenn zu
  staph.[1,7]

mortification/Kränkung

uraemic
urémiques
urämische
  apis[3], apoc., ars.[3], **carb-ac.**[8], chlf.[15],
  cic.[8], crot-h., **cupr.**, cupr-ar., **dig.**,
  glon.[8], hell.[8], hydr-ac., **KALI-BR.**[2, 8],
  kali-s., merc-c., **mosch.**, oena.[8],
  op.[8], pilo.[8, 12], **plb.**, stram.[7], **ter.**,
  urt-u.[8, 12], **verat-v.**[3]

vaccination, after
vaccination, par
Vakzination, nach
  SIL., thuj.[8]

vexation, after
contrariété, par
Ärger, durch
  agar.[6], ars., bell., **calc.**, camph.,
  cham.[6], **CUPR., ign., ip.**, nux-v.,
  staph.[1, 7], sulph., verat.[6], zinc.[6]

anger/colère/Zorn

vomiting, during
vomissement, pendant le
Erbrechen, bei
  aeth.[6, 8], **ant-c.**[2], **CUPR.**[2], guar.,
  ip.[2], oena.[2], op., upa.[8]

  am.
    agar.

waking, on
réveil, au
Erwachen, beim
  bell., lyss.[2], **ign.**[2]

warm bath agg.
bain chaud agg.
warmes Bad agg.
   apis, glon., nat-m., op.

warm room, in[1']
chambre chaud, dans une
Zimmerwärme, bei
   op.

water, at sight of
eau, à la vue de l'
Wasser, beim Anblick von
   bell., LYSS., STRAM.

waving of arms[9]
agitation des bras, avec
Fuchteln der Arme, mit
   cyt-l.

weakness, during
faiblesse, au cours de
Schwäche, bei
   hura[11], kali-c.[6]

   weakness-c./faiblesse-c./
   Schwäche-K.

   nervous
   nerveuse
   nervöser
      sep.

wet, from becoming
mouillant, en se
Naßwerden, durch
   calc., cupr., rhus-t.

worms, from
vers, par
Würmer, durch
   art-v.[2], asaf.[4], bar-m.[2], bell.[2], cham.[2],
   cic.[2, 8], CINA, cupr.[6], cupr-o.[6],
   hyos., ign., indg.[2, 6, 8], kali-br.[6, 8],
   sabad., santin.[8], sil., spig.[8], stann.,
   stram.[2], sulph.[8], tanac.[8], ter.,
   teucr.[8]

yawning
baillant, en
Gähnen, beim
   graph.

CONVULSIVE movements
CONVULSIFS, mouvements
KRAMPFARTIGE Bewegungen
   acon., agar., alum., alum-p.[1'], ang.[3],
   ant-t., apis, arg-n., arn., ars., ars-i.,
   asaf., bar-c., bar-i.[1'], BELL., brom.[3],
   bry., bufo, cact., calc., calc-i.[1'],
   camph., cann-s., canth., caust.,
   CHAM., chin-s., CIC., cina, COCC.,
   coff., con., croc., CUPR., cupr-ar.,
   dig., dulc., hell., HYOS., IGN., iod.,
   IP., kali-ar., lach., laur., lyc.,
   m-arct.[3], mag-p., meny., merc.,
   mosch., mygal., nat-c., nux-m.,
   nux-v., olnd., OP., phyt.[3], plb., petr.,
   ph-ac., phos., plat., ran-b.[3], ran-s.,
   rheum, rhus-t., ruta, sabad., samb.,
   SEC., spig., spong., squil., stann.,
   staph., STRAM., sulph., tab.[3],
   tarent., verat., zinc.

beginning in extremities[3]
commençant dans les membres
beginnen in den Gliedern
   verat.

face[3]
face, dans la
Gesicht, im
   dulc.

COPPER fumes agg.
CUIVRE, agg. par des vapeurs de
KUPFERDÄMPFE agg.
   camph., ip., lyc., merc., nux-v., op.,
   puls.

vessels of, agg.[7]
récipient de, agg.
Kupfergefäße agg.
   hep.

CORYZA am. general symptoms[3, 7]
CORYZA am. symptômes généraux
SCHNUPFEN am. Allgemeinsymptome
   thuj.

suppressed c. agg.[3]
supprimé agg.
unterdrückter agg.
   acon.[2], am-c., **am-m.**, ambr., ars.,
   BRY., calad., **CALC.**, carb-v., caust.,
   cham., **chin.**[3, 12], cina, con., **dulc.**[3, 6],
   fl-ac., graph., hep., ip., **kali-bi.**[3, 6],
   kali-c., kreos., **LACH.**[2, 3, 6], laur.,
   lyc., mag-c., mag-m., mang., merc.,
   mill.[6], nat-c., nat-m., **nit-ac.**, nux-m.,
   NUX-V., par., petr., phos., **puls.**,
   rhod., sabad., samb., sars., **sep.**,
   sil., spig., spong., stann., stram.,
   sul-ac., **sulph.**[3, 6], teucr., thuj.,
   verat., zinc.

COVERS agg., intolerance of [3, 6]
COUVERTURES agg., intolérance des
BETTDECKEN agg., werden nicht
ertragen
   acon., aloe, **apis**, asar., **camph.**,
   cham., ferr., ign.[3], **iod.**, kali-i., led.,
   med.[7], merc.[16], mur-ac., op., phos.,
   puls., rhus-t., **sec.**, **sulph.**, tab.[3],
   verat.

*clothing-intolerance/vêtements-
   intolérance/Kleidung – nicht
   ertragen
   warm-wraps/chaud-habits/Wärme-
   Umhüllung*

am. and desire for[3, 6]
am. et désir de
am. und Verlangen nach
   ars., aur., bell.[6], clem., colch., **hep.**,
   nux-v., **puls.**, rhus-t., **samb.**, sil.,
   squil., **stront-c.**, tub.[3]

aversion to[3]
aversion pour
Abneigung gegen
   calc-s., camph., led., sec.

kicks off[6]
repousse
stößt B. weg
   BRY.[7], camph., **cham.**, iod.

in coldest weather[7]
quand il fait très froid
bei kältestem Wetter
   hep., sanic., sulph.

CRAMPS of muscles (1897)
CRAMPES musculaires
MUSKELKRÄMPFE
   acon., agar., alum., am-c., am-m.,
   ambr., **ANAC.**, **ANG.**[3], arg-m., **arn.**,
   ars., asaf., asar., aur., bar-c., **BELL.**,
   bism., bor., bov.[3], bry., bufo[3],
   CALC., camph., **cann-s.**, caps.,
   carb-an., carb-v., carbn-s.[11], **cast.**[2],
   caust., cham., chin., cic., cimic.[3, 6],
   CINA, clem., **cocc.**, colch., **coloc.**,
   con., croc., cupr., dig., dios., dros.,
   dulc., euph., **euphr.**, ferr., gels.,
   glon., **graph.**, hell., hep., hyos., **ign.**,
   iod., ip., **iris**[2], jab., **kali-br.**[2], **kali-c.**,
   kali-n., kreos., lach., **LYC.**, mag-c.,
   mag-m., **mag-p.**[3, 6], mang., meny.,
   MERC., mez., mosch., **mur-ac.**,
   nat-c., nat-m., **nit-ac.**, nux-m.,
   nux-v., olnd., **op.**[2, 3, 6], par., **petr.**,
   ph-ac., phos., phyt.[3, 6], **plat.**, **plb.**,
   puls.[3, 6], ran-b., rheum[3], rhod.,
   rhus-t., ruta, sabad., samb., sang.[3],
   sec., **SEP.**, **SIL.**, **spig.**, **spong.**, squil.,
   stann., staph., stram., stront-c.,
   sul-ac., **SULPH.**, tab.[2, 3, 6], **thuj.**,
   valer., verat., **verb.**, vib., viol-o.,
   viol-t., zinc.

night on waking[16]
nuit au réveil
nachts beim Erwachen
   sulph.

CROSSING of limbs agg.[3]
CROISER les membres agg.
KREUZEN der Glieder agg.
   agar., alum., ang., arn., **asaf.**, aur.,
   bell., bry., **dig.**, kali-n., laur., lyc.,
   mur-ac., nux-v., phos., plat., rad.,
   rheum, rhod., **rhus-t.**, squil., valer.,
   verb.

am.[3]
   abrot., ant-t., rhod., **SEP.**

CYANOSIS
CYANOSE
ZYANOSE

absin.[11], acetan.[12], acon., agar., alum., **am-c.**, amyg.[11], ang.[3], anil.[11], **ant-ar.**[6], ant-c., **ant-t., arg-n.**, arn., **ars.**, asaf., asar., aur., bar-c., **bell.**, ben-n.[11, 12], bism., both.[11], bry., calc., calc-p.[3], **CAMPH.**, canth.[3], carb-an., **CARB-V.**, carbn-o.[11,] caust., cedr., cham., chel., chin., chin-ar., cic., cina, cocc., cod.[11], **con., crot-h**[6], **CUPR.**, cupr-ar.[6], **DIG.**, dros., ferr., glon.[3, 11], hep., **hydr.-ac.**[6, 11], hyos., ign., iod.[3], **ip.**, kali-c.[3], **kali-chl.**, kali-n.[11], **LACH., LAUR.**, led., lyc., mang., merc., merc-c.[3], meth-ae-ae.[11], mez.[3], mosch., mur-ac., **naja**, nat-m., nat-ns.[12], nit-ac., nux-m., nux-v., **OP.**, ox-ac.[3, 6], petr.[11], ph-ac., phenac.[12], phos., phyt.[3], plb., puls., ran-b., **rhust-t.**, ruta, sabad., **samb.**, santin.[11], sars., **sec.**, seneg., sil., spong., staph., stram., stry.[11], sul-ac., sulfon.[12], sulph., thuj., **VERAT., VERAT-V.**[3, 6], vip[11], xan., zinc.[3]

fever, during[11]
fièvre, pendant la
Fieber, bei
arund., crot-h.

infants, in
petits entfants, chez les
Kleinkindern, bei
arn., ars., **bor., cact., camph., carb-v.**, chin., **DIG., LACH., LAUR., naja**, op., **phos.**, psor., rhus-t., sec., sulph.

DARKNESS agg.[3]
OBSCURITÉ agg.
DUNKELHEIT agg.

acon., **am-m.**, anac., ang., arg-n.[3], **ars.**[3, 8], bar-c., **CALC.**[3, 8], camph., **cann-s., carb-an.**[3, 8], **carb-v.**[3], caust.[3], con., **gels.**[3], **lyc.**[3], nat-m., phos.[8], **plat., PLB.**, puls.[3], **rhus-t.**, staph., **STRAM.**[3, 6, 8], **stront-c.**, sul-ac., valer.[3], zinc.[6]

am[2, 3]

acon.[2, 3, 6], agar., agn.[3], am-c., **am-m., anac.**, anh.[9, 14], **ant-c.**, arn., **ars., asar.**, bar-c., **bell.**[2, 3, 6, 7], **bor.**, bry., **CALC.**[2, 3, 6], camph., carb-an., **caust., cham., chin.**[2, 3, 6], cic., **cina, clem.**, coc-c.[2], coca[8], cocc.[3], **coff.**, colch., **CON.**[2, 3, 8], croc., dig., dros., **EUPHR.**[2, 3, 6, 8], **GRAPH.**[2, 3, 6, 8], **hell., hep.**, **hyos.**[2, 3, 6], **ign.**, kali-c., kali-n., lach., **laur., lyc.**, mag-c., **mag-m.**, **mang., merc.**, mez., mur-ac., **nat-c.**, nat-m., **nit-ac.**, nux-m., **nux-v.**, petr., **ph-ac., PHOS.**[2, 3, 8], **puls.**, rhod., rhus-t., ruta, **sang.**[8], **sars.**, sel., **seneg., sep.**[2, 3], **sil.**[2, 3], **spig.**, staph., **stram., sulph.**, tarax.[3], tarent.[2], thuj., valer., verat., zinc.

DEATH APPARENT; asphyxia (1897)
MORT APPARENTE, état de; asphyxie
SCHEINTOD, drohende Erstickung

acet-ac., acon.[3], ant-t., arn., **bell.**, **carb-v., carbn-s.**[2], chin., **cochl.**[2], **coff.**, coloc., crot-h.[4], hydr-ac.[4], laur., merc., nit-ac., **op.**, ph-ac., phos., **rhus-t.**[2], sin-n.[2], stram., sul-h.[12], tab.[2]

carbon monoxide, poisonning from[4]
carbone, empoisonnement par
monoxyde de
Kohlenmonoxyd, Vergiftung durch
acon., bell., op.

coal gas/gaz/Gasvergiftung

drowned persons, of[4]
noyés, des
Ertrunkenen, bei
lach.

frozened persons, of[4]
gelées, des personnes
Erfrorenen, bei
acon., ars., bry., carb-v.

haemorrhages, after[4]
hémorrhagies, après
Blutungen, nach
chin.

hanged, strangled persons, of[4]
pendues, étranglées, des personnes
Erhängten, Erdrosselten, bei
op.

injuries, after[4]
traumatismes, après
Verletzungen, nach
arn.

lightning-stroke, after[4]
coup de foudre, après
Blitzschlag, nach
lach., nux-v.

neonatorum, asphyxia
nouveau-nés, asphyxie des
Neugeborenen, der
acon., am-c.[3, 6, 8], **ant-t., arn.,**
bell.[3, 6], **CAMPH.,** chin., crot-h.[3, 6],
hydr-ac.[3, 6, 8], hyos.[3, 6], **laur.,**
op., sul-h.[8], upa.[8], vip.[3, 6]

DEBAUCH, agg. **during**[3]
DÉBAUCHE, agg. **pendant** une
AUSSCHWEIFUNG, Schlemmerei, agg.
während einer
acon., bell., **op.**

after a, agg.[3]
après une, agg.
nach einer, agg.
acon., agar., **am-m.,** ang., **ant-c.**[3, 6],
arg-m., ars.[6], bell., **bry.**[3, 6], calc.,
CARB-V.[3, 6], chin., cocc., **coff.**[3, 6],
dulc., **ip.**[3, 6], kali-c., kali-n., kreos.,
lach.[3], **laur.,** nat-c.[3, 6], nat-m.,
nit-ac., nux-m., **NUX-V.**[1', 3, 6, 7],
OP., ph-ac., phos., **puls.**[3, 6], rheum,
rhus-t., samb., sars.[1'], **spong.,** squil.,
staph.[6], **stram.,** sul-ac.[3], sulph.[3, 6],
teucr., valer.

ailments from[12]
troubles à la suite d'une
Beschwerden infolge von
arg-n., carb-v., dig., nux-v., sel.

eating–overeating/manger–
se gaver/Essen–Überessen

feeling as after[11]
sensation d'avoir fait la bombe
Gefühl wie nach einer
caj., conin., kreos., lyc., op., ox-ac.

DENTITION, difficult*
DENTITION difficile
DENTITIO difficilis
ACON.[2, 3, 8, 12], aeth.[2, 8, 12], am-c.[3],
ant-c.[2], ant-t.[2], apis[2], arn[2],
ARS[2, 3], arund.[12], bell.[2, 3, 8], bism.[2],
BOR.[2, 3, 8, 12], bry.[2, 3, 12], CALC.,
calc-f.[10], CALC-P., canth.[2],
caust.[2, 8, 12], CHAM., cheir.[8], chlol.[2],
chlor.[12], cic., cimic[12], cina[2, 3, 12],
coff.[2, 3, 7, 8, 12], colch.[2, 3], coloc.[2],
cupr., dol.[2, 12], dulc.[2], ferr.[2, 3],
ferr-p.[2, 6], gels.[2, 6, 8, 12], graph[2],
hecla[8, 12], hell.[2], hep., hyos.[2], ign.,
ip[2, 3], kali-br.[8], kreos., lyc.[2],
mag-c.[2, 3], MAG-M.[2, 3, 12],
mag-p.[2, 8, 10, 12], meli.[2], merc.[2, 3, 8, 12],
merc-c.[3], mill.[12], nat-m.[12], nit-ac.[3],
nux-m.[2, 3], NUX-V.[2, 3, 8], op.[3],
passi.[8, 12], phys.[2, 12], phyt., plat.[12],
plect.[12], podo., psor[2], puls.[3, 8],
rheum, rhus-t.[2, 3], scut.[12], sec., sep.,
SIL., sol-n.[8], stann., STAPH.[2, 8, 12],
stram.[2, 3], sul-ac.[2], SULPH.[2, 3, 8],
syph.[12], ter.[8, 12], til.[12], tub.[3], tub-k.[12],
verat.[2], zinc.[2, 3, 8, 12], zinc-br.[8, 12]

convulsions–d./Konvulsionen–
Zahnen
weakness – d./faiblesse – d./
Schwäche – Zahnen

Vol. III: *sleeplessness–d./*
insomnie–d./Schlaflosigkeit–
Zahnung

ailments from[12]
troubles à la suite de
Beschwerden infolge von
cham., mag-c., mag-p., rheum,
stann., staph.

wisdom teeth
dents de sagesse, des
Weisheitszähnen
calc., cheir., ferr-pic.[7], fl-ac.,
mag-c., SIL.[1, 7]

diarrhoea, with
diarrhée, avec
Durchfall, mit
  acet-ac.[8], **acon., aeth., apis,** apoc.[6, 7],
  arg-n., ars., arund.[8], **bell.,** benz-ac.,
  bor., CALC., calc-a.[8], **calc-p.,** canth.,
  carb-v., **CHAM.,** chin., **cina, coff.,**
  colch., **coloc.,** corn., cupr., **DULC.,**
  FERR., ferr.-ar., **gels.,** graph., hell.,
  hep., ign., **ip.,** jal.[8], **kreos., mag-c.,**
  mag-p.[2], **merc.,** nux-m., olnd.[8],
  ph-ac., **phyt.**[2, 8], **podo., psor.,**
  RHEUM, sep., **SIL.,** sul-ac., **sulph.,**
  zinc.

  slow
  lente
  langsame Zahnung
    aster.[14], **CALC.,** calc-f.[6], **CALC-P.,**
    fl-ac., mag-c., mag-m., merc.[6],
    nep.[14], phos.[6], **SIL.,** sulfa.[14], **sulph.**[6],
    thuj.[6], **tub.**[7]

DESCENDING agg.
DESCENTE agg., mouvement de
ABWÄRTSBEWEGUNG agg.
  acon., alum., am-m., **arg-m.,** bar-c.,
  bell., berg[3], **BOR.,** bry., canth.,
  carb-v.[3], **coff., con., ferr.,** GELS.[3, 8],
  lyc., meny., nit-ac., phys.[3], plb.,
  rhod., rhus-t., **ruta,** sabin., sanic.[3, 8],
  sep.[3], **stann.**[1, 7], stram.[3], sulph.,
  verat., verb.

  am.[2]
    acon., alumn., am-c., anac., **ang.,**
    ant-c., **arg-m.,** arn., **ARS.,** asar.,
    aur., bar-c., bell., **bor., BRY.,** calc.,
    cann-s., canth., carb-v., caust.,
    chin., coff., **cupr.,** dig., dros., **euph.,**
    graph., hell., hep., **hyos., ign.,**
    kali-c., **kali-n., lach.,** led., **lyc.,**
    mag-c., mag-m., **meny., merc.,**
    mosch., mur-ac., **nat-c.,** nat-m.,
    nit-ac., nux-m., **nux-v., par., petr.,**
    ph-ac., phos., plat., plb., ran-b.,
    rhus-t., ruta, sabad., **seneg., sep.,**
    sil., **spig.,** SPONG.[2, 8], **squil., stann.,**
    staph., sul-ac., **sulph., tarax., thuj.,**
    verb., **zinc.**

DEVELOPMENT, arrested[3]
ENTWICKLUNGSSTILLSTAND
ENTWICKLUNGSHEMMUNG
  agar., bac.[8], **bar-c.**[1, 3, 8], bor.[1], **calc.**[8],
  CALC-P.[3, 8], caust.[8], chin., cupr.[11],
  des-ac.[14], kali-c., kreos.[8], lac-d.[8],
  med.[8], nat-m.[1, 3, 8], nep.[14], ph-ac.[3, 8],
  phos., pin-s.[8], **sil.**[3, 8], sulfa.[14], sulph.,
  thyr., vip.[11]

DIARHOEA am.
DIARRHÉE am.
DIARRHOE am.
  abrot.[1], bry.[7], nat-s.[1], ph-ac.[1, 7],
  zinc.

  yellow am.[9]
  jaune am.
  gelbfarbene am.
    saroth.

DISCHARGES am.[3]
ÉCOULEMENT am.
ABSONDERUNGEN,
  Ausscheidungen am.
  ars., **bry.**[3, 6], calc., camph., cimic.[3, 6],
  cupr.[6], dulc.[6], graph.[6], ip., **LACH.**[3, 6, 8],
  lyc., mosch.[6, 8], nux-v.[3, 6], ph-ac.,
  PULS.[3, 6], rhus-t., sep.[3, 6], sil., stann.[8],
  SULPH.[3, 6], thuj.[6], verat., zinc.[3, 6, 8]

DISTENTION blood vessels
DISTENTION des vaisseaux sanguins
ERWEITERUNG der Blutgefäße
  acon., aesc.[3], agar., alum., alum-p.[1],
  alum-sil.[1], **am-c.,** ambr.[3], ant-t.[3],
  apoc.[1], **arn.,** ars., aur.[3], aur-m.[7],
  aur-s.[1], **bar-c., bar-m.,** bar-s.[1],
  BELL., bov.[3], bry., calc., calc-f.,
  calc-sil.[1], **camph., carb-v., carbn-s.,**
  caust.[3], celt.[11], **chel., CHIN.,**
  chin-ar., **chin-s.,** cic., clem.[3],
  cocc.[3], coloc., con., **croc.,** cycl., dig.,
  FERR., ferr-ar., ferr-i.[1], ferr-p.,
  fl-ac.[3], **graph., ham.,** hep.[3], **HYOS.,**
  kreos.[3], **lac-d.**[7], lach., laur.[3], **led.,**
  lil-t.[3], lyc., mag-c.[3], meny., merl.,
  mosch., nat-c.[3], nat-m., nit-ac.[1],

nux-v., olnd., op., ph-ac., **phos.,**
pilo.[11], **plb., podo., PULS.,** rheum[3],
rhod., rhus-t., ruta[3], sars., sec., sel.[3],
sep., sil., spig., **spong.,** staph.,
stront-c., sul-ac.[3], **sulph., THUJ.,**
vip., zinc.

evening
soir
abends
PULS.

fever, during
fièvre, pendant la
Fieber, im
agar., bell., camph., **CHIN.,** chin-s.,
HYOS., LED., PULS.

motion, on[16]
mouvement, au
Bewegung, durch
spong.

DOUBLING UP of the body[3, 6]
PLIÉ EN DEUX, corps
ZUSAMMENKRUMMEN des Körpers
acon.[3], aloe[3], ant-t., **ars., calc.[3],**
caps.[3], caust., cham.[3], chin., cimic.,
cocc., coloc., dros.[3], graph.[3],
kali-c.[3], li-t.[11], lyc.[3], mag-c.[3], mag-p.,
merc-c.[3], pareir.[3], plb.[3], puls.[3],
rheum[3], rhus-t., sabin., sec., **sep.[3],**
sin-n.[11], sulph., thuj.[3]

bending-double/plier-en deux/
Sichbiegen – Sichkrümmen
bent holding/parties pliées/Beuge-
haltung

DRAWING UP the limb, flexing **agg.[3]**
REMONTÉ, fléchi **agg.,** membre
ANZIEHEN des Gliedes **agg.**
agar., alum., am-m., anac., **ant-t.,**
asar., bell., bor., carb-an., carb-v.,
cham., chel., chin., coff., dig., dros.,
dulc., ferr., guaj., hep., ign.,
kali-c., mag-c., merc., mur-ac.,
nat-m., nux-m., nux-v., olnd., par.,
petr., plat., puls., rheum, rhod.,

RHUS-T., sabad., sabin., **SEC.,**
stann., staph., thuj., verb., zinc.

am.
alum., am-c., am-m., anac., ang.,
ant-c., arg-m., arn., aur., bar-c.,
bell., bov., **bry., CALC.,** cann-s.,
caps., carb-v., caust., cham., **chin.,**
cina, clem., **coloc.[6],** con., croc.,
crot-h.[3, 6], dig., dros., dulc., ferr.,
graph., guaj., **hep.[3, 6],** ign., kali-c.,
lach.[3, 6], laur., lyc., **mang., meny.,**
merc., mur-ac., nat-m., nux-v.,
petr., phos., plat., plb., puls., rheum,
rhus-t., **ruta,** sabin., sel., **SEP.[3, 6, 8],**
sil.[3, 6], spig., spong., stann., staph.,
SULPH.[3, 8], THUJ.[3, 8], valer., verat.

DRINKING agg.[3]
BOIRE agg.
TRINKEN agg.
acon.[2], **aeth.[3, 6],** anac., **arg-n.[3],**
ars.[3], aur.[2], **bell.[3, 7, 8], bry., CALC.[3],**
CANTH.[3], caps.[3], cham., **chin.[3],**
cina[3, 6], cocc.[2, 3, 4], colch., coloc.[3],
con.[3], **crot-t.[3, 6],** cupr., dig.[2],
eup-per.[6], ferr.[3, 6], gink-b.[14], grat.[6],
hell.[4], **hyos.[3, 4, 6],** ign., **IOD.[3],**
kali-c.[3], **LACH.,** laur., med.[2],
merc.[2, 3], merc-c.[3], nat-ar.[2], nat-m.,
nux-v.[3, 6], phos., phyt., podo.[3],
puls.[2], rhus-r.[3], rhus-t., sabad.,
sabin., **sel.[2],** sep., **sil.[3],** squil.,
stann.[3], stram.[3, 6], sul-ac.[3], **verat.[3]**

after d. agg.[3]
après avoir bu agg.
nach dem T. agg.
acon., ambr., anac., ang., ant-t.,
arn., **ARS.,** asaf., asar., aur., **bell.,**
bry., cann-s., **canth.,** caps.,
CARB-V., caust., cham., **chin.,**
cic., cina, **cocc.,** colch., coloc.,
con., **croc.,** cupr., dros., **ferr.,**
graph., hell., **hep.,** hyos., ign., ip.,
kali-c., lach., laur., lyc., **MERC.,**
mez., mosch., mur-ac., **NAT-C.,**
nat-m., nit-ac., **NUX-V.,** op., petr.,
ph-ac., phos., plb., **PULS.,** rhod.,
rhus-t., ruta, sabad., sabin., sec.,
sel., sep., **SIL.,** spig., squil.,

staph., stram., **SUL-AC.**[3, 6],
SULPH., tarax., teucr., thuj.,
verat.

am.[3, 6]
acon., alum.[3], bapt.[3], bar-c.[3],
bism.[3], brom.[3], **bry.**[3], carb-an.[3],
CAUST., cist., coc-c.[3], crot-h.[3],
cupr.[3], ferr.[3], graph.[3], ip.[3],
lac-c.[3], lob., lyc.[3], mosch.[3],
nat-m.[3], nit-ac.[3], nux-v.[3], olnd.[3],
phos., psil.[14], psor., rhus-t.[3], sep.[3],
sil., spig.[3], **spong.**[3], sulph.[3],
tarax.[3]

aversion to drink in spite of thirst[6]
aversion de b. malgré la soif
Abneigung, zu t. trotz Durst
cann-i., canth., stram.

rapid, hasty, agg.[3, 6]
hâtivement agg., b.
schnelles T. agg.
ars., **hell.**[6], hep.[6], ip., nat-m.,
NIT-AC., nux-v., SIL., sulph.,
verat.[6]

DROPSY from **abuse of quinine**[8]
HYDROPISIE par l'**abus de quinine**
WASSERSUCHT durch **Chinin-**
mißbrauch
apoc.

albuminuria, with[2]
albuminurie, avec
Albuminurie, mit
AUR-M.[1, 2]**, chin., eup-pur., helon.,**
hep.

alcoholism, from[8]
alcoolisme, par
Alkoholismus, durch
ars., fl-ac.[1, 8], sulph.

eruption, from suppressed[2]
éruption supprimée, par
Hautausschlag, durch unterdrückten
APIS, apoc., **ars.,** asc-c., dig., dulc.[8],
hell., sulph.

exanthema, from suppressed[3]
exanthème supprimé, par
Exanthem, durch unterdrücktes
apis[8], ars., hell.[3, 8], rhus-t., sulph.,
zinc.[8]

external
externe
äußere
abel.[14], acet-ac., acetan.[8],
acon.[3, 8], adon.[3, 6], adren.[6], aeth.[2],
aether[8], agar., alco.[11], all-c.[2],
am-be.[6], am-c.[3], ambr.[3, 6],
ammc.[2]**, anac-oc.**[2]**, anag.**[2],
ANT-C., ant-t., anthraci.[2], **APIS,**
apoc., arn.[8], **arg-n.**[1, 2]**, ARS.,**
ars-i., **ARS-S-F.**[2]**, asaf.**[2]**, asc-c.,**
asc-t.[2]**, aspar.**[2], aur., aur-ar.[1],
aur-i[1]', **aur-m., aur-m-n.**[2], aur-s.[1]',
bar-m.[2]**, bell.,** bism., bor-ac.[12],
bov.[3, 6], **brom.**[2], bry., cact.,
cain.[7,8], **caj.**[2], calad., **calc., calc-ar.,**
calc-p.[3], **calc-s.**[2], calc-sil.[1]',
camph., cann-s.[3], **canth.,**
carb-v.[2], **carbn-s., card-m.,** casc.[2],
cedr., cham.[2, 11], chel., **chen-a.**[2],
chim.[2]**, CHIN., chin-ar., CHLOL.**[2],
cinnb., cinnm.[2], coca, **coch.**[2],
coff.[3, 6], **COLCH., coll.,** coloc.,
con., conv., convo-a.[4], cop.,
cortiso.[14], **crat.**[3, 6, 8]**, crot-h., DIG.,**
dulc., elat.[2, 8], erig.[2], eup-pur.,
euph., **ferr.,** ferr-ar., **ferr-i.,** ferr-p.,
ferr-s.[2], **fl-ac.**[1, 2]**, form.**[2], frag.[12],
gamb.[2]**, GRAPH., grat.**[2], guaj.,
ham.[2]**, HELL., helon.**[2]**, hep.**[2, 4],
hippoz.[2, 12], hom.[12], **hydr.**[2], hyos.,
iber.[2], **ictod.**[2]**, IOD.,** iris[2], jat-m.[12],
just.[3], kali-ar., **kali-c.,** kali-chl.[12],
kali-i., kali-m.[2], kali-n., kali-p.,
kali-s., **kalm.**[2, 3], kreos.[4], **lac-d.,**
lact.[2], **lach.,** lat-k.[12], **laur.**[2, 3]**, led.,**
lept.[2], **liat.**[3, 7, 8], lith-c.[3, 6], lob.[3],
lyc., lycps.[3, 6], mag-m.[3, 6], **MED.,**
MERC.[1, 7]**, merc-c.**[2, 8], mez.,
mur-ac., **naja**[2], nat-ar., nat-c.,
nat-m.[1'-3, 12], nat-s.[1', 2], nat-sal.[12],
nit-ac., nux-m., OLND., OP.,
oxyd.[8], ped.[12], phos., pic-ac., plat.,
plb., prun.[2, 3, 6-8]**, psor.**[2]**, puls.,**
pyrog.[3, 6], ran-b.[2], rauw.[14], reser.[14],
rhod., rhus-t., **ruta,** sabad.[2],

sabin., **sal-ac.**[2, 6], **samb.**, sars.,
sec., senec.[1'], **seneg., sep.**, sil.,
solid.[3, 6], **SQUIL.**, staph.[3], stram.,
stront-c.[3, 4], stroph-h.[6], **sulph.**,
TER., teucr., thyr.[7, 12], til.[3], toxi[12],
uran-n.[2, 8], urea[11], **urt-u.**[2, 3],
verat., verat-v.[2], **verb.**, vesp.[12],
vip.[3, 4, 6], zinc., **zing.**[2]

morning
matin
morgens
   chin., **nat-c.**

forenoon[3]
matinée
vormittags
   apoc., aur., just., kali-chl., phos.,
   sep., sil.

old people, in[7]
personnes âgées, chez les
Alter, im
   KALI-C.

serum oozing, with[8]
sérum suintant, avec
Serumaustritt, mit
   ars., lyc., rhus-t.[3, 8]

haemorrhage, after[3]
hémorrhagies, après
Blutungen, nach
   apoc., chin.

heart disease, from[2]
cœur, par affection du
Herzkrankheiten, durch
   adon.[8], aml-ns., **apis**[2, 8], **apoc.**[2, 8],
   arn.[8], **ARS.**[2, 8], **ars-i.**[8], asc-c.[8],
   AUR-M.[1', 2, 8], **bry., cact.**[2, 8], **calc-p.**,
   chin-ar., **chlol.**, coffin.[8], **colch.**[2, 6],
   COLL.[2, 7, 8, 12], **conv.**[8], cop., crat.[8],
   crot-h., **dig.**[2, 8], **digin.**[8], **fl-ac.**, hell.,
   iod.[8], kali-c.[1'], **kali-m.**, kalm.[8],
   LAC-D.[1', 2], **LACH.**, liat.[8], **LYC.**[1', 2],
   lycps.[6], merc-d.[8], merc-sul., **nat-m.**,
   ph-ac., phos., **prun.**, rauw.[14], **sep.**,
   squil., stroph-h.[8, 12], ter.

internal
interne
innere
   acet-ac.[6, 8, 12], acetan.[8], **acon.**[3, 4, 8, 12],
   adon.[6, 8, 12], agn., alco.[11], am-be.[8, 12],
   am-c., ambr., ampe-qu.[8, 12], anag.[12],
   ant-ar.[6], ant-c., **ant-t.**, anthraco.[4],
   APIS, apisin.[6], **apoc.**, apoc-a.[12],
   arg-m., arg-n.[11], arg-p.[8], arn., **ARS.**,
   ars-i., asc-c.[8, 12], aspar.[12], aur.,
   aur-ar.[1'], aur-i.[1'], **aur-m., bar-m.**[4],
   BELL., benz-ac.[8], blatta[6],
   blatta-a.[8, 12], brass.[8, 12], **bry.**, bufo[12],
   cact.[8, 12], **cain.**[8, 12], caj.[12], **calc.**,
   calc-ar.[6, 8, 12], calc-s.[12], camph.,
   cann-s., canth., caps., carb-v.,
   CARD-M., casc.[12], chel.[4], chen-a.[12],
   chim.[12], **CHIN., chin-ar.**, chin-s.[12],
   chlol.[12], cina, cit-l.[12], coca[11], coch.[8],
   coffin.[8], **COLCH.**, coloc., **con.**,
   conv.[6, 8], cop.[8], **crat.**[6, 8], crot-h.[4],
   DIG., dulc., elat.[8, 12], equis.[12],
   ery-a.[12], euonin.[12], eup-pur.[6, 8, 12],
   euph., **ferr.**, ferr-ar., ferr-i.[1'],
   ferr-p., **fl-ac.**[6, 8, 12], form.[12], gali.[8],
   graph.[6, 12], grat.[12], guaj., **HELL.**,
   hep., hyos., iber.[12], ictod.[12],
   ign.[3], iod., **ip.**, iris[8], iris-g.[8,12],
   jatr.[8], junc-e.[12], **juni-c.**[6, 8, 12],
   kali-a.[6, 8, 11, 12], **kali-ar.**, kali-bi.[6],
   kali-bit.[6], **kali-c., kali-i.**[6, 8, 12],
   kali-m.[12], **kali-n.**[4, 6, 8], kali-p.,
   kali-s., **kalm.**[6, 12], lac-d.[8, 12], lach.,
   lact., laur., **led., liat.**[8, 12], lith-c.[6],
   lyc., lycps.[6], med.[1'], **merc.**,
   merc-c.[6], merc-d.[6, 8], merc-sul.[6, 12],
   mez., mur-ac., nat-a.[6], nat-m.[1', 12],
   nast.[8], nit-ac., **nit-s-d.**[6, 8],
   nux-m.[11], nux-v.[3], olnd.[4], onis.[8],
   op.[3, 4, 11], **oxyd.**[8, 12], ph-ac.,
   phase.[6, 8, 12], phos., **pilo.**[8], **plb.**[4, 12],
   prim-v.[12], prun.[6, 8, 12], psor.[8], puls.,
   querc.[8], ran-b.[12], **rhod.**[4], **rhus-t.**,
   ruta[4], sabad., **sabin.**[4], sacch.[11, 12],
   samb., **samb-c.**[8], sanic.[12], sars.,
   sec.[4], senec.[12], **seneg., sep.**, sil.,
   sol-n.[8], **solid.**[6, 8], spig., spong.,
   squil., stann., stigm.[12], stram.,
   stroph-h.[6, 8, 12], stry-ar.[8], sul-i.[1'],
   SULPH., tarent.[11], **ter.**[1], teucr.,
   teucr-s.[8], thlas.[8, 12], thyr.[12], toxi.[8],
   ur-ac.[8], urea[12], urea-n.[6], urt-u.[6],

verat., vesi.[12], vince., viol-t., zinc.[3],
zing.[12], ziz.[12]

joints, of[6]
articulations, des
Gelenke, der
apis, arn., **bry.**, canth., cedr., chin.,
chin-s, iod., kali-m., **ran-b.**, samb.

kidney disease, from[8]
rénale, par affection
Nierenkrankheiten, durch
ampe-qu., ant-t., **apis.**[2, 6, 8],
apoc.[1', 6, 8], **arg-n.**[6], ars.[6], **asc-c.**[2, 8],
aspar., aur.[6], **calc-p.**[2], **chim.**[2, 8],
COLCH.[2, 6], coloc.[2], crot-h.[2], **dig.**,
digin., eup-pur.[2, 6, 8], **hell.**[6], helon.,
lac-d., liat.[8, 12], **merc.**[6], **merc-c.**,
merc-d., nit-ac.[6], phos.[6], plb.,
rauw.[14], **sal-ac.**[2], senec.[1'], **solid.**[6],
ter.[6, 8], ur-ac.

liver disease, from[2]
foie, par affection du
Leberkrankheiten, durch
apoc.[8], ars.[8], ars-s-f.[1'], asc-c.[8], aur.[8],
AUR-M.[1', 2], **CALC.**, card-m.[1', 2, 8],
cean.[8], chel.[8], **chim.**[2, 8], chin., cop.,
cupr., **ferr.**, **fl-ac.**[1', 2], iris, kali-ar.[1'],
kali-m., lac-d.[1', 8], **LACH.**, lept.,
liat.[8], **LYC.**[1', 2, 8], merc., merc-sul.,
mur-ac.[8], **nat-m.**, **nux-v.**, polym.[8],
tarax.[9]

motion am.[16]
mouvement am.
Bewegung am.
nat-c.

newborn, in[8]
nouveaux-nés, chez les
Neugeborenen, bei
apis, carb-v., coffin., dig., lach.

overexertion agg.[3]
exercice excessif agg.
Überanstrengung agg.
apis

painful[16]
douloureuse
schmerzhafte
dulc.

pregnancy, in[2]
grossesse, pendant la
Schwangerschaft, in der
apis, apoc., ars., aur-m., colch.,
dig., dulc., hell., helon., **jab.,** lyc.,
merc.[11], merc-c., sanic.[12], uran-n.

scarlatina, after[2]
scarlatine, après
Scharlach, nach
acet-a., acon.[8], **ambr., APIS**[2, 8],
apoc.[8], **ARS.**[2, 8], **asc-c.**[2, 8],
AUR-M.[1', 2], bar-c., **bar-m.**[1', 2], **calc.,**
colch.[1', 2, 8], coloc., cop., **crot-h.,**
dig.[8], **dulc.**[2, 8], **HELL.**[2, 8], **hep.**[2, 8],
juni-c.[8], **LACH.**[2, 8], merc.[2], **nat-m.,**
nat-s., **phos.**[1', 2], pilo.[8], squil.[8],
stram.[2, 12], **TER.**[2, 8], verat-v., zinc.

spleen disease, from[8]
rate, par affection de la
Milzkrankheiten, durch
cean., **LACH.**[2], liat., querc.[8, 12],
squil.[8, 12]

thirst, with[8]
soif, avec
Durst, mit
acet-ac., acon., **apoc.**[1', 8], ars.

without[8]/sans/ohne
apis, hell.

urine, with supressed[1]
urine supprimée, avec
Urin, mit unterdrücktem
aral-h., **hell.**[2, 8]

weakness-dropsy/faiblesse-hydro-
pisie/Schwäche – Wassersucht

DRY sensation **in internal parts**[3]
SÉCHERESSE des **parties internes,**
sensation de
TROCKENHEIT innerer Teile, Gefühl
von
acon., ALUM.[3, 6], am-m., arg-m.,
arn., ars.[3, 6], **asaf.**[3, 6], **asar.,** bar-c.[3, 6],
bell.[3, 6], **bry., calad.,** camph.[3, 16],
cann-i.[6], cann-s., canth., caps.,
carb-v., caust., chin., cic., cina,

cinnb.[3, 6], cocc., coff., con.[3, 6], croc.,
dros., euph., ferr., ign., kali-c.,
m-arct., m-aust., meny., merc.,
mez., mosch., **nat-m.**[3, 6], **NUX-M.**[3, 6],
nux-v., olnd., par., petr., phos.[3, 6],
plb., **puls.**[3, 6], rheum, **RHUS-T.**[3, 6],
ruta, sabad., sec.[3, 6], seneg., sil.[3, 6],
spig., squil., stann., staph., **stram.**[3, 6],
sul-ac., sulph.[3, 6], tarax., teucr.,
thuj.[3, 6], valer., **verat.**, viol-o.,
viol-o., viol-t., **zinc.**[3, 6]

joints, in[3, 6]
articulations, des
Gelenke, der
  canth., croc., **lyc.**, m-arct.[3],
  NUX-V., ph-ac., **PULS.**

dry weather see weather–dry

**DRYNESS of usually moist internal
  parts**[3]
**SÉCHERESSE de parties internes en
  général humides**
**TROCKENHEIT gewöhnlich feuchter
  innerer Teile**
  acon.[3, 6], agar., agn., alum., am-c.,
  am-m., ambr., anac., ang., ant-c.,
  ant-t., apis[3, 6], arg-n.[3, 6], arn., **ars.**[3, 6],
  asaf., asar., atro.[6], aur., **bar-c.**[3, 6],
  BELL.[3, 6], bor., bov., bry., **CALAD.**[3, 6],
  CALC.[3, 6], **camph.**[3, 6], **cann-i.**[6],
  CANN-S., canth.[3, 6], caps., carb-ac.,
  carbn-o., caust.[3, 6], **cham.**, chel., chin.,
  cic., cina, clem., cocc.[3, 6], coff., colch.,
  con.[3, 6], cor-r.[6], croc.[3, 6], cupr., cycl.,
  dig., dros., dulc., euph., euphr., ferr.,
  gels.[3, 6], **graph.**[3, 6], guaj., hell., hep.,
  hist.[9], **hyos.**, ign., iod., ip., **kali-bi.**[3, 6],
  kali-i.[3, 6], kali-n., kreos., lach., laur.,
  led., **lyc.**, mag-m., **mang.**, meny.,
  merc., mez., mosch., mur-ac., nat-c.,
  NAT-M.[3, 6], **nit-ac.**[3, 6], NUX-M.[3, 6],
  nux-v.[3, 6], olnd., op., **par., petr.,** ph-ac.,
  PHOS.[3, 6], plat., plb., **puls.**[3, 6], ran-b.,
  ran-s., rheum, **rhod., rhus-t.**[3, 6], ruta,
  sabad., sabin., samb. sang.[3, 6], sars.,
  sec., sel., **SENEG.**[3, 6], **SEP.**[3, 6], **sil.,**
  spig., spong., squil., stann., staph.,
  stram.[3, 6], **stront-c.**, sul-ac., **sul-i.**[3, 6],

SULPH.[3, 6], tarax., **thuj., verat.**[3, 6],
verat-v.[3, 6], **zinc.**

DUST in internal parts, feeling of[3]
**POUSSIÈRE dans les parties internes,
  sensation de**
STAUB in inneren Teilen, Gefühl von
  am-c., ars., **bell., CALC.**, chel.,
  cina, cocc., crot-c., dros., hep.,
  ign., ip., op., **ph-ac.**, plat., rheum,
  sulph., teucr., zinc.

DWARFISHNESS
NANISME
ZWERGWUCHS
  ambr.[3], aster.[14], bac.[12], **BAR-C.,**
  bar-m., bor.[7], calc., **CALC-P., carbn-s.,**
  carc.[9], **con.**[3], iod., lyc., mag-m.[3, 6],
  med., merc., merc-pr-a.[12], nat-m.[7],
  nep.[14], **ol-j.**, op.[3], ph-ac.[7], sec., **sil.,**
  sulfa.[14], **SULPH., SYPH.**[1', 2, 3, 7],
  thyr.[12], **tub.**[2, 7], zinc.

EATING, before
MANGER, avant
ESSEN, vor dem
  acon., alum., am-c., am-m., **ambr.,**
  anac., ang.[3], arn., ars., **ars-i.,**
  ars-s-f.[1'], bar-c., bar-i.[1'], bell., **bov.,**
  bry., **calc.**, calc-i.[1'], **cann-s.,**
  carb-an., carb-v., carbn-s., caust.,
  cham., **chel., chin.**, colch., **croc.,**
  dulc., euphr., **ferr., FL-AC.**[3], **graph.,**
  hell, hep., **ign., IOD.,** kali-c., **lach.,**
  LAUR., mag-c., mang., meny.,
  merc., mez., mosch., **NAT-C.,**
  nat-p., nit-ac., nux-v., olnd., petr.,
  PHOS., plb., puls., ran-b., **rhus-t.,**
  sabad., sabin., sars., seneg., sep.,
  sil., spig., squil., stann., staph.,
  stront-c., sulph., tarax., valer.,
  verat., verb.

while
en mangeant
beim
  aloe, alum., **AM-C.**, am-m.,
  ambr., anac.[3], ang.[3], ant-c., ant-t.,

arg-m., arn., ars., aur., aur-ar.[1]',
aur-s[1]', **bar-c.**, bar-s.[1]', bell.,
bism., **bor.**, bov., **bry.**, **calc.**,
calc-f.[7], calc-sil.[1]', cann-s.,
canth., **carb-ac.**, **CARB-AN.**,
CARB-V., **carbn-s.**[1], **caust.**,
cham., chin., **cic.**, clem., **cocc.**,
coff., colch., **CON.**, cycl., dig.,
dros., dulc., euph., ferr., **graph.**,
hell., **hep.**, ign., iod., kali-bi.[3],
KALI-C., kali-n., kali-p., lach.,
laur., led., **lyc.**, mag-c., **mag-m.**,
mang., merc., mur-ac.[3], **nat-c.**,
nat-m., **NIT-AC.**, nux-m., nux-v.,
olnd., petr.[1], ph-ac., **phos.**, plat.[3],
plb., **puls.**, ran-b., ran-s., rauw.[14],
rhod., rhus-t., **rumx.**, ruta,
sabin., samb., sars., sec., **sep.**,
sil., spig., spong., squil., staph.,
stram., sul-ac., **SULPH.**, tarax.,
teucr., thuj., valer., verat.,
verb.[3], zinc.

am.
aloe, **alum.**, **alumn.**[2], am-m.,
ambr., **ANAC.**, aq-mar.[14], arn.,
aur., **auran.**[2], bar-c.[4], bell.,
buth-a.[14], cadm-met.[14], cadm-s.,
calc-p., cann-i., **caps.**, carb-an.,
carb-v., cham., **chel.**, chin.,
cimic.[14], cocc., **croc.**, cur.[2],
cyn-d.[14], dig., dros., ferr., fl-ac.[7],
graph., **IGN.**, iod., **LACH.**, laur.,
led., lyc., mag-c., mang., merc.,
methys.[14], **mez.**, nat-c., nit-ac.,
nux-v., onop.[14], par., perh.[14],
ph-ac., phos., phyt.[3], plat.[2, 3],
prot.[14], puls., rheum, rhod.,
rhus-t., sabad., sabin., **sep.**, sil.,
spig., spong., squil., stann.,
staph., sul-ac., sulph., tarax.,
thymol.[14], v-a-b.[14], **ZINC.**

after
après avoir mangé
nach dem
abies-n., acon., aesc.[8],
AETH.[3, 8], **agar.**, agn., all-c.,
ALOE, alum., alum-p[1]',
alum-sil.[1]', am-c., **am-m.**, ambr.,
ANAC., ang.[3], ant-c., ant-t.,
apis, apoc., arg-m.[3], **arg-n.**, arn.,

ARS., **ARS-S-F.**[1]', arum-t.[2],
asaf., asar., aur., aur-ar.[1]',
aur-s.[1]', **bar-c.**, bar-i.[1]', bar-s.[1]',
bell., **bism.**, bor., bov., **BRY.**,
bufo, cain., calad., **CALC.**,
calc-i.[1]', **CALC-P.**, calc-sil.[1]',
camph., cann-s., canth., caps.,
carb-an., **carb-v.**, **carbn-s.**,
CAUST., **cham.**, **chel.**, **chin.**,
chin-s.[2], chion.[8], chloram.[14],
cic., cina, cinnb.[1]', clem.,
coc-c., **cocc.**, **coff.**, colch.,
COLOC., **CON.**, croc., **crot-t.**,
cycl., dig., dros., dulc.,
eup-per., euph., euphr., **ferr.**,
ferr-ar., **ferr-i.**, ferr-p., **gran.**,
graph., grat., guat.[9, 14], hell., hep.,
hyos., ign., **indg.**, iod., ip., **jug-r.**,
kali-ar., **KALI-BI.**, **KALI-C.**,
kali-m.[1]', kali-n., kali-p., kali-s.,
kali-sil.[1]', kreos., **LACH.**, laur.,
led., **LYC.**, mag-c., mag-m.,
manc.[2], mang., meny.[3], meph.[3],
merc., **mez.**, mosch., mur-ac.,
nat-ar., **nat-c.**, **NAT-M.**, nat-s.,
nat-sil.[1]', **nit-ac.**, **nuph.**[2], nux-m.,
NUX-V., ol-an.[8], olnd., op.,
ox-ac., par., **petr.**, ph-ac., **PHOS.**,
phyt., plat., plb., **podo.**, **psor.**,
ptel., **PULS.**, **ran-b.**, ran-s.,
raph.[2], rauw.[14], **rheum**, rhod.,
rhus-t., **RUMX.**, ruta, sabad.,
sabin., samb., sang., sars., sec.,
sel., **seneg.**, **SEP.**, **SIL.**, spig.,
spong., squil., stann., staph.,
stront-c., stry.[8], sul-ac., sul-i.[1]',
SULPH., **tarax.**, teucr., thea[8],
thuj., tril., trom.[1], valer., verat.,
verb., viol-t., **ZINC.**, zinc-p.[1]'

agg. long after e.[3]
agg. longtemps après avoir m.
agg. lange nach dem E.
grat., kali-i., kreos., murx., **phos.**,
PULS.

am.
acet-ac.[8], acon., agar.[2],
aloe, alum., alumn., am-c.,
am-m., ambr., amor-r.[14], **anac.**,
ang.[2, 3], arn., ars., ars-i., **aster.**[2],
bar-c., bar-i.[1]', bell-p.[14], **bov.**,

brom., **bry.**, buth-a.[9, 10],
cadm-met.[9, 10], cadm-s.[8], calc.,
calc-f.[10, 14], calc-i.[1'], **calc-s.**,
cann-i.[2], **cann-s.**, caps.[8], carb-an.,
carbn-s., **caust.**, cham., **chel.**,
chin., cimic.[8], cist.[6, 8], con.[3, 8],
cupr.[3, 8], dicha.[10, 14], dios., euphr.,
ferr., ferr-a.[8], fl-ac., gamb., goss.[7],
graph., guat.[9], hed.[9, 10], hell.,
hep., hom.[8], **ign., IOD.**, kali-bi.,
kali-br., kali-c., **kali-p.**[8], **kali-s.**,
kalm.[6], kreos.[2], lac-ac.[2, 6], lach.,
laur., lith-c., lyss.[2], mag-c.[3],
mag-m., mand.[10], mang., med.[7],
meny., merc., mez., mosch.,
NAT-C., nat-m.[3, 8, 16], **nat-p.**,
nicc., nux-v., **onos.**, ox-ac.[3],
paeon., petr., **PHOS.**, pip-n.[8],
plan., plat.[2], plb.[3], **psor.**[8], **puls.**,
ran-b., rhod., rhus-t., **sabad.**,
sars., **SEP.**, sil., spig., **SPONG.**,
squil., stann., **stront-c.**, sul-i.[1'],
sulph.[1'], verat., zinc.[3, 6, 8],
zinc-p.[1']

fast
vite
schnelles
　　ars., **ip.**, led., **nux-v.**, sulph.

overeating agg.[3, 6]
trop manger agg.
Überessen agg.
　　acon.[3], aeth.[3], alum.[3],
　　ANT-C.[3, 6, 8], **ant-t.**, arg-n.[7],
　　arn.[3], ars.[3], asaf.[3], bry.[3], calc.[3],
　　carb-v., caust., chin.[3], **coff.**[3, 6, 7],
　　hep.[3], ign.[3], **IP., lyc.**[3], mag-c.[3],
　　nat-c., nat-p.[3], nux-m.[3],
　　nux-v.[3, 6, 8], **PULS.**[3, 6, 8], staph.,
　　sulph.[3], tub.[1']

ailments from[12]
troubles à la suite de
Beschwerden infolge von
　　all-s., ant-c., bry., dios., nux-m.

children, in[3, 6]
enfanzs, chez les
Kindern, bei
　　aeth., nat-p.

satiety, to
satiété, à
Sättigung, bis zur
　　bar-c., bar-s.[1'], **calc.**, carb-v.,
　　chin.[3], **LYC.**, nat-c., nat-m.,
　　nux-v., phos.[16], **PULS.**, sep., sil.,
　　sulph., zinc.[16]

　　am.
　　ars., **iod.**, phos.

small quantity agg., of a[3]
petites quantités, agg., par
kleinen Menge agg., einer
　　alet., am-c., arg-n., bar-c., bell.,
　　BRY., canth., carb-an., **carb-v.**,
　　chin., con., crot-t., cycl., ferr.,
　　hep., **ign.**, kali-bi., **kali-c.**, kali-s.,
　　led., lil-t., **LYC.**, merc., nat-m.,
　　nat-p., **NUX-V.**, petr.[3], **PHOS.**,
　　puls., rhod., rhus-t., sars., **sep.**,
　　sulph., thuj., verat., zinc.

　　am.[9, 14]
　　guat.

EFFICIENCY increased[6]
EFFICIENCE augmentée
LEISTUNGSFÄHIGKEIT erhöht
　　agar., ars., coca, coff., kola, lach.,
　　nat-p., op., pic-ac., pip-m., stram.

vigor–increased/vigeur–augmentée/
　　Kräfte–Zunahme

ELECTRIC STATES, ailments from[12]
ÉTATS ÉLECTRIQUES, troubles à la
　　suite d'
ELEKTRIZITÄT, Beschwerden infolge
von
nat-c.

ELECTROSHOCK, ailments from[12]
ÉLECTROCHOC, troubles à la suite d'
ELEKTROSCHOCK, Beschwerden
infolge von
morph.

ELEPHANTIASIS[8]
ÉLÉPHANTIASIS
ELEPHANTIASIS

anac.[8, 12], **ars.**, calo., card-m., **elae.**, graph., ham., hell.[2], hippoz.[12], **hydr.**, iod., lyc., **myris.**, sil.[8, 12], still.[2, 12]

arabum[12]
Arabes, des
arabum (Filariasis)

ars., elae., **hydrc.**[2, 12], myris., **sil.**[2]

EMACIATION
AMAIGRISSEMENT
ABMAGERUNG

ABROT., acet-ac., adren.[7], **agar.,** alco.[11], **alet.**[2, 12], **alum.,** alum-p.[1'], alum-sil.[1'], alumn., am-c., am-caust.[11], am-m., **ambr.,** ambro.[12], anac., ant-c., ant-i.[8], ant-t., **apis,** apoc.[1', 11], aq-mar.[14], **arg-m., arg.-n.,** arn., **ARS., ARS-I.,** ars-met.[2, 11], ars-s-f.[1'], arum-i.[11], asc-t., astra-e.[14], **aur.**[2], aur-ar.[1'], aur-m., bar-a.[11], **BAR-C.,** bar-i.[1'], **bar-m.,** bar-s.[1'], **bell.**[2], ben-n.[11], benz-ac.[2, 11], beryl.[14], bism.[3], bor., both.[11], brach.[2, 11], **brom.**[1', 2], **bry., bufo,** buni-o.[14], **cact., CALC.,** calc-ar.[6], calc-f.[10, 14], calc-hp.[6], **CALC-I.,** calc-m.[11], **calc-p., calc-sil.**[1', 8], **camph.,** cann-s.[11], **canth., caps.**[2], **carb-an.**[2, 3, 6, 8], **carb-v.,** carbn-o.[11], **carbn-s.,** carl.[11], **caust.**[2, 3, 6, 8, 12], **cench.**[1'], cere-b.[11, 12], **cetr.**[2, 8], **cham., chel., CHIN.,** chin-ar., chin-s.[2, 4, 11], chlol.[11], **chlor., chion.,** cic.[14], cimic.[10], cina, **cist.**[2, 6], **clem.,** cob-n.[14], coca[2, 11], **cocc., colch.,** **coloc.,** con., cor-r., **crot-c.,** crot-t., cub.[2, 11], cund.[2, 6], **cupr.,** dig., digin.[11], dros., dulc., echi.[11], euphr.[2], **FERR., ferr-ar., ferr-i.,** **ferr-m.,** ferr-p.[8], **fl-ac.,** fuc.[11], **gamb.**[2], gels.[11], glyc.[8], gran.[4, 11], **GRAPH., guaj.,** hed.[10], **HELL.,** **helon., hep., hippoz.,** hura[11], **hydr.,** **ign., IOD., ip.,** jug-c.[11], **kali-ar.,** kali-bi., **kali-br.**[2, 6, 11], **kali-c.,** **kali-i., kali-p.,** kali-s., **kali-sil.**[1'],

kali-t.[11], **kreos.,** kres.[10, 13, 14], **lac-ac.**[2], lac-c.[2], **lac-d.**[2], **lach.,** lat-k.[11], **laur.**[2], led.[3, 8], lil-t.[11], **lith-c.**[2], luf-op.[10, 14], **LYC.,** lycps.[2], lyss.[2], mag-c., mag-m., mag-p.[12], mang.[3, 6, 8], med.[1', 7], **merc.,** **merc-c.**[8, 11], mez., moly-met.[14], morph.[11], **mur-ac.**[2, 3, 6, 11, 16], myos-a.[6], **myos-s.**[2], naja[11], **nat-ar.,** **nat-c., NAT-H., NAT-M., nat-n.**[6], **nat-p., nat-s.,** nat-sil.[1'], **nicc.**[2], **NIT-AC.,** nit-s-d.[6], nuph.[11], nux-m., **NUX-V., ol-j., op.,** ox-ac.[11], parathyr.[14], pers.[14], **petr., ph-ac.,** phel.[2], **PHOS., phyt.**[6, 8], pic-ac.[2], pin-s.[6], pip-m.[11], **plan.**[2], **PLB.,** **plb-a.**[8], plb-i.[8], **podo.**[2], **psor., puls.,** pyrog.[3, 6], raph.[4, 11, 12], **rheum**[2], rhus-g.[11], **rhus-t.**[3, 8], rhus-v.[4, 11], ric.[8], **rumx.**[2], ruta, sacch.[11], samb., **sanic.**[3, 8, 12], saroth.[14], **sars., sec.,** **SEL., senec.**[2], sep., **SIL.,** spig., spong., **STANN., stann-i.**[6], staph., still.[11], **stram., stront-c.,** **sul-ac.**[1', 2, 6, 11], sul-h.[11], sul-i.[1'], sulfa.[14], **SULPH.,** sumb., **syph.**[1'-3, 7, 8], tab.[3, 4, 11], **tarent., ter.,** **teucr.**[2], thal.[10, 11, 14], **ther.**[2, 7], **thuj.**[2, 3, 6, 8, 11], thuj-l.[14], thyr.[3, 14], **TUB.,** tub-r.[14], uran., uran-n.[6], vanad.[7, 8], **verat., verat-v.**[2], vesp.[11], vip.[4, 6], voes.[11], x-ray[14], **zinc.**[1'-3, 6, 8, 12], zinc-m.[11, 12], zinc-val.[12]

cachexia/cachexie/Kachexie

affected parts, of
affectées, des parties
leidender Teile

ars., bry., calc.[3], **carb-v., caust.**[8], cupr.[16], dulc., **GRAPH., LED., lyc.,** **mez.,** nat-m., **nit-ac.,** nux-v., ph-ac., **phos., plb., PULS., SEC.,** sel., sep., sil.

appetite with e., ravenous
boulimie, avec
Heißhunger, mit

abrot., acet-ac.[8], ars.[3], ars-i.[8], bar-c.[6, 8], bar-i.[1'], **CALC.,** calc-f.[14], chin.[6], cina[3], con.[8], **IOD.,** luf-op.[14],

lyc.[3, 6], **NAT-M., PETR., phos.,**
psor., sanic.[6-8], sil.[6], **sulph.,** thyr.[8],
tub., uran.[7], uran-n.[6]

children, in
enfants, chez les
Kindern, bei
  abrot., ars-i., **bar-c., bar-i.**[1, 7],
  CALC., calc-p., caust., **chin.,**
  CINA, IOD., lyc., **mag-c.,**
  NAT-M., nux-v., petr., **sil.,**
  sul-i.[1'], **sulph.**

cancerous see cancerous–cachexia

children, in; marasmus
enfants, chez les; marasme
Kindern, bei; Marasmus
  abrot., **ACET-AC.**[2, 7], aeth.[2], alum.,
  ant-c., **apis**[2], **arg-n.,** arn.[4], **ARS.,**
  ARS-I., ars-s.[8], ars-s-f.[12], **ARUM-T.**[2],
  aur.[3], bac.[8], bar-c., bell.[4], **CALC.,**
  CALC-P., calc-sil.[1', 7, 8], **carb-v.,**
  caust., cham.[4], chin., cina, coca[12],
  con.[7], **ferr.**[1', 2, 4], hecla[7], hep.[4], **hydr.,**
  IOD., kali-c., kali-i.[12], **kreos.,** lyc.,
  mag-c., med.[1'], **NAT-M., nux-m.,**
  nux-v., ol-j., op., petr., **phos., plb.,**
  podo.[2, 8], **psor., puls., sanic.**[7, 8], sars.,
  sep., SIL., staph.[2], sul-i.[1'], **sulph.,**
  ther.[2], thyr.[8], **tub.**[7, 8]

downwards, spreads
de haut en bas, s'étend
von oben nach unten
  calc.[1', 7], cench.[1'], lyc., nat-m.,
  psor.[1'], sanic.[3, 6], sars.

grief, after
chagrin, par
Kummer, durch
  petr., ph-ac.

insanity with
folie avec
Geisteskrankheit mit
  arn., ars., calc., chin., graph., lach.,
  lyc., nat-m., nit-ac., nux-v., phos.,
  puls., sil., sulph., verat.

loss of animal fluids, from
perte de fluides vitaux, par
Verlust von Körpersäften, durch
  CHIN., LYC., SEL.

old people
personnes âgées, chez les
Alter, im
  ambr., anac.[3, 6], **BAR-C.,** carb-v.[3, 6],
  chin.[3], chin-s.[4], **fl-ac.**[3, 6], **IOD., LYC.,**
  nit-ac.[3, 6], op.[3], rhus-t.[3, 6], **sec., sel.,**
  sil.[7]

pining boys
jeunes garçons dans un état de
  langueur, chez des
Jugendlicher in einem Zustand der
  Entkräftung
  AUR., LYC., nat-m., **ph-ac.**[2], **TUB.**

children–delicate/enfants–maladifs/
  Kindern–zarte

single parts, of
parties isolées, de
einzelner Teile
  bar-c.[3], bry., calc., caps., carb-v.,
  caust.[3], con., dulc., graph., **iod.,**
  led., **mez.,** nat-m., nit-ac., ph-ac.,
  plb.[3], **puls.**[3], sec.[3], **sel.,** sil., **sulph.**[3]

upwards
de bas en haut, s'étend
von unten nach oben
  abrot., arg-n.

EMISSIONS agg., SEMINAL＊
PERTES SÉMINALES agg.
SAMENVERLUSTE agg.
  abrot.[6], agar., **alum.,** ars., aven.[6],
  bar-c., bor., bov., bufo[6], **calc.,**
  cann-i.[6], cann-s., carb-ac.[6],
  carb-an., carb-v., **caust.**[1, 5], **chin.,**
  cob., con.[5, 6], dig., ferr-br.[6], **iod.,**
  KALI-C., led., **lyc.,** merc., mez.,
  nat-c., **NAT-P., NUX-V.,** petr.,
  ph-ac., phos., pic-ac., plat.[6], **plb.,**
  psor., puls., ran-b., rhod., sabad.,
  SEL., SEP., sil., stann.[6], **staph.,**
  stram.[6], **sulph.,** thuj.

ailments from[12]
troubles à la suite de
Beschwerden infolge von Samenverlusten
staph.

am.[2]
agn., calc-p., **lach., zinc.**[2, 7]

EMPTINESS, sensation of (Kent 1897)
VIDE, sensation de
LEERE, Gefühl von
alum.[3], am-c.[3], am-m[3], ant-c.[3],
ant-t.[3], arg-m[3], arn.[3], astra-m.[12],
aur.[1', 3, 6], bar-c.[3], bry.[3], calad., calc.[3],
caps.[3], carb-an.[3], carb-v.[3], caust.[3],
cham.[3], **chin.**[3], cina[3], **COCC.,** coff.[3],
coloc.[3], croc.[3], cupr.[3], dig.[3, 6], dulc.[3],
euph.[3], glon.[3, 6], graph.[3], hep.[3],
hydr.[3, 6], **IGN.,** iod.[3], ip.[3], **KALI-C.,**
kali-n.[3], lach.[3], laur.[3], **LYC.,**
mag-c.[3], mang.[3], med.[3], meny.[3],
merc.[3], mez.[3], **mur-ac.,** nat-c.[3],
nat-m.[3], nux-v.[3], olnd., op.[3], par.[3],
petr.[3, 6], **PHOS.**[3, 6], plat.[3], plb.[3],
podo.[3, 6], **PULS.,** rhus-t.[3], ruta[3],
sabad.[3], **SARS.,** seneg.[3], **SEP.,** spig.[3],
squil.[3, 6], **STANN.,** staph.[3], stram.[3],
sul-ac.[3], **sulph.,** tab.[3, 6], tell.[3],
teucr.[3], verat.[3], verb.[3], vib.[6], vinc.[12],
zinc.[3, 6], **zing.**

fainting, with sensation of
(Kent 1897)
évanouissement, avec sensation d'
Ohnmacht, mit Gefühl von
SEP.

general[11]
général
allgemeiner
ail., apoc., aur.[3, 11], cob-n.[9],
hydr-ac., kali-c.[3, 11], merc., SEP.,
zing.

EXERTION agg., physical
EXERCICE physique **agg.**
ANSTRENGUNG agg., körperliche
acon., **agar.,** agn.[1', 7], allox.[14],
ALUM., alum-p.[1'], alum-sil.[1'],

alumn., am-c., am-m., **ambr.,**
ammc.[4], **anac.,** ant-c., **ant-t.,**
apis, apoc., **arg-m., arg-n.,**
arist-cl.[9], **ARN., ARS., ARS-I.,**
ars-s-f.[1'], asaf., asar., aur., aur-ar.[1'],
aur-i.[1'], aur-m[1'], aur-s.[1'], **bar-c.,**
bar-i.[1'], **bar-s.**[1'], bell-p.[10], **benz-ac.,**
berb.[3], beryl.[14], **bol-la.,** bor.,
bov., brom.[3], **BRY.,** buni-o.[14],
buth-a.[9, 10, 14], **cact., CALC.,**
calc-ar.[1'], calc-c-f.[9, 10, 14], **calc-p.,**
CALC-S., calc-sil.[1'], **cann-s.,**
carb-an.[3], **carb-v., caust., chel.,**
chin., chin-ar., chin-s.[4], cic., cina,
coca[6, 12], **COCC.,** coff., **colch.,**
CON., croc., **crot-h.,** cur.[6], cycl.,
DIG., dulc.[1'], erig.[10], euphr., **ferr.,**
ferr-ar., FERR-I., ferr-p., fl-ac.[3],
flor-p[14], **GELS.,** graph., **guaj., ham.,**
hell., **helon., hep.,** ign., **IOD.,** ip.,
kali-ar., kali-bi., kali-c., kali-m.[1'],
kali-n., **kali-p.,** kali-s., kali-sil[1'],
kalm., kreos., lac-d.[7], **lach.,** lact.[4],
LAUR., led., lil-t., **lob., lyc.,**
lycps., m-arct.[4], mag-p.[1'], meny.,
merc., merc-c., mur-ac., murx., naja,
NAT-AR., NAT-C., NAT-M., nat-p.,
nat-sil.[1'], nit-ac., nux-m., **nux-v.,**
olnd., **ox-ac.,** paro-i.[14], petr.[4], **ph-ac.,**
phos., PIC-AC., plat., **plb., podo.,**
prot.[14], **psor., puls., rheum,** rhod.,
RHUS-T., ruta, sabad., **sabin.,**
sacch-l.[12], **sang.,** sarcol.-ac.[9], sars.,
sec., **SEL., SEP.,** sil., sol-n., **SPIG.,**
SPONG., squil., **STANN., STAPH.,**
stront-c.[3], stroph-h.[3], stroph-s.[14],
sul-ac., sul-i.[1'], **SULPH.,** tab.[3],
tarent., tax.[14], tell.[14], **thuj., tub.,**
v-a-b.[14], **valer.,** verat., **zinc.,**
zinc-p.[1']

ailments from[12]
troubles à la suite d'
Beschwerden infolge von
agar., alum., ars., calc., carb-an.,
carb-v., cimic., cocc., con., epiph.,
kali-c., mill., nat-c., ovi-p., rhus-t.,
ruta, sanic., scut., sel., sil., sulph.,
ter.

am.

agar.[3], alumn.[8], brom.[8], canth.,
cycl.[3, 6], fl-ac.[3, 7], helon.[6], **hep.**[3], **ign.**,
kali-br.[3], kali-c.[14], **LIL-T.**[3, 6], nat-m.,
phys.[3], plb., rauw.[9, 14], **RHUS-T.**,
SEP., sil., stann., thlas.[3], tril.

in open air[9]
en plein air
im Freien
rauw.

impossible/unmöglich
calc-i.[1']

EXOSTOSES
EXOSTOSEN

am-c.[4], **arg-m., AUR., AUR-M.,** calc.,
CALC-F., calc-p.[2], crot-c., daph.[12],
dulc., ferr-i.[2], **fl-ac.,** graph.[2], hecla,
kali-bi.[7, 8, 12], **kali-i.,** lap-a.[7, 8],
maland.[7, 8], **MERC.**[2, 3, 7, 8, 11], **merc-c.,**
merc-p.[8], **mez., nit-ac.,** ph-ac.[3, 4],
PHOS., plb.[4, 12], **puls.,** rhus-t., **ruta,**
sars.[2], **SIL.,** staph.[1'], still.[7, 8], sul-i.[3],
sulph., syph.[1', 3, 7], **zinc.**[4, 7, 8], zinc-m.[7]

FAINTNESS, fainting
ÉVANOUISSEMENT, défaillance
OHNMACHT

abies-c., acet-ac., acetan.[8, 12],
ACON., aesc., aeth.[6], aether[11],
agar., agar-em.[11], alco.[11], alet.[8],
all-c., aloe[6], **alum.,** alum-p.[1'],
alum-sil.[1'], alumn., am-br.[11], am-c.,
am-m., ambr., **aml-ns.**[2, 8],
amyg.[2, 11, 12], anac., ant-c., ant-m.[2],
ant-t., apis, **apoc.**[6], apom.[7, 11],
arg-n., arn., ARS., ars-h., **ars-i.,**
ars-s-f.[1', 11], ars-s-r.[2, 11], asaf., asar.[2],
atro., bapt., bar-c., bar-i.[1'], **bar-m.,**
bar-s.[1'], bell., ben-n.[11], benz-ac.,
berb., beryl.[9], bism.[6], bol-la.[11],
bol-s.[11], bor., **both.**[11], bov., brom.[1'],
BRY., bufo, cact., **CADM-S.**[3], calad.,
calc., calc-ar.[1'], calc-i.[1'], calc-m.[11],
calc-p., calc-sil.[1'] calo.[11], **camph.,**
cann-i., **cann-s., canth.,** carb-ac.,
carb-v., carbn-o., carbn.s., carl.[11],

cass.[11], cast.[2], cast-eq., **CAUST.,**
cedr., cench., cere-s.[11], **CHAM.,**
chel., chim., **CHIN., chin-ar.,** chin-s.,
chlol., chlor.[1], cic., **cimic.,** cina,
cinnm.[2], cinch.[11], cit-v.[12], **COCC.**[1, 7],
coch.[2], coff.[6], colch., **coll., coloc.,**
con., conin.[11], conv.[6], convo-d.[11],
cot.[11], croc., **crot-c., CROT-H.,**
crot-t., culx.[1'], cupr., cupr-a.,
cupr-ar.[2, 11], cupr-s., cur., cycl.,
cyt-l.[9, 11], **DIG.,** digin.[11], digox.[11],
dios., dros., dubo-h.[11], dubo-m.[11],
dulc., elaps, ery-a.[11], eucal.[2, 11],
eup-pur., **euph.**[2, 11], euph-c.[11], **ferr.,**
ferr-ar., ferr-i., ferr-p., **form.,**
gamb., gels., gent-c.[11], **GLON.,**
gran.[11], **graph.,** grind., hedeo.[11],
hell., hell-f.[11], **HEP.**[1, 7], hippoz.,
hura, **hydr.**[1', 12], hydr-ac., **hyos.,**
IGN., IOD., iodof.[2], **IP.**[1, 7], iris,
jab., jal., jasm.[11], jug-c., kali-ar.,
kali-bi., kali-br., kali-c., kali-cy.,
kali-m.[1'], kali-n., kali-ox.[11], kali-p.,
kali-sil.[1'], **kalm., kreos.,** lac-ac.,
lac-d.[2], **LACH.,** lat-k.[11, 12], **laur.,**
led., lept., **lil-t., lina.**[8, 12], lob.[12],
luf-act.[11], lup.[11], **lyc.,** lycps.[2], lyss.,
mag-c., **mag-m.,** magn-gl.[12],
magn-gr.[12], manc., mang., merc.,
merc-c., merc-cy., merc-d.,
merc-i-f.[3], merc-ns.[11], merc-pr-r.[11],
mez., mom-b.[11], **MOSCH.,** mur-ac.,
naja, narc-po.[11], narc-ps.[11],
nat-hchls., nat-m., nat-ns.[12],
nat-p.[11], nit-ac., nitro-o.[11], **NUX-M.,**
NUX-V., oena., ol-an., olnd., **op.,**
ox-ac., paeon.[2], pana.[11], parth.[12],
petr., ph-ac., phase.[8], **phos.,** phys.,
phyt.[2, 3, 11], picro.[11], pip-m.[11], plan.,
plat.[6], **PLB., PODO., psor.,** ptel.,
PULS., puls-n.[11], ran-a.[11], ran-b.,
ran-s., raph.[11], rhodi.[11], rhus-t.,
rob., ruta, sabad., sacch.[11],
sal-ac.[2], **sang.,** sapin.[11], **sars.,** sec.,
senec.[12], **seneg., SEP.,** sieg.[10], **sil.,**
sin-n., sol-t.[11], sol-t-ae., **spig.,**
spong.[8, 12], stann.[2, 6], staph.,
STRAM., stroph-h.[3], stry., sul-ac.,
sul-i.[1', 11], **SULPH., SUMB., tab.,**
tanac.[11], tarent., tax., **ter.**[2, 11], thea[11],
ther., thuj., thyr.[8, 12], til., **tril.**[6, 8],
tub.[1'], uran-n.[2], ust., valer., **VERAT.,**

verat-v., verin.[11], vesp., **vib.**,
viol-o., vip., wies.[11], zinc., zinc-m.,
zinc-p.[1'], zing.

Vol. I: *unconsciousness/incon-
science/Bewußtlosigkeit
convulsions-consciousness/convul-
sions-conscience/Konvulsionen-
Bewußtsein*

collapse/collapsus/Kollaps

morning
matin
morgens
    alumn., **ARS.**, bor.[4, 16], **carb-v.**,
    cocc., con., culx.[1'], dios., kali-c.[4],
    kali-n.[4], **kreos.**, lach.[4], med.,
    nat-m., nit-ac.[4], **NUX-V.**, petr.[4],
    plb., puls., **sang.**, sep.[4], staph.[4],
    stram., stry., **SULPH.**

7 h
    dios.

8 h[11]
    dios., ped.

8–9 h
    phos.

air, in open
air, en plein
Freien, im
    mosch, nux-v.

bed, in[2]
lit, au
Bett, im
    carb-v.[16], **con.**

eating, before
manger, avant
Essen, vor dem
    calc.

    during
    en mangeant
    beim
        lach.

am.
    nux-v.

house, on entering
appartement, en entrant dans l'
Hauses, beim Betreten des
    petr.

rising, on
levant, en se
Aufstehen, beim
    BRY., calc.[16], **CARB-V.**,
    COCC.[1, 7], **iod., kreos.**[1], **lac-d.**[7],
    lach., nat-m.[16], petr.[4], sep.

quickly from stooping or turn-
    ing head
rapide e. en se baissant ou en
    tournant la tête rapidement
schnell vom Bücken oder beim
    schnellen Kopfdrehen
    sang.

stool, during
selle, pendant la
Stuhlgang, beim
    phys.

waking, on[11]
s'éveillant, en
Erwachen, beim
    graph.

forenoon
matinée
vormittags
    kali-n.[4], phos., sep., staph.,
    stram.

9 h[11]
    ped.

10 h[14]
    ven-m.

    in phthisis[2, 7]
    dans la phtisie
    bei Phthisis
    kali-c.

11 h
  ind., **lach.**, **SULPH.**

11–12 h[6]: zinc.

standing erect, on
debout, en étant
Aufrechtstehen, beim
  dios.

walking in open air, on
marchant en plein air, en
Gehen im Freien, beim
  lycps.

noon[16]
midi
mittags
  bov., cic.

afternoon
après-midi
nachmittags
  anac., **asar.**, bor., dios., phys.[11],
  seneg.[4], sulph.

13 h
  lycps.

14 h after chill
14 h après les frissons
14 h nach Fieberfrost
  gels.

16 h after mental exertion[11]
16 h après travail intellectuel
16 h nach geistiger Anstrengung
  rhodi.

17.30 h
  nux-m.

evening
soir
abends
  aesc-g.[7], alet., am-c., asaf.,
  calc.[1, 7], coff.[4], glon., **hep.**,
  kali-n.[4, 16], **lac-d.**[2, 7], lach.[4], lyc.,
  lycps., mosch., **nat-m.**[1, 7], nux-v.,
  phos., rhus-t.[4], **sep.**

18 h
  glon.

19 h
  lycps., seneg.

20–21 h
  nux-v.

21 h
  mag-m., meli., rhus-t.

cardiac depression, from
cardiaque, par faiblesse
Herzschwäche, durch
  lycps.

exertion, on
exercises physiques, par
Anstrengung, durch
  nat-m.

stiffness of fingers and arms, with[16]
raideur des doigts et des bras, avec
steifen Fingern und Armen, mit
  petr.

stool, during[11]
selle, pendant la
Stuhlgang, beim
  sars.

undressing, on
deshabillant, en se
Ausziehen, beim
  chel.

night
nuit
nachts
  am-c., ars.[4], bar-c., calc.[4],
  carb-v.[4], dios.[11], graph.[4],
  mosch.[1, 7], nit-ac., nux-m.,
  nux-v.[2, 4, 7], sep.[4], **sil.**, ther.,
  vip.[4]

midnight
minuit
Mitternacht
  sep.

3 h
  dios.

abortion, after[11]
avortement, par
Abort, nach
  rosm.

Addison's disease, in[2]
maladie bronzée, pendant la
Addison' Syndrom, beim
  calc.

after-pain, after every
tranchées utérines, après chaque
Nachwehe, nach jeder
  hep., **nux-v.**

agg. after f.[3]
agg. après un é.
agg. nach einer O.
  acon., ars., chin., **mosch.,** nux-v.,
  op., sep., stram.

air, in open
air, en plein
Freien, im
  mosch.[2, 4], nit-ac.[16], **nux-v.**[2]

  am.[11]
    bor.[4], crot-c., dios., trif-p.

amenorrhoea, in[2]
aménorrhée, pendant l'
Amenorrhoe, bei
  glon.

anaemia, in[2]
anémie, par
Anaemie, durch
  acet.-ac.[1'], ferr-i.[1'], **mosch., spig.**

anger, after
colère, par
Zorn, durch
  cham.[7], gels., **nux-v.**[2, 5], phos.[5],
  staph.[2, 5], vesp.[1']

angina pectoris, in[2, 7]
angine de poitrine, par
Angina pectoris, durch
  arn.[2], **hep., spong.**

cardiopathy/cardiopathie/
  Herzleiden
heart/cœur/Herzdruck
pain–heart/douleurs–cœur/
  Schmerzen–Herz

  praecordial, anguish with[2], [7]
  angoisse précordiale avec
  Herzangst mit
    aml-ns., merc-i-f.[7], plb.[11], tab.

anguish, after[2]
angoise, après
qualvoller Angst, nach
  nux-v., verat.

ascending hill, on
ascension d'une colline, par l'
Steigen auf einen Hügel, beim
  agar.

  mountains, on[7]
  montagne, d'une
  Bergsteigen, beim
    coca

  stairs
  escaliers, des
  Treppensteigen, beim
    aether[7, 11], **anac.,** iod., lycps.,
    plb.

asthma, from[7]
asthme, par
Asthma, durch
  ars., atro.[2], berb., kreos., lach.,
  morph.

bed, in
lit, au
Bett, im
  caust., dios.

bending head backwards am.[15]
fléchir la tête en arrière am.
Rückwärtsbeugen des Kopfes am.
  ol-an.

blood, at sight of
sang, à la vue du
Blut, beim Anblick von
  ALUM.[7], nux-m., **verat.**[7]

Vol. I: *blood–wounds/sang–plaies/*
Blut–Wunden
unconsciousness–blood/
inconscience–sang/Bewußtlosig-
keit–Blut
f.–wounds/é.–blessure/O.–Wunden

blowing an instrument, when[16]
soufflant dans un instrument, en
Blasen eines Instrumentes, beim
kali-n.

breakfast, before[2]
petit déjeuner, avant le
Frühstück, vor dem
calc.

after/après le/nach dem
bufo, naja

breath am., deep
respiration profonde am.
Tiefatmen am.
asaf.

cardiopathy, in[2, 7]
cardiopathie, par
Herzleiden, bei
arn.[7], ars., cact., chel., dig., kali-p.,
lycps., **spig.**

angina pectoris/angine poitrine/
Angina pectoris
palpitation/palpitations/Herz-
klopfen

weakness of heart, from[15]
cardiaque, par faiblesse
Herzschwäche, durch
ars., dig., hydr-ac., lach., laur.,
verat.

chill, before[2, 7]
frissons, avant les
Fieberfrost, vor
ars.

during/pendant les/während
acon.[7], ars., asar., **calc.**[2, 7],
calen.[4], coloc.[7], kali-c.[4], morph.[7],
sapin.[7, 11], **SEP.,** stram.[2, 7],
valer.[2, 7]

chilliness with[2]
frilosité avec
Frösteln mit
zing.

church, in[2, 7, 11]
église, à l'
Kirche, in der
ign.[1', 7], merc-i-f.

crowded room/chambre remplie de
monde/überfüllten Zimmer
kneeling/s'agenouille/Knien

climacteric period, during[2, 7]
ménopause, pendant la
Klimakterium, im
ACON., chin.[6], cimic.[6, 8], cocc.,
coff., crot-h.[8], ferr.[8], glon.[6, 8],
hydr-cy., kali-c., LACH.[2, 6-8],
mosch., nit-ac.[6, 8], nux-m.[6, 8], nux-v.[6],
phys.[2], sep.[6, 8], sulph.[2, 6-8], tab.[6],
tril.[8], valer., **verat.,** viol-t.

close room, in
chambre close, dans une
engen, geschlossenen Raum, im
acon.[1, 7], asaf., ip., **lach., PULS.,**
tab., vesp.[1']

coition, during[8]
coït, pendant le
Koitus, beim
murx., orig., **plat.**[6, 8]

after/après le/nach
AGAR., ASAF.[1, 7], dig., nat-p.,
sep.

clothes, from tight[16]
vêtements serrés, par
Kleidung, durch enge
kali-n.

cold, from taking
refroidissement, par
Erkältung, durch
petr., **sil.**

water am.
l'eau froide am.
kaltes Wasser am.
 glon., vip.[4]

weather, from
temps froid, par
Wetter, durch kaltes
 sep.

coldness of skin, with[2]
froide, avec peau
kalter Haut, mit
 camph., carb-v., **chin., laur.,**
 mosch., **tab., verat.**

colic, during intestinal[2]
colique intestinale, pendant la
Darmkolik, während einer
 asaf., **cast., coll.**[7] **coloc.,** hydr.[7],
 manc., nux-m., stram.

constriction of chest, with
constriction de la poitrine, avec
Zusammenschnüren der Brust, mit
 acon., ars.[16]

convulsions, after[2]
convulsions, après
Konvulsionen, nach
 ars-s-f., **verat.**

cough, during
toux, pendant la
Husten, bei
 ars., cadm-s., cina, coff., **cupr.,**
 ip.[15], **phos.**[2, 7, 15]

between spells[2, 7]
pendant les accès
zwischen den Anfällen
 ant-t.

crowded room, in
chambre remplie de monde, dans une
überfüllten Zimmer, im
 am-c., ambr., **ars.,** bar-c., con.,
 ign.[1, 7] **lyc.,** nat-c., **nat-m.,**
 nux-m.[1, 7] **nux-v.**[1, 7] **phos.,** plb.,
 PULS., sulph.

church/église/Kirche

street
rue très fréquentée, dans une
Straße mit vielen Menschen, auf
 einer
 asaf.

dark places, in
endroits sombres, dans des
dunklen Orten, an
 stram.

diarrhoea, before
diarrhée, avant la
Diarrhoe, vor
 ars., sulph., sumb.

during[7]/pendant la/während
 ars., crot-t.[2], **cupr-a.**[2] **nux-m.**[2]
 paeon., podo., **puls.**[2] verat.

after/après la/nach
 aloe[6], ars., colch.[6], **NUX-V.**[2, 7]

*collapse-diarrhoea/collapsus-
 diarrhée/Kollaps-Diarrhoe*

dinner, during
déjeuner, pendant le
Mittagessen, beim
 asaf., lyc., **mag-m., nux-v.**

after, when taking exercise in open
 air
après le, en prenant de l'exercice
 en plein air
nach dem M. beim Gehen im Freien
 am-m., **kali-c.**[2, 7] **nux-v.**[2, 7]

diphtheria, in[2, 7]
diphtérie, pendant la
Diphtherie, bei
 brom., **canth.,** kali-m.[7], lach.[7],
 sulph.

discouraged, when
découragé, quand il est
entmutigt, wenn
 ars.

drowsy, with
somnolence, avec
Schläfrigkeit, mit
 ars.

drug, on thinking of
remèdes, en pensant aux
Arzneimittel, beim Denken an
    asaf.

eating, before
manger, avant
Essen, vor dem
    asaf., bufo., ind., phos., ran-b.[1],
    sulph.

    hunger/faim/Hunger

    after
    après avoir mangé
    nach dem
        bar-c., bufo, **caust.**[1, 7], dios.[2, 7],
        kali-bi.[2, 7], kali-c.[2, 7], **mag-m.,**
        nux-v., ph-ac., plan., sang., sil.[3],
        sul-ac.[3]

egg, on smelling freshly beaten
œufs fraîchement battus, par
    l'odeur d'
Ei, beim Geruch von frisch geschlage-
    nem
    colch.

emission, after seminal
pertes séminales, après
Samenverlust, nach
    ASAF., ph-ac.

epistaxis, from [2, 7]
épistaxis, par
Nasenbluten, durch
    acon., cann-s., croc.[7], crot-h., **ip.,**
    lach.

    before[2, 7]/avant/vor
    carb-v.

    with[7, 15]/avec/mit
        calc.[3], cann-s.[3], carb-v.[15], croc.,
        lach.

eructation, from
renvois, par
Aufstoßen, durch
    arg-n., CARB-V.[2, 7], **nux-v.**[2, 7]

after/après/nach
    arg-n.[2, 7], **nux-v.**
    am.
        mag-m.

excitement, on
excitation, par
Erregung, durch
    acon.[1, 7], am-c., **asaf.,** aster.[7],
    camph., **caust., cham.,** cocc.[3],
    COFF., IGN., kali-c.[3], **LACH.,**
    mosch.[6], **nat-c., nux-m., OP., ph-ac.,**
    SUMB., verat.[1, 7], vesp.[1']

exertion, on
exercices physiques, par
Anstrengungen, bei
    arn.[7], ars., calc., **calc-ar.**[2], **carb-v.,**
    caust., cocc., ferr.[1'], hyper., **iod.**[2],
    lach.[2], **lob.**[2, 7], mosch.[6], nat-m.,
    nux-v., plan., plb., **rhus-t.**[7], **senec.,**
    SEP., sulph., **ther., verat.**

eyes closing agg.[3]
yeux agg., fermer les
Augenschließen agg.
    ant-t.

face, with blue[7]
face bleue, avec
Gesichtsfarbe, mit blauer
    morph.

    pale[2]
    pâle
    blasser
        acon.[7], berb.[7], **cimic., ip.,**
        LACH.[2, 7], **lob.,** nat-m.[7], nux-v.[7],
        puls.[7], **stram., tab.**

    red
    rouge
    roter
        acon.[7], **ptel.**[2]

falling, with[2, 7]
chute, avec
Fallen, mit
    ars., camph., stram.

backward[2, 7]
en arrière
rückwärts
    lac-d.

to left side[2, 7]
à gauche
nach links
    mez.

fasting am.[1']
jeûner am.
Fasten am.
    alum-sil.

fever, before[4]
fièvre, avant la
Fieber, vor
    ars.

    during/pendant la/im
      acon., arn., ars.[4], bell.,
      eup-per.[2], **ign.**[2, 7], nat-m.,
      nux-v., op., **phos.**, **puls.**[2], **SEP.**

    intermittent[2, 7]
    intermittente
    intermittierenden
      phos.

    puerperal[2, 7]
    puerpérale
    Puerperalfieber
      cimic., **coloc.**

    after[2, 7]/après la/nach
      sal-ac.

frequent
fréquent
häufig
    ARS., **bapt.**[2, 7], **camph.**[2, 7],
    carbn-s.[2, 7], **hyos.**[2, 7], **merc.**[2],
    merc-cy.[2, 7], **murx.**[2, 7], **op.**[2, 7], phos.,
    SULPH.

fright, after
frayeur, par
Schreck, durch
    ACON., gels., ign., lach., nux-v.[5],
    OP., phos.[5], staph.[5], verat.[1, 7]

fruit am., acid
fruits acides am.
Obst am., saures
    naja

gastric affections, in[2]
gastriques, dans les affections
Magenerkrankungen, bei
    alumn., **ARG-N.**[2, 7], bufo, dios.,
    dor.[2, 7], elaps, **kali-bi.**[2, 7], **mag-m.**,
    mez., **nat-s.**[2, 7], sang., **SULPH.**

pain-stomach/douleurs-estomac/
Schmerzen – Magen

grief, from[7]
chagrin, par
Kummer, durch
    ign., staph.

haematemesis, from[7]
hématémèse, par
Bluterbrechen, durch
    ARS.

haemoptysis, after[16]
hémoptysie, après
Haemoptysis, nach
    sil.

haemorrhages, nose bleeding, from[2]
hémorhagies, saignement de nez, par
Blutungen, Nasenbluten, durch
    acon., cann-s., crot-h., **ip.**, **lach.**

    post partum[2, 7]
      cann-s., **croc.**, **IP.**[7], **TRIL.**[7]

    rectum[2, 7]
    rectale
    rektale
      ign., nux-v.

    uterine[2, 7]
    utérine
    Uterusblutungen
      apis, **CHIN.**, **coc-c.**[7], kreos.,
      merc., **phys.**, tril.[12]

headache, during
maux de tête, pendant les
Kopfschmerzen, bei
    ars.[11], **calc.**[2, 7], **carb-v.**[2, 7], cast.[2],

gels.[2, 7], glon., graph.[7], hippoz.[2], lyc.[7, 16], mez.[16], mosch.[3, 7], nat-m.[7], **sil.**[2, 7], stram., **sulph.**[2, 7], **ter.**[2], verat., zing.

heart, with pressure about
cœur, avec pression sur le
Herzdruck, mit
cimic., **manc.**[2], petr., plb.

*angina pectoris/angine de poitrine/
   Angina pectoris
cardiopathy/cardiopathie/
   Herzleiden
pain–heart/douleurs–cœur/
   Schmerzen–Herz*

heat, with flushes of[2]
bouffées de chaleur, pendant des
Hitzewallungen, mit
crot-t., sep.[15], **SULPH.**

heat then coldness, with
chaud, puis de froid, avec sensation de
Hitze, dann Kälte, mit
   SEP.

from[7]/par/durch
   ant-c.[2], berb., nux-v., petr.

heated, when[3, 4]
échauffant, en s'
Erhitzung, bei
   tab.

hunger, from
faim, par la
Hunger, durch
   cocc.[2, 7], crot-c.[7, 11], culx.[1'], **phos., sulph.**

hysterical
hystérique
hysterische
   acon.[8], am-c.[1', 7], arn.[2, 7], ars., asaf.[8], cench.[1'], **cham.,** cimic., **COCC.,** cupr.[8], **dig.**[2, 7], **IGN.,** kali-ar.[1'], lac-d., lach.[8], **mosch., nat-m., nux-m., nux-v.,** puls., **sep.**[2], stict.[2], sumb., ter.

injury, from shock in[2]
choc traumatique, au cours de
Verletzungsschock, beim
   arn.[4], atro., **camph., cham.,** dig., **hyper.**

wounds/blessure/Wunden

concussion of brain, from[2, 7]
commotion cérébrale, par
Gehirnerschütterung, durch
   hyos.

kneeling in church, while
s'agenouille à l'église, quand il
Knien in der Kirche, beim
   SEP.

church/église/Kirche

labor, during
accouchement, pendant l'
Entbindung, während der
   cimic., cinnm.[2, 7], **coff., NUX-V., PULS., SEC., verat.**

after[7]/après l'/nach der
   cann-s., croc.

leucorrhoea, with[2]
leucorrhée, avec
Fluor, mit
   bar-c., cycl., **lach., nux-m.,** sulph.

lights, from being in a room with many
lumières, en étant dans une chambre éclairée de nombreuses
Lichtern, durch Aufenthalt in einem Raum mit vielen
   nux-v.

listening to reading, from[11]
écoutant quelqu'un qui lit, en
Zuhören bei einer Lesung, durch
   agar-em.

looking steadily at any object
  directly before eye
regardant fixement un objet se trou-
  vant immédiatement devant les
  yeux, en
Sehen auf einen Gegenstand direkt
  vor dem Auge, durch angestrengtes
  sumb.

  upward[3]
  vers le haut, en
  Hochsehen, beim
    tab.

loss of fluids, from
perte de fluides vitaux, par
Säfteverluste, durch
    ars.[7], bar-c.[4], **carb-v.**[2, 7], **CHIN.,**
    IP.[7], kreos.[7], merc.[7], nux-m.[7],
    nux.v.[7], **PH-AC.**[1, 7], **TRIL.**[1, 7],
    verat.[2, 7]

  blood
  sang
  Blutverluste
    chin.[6], ferr.[1'], **ip.**[6], op.[1', 6], tril.[6]

lying, while
couché, en étant
Liegen, im
    berb.[2, 7], calad., **CARB-V.**[2, 7],
    caust.[4], iod., lyc., sulph.

  am.
    alumn., dios., hedeo[7]., **merc-i-f.,**
    nux-v.

  after
  après s'étre étendu
  nach dem
    calad., mag-c.

  on the side, while
  sur le côté, en étant
  auf der Seite, im
    lyc., sil.

meditating, mental exertion, from
intellectuel, par travail;
  en réfléchissant
geistige Anstrengung, durch
    calad., **calc.**[2], coff.[2, 7], **nux-v.**[2, 7],
    par.[2]

meningitis, in[2]
méningite, dans la
Meningitis, bei
    ant-t., **dig., glon.**

menses, before
menstruation, avant la
Menses, vor den
    am-c.[6], cimic.[2], cocc., lach., **lyc.,**
    murx., nat-m.[2, 6, 7, 16], **nux-m.,**
    nux-v., **sep., thuj.**

  during
  pendant la
  während der
    acon.[2], apis, berb., **calc.**[1, 7],
    cham., chin.[4, 6], cimic., **cocc.,**
    glon.[2, 6, 7], **ign., LACH.,**
    lyc.[3, 4, 6], mag-m., **mosch.,**
    murx.[7], nat-m., nux-m.,
    NUX-V., plb., **puls.,** raph.,
    sars., SEP., sulph., uran-n.[2, 7],
    verat., **vib.**[2], wies.[7, 11]

  from pain
  par des douleurs
  durch Schmerzen
    cocc.[2, 7], kali-s., **lap-a.,**
    nux-v.[2, 7], sars.[2, 7], sep.[2, 7]

  after
  après la
  nach den
    chin.[1, 7], lach., lyc.[1, 7]

  suppressed, from[8]
  supprimée, par la
  unterdrückte, durch
    cocc.[4], kali-c., **nux-m.,** op.

metrorrhagia with[8]
métrorrhagies avec
Metrorrhagien mit
    apis, chin.[4, 8], ferr-m., **tril.**

moving, on
mouvement, au
Bewegung, durch
    ARS., BRY.[2], **COCC.**[1, 7], croc.[7],
    cupr., cupr.a.[11], **hyos.**[2, 7], kali-c.,
    lob.[7], nat-hchls.[11], **nit-ac.,**

nux-v.[4], phys., spig.[7], **SPONG.,
verat.**

am.
  jug-c.

quickly
rapide
schnelle
  samb., sumb.[11]

music, on hearing
musique, en écoutant
Musik, beim Hören von
  cann-i., sumb.

mydriasis, with[7]
mydriase, avec
Mydriasis, mit
  morph.

nausea, before[11]
nausée, avant la
Übelkeit, von der
  dig., glon., **verat.**[2]

during/pendant la/bei der
  ail.[11], alum., alumn.[2], ang.[2, 7],
  arg.n., ars.[11], calad.[2, 7], calc.,
  carb-an.[7], carbn-s., caust.[7],
  cham., chel., **COCC.,** coff-t.[11],
  fago., **glon.,** graph., **IP.**[2, 7],
  kali-c.[2, 7], **LACH.,** lob.[2, 7], nat-m.,
  NUX-V., op., petr.[7], picro.[7, 11],
  plan.[2, 7], sep.[11], sul-ac., sulph.,
  tab.[2, 7], valer.[2, 7], verat.,
  vesp.[2, 7, 11]

after/après la/nach der
  kali-bi.

nervous[1']
neurasthénique
neurasthenische
  cench.

noise, from
bruit, par le
Geräusche, durch
  ant-c.[1'], asaf., bor.[1'], lyc.[1'], merc.,
  nat-m.[1']

numbness, tingling, with[7]
engourdissement et picotement, avec
Taubheit, Prickeln, mit
  ACON.[2], bor., nat-m., nux-v.

odors, from
odeurs, par
Gerüche, durch
  ign., **NUX-V., PHOS.**[1, 7], sang.[11]

  Vol. I: *sensitive-odors/sensible-
  odeurs/empfindlich – Gerüche*

cooking food, of
nourriture cuite, de
kochender Speisen
  COLCH., ip.

eau de Cologne am.[7, 11]
  sang.

eggs, of[2]
œufs, des
Eiern, von
  colch.

fish, of
poisson, de
Fisch, von
  colch.

flowers, of
fleurs, de
Blumen, von
  PHOS.[1, 7], sang.

perfume or vinegar, of[2, 7]
parfum ou vinaigre, de
Parfüm oder Essig, von
  agar.

operations, on talking of[7]
opérations, en entendant parler d'
Operationen, beim Gespräch über
  alum.

pain, from
douleurs, par
Schmerzen, durch
  acon.[2, 3, 7], apis, ars.[3, 5], asaf.,
  bism.[7], bol-la.[7, 11], **cham., cocc.,**
  coff.[3], coloc., **gels.**[2, 7], **HEP.**[1, 7],

iod.[3], **nux-m., nux-v.,** phos.[7],
phyt., ran-s.[3], sil.[3], stroph-h.[3],
valer., verat.[1, 7], vib.[3], vip.[3]

Vol. I: *sensitive-pain/sensible-*
douleurs/empfindlich –
Schmerzen

abdomen, in
abdomen, dans l'
Abdomen, im
   cocc., coll.[7], plb., stram.[7]

anus, in[16]
anus, dans l'
Anus, im
   sulph.

ear, in
oreilles, dans les
Ohr, im
   cur., hep., merc.

head, in[16]
tête, dans la
Kopf, im
   mez.

heart, in
cœur, dans le
Herz, am
   arn.[1] (non: aur.), **cact.**[2, 7], **LACH.,**
   manc.[2]

angina pectoris/angine de
poitrine/Angina pectoris
heart/cœur/Herzdruck

prick of a needle, from[16]
piqûre d'aiguille, par
Nadelstich, durch
   calc.

sacrum, in[11]
sacrodynie
Kreuz, im
   dios., hura

spermatic cords, in[2, 7]
cordons spermatiques, dans les
Samensträngen, in
   calc-ar.

stomach, in
estomac, dans l'
Magen, im
   ars.[2, 7], **BISM., coll.,** cupr-s.[2],
   dios.[2], **nux-v.,** puls., ran-s.,
   sin-n.[2], **sulph.**[2]

gastric/gastriques/Magen-
erkrankungen

stool, during[2, 7]
selle, pendant la
Stuhlgang, während
   cocc.

teeth, in
dents, dans les
Zähnen, in den
   chin., **puls.,** verat.

testicles, in[2, 7]
testicules, dans les
Hoden, in den
   laur.

palpitations, during
palpitations, pendant
Herzklopfen, bei
   ACON.[2, 7], **am-c.**[2, 7], arg-n.[15],
   beryl.[9], cact., cimic., **cocc., hydr.**[2],
   iod., kalm.[2], **LACH., manc.**[2],
   NUX-M., petr., sul-i.[1'], **verat.**

after[15]/après/nach
   am-c.

periodical
périodique
periodische
   cact., **coll.**[2], fl-ac., lyc., nit-ac.[4],
   staph.[4]

every day[2, 7]
chaque jour
täglich
   hydr.

perspiration, during
transpiration, pendant la
Schweiß, bei
   agar., ant-t.[2], apis, **ars., calc.**[2],
   carb-v., hyos., **ign., lob.**[2],
   morph.[7], **sep.**[2]

cold, with[2]
froide, avec
kaltem, mit
   bry., camph., caps., carb-v.,
   chin., DIG., hydr., lach.[7], **tab.,**
   ther., **verat.**[2, 7]

am.[2, 7]
   olnd.

after/après la/nach
   apis[2, 7], arn.[3, 11], **chin.**[7], sal-ac.[2]

suppressed foot sweat, from[2, 7]
supression de la t. des pieds, par
Unterdrückung von Fußschweiß,
durch
   sil.

pregnancy, during
grossesse, dans la
Schwangerschaft, in der
   bell., kali-c.[7], **nux-m., nux-v.,**
   puls., sec., **sep., verat.**[2]

slightest motion of child, from[2, 7]
moindre mouvement de l'enfant,
   par le
leichteste Kindsbewegung, durch
   die
   lach.

pressure in waist, by
pression à la taille, à la ceinture, par
Druck in die Lenden, durch
   lac-c.[2, 7], **merc.**[7]

prolonged
prolongé
lang anhaltende
   hydr-ac., laur.

puerperal
puerpéral
Kindbett, im
   coloc.[2, 7], cimic.[7]

pulse, with imperceptible[2, 7]
pouls imperceptible, avec
Puls, mit nicht wahrnehmbarem
   chin., crot-h., morph.[7]

irregular[2, 7]
irrégulier
unregelmäßigem
   DIG., morph.[7]

slow[2, 7]
lent
langsamem
   DIG.

raising arms above head
élevant les bras au dessus de la tête,
   en
Heben der Arme über den Kopf, beim
   lac-d., lach., spong.

the head
la tête, en relevant
des Kopfes
   apoc., **bry.,** ip.

read, when attempting to, while
   standing
lire étant debout, en essayant de
lesen, beim Versuch, im Stehen zu
   glon.

reading, after
lu, après avoir
Lesen, nach dem
   asaf., cycl., tarax.

restlessness, after
agitation, après
Ruhelosigkeit, nach
   calc.

riding, while
à cheval, en étant
Reiten, beim
   berb., cocc.[7], grat., **sep.,** sil.

after[11]
après une course
nach dem
   berb., sep.

rising, on
levant, en se
Aufstehen, beim
   acon.[7], ambr., **bry.,** calad., **calc.**[2, 7],
   cere-b.[11], chel., crot-h., cupr., ind.,

iod.[2], **lach.**[2, 7], merc-i-f.[3], phyt.[3],
plb., ran-a.[11], vac.[2, 7], vario.[2, 7],
verat-v.[2, 3, 7], vib.[3]

sitting up/assis/Sitzen

from bed, on
sortant du lit, en
Bett, aus dem
    acon., apoc.[1'], berb.[4], **BRY.,**
    calad., **calc.**[2], **carb-v., cina,**
    colch.[15], **iod.**[1, 7], nat-m.[16], op.,
    PHYT., rhus-t., rob., sep.,
    trom.[11]

from a seat, on
d'un siège, en se
Sitz, von einem
    carb-v.[16], staph., sumb., trom.

after[2]
après s'être levé
nach dem
    CARB-V., iod.

running up stairs
montant rapidement des escaliers, en
hinaufläuft, wenn er Treppen
    sumb.

scolding, from[7]
grondé, étant
Schelte, durch
    mosch.

sexual excesses, after
sexuels, après excès
sexuellen Ausschweifungen, nach
    dig.[2], ol-an.[6]

shock, from[2]
choc, par
Schock, durch
    atro.

sitting, while
assis, étant
Sitzen, beim
    iod., kali-n., nat-s., nux-v.[4]

down, on[4]
s'asseyant, en
Hinsetzen, beim
    bov., kali-n.

up, from
levant, en se
Aufsitzen, beim
    ACON., arn., **BRY.,** carb-v.,
    chin.[6], **dig.**[6], dios., **ip., nux-v.,**
    PHYT.[1, 7], **ran-b.**[2, 7], **sep.**[2, 7],
    sulph., verat-v., **vib.,** vip.[6]

rising/levant/Aufstehen

suddenly
rapidement
plötzlichen
    ery-a., **verat-v.**

upright, while[7]
tout droit
Aufrechtsitzen
    acon., calad.

sleep, after[2, 7]
sommeil, après le
Schlaf, nach dem
    CARB-V.

followed by, f.[2, 7]
suivi de, é.
gefolgt von, O.
    nux-m.

loss of, by[2, 7]
manque de, par
Schlafmangel, durch
    syph.

sleeping on left side
s'endort à gauche, s'il
Schlafen auf der linken Seite, beim
    asaf.

smoking, on
fumant, en
Rauchen, beim
    ign.[2, 7], **ip.**[2, 7], sil.

after
après avoir fumé
nach dem
  caust.[2, 7], lob.[2]

snoring, with[7]
ronflement, avec
Schnarchen, mit
  stram.

speaking, from
parlant, en
Sprechen, durch
  ars.

standing, while
debout, étant
Stehen, beim
  ALUM., ALUMN.[2], apis, berb.[4],
  bry., cur.[7], dig., dios.[11], glon.[11],
  kali-n.[4], lil-t., lyc.[4], nux-m.,
  nux-v., phyt., rhus-r., sil., sulph.,
  zinc.

in church during menses
à l'église pendant la menstruation
in der Kirche während der Menses
  lyc., nux-m., puls.

prolapse of uterus, from[7]
prolapsus de l'utérus, par
Uterusprolaps, durch
  lil-t.

urinating, while[2, 7]
uriner, pendant
Urinieren, beim
  acon.

starting at something falling to the
  floor, from[11]
tressaillement en entendant tomber
  qc. sur le plancher, par
Auffahren beim Fallen von irgend
  etwas auf den Boden, durch
  merc.

stomach, sensation of something
  rising from
estomac, avec la sensation de qc. qui
  monte depuis l'
Magen, Gefühl, als ob etwas aufsteigt
  vom
  am-br., CALC.[2, 7]

stool, before
selle, avant la
Stuhlgang, vor dem
  ars., dig., glon., puls., sars.,
  sulph.[2], sumb.

during/pendant la/während
  aloe, bor.[2, 7], colch.[2, 7], coll.,
  crot-t.[7], dulc., dios., nux-m.,
  ox-ac., petr.[2, 7], plan.[2, 7], puls.[1, 7],
  sars.[1, 7], spig.[4, 7], stann.[6], sulph.,
  verat.[2, 7], verat-v.[6]

after/après la/nach dem
  aloe[2, 7], apis[2, 7], ars., ars-s-f.[1'],
  bol-la.[2, 7], calc.[1, 7], cocc., colch.,
  CON., crot-t.[2], cur., dig.[2, 7], dios.,
  hydr.[2, 7], kiss.[11], lyc., morph.,
  nat-s., nux-m., phos.[1], phyt.,
  plan., PODO., sarr.[2, 7], sulph.,
  ter., verat.

am. by[11]/par/durch
  rhodi.

odor of, from
odeur de la, par
Stuhlgeruch, durch
  dios.

urging, from
besoin de, par
Stuhldrang, durch
  cocc.

stooping, on
baissant, en se
Bücken, beim
  elaps, sumb.

storm, before a[11]
tempête, avant une
Sturm, vor einem
  petr.

sudden
soudain
plötzliche
 ant-c.[1'], camph.[7], cham.[12],
 hydr-ac.[6], kali-cy.[7], **phos.**, podo.[6],
 ran-b.[1', 6, 7], rhus-t., **sep.**, valer.[6]

summer heat, from
chaleur de l'été, par la
Sommerhitze, durch
 ant-c., ip.

tendency to[2, 11]
tendance aux évanouissements
Tendenz zur
 aether, carbn-o., carbn-s., colch.,
 cupr-s., dig., elpas, euph., iod.[4],
 kali-ox., **magn-gl.**, nux-m.[4], ol-an.,
 sol-t-ae., sulph., **sumb.**[7], tab., thea,
 verat.[4]

temples with both hands, on rubbing
tempes avec les deux mains, en se
 frottant les
Schläfen mit beiden Händen, beim
 Reiben der
 merc.

tetanic spasm, before[11]
tétanique, avant spasme
tetanischem Spasmus, vor
 sul-h.

 after[11]/après/nach
 nux-v.

thunderstorm, before
orage, avant un
Gewitter, vor
 petr., sil.

transient[2, 7]
passager
schnell vorübergehende
 mur-ac., nux-m.

trembling, with[7]
tremblements, avec
Zittern, mit
 asaf.[11], caust.[6], **lach.**[2], nux-v., petr.

trifles, from
futilités, par des
Kleinigkeiten, bei
 sep., sumb.[7]

turning the head, on
tournant la tête, en
Drehen des Kopfes, beim
 ery-a.[11], ptel.

urinating, during[6]
uriner, pendant
Urinieren, während
 stann.

 after/après/nach
 ACON., all-c., med.

uterine affection in[2]
utérine, dans une affection
Uteruserkrankung, bei
 cimic.[2, 7], cocc., **murx.**

vomiting, before[2]
vomissement, avant
Erbrechen, vor
 ARS., crot-h., **IP.**

 with[2, 7]/avec/mit
 agar.[2], apom.[7], crot-t.[11], **IP.,**
 kali-c., nit-ac.[16], **phyt., TAB.,**
 VERAT.

 after/après/nach
 ARS., bism.[6], **cocc.**[2], dig., elaps,
 gamb., kali-c.[16], **NUX-V.**[2], **stict.**[2],
 verat.[2]

waking, on
réveil, au
Erwachen, beim
 CARB-V., dios., graph., lach., ptel.,
 ther.[4]

walking, while
marchant, en
Gehen, beim
 aether[7, 11], arn., **ars.,** berb.[4], bov.,
 con.[2], cur., dor., ferr., get.[11],
 merc.[5], nat-s., **verat-v.**

after
après la marche
nach dem
    berb., **con.**[2, 7], nux-v.[4, 7], paeon.

continuing am.
continuée am., une marche
andauerndes G. am.
    anac.

downstairs, from going
descendant, en
Herabgehen, durch
    ery-a.[11], stann.[2, 7]

in open air
en plein air
im Freien
    berb.[4], bor.[4], caust.[16], lycps.,
    mosch.[4], seneg., sep.

    am.[4]
    am.-c.

rapidly am.
à pas rapides am.
schnelles G. am.
    petr.

after
après la marche
nach G.
    nux-v.

upstairs, from going[2, 7]
en montant des escaliers
Heraufgehen, durch
    anac.

warm bath from
chaud, par un **bain**
warmes Bad, durch ein
    lach.

warm room, in
chaude, dans une **chambre**
warmen Zimmer, im
    acon., ant.-c.[2, 7], calc-i.[1'], **ip.,**
    kreos., **lach., LIL.-T.**[1], lyc., **nat-m.,**
    nux-v., **PULS., SEP.,** spig., tab.,
    trif-p.[7, 11], vesp.[1']

water on, am. by dashing cold[11]
eau froide, am. quand on l'asperge d'
Wasser am., Bespritzen mit kaltem
    glon.

weakness, from[2, 7]
faiblesse, par
Schwäche, aus
    ant-t.[4], **ars.**[2], **carb-v.**[3, 4], caust.[4],
    chin.[3], **coca, ferr., hydr.**[2], lach.[2],
    nux-m.[3], nux-v.[3], ran-b.[2], **sang.,**
    verat.[2, 3], **zing.**

loss of fluids/perte de fluides/
    Säfteverluste

wet, after getting
mouillé, après être
Naßwerden, nach
    sep.

wine agg.[11]
vin agg., le
Wein agg.
    sumb.

wounds, from slight
blessure, par la moindre
Wunden, durch kleine
    verat.[1, 7]

writing, after
écrit, après avoir
Schreiben, nach
    calad., **calc.**[2], mosch., op.

FANNED, desire to be[3]
ÉVENTÉ, désir d'être
ANGEFÄCHELT zu werden, **Verlangen**
    apis, ars., bapt., **CARB-V.**[1', 3, 6, 7],
    caust., chin.[3, 6], chlol.[7], chlor., glon.[1'],
    kali-n., lach., lyc., med.[1', 3], nux-m.,
    puls., **sec.**[3, 6], sulph.[2], tab., zinc.

being, am.[3, 8]
étant, am.
zu werden am.
    ant-t.[3], apis.[3], **arg-n.,** bapt.[3],
    CARB-V., chin., crot-h.[3], ferr.[3],
    hist.[14], kali-n.[3], lach., med., sec.[3],
    xan.[3]

sensation see air–draft–sensation

FASTING, while
JÉUNE, au cours du
FASTEN, beim
 acon.[3], aloe, alum., am-c., **am-m.**[1],
 ambr., anac.[1], ars., **bar-c.,** bar-i.[1]',
 bov.[3], bry.[3], cact.[3], **CALC.,** calc-i.[1]',
 cann-i.[3], canth.[3], **carb-ac., carb-an.,**
 carb-v., caust., **chel.,** chin., cina,
 coc-c., CROC., ferr., ferr-p., **graph.,**
 hell., **hep.,** ign., **IOD., kali-c.**[1], **kreos.,**
 LACH., laur., lyc., mag-c., mag-m.,
 merc., **mez.,** nat-c., nat-p.[1]', nit-ac.,
 nux-v., petr., **phos., PLAT., PLB.,**
 puls., **RAN-B.,** rhus-t.[3], **rumx.,**
 sabad., SEP., spig., **STAPH., sulph.,**
 TAB., tarax., teucr., **valer.,** verat.,
 verb.

agg. (1897)
 acon., aloe, alum., am-c., am-m.,
 ambr., anac., ars., bar-c., bov., bry.,
 cact.[3], **CALC.,** cann-s., canth.,
 carb-ac., carb-an., carb-v., cast.[3],
 caust., **chel.,** chin., cina, coc-c.,
 CROC., ferr., ferr-p., gran.,
 graph., hell., hep., **ign., IOD.,**
 kali-c., kreos.[3], **lach.,** laur., lyc.,
 mag-c., mag-m., merc., mez., **nat-c.,**
 nit-ac., nux-v., petr., phos., **plat.,**
 plb., **psor.,** puls., **ran-b.,** ran-s.,
 rhod., rhus-t., **rumx., sabad., sep.,**
 spig., STAPH., stront-c., sulph.,
 tab., tarax., teucr., valer., verat.,
 verb.

ailments from[12]
troubles à la suite de
Beschwerden infolge von
 dios.

am. (1897)
 agar., alum., alum-sil.[1]', am-m.,
 ambr., anac., ant-c., arn., ars., asaf.,
 bar-c., bell., bor., **bry.,** calc.,
 calc-sil.[1]', caps., carb-an., carb-v.,
 caust., CHAM., chin., cocc., **CON.,**
 cycl., **dig.,** euph., ferr., graph., hell.,
 hep., hyos., ign., iod., **kali-c.,**

 kali-n., kali-p.[1]', kali-s.[1]', lach.,
 laur., lyc., mag-c., mang., nat-c.,
 NAT-M., nit-ac., **nux-m.,** nux-v.,
 par., petr., **ph-ac.,** phos., plb., puls.,
 rhod., rhus-t., sabin., sars., sep.,
 sil., stann., stront-c., sul-ac., sulph.,
 thuj., valer., verat.[3], **zinc.**

fat people see obesity

FATTY DEGENERATION of organs[8]
DÉGÉNÉRESCENCE GRAISSEUSE
 des organs
FETTIGE DEGENERATION der Organe
 ars., **AUR.**[2, 8], **calc-ar.**[2], **cupr.,** kali-c.,
 lac-d.[2], **PHOS.**[2, 8], vanad.

FEATHER-BED agg.
LIT DE PLUMES, agg. dans un
FEDERBETT agg.
 asaf., cocc., **coloc.,** led., lyc., **MANG.,**
 merc., psor., sulph.

FEEL every muscle and fibre of her
 right side, as if she could
SENTIR tous les muscles et les fibres
 de son côté droit, comme si elle
 pouvait
FÜHLEN, als könnte sie jeden Muskel
 und jede Sehne der rechten Seite
 sep.

FEMALES' disease[3]
FEMMES, maladies des
FRAUENLEIDEN
 acon.[3, 4], agar., am-m., ambr., ang.,
 ant-t., apis[3], arn., ars.[4], asaf.,
 BELL.[3, 4], bor., **bry., CALC.**[3, 4],
 camph., canth., **CAPS., caust.,**
 CHAM.[3, 4], **chin.**[3, 4], cic., cimic.[3], clem.,
 COCC.[3, 4], **con.**[3, 4], **CROC.,** cupr., dig.,
 euph., ferr., fl-ac., graph., hell., **hyos.,**
 ign.[3, 4], iod., ip.[3, 4], kali-c., lach.[3, 4],
 laur., led., mag-c.[3, 4], mag-m.[4], mang.,
 merc., merc-c., **mosch.**[3, 4], mur-ac.,
 nat-c., **nat-m.,** nux-m.[3, 4], nux-v., op.,

perh.[14], **PLAT.**[3, 4], plb., **PULS.**[3, 4],
rheum, **rhus-t.**, sabad., **SABIN.**[3, 4],
sec., sel., seneg., **SEP.**[3, 4], sil., spig.,
spong., stram., sul-ac., sulph., thuj.,
valer., verat., viol-o., vip.[3]

FEVER agg., **before**[3]
FIÈVRE agg., **avant** la
FIEBER agg., **vor**
    acon., ant-c., ant-t., **arn., ARS.,**
    bar-c., bell., bry., calc., caps.,
    carb-v., caust., **CHIN., cina,** cocc.,
    ferr., graph., hep., hyos., ign., **ip.,**
    kali-c., kali-n., lach., lyc., mag-c.,
    merc., nat-c., nat-m., nit-ac., nux-v.,
    ph-ac., phos., **PULS.,** rhod., **rhus-t.,**
    ruta, sabad., sabin., samb., sep., sil.,
    spig., **sulph., verat.**

during, agg.[3]
pendant la, agg.
im, agg.
    acon., agar., alum., am-c., am-m.,
    ambr., anac., ang., **ant-c.,** ant-t.,
    arn., **ARS.,** aur., bar-c., bell., bor.,
    bov., **bry.,** calad., **calc.,** canth.,
    caps., carb-v., caust., **cham., CHIN.,**
    cina, cocc., coff., con., croc., dig.,
    dros., dulc., euph., **ferr.,** graph.,
    hell., hep., hyos., ign., iod., **ip.,**
    kali-c., kali-n., kreos., lach., laur.,
    led., **lyc.**[3, 12], mang., merc., mez.,
    mosch., mur-ac., nat-c., **nat-m.,**
    nit-ac., nux-m., **NUX-V., op.,** petr.,
    ph-ac., **phos.,** plat., **puls.,** ran-b.,
    rheum, rhod., **rhus-t.,** ruta, sabad.,
    samb., sars., sec., **SEP.,** sil., spig.,
    staph., stram., stront-c., sul-ac.,
    sulph., tarax., teucr., thuj., valer.,
    verat., zinc.

after, agg.[3]
après la, agg.
nach, agg.
    ant-c., ant-t., arn., **ARS., bell.,** bry.,
    carb-v., **CHIN.,** cina, dig., **hep.,**
    kali-c., nat-m., **nux-v.,** phos., puls.,
    sep., sil., verat.

convalescence/Rekonvaleszenz

FISTULAE[12]
FISTULES
FISTELN
    alum., aur-m., bac., bar-m.,
    berb.[3, 12], bry.[6], bufo[2], cact.,
    CALC.[3, 6, 12], **calc-f.**[3, 6], calc-hp.[6],
    calc-p.[3, 6, 12], calc-s.[6, 12], **calen.,**
    carb-v.[6], **caust.**[3, 12], con.[6], cop.,
    cund., eucal., **fl-ac.**[3, 6-8, 12], **hep.**[2, 6],
    hydr., iris, kreos.[6], lach.[6], **lyc.**[3],
    maland., mez.[1'], **nat-s.**[2],
    nit-ac.[3, 6, 8, 12], ol-j., petr.[3, 6, 12],
    phos.[1', 2, 3, 6, 12], puls.[3, 6], pyrog.,
    querc., **SIL.**[1', 2, 3, 6, 8, 12], stront-c.[6],
    sulph.[1', 3, 6], syph.[1'], thuj.[6], **tub.**[6],
    tub-k.[12]

abscesses/abcès/Abszesse

bones, of[6, 10]
os, des
Knochenfisteln
    ang., **asaf.,** aur.[6], bufo[2],
    calc-f.[3, 6, 7, 10], calc-hp.[3, 6], calc-p.[10],
    calc-sil.[10], fl-ac.[10], **hep.**[2, 3, 6], lyc.[6],
    merc.[6], **nat-s.**[2, 12], **ol-j.**[2], phos.[3, 6, 10],
    SIL.[3, 6, 10]

glands, of
glandes, des
Drüsenfisteln
    cist.[6], lyc.[6], merc.[6], nit-ac.[6], **phos.,**
    phyt.[6], **sil., sulph.**

joints, of
articulations, des
Gelenkfisteln
    calc., hep., ol-j., **PHOS., SIL.,** sulph.

operation of, after[1']
opération de fistule, après
Fisteloperation, nach
    berb., calc., calc-p.[1', 12], caust.,
    graph., sil., sulph., thuj.

ulcers of skin with
ulcères de la peau avec
Hautgeschwüre mit
    agar., ant-c., ars., **asaf.,** aur., bar-c.,
    bell., berb.[3], **BRY., CALC., calc-f.**[3],
    calc-m.[6], **calc-p.,** calc-s., carb-ac.,
    carb-v., carbn-s., **CAUST.,** chel.,

cinnb., clem., **con., fl-ac., hep.,
hippoz.**, kreos., **lach.**[4], led., **LYC.,
merc., mill.**[2], nat-c., **nat-m.**, nat-p.,
nit-ac., petr., ph-ac.[3, 4], **PHOS.,
PULS.,** rhus-t., ruta, sabin., sel.,
sep., **SIL.,** stann.[4], **staph.,** stram.,
sulph., ter.[3], **thuj.**

FLABBY feeling
MOLLESSE, sensation de
ERSCHLAFFUNG, Gefühl der
acon., agar., am-m., ambr., ant-t.,
arg-m., arn., **ARS.,** asar., **bar-c.,**
bell., bov., bry., **CALC., calc-p.,**
calc-s., calc-sil.[1'], canth., **CAPS.,**
carb-an., carb-v., **CAUST., cham.,
chel.,** chin., chin-ar.[1'], cic., cina,
clem., coff., **CROC., cycl., dig.,**
euph., euphr., **ferr., fl-ac.,** graph.,
hep., **IGN.,** iod., **ip., kali-ar., kali-c.,**
kali-n., kali-p., kali-s., laur., **LYC.,**
mag-c., mag-m., meny., merc.,
mosch., mur-ac., **NAT-C.,** nit-ac.,
nux-m., **nux-v.,** olnd., par., petr.,
PHOS., plat., psor., puls., rhod.,
rhus-t., **sabad.,** sabin., seneg., **sep.,**
sil., spong., **staph.,** stront-c.,
SULPH., tarax., teucr., tril.[12], thuj.,
VERAT., zinc.

*relaxation–physical/relâchement–
physique/Erschlaffung,
körperliche*

hard parts, in
parties dures, des
festen Teilen, in
bar-s.[1'], caust., **merc.,** mez., **nit-ac.,**
nux-m.

**internally
interne
innerlich**
calc., kreos., **SEP.**

foggy weather see weather–foggy

**FOOD and DRINKS
ALIMENTS et BOISSONS
SPEISEN und GETRÄNKE**

alcohol agg.*
alcool agg.
Alkohol agg.
  acon., **agar.,** agav-t.[14], aloe[6],
  alum., alumn., **am-c.**[3], am-m.,
  anac., ang.[3], **ant-c.,** apom.[8],
  aran-ix.[10, 14], **arg-n.,** arn., **ARS.,
  ASAR.,** aur.[8, 12], **BAR-C., bell.,**
  berb.[2], bor., bov., cadm-s.,
  calc., calc-ar., calc-f.[10],
  calc-sil.[1'], **cann-i.**[8], **carb-ac.**[13],
  carb-an., **carb-v., carbn-s.,**
  card-m.[8], caust., **chel., chin.,**
  chlol., cimic.[3, 8], **coca**[2, 8], cocc.,
  coff., colch.[8], **con.,** cortiso.[9],
  crot-h., dig., eup-per.[8], **ferr.**[2],
  ferr-i.[12], fl-ac.[1', 3, 7], gels., **glon.**[2, 6],
  gran.[12], grat.[1'], guar.[12], hed.[9],
  hell.[3], hep., hydr.[8], hyos., **ign.,** ip.[8],
  kali-bi., **kali-br.**[2], **LACH.,** laur.,
  led., lob.[8], **lyc.,** mand.[9, 10, 14],
  merc.[2, 3, 4], naja, **nat-c., nat-m.,**
  nux-m., **NUX-V., OP.,** petr.,
  phos.[3], phyt.[7], **puls.,** querc.[8],
  RAN-B., rhod., rhus-t., ruta,
  sabad., **sang., SEL.,** sep., **sil.,**
  spig., **stram.,** stront-c., stroph-h.,
  stry.[8], **SUL-AC., SULPH.,**
  syph.[2, 7], tab., thuj., verat., zinc.

easily intoxicated
enivré facilement par
leicht betrunken
  CON.[2, 7, 11, 12], naja[11], **zinc.**[2]

  beer/bière/Bier

ailments from[12]
troubles à la suite d'
Beschwerden infolge von
  agar., ars., aur., bry., cadm-s.,
  calc., carb-v., chin., crot-h., dig.,
  gels., lach., led., lob., nux-m.,
  nux-v., op., querc., ran-b., sel.,
  sep., stroph-h., sulph., ter., verat.

am.
  dicha.[10], gels.[7]

aversion/Abneigung
ail.[2], alco.[11], ang.[3], ant-t., ars.,
ars-met.[2, 11], bell., bry.[6], calc.[13],
calc-ar.[13], carb-v.[13], cham.[6], chin.[6],
cocc.[6], **hyos.**, ign., lec.[13], manc.,
mand.[10, 14], merc., nux-v., ph-ac.,
phos.[13], phyt.[7], psor.[13], **rhus-t.**,
sil.[8], spig.[6], spong.[6], stram.,
sul-ac.[13], sulph.[6, 13], zinc.[6]

desire/désir/Verlangen
acon., agav-t.[14], ail.[6], alco.[11],
aloe, am-c., ant-t., arg-m.[3], arn.,
ARS., ars-i., ASAR., aster.,
aur., aur-ar.[1'], aur-i.[1'], bov.,
bry., bufo, calc., **calc-ar.,**
calc-s., **CAPS.,** carb-ac.[3, 8],
carb-an., **carb-v.**[3, 6, 8], chin.,
cic., **coca**[2, 6, 8, 13], cocc.[8],
CROT-H., cub., cupr.,
ferr-p.[8, 13], fl-ac., gins., hell.,
hep., iber.[2], ign.[3], **iod.,**
kali-bi.[8, 13], **kreos.,** lac-c.,
LACH., lec.[8], **led., lyc., med.,**
merc., mosch.[2, 3, 8, 13], **mur-ac.,**
naja, nat-m.[3], nat-p., nux-m.[3],
NUX-V., olnd.[6], **op., phos.,**
plb., **psor., puls.,** rhus-t.[3], **sel.,**
sep., sil.[3], sol-t-ae., **spig.,**
staph., stront-c.[8, 13], stry-n.[7],
sul-ac., SULPH., sumb., **syph.,**
tab., ter., ther., **tub.,** ziz.[2]

disgust for, but[14]
dégoût d', mais
Widerwillen gegen, aber
thiop.

menses, before
menstruation, avant la
Menses, vor den
SEL.

ale agg.[2]
bière blonde anglaise agg.
englisches helles Bier agg.
gamb., spong., sulph.

beer/bière/Bier

aversion/Abneigung
ferr., **NUX-V.**

desire/désir/Verlangen
ferr-p., **med., sulph.**

almonds, desire for
amandes, désir d'
Mandeln, Verlangen nach
cub.

anchovies, desire for[3]
anchois, désir d'
Sardellen, Verlangen nach
verat.

herring/hareng/Hering
sardines/Sardinen

apples agg.[3]
pommes agg.
Äpfel agg.
alum., ant-t.[3, 7], arg-n., ars.[5],
ars-i.[3], bor.[16], chin.[5], con., mang.[16],
merc-c., nat-s., ox-ac.[1'], phos.,
puls., rumx., sep., sulph.[5], thuj.

am.[11]
ust.

aversion/Abneigung
ant-t.[13], guaj.[13], lyss.

desire/désir/Verlangen
aloe, ant-t., fel[11], **guaj.,** menth.[6],
sulph., tell.

aromatic drinks agg., smell of[3]
aromatiques agg., odeur des boissons
aromatischer Getränke agg., Geruch
agn., puls.

desire/désir/Verlangen
anan.

ashes, desire for
cendres, désir de
Asche, Verlangen nach
tarent.

indigestible things/indigestes,
choses/Unverdauliches

bacon am.
lard am.
Speck am.
    ran-b., ran-s.

aversion[12]/Abneigung
    rad-br.

desire/désir/Verlangen
    ars.[6, 7, 13], calc.[3], **calc-p.**, cench.,
    mez., rad-br.[3], **sanic.**, tell.[14], **tub.**

fat ham/gras, jambon/fettem
    Schinken

bananas, aversion to
bananes, aversion des
Bananen, Abneigung gegen
    bar-c.[2], elaps

desire/désir/Verlangen
    ther.

beans and **peas** agg.
fèves et **pois** agg.
Bohnen und **Erbsen** agg.
    ars., **BRY.,** **calc.,** carb-v., chin.,
    cupr., erig.[10], hell., kali-c., **LYC.,**
    nat-m., **petr.,** phos.[3], puls., sep., sil.,
    sulph.[5], verat.

beef, aversion to
bœuf, aversion de
Rindfleisch, Abneigung gegen
    crot-c., merc.[7], ptel.[7]

smell[11]/odeur/Geruch
    ptel.

beer agg.
bière agg.
Bier agg.
    act-sp.[2, 7], acon., **aloe,** alum.[3],
    ars., asaf., bapt.[2, 3, 7], bell., **bry.,**
    cadm-s., calc-caust.[6], carbn-s.,
    chel., chin., chlol., chlor.[13],
    coc-c., cocc.[3], coloc., crot-t.,
    euph., **ferr.,** fl-ac.[3], ign.,
    kali-bi., kali-m.[2], **led.,** lyc.[1, 7],
    merc-c.[3], mez., mur-ac.,
    nux-m.[8], **NUX-V.**[1, 7], **puls.**[1, 7],
    rhus-t., sec.[3], sep., **sil.**[1, 7],

stann., staph., stram., **sulph.**[1, 7],
teucr., **thuj.**[2, 3, 7], **verat.**[1, 7]

ale/bière blonde/englisches
    helles Bier

easily intoxicated[2, 7]
facilement intoxiqué par
leicht betrunken
    chim., coloc., ign.[6], kali-m.

new[7]
nouvelle
junges
    chin., lyc., puls.

smell[3, 4]/odeur/Geruch
    cham.

ailments from[12]
troubles à la suite de
Beschwerden infolge von
    kali-bi., rhus-t., thuj.

bad[12]/mauvaise/schlechtem
    nux-m.

am.
    aloe[3, 6], mur-ac.[2, 7], **verat.**[3]

aversion/Abneigung
    alum., alum-p.[1'], asaf., atro.,
    bell., bry., calc., carbn-s.[11],
    cham., CHIN., clem., **cocc.,**
    crot-t., **cycl., ferr., kali-bi.**[13],
    merc.[1'], nat-m., **nat-s., NUX-V.,**
    pall., ph-ac., **phos.,** puls.[3, 8, 13],
    rhus-t., sang.[3], sep., spig.,
    spong., **stann., sulph.**

morning/matin/morgens
    nux-v.

evening/soir/abends
    bry., nat-m., sulph.

smell[11]/odeur/Geruch
    cham.

desire/désir/Verlangen
ACON., agar., aloe, am-c.,
ant-c., ant-t.[11], arn., ars., asar.,
bell., bry., calad., calc., camph.,
carbn-s., **caust.,** chel., chin.,
cic.[14], coc-c., **cocc.,** cod.[11],
coloc., cupr., dig., digin.[11],
graph., kali-bi., kali-i.[13], **lach.,**
mang., med.[7], **merc.,** mosch.,
nat-ar., **nat-c., nat-m.,** nat-p.,
nat-s., NUX-V., op., **petr.,**
ph-ac., **phel.,** phos., psor., **puls.,**
rhus-t., sabad., sep., **spig.,**
spong., staph., stram., **stront-c.,**
stroph-h.[3], **SULPH.,** tell.,
zinc.[1, 7]

morning[11]/matin/morgens
nux-v., phel., **puls.**[2, 7]

forenoon[11]/matinée/vormittags
agar., phos.

afternoon[11]/après-midi/nach-
mittags
psor., sulph.

evening/soir/abends
coc-c.[11], **kali-bi.**[11], mang.[11],
med.[7], nux-v.[11], sulph.[11],
zinc.[1, 7]

bitter[8]/amère/bitterem
aloe, cocc., **kali-bi.,** nat-m.,
nux-v., puls.

chill, during[2, 11]
frissons, pendant les
Fieberfrost, bei
ant-c., **nux-v.**

colic, after[11]
colique, après la
Kolik, nach
ph-ac.

fever, during[11]
fièvre, pendant la
Fieber, im
acon.[2, 11], nux-v., puls.

after[11]/après la/nach
puls.

thirst, without[2, 7]
soif, sans
Durst, ohne
calad.

biscuit, desire for
biscuit, désir de
Keks, Verlangen nach
plb.

bitter drinks, ailments from
amères, désir de boissons
bitteren Getränken, Verlangen nach
acon., aloe[13], cod.[7, 11], dig., **nat-m.,**
ter., ther.[13]

bitter, food, ailments from[12]
amers, troubles à la suite d'aliments
bitteren Speisen, Beschwerden
infolge von
nat-p.

desire/désir/Verlangen
cod.[2], dig., graph.[3, 6], **nat-m.,**
nux-v.[1', 7], sep.[1']

brandy, whisky agg.
eau de vie, whisky agg.
Weinbrand, Whisky agg.
agar., **ars.,** ars-met.[2], bell.,
calc., carb-ac.[13], chel.[3, 6, 13],
chin., cocc., fl-ac.[3], hep., hyos.,
ign., lach., laur., **led.,** med.[7],
NUX-V., OP., puls., **ran-b.,**
rhod., **rhus-t.,** ruta, spig.,
stram., sul-ac., **SULPH.,** verat.,
zinc.

and wine am.[2]
et vin am.
und Wein am.
sul-ac.

ailments from bad[12]
troubles à la suite de mauvaise
Beschwerden infolge von
schlechtem
carb-v.

am.
prot.[14], sel.[3, 6]

aversion/Abneigung
 ant-t.[2], **carb-ac.**[2, 11], ign., lob.[13],
 lob-e.[8], **merc.,** ph-ac.[3, 6],
 rhus-t., stram.[13], zinc.

brandy drinkers, in
buveurs d'eau-de-vie, chez les
Schnapstrinkern, bei
 arn.

desire (+ Kent 1897)/désir/
Verlangen
 acon., **agar.,** ail., alum., am-m.,
 anac., **ant-c.,** arg-n., **arn., ars.,**
 ars-met., asar.[6], aster., **bell.,** bor.,
 bov., bry., bufo, cadm-s., **calc.,**
 carb-ac., **carb-an.,** carb-v.,
 carbn-s., caust., **chel., chin.,** cic.,
 coc-c.[13], coca, **cocc., coff.,** con.,
 crot-h., cub., ferr-p., fl-ac., gels.,
 hep., hyos., **ign., LAC-C., LACH.,**
 laur., **led., LYC., med.**[7], merc.,
 mosch., mur-ac., **nat-c., nat-m.,**
 nux-m., NUX-V., olnd., **OP.,**
 petr., phos., puls., **RAN-B., rhod.,**
 rhus-t., ruta, sabad., **sel., sep.,**
 sil., spig., staph., stram., stront-c.,
 sul-ac., SULPH., ther., **verat.,**
 zinc.

bread agg.
pain agg.
Brot agg.
 ant-c., bar-c., BRY., carb-an.,
 caust., chin., cina[2, 3], clem., coff.,
 crot-h., crot-t., cupr.[13], **hydr.**[2, 6, 8],
 kali-c., lith-c.[13], **lyc.**[2, 8], merc.,
 nat-m., nit-ac., nux-v., olnd.,
 ph-ac., phos., **PULS.,** ran-s.,
 rhus-t., ruta, **sars.,** sec., **sep.,**
 staph., sul-ac., **sulph.,** teucr.,
 verat.[2, 3], **zinc.,** zinc-p.[1'], zing.

black, agg.
noir agg.
Schwarzbrot agg.
 bry., ign., **kali-c., lyc.,** nat-m.,
 nit-ac., nux-v., **ph-ac.,** phos.,
 puls., sep.[3], sulph.

butter agg., and
tartine de beurre agg.
Butterbrot agg.
 acet-ac.[2], carb-an., caust., **chin.,**
 crot-t., cycl., meny., nat-m.,
 nat-s.[3], **nit-ac.,** nux-v., phos.,
 PULS., sep., sulph.

ailments from[12]
troubles à la suite de
Beschwerden infolge von
 nat-m., zing.

am.[2, 3]
 caust., lact.[13], laur., **nat-c.**[2, 3, 13],
 phos.

aversion/Abneigung
 agar., aphis[8, 13], **CHIN., con.,**
 corn.[11], cur., **cycl.,** elaps,
 ferr-ar.[13], hydr.[13], ign., **kali-c.,**
 kali-p., kali-s., **lach.**[1, 7], lact.,
 lil-t., **lyc., mag-c.**[1, 7], manc.,
 meny., **NAT-M., nat-p., nat-s.,**
 nit-ac., nux-m.[11], **nux-v.,** ol-an.,
 ph-ac., phos., puls., **rhus-t.**[1, 7],
 sep., sulph.[1, 7], tarent.

black/noir/Schwarzbrot
 kali-c., lyc., merc.[6],
 nat-m.[3, 6, 11, 16], **nux-v.**[1, 7],
 ph-ac.[3, 6, 16], puls., sulph.

butter, and
tartine de beurre
Butterbrot
 cycl.[1, 7], **mag-c.**[1, 7], meny.,
 nat-p., sang.[3]

pregnancy, during[2, 7]
grossesse, dans la
Schwangerschaft, in der
 ant-t.[16], laur.[16], **sep.**

rye bread[7]
pain de seigle
Roggenbrot
 lyc., nux-v.

desire/désir/Verlangen
 abrot., aloe, am-c., **ars., aur.,**
 aur-ar.[1'], **bell.**[1, 7], bov.,

cann-i.[11], con., **cina, coloc.,**
cub., **ferr.,** ferr-ar., ferr-m.[13],
grat., hell., hydr., ign., lyc.[13],
mag-c., merc., nat-ar., **nat-c.**[1'],
nat-m., ol-an.[11], op., **plb.,**
puls.[1, 7], sec., sil., staph.,
stront-c., sumb.

evening/soir/abends
cast.[11], tell.[14]

boiled in milk
bouilli dans du lait
gekocht in Milch
abrot.

butter, and
tartine de beurre
Butterbrot
agar., **bar-m.**[13], bell., **ferr.,**
grat., hell., hydr., ign., **mag-c.,**
MERC., merc-sul.[2], puls.,
stront-c.[3]

dry/rassis/altbackenem
aur.[3], **bar-m.**

only/seulement/trockenem
bov., grat.

rye bread
pain de seigle
Roggenbrot
ars., carl., **ign.**[1, 7], plb.

white/blanc/Weißbrot
aur.[3], bar-m.[3']

broth agg.
bouillon agg.
Fleischbrühe agg.
mag-c.

sensitive to the smell of
sensible à l'odeur de
empfindlich gegen den Geruch
von
COLCH.

aversion[2, 3, 11]/Abneigung
arn.[1'-3 11], **ars.**[2, 3], bell.[2, 3],
cham., graph.[2, 3, 11, 16], kali-i.[11],
rhust-t., sil.[7, 16]

desire[1']/désir/Verlangen
mag-c.

buckwheat agg.
sarrasin agg.
Buchweizen agg.
ip., **phos.**[2, 3], **PULS.,** sep.[2, 3], verat.

butter agg.
beurre agg.
Butter agg.
acon., ant-c., ant-t., **ars.,** asaf.,
bell., carb-an., **CARB-V.,** caust.,
chin., colch., **cycl.,** dros., euph.,
ferr., ferr-ar., hell., hep., ip.,
mag-m., meny., merc-c.[3], nat-ar.,
nat-c., nat-m., nat-p., nit-ac.,
nux-v., **phos., ptel., PULS., sep.,**
spong., sulph., **tarax., tarent.**[13],
thuj.

bread–butter/pain–tartine de
beurre/Brot–Butterbrot

ailments from[12]
troubles à la suite de
Beschwerden infolge von
carb-v.

aversion/Abneigung
ars., carb-an.[13], carb-v., **CHIN.,**
cycl., hep.[8], mag-c., meny., **merc.,**
nat-m.[13], petr., **phos.,** prot.[14],
ptel.[1], **PULS.,** sang.

desire/désir/Verlangen
all-s., ferr.[3, 8], ign.[3], mag-c.[3],
mand.[9], merc., nit-ac.[6], prot.[14],
puls.[3]

buttermilk agg.[3, 16]
lait de beurre agg.
Buttermilch agg.
puls.

aversion[13]/Abneigung
cina

desire[3]/désir/Verlangen
ant-t., chin-s., chion., elaps[3, 8, 13],
sabal., thlas.

cabbage agg.
chou agg.
Kohl agg.
    ars., **BRY.,** calc., carb-v., **chin.,**
    cupr., erig.[10], hell., kali-c., **LYC.,**
    mag-c., nat-m., **nat-s., PETR.,**
    phos.[3], podo.[1'], **puls.,** sep., sil.,
    sulph.[5], verat.

  ailments from[12]
  troubles à la suite de
  Beschwerden infolge von
    petr.

  aversion[13]/Abneigung
    bry., carb-v., cocc., kali-c., lyc.,
    petr.

  desire[3]/désir/Verlangen
    acon.[11], **acon-l.**[7], alum.[13], **CIC.,**
    con.

carrots agg.
carottes agg.
Karotten agg.
    calc., **lyc.**

cereals, aversion to
céréales, aversion des
Getreideprodukte, Abneigung gegen
    ars., phos.

charcoal, desire for
charbon de bois, désir de
Holzkohle, Verlangen nach
    alum., **calc.**[2, 8, 13]**,** cic., con.,
    ign.[8, 13], nit-ac., nux-v., **psor.**[8, 13]

    indigestible/indigestes/Unver-
      dauliches

  chlorosis, in[7]
  chlorose, au cours de
  Chlorose, bei
    alum.

cheese agg.[2, 3, 6]
fromage agg.
Käse agg.
    arg-n.[5], ars.[3, 6], coloc.[2, 3, 6, 8],
    nux-v., phos.[3], ptel., sanic.[3],
    sep.[3], staph.[5]

  old ch. agg.
  vieux f. agg.
  alter K. agg.
    ars., bry., coloc., hep.[3], nux-v.[3],
    ph-ac., **ptel., rhus-t.,** sanic.[3],
    sep.[3]

  spoiled ch. agg.[6]
  avarié agg.
  verdorbener K. agg.
    ars., bry.[3, 6], ph-ac., rhus-t.

  ailments from[12]
  troubles à la suite de
  Beschwerden infolge von
    nit-s-d.

  aversion/Abneigung
    arg-n.[5, 7]**, chel.,** chin.[3], **nit-ac.**[5, 7]**,**
    olnd.[1, 7]**, staph.**[5, 7]

    Gruyère[5, 7]/Greyerzer
    merc., sulph.

    Roquefort[5, 7]
    hep.

    strong[5, 7]
    fort
    scharfen
    hep., nit-ac.

  desire/désir/Verlangen
    arg-n., aster., calc-p.[10], **cist.,**
    coll.[13], ign., mand.[9, 10, 14],
    mosch., puls., sep.[3, 6]

    strong
    fort
    scharfriechendem
    arg-n., aster., ign.[6]

cherries, desire for
cerises, désir de
Kirschen, Verlangen nach
    chin.

chicken agg.[1']
poulet agg.
Hühnerfleisch agg.
    bac.[7], bry.

  aversion[7]/Abneigung
    bac.

chocolate agg.[2, 3, 5, 7]
chocolat agg.
Schokolade agg.
　　bor.[2, 7], bry.[2, 3, 7], calad.[2, 7],
　　caust.[2, 3, 7], coca[3], kali-bi.[3], lil-t.[3],
　　lith-c.[2, 7], **LYC.**, ox-ac.[3], prot.[14],
　　puls.

　　aversion/Abneigung
　　　osm., prot.[14], tarent.

　　desire/désir/Verlangen
　　　arg-n.[7], calc.[7], **carc.**[7], lepi., lyss.,
　　　sep.[7]

cider agg.
cidre agg.
Apfelwein agg.
　　aster.[14], phos.[3]

　　am.[3]
　　　bell.

　　desire/désir/Verlangen
　　　ben., benz-ac.[13], puls.[3], sulph.

cloves, desire for
clous de girofle, désir de
Gewürznelken, Verlangen nach
　　alum., chlor.

coal, desire for
charbon, désir de
Kohle, Verlangen nach
　　alum., calc., cic.[1, 7], ign.[13], psor.[13]

　　*indigestible/indigestes/Unverdau-
　　　liches*

cocoa, aversion to
cacao, aversion du
Kakao, Abneigung gegen
　　osm.[2, 11], tarent.[2]

coffee agg.
café agg.
Kaffee agg.
　　aeth., agar.[3], alet.[6], all-c.,
　　anac.[14], ars., arum-t., aster.,

　　aur-m.[1', 2], bell., bov., bry.,
　　cact., calc., **calc-p.**, cann-i.[8, 13],
　　CANTH., caps., carb-v., caul.[2],
　　CAUST., CHAM., chin.[2, 3], cist.,
　　clem.[7], **cocc.**, coff.[13], colch.,
　　coloc.[2, 3, 13], cycl., fl-ac., form.,
　　glon., grat., guar.[8, 12], **hep.**,
　　IGN., ip., kali-bi., kali-c.[8, 13],
　　kali-n., **lyc.**, mag-c.,
　　mand.[9, 10, 14], mang., **merc.**,
　　nat-m., **nat-s.**, nit-ac., **NUX-V.**,
　　ox-ac., **ph-ac.**, plat., psor.[8, 13],
　　puls., rhust-t., sep., stann.[14],
　　stram., sul-ac., sulph., **thuj.**,
　　vinc.

　　hot[13]/très chaud/heißer
　　　caps.

　　smell of c. agg.
　　odeur de c. agg.
　　Kaffeegeruch agg.
　　　fl-ac.[3], lach.[3], **nat-m.**[3], osm.[3],
　　　sul-ac., tub.[3]

　　sensitive to the
　　sensible à l'
　　empfindlich gegen den
　　　arg-n., lach., sul-ac.

　　climacteric period, during
　　ménopause, pendant la
　　Klimakterium, im
　　　LACH.[7], **sul-ac.**[2]

ailments from[12]
troubles à la suite de
Beschwerden infolge von
　　grat., nux-v., ox-ac., thuj.

am.
　　acon., agar., aran-ix.[10], arg-m.,
　　ars., brom.[3, 6], cann-i., canth.,
　　CHAM., chel.[2, 3, 6], **coloc.**,
　　dicha.[10], eucal., **euph.**[13], euphr.,
　　fl-ac.[8, 13], glon.[3], hyos., **ign.**[3],
　　lach., levo.[14], mag-c.[16], mosch.[3],
　　nux-v.[3], op., phos.,

　　aversion/Abneigung
　　　acon.[13], alum-sil.[1'], **bell., bry.,**
　　　CALC., calc-s., carb-v.,

caust.[13], **cham.**, chel., **chin.**,
cinnb.[3], coc-c., **coff.**, con.[13],
dulc., fl-ac., kali-bi.[2], kali-br.,
kali-i.[13], kali-n., lec.[13], lil-t.,
lol.[3, 6], **lyc.**, mag-p., mand.[9],
merc., nat-c., **nat-m., NUX-V.,**
osm., ox-ac., ph-ac., **phos.**,
phys., puls.[7, 16], rheum, rhus-t.,
sabad., **spig., sul-ac., sulph.**[13]

morning[11]/matin/morgens
lyc.

noon[11]/midi/mittags
ox-ac.

smell[16]
odeur
Kaffeegeruch
sul-ac

sweetened[2]/sucré/gesüßten
aur-m.

unsweetened[3, 11]/sans sucre/
ungesüßten

desire/désir/Verlangen
alum., alum-p.[1'], **ANG.**, arg-m.,
arg-n., **ars.**, ars-s-f.[1'], aster.,
aur., aur-ar.[1'], aur-s.[1'], bell.[3],
bry., calc.[5], calc-p., **caps.,**
carb-v., cham., chel., **chin.**,
chin-s.[5], colch., **con., fl-ac.**[3, 6],
gran., grat.[12], kali-i.[13], lach.,
lec., lepi.[11], lob., **mez.**, mosch.,
nat-m., **nux-m.**, nux-v., paull.[11],
ph-ac., puls.[5], sabin., **sel.**,
sol-t-ae., stroph-h.[3], sulph.,
xan.[3]

beans of[6]/grains de c./Kaffee-
bohnen
chin.[2, 6, 7], nux-v., sabin.

black[2, 7, 11]/noir/schwarzem
mosch.

burnt/torréfié/geröstetem
alum., chin.

dysmenorrhoea, in[2, 7]
dysménorrhée, pendant la
Dysmenorrhoe, bei
lach.

ground of[6, 7]/marc de/Kaffeesatz
alum.

strong/fort/scharfriechendem
bry.[2, 7], mosch.[7]

which nauseates
qui lui provoque des nausées
verursacht Übelkeit
caps.[1, 7]

cold drink, cold water agg.
boissons froides, eau froide agg.
kalte Getränke, kaltes Wasser agg.
agar., **all-s.**[2], allox.[9], **alum.,**
alum-p.[1'], alum-sil.[1'], **alumn.**[2],
anac., **ant-c.**, apis, **apoc.**, arg-n.,
ars., ars-s-f.[1'], aur-ar.[1'], **bell.,**
bell-p.[7], bor., bry.[1'], cadm-s.[1'],
calad.[8], calc., calc-p.,
calc-sil.[1'], camph.[3], **CANTH.,**
caps.[1'-3], carb-an., **carb-v.,**
cham.[2, 3], **chel., chin.**[2, 3], clem.,
cocc., coloc., con.[2, 6], **croc.,**
crot-t.[8, 13], cycl.[8, 13], **dig.**, dros.[8],
dulc., elaps[8], **FERR.**, ferr-ar.,
ferr-m.[13], ferr-p.[1'], **graph.,**
grat., hep.[3], hyos., **ign.**, kali-ar.,
kali-c., kali-i., kali-m.[1'], kali-p.,
kali-sil.[1'], **kreos.**[2, 6], lach.[6],
lept.[3], lob.[3, 8], **lyc., mag-p.,**
mang., merc., mur-ac., nat-ar.,
nat-c., nat-p., nat-sil.[1'], nit-ac.[6],
nux-m., nux-v., oci-s.[9], op.[3],
ph-ac., puls., rauw.[9], **rhod.,**
RHUS-T., sabad.[8, 13], sars.,
SEP.[3, 6], **sil., spig.**, spong.[3, 8, 13],
squil.[3, 6], staph.[3], stram.,
sul-ac., sulph., tarent., teucr.,
thuj., verat.

heated, when
échauffé, étant
erhitzt, wenn
bell-p.[7, 9, 12], **bry.**[1', 7], **kali-ar.,**
kali-c., nat-c., rhus-t.[1', 7], samb.

hot weather, in
chaud, quand il fait
heißem Wetter, bei
bry., kali-c., nat-c.

am.
acon.[3, 6], acon-f., all-c., aloe,
ambr., anac., **ant-t.,** apis, arg-n.[3],
ars., **asar.,** aster.[14], **BISM.,** bor.,
brom.[3, 6], **BRY.,** calc., cann-s.[3],
carb-ac.[2], **CAUST.,** cham., **clem.,**
coc-c., coff., **cupr., fl-ac.**[3], **jatr.**[8],
kali-c., laur., meph.[14],
moly-met.[14], **onos.,** op.[3], **PHOS.,**
phyt.[3, 6], pic-ac.[8], **puls.,** sel.[14],
SEP., stann.[14], sumb., tab.[3], thuj.,
trios.[14], verat., zinc., zinc-p.[1']

aversion to cold drinks
aversion des boissons froides
Abneigung gegen kalte Getränke
acon.[3], alum-p.[1'], ant-t.[13],
arn.[13], **ars.**[13], bram.[6], calad.,
calc-ar.[13], carb-an.[11], chel.[3, 6],
dig.[13], elaps[13], kali-i.[13], mag-c.[7],
nat-m.[13], nat-s.[13], nux-v.[13],
onos.[13], phel.[13], phos.[13], phys.,
stram.[13], **verat.**[13]

cold water, to
eau froide, d'
kaltes Wasser, gegen
bell., brom., bry., **calad.,**
canth., caust., chel., chin.,
chin-ar., lyss.[1], nat-m., nux-v.,
phel., phos[13], phys., puls.[13],
rhus-t.[13], **SABAD.**[13], **stram.,**
sulph.[13], tab.

desire/désir/Verlangen
abel.[14], achy.[14], **ACON.,** agar.,
agar-em.[8], ail., allox.[9], **alum.**[13],
alumn., am-c., am-m.[3], **ang.,**
ant-t., apis[3], apoc.[1', 8], **arg-n.,**
arn., **ARS.,** arum-t.[2], asim.,
asaf., aster., aur., aur-ar.[1'],
aur-s[1'], **bell.,** bism., bor.[13],
bov., BRY., cadm-s.[1', 7], **calc.,**
calc-ar., calc-s., camph.[2],
cann-i., cann-s.[3], **caps.,**
carbn-s., **caust.,** cedr., **cench.,**
CHAM., chel., **CHIN., chin-ar.,**

cimic., **CINA,** cinnb., clem.,
coc-c., **cocc.,** colch., corn.[2],
croc., cub., **cupr., cupr-a.**[2],
dig., **dulc.,** echi., **EUP-PER.,**
euph., fl-ac., **glon., graph.,**
hell., ign.[3], kali-bi., kali-m.[3],
kali-n., **kali-p., kali-s.,** lap-a.,
led., lyc., lycps., mag-c.,
mag-p.[3], manc., **MERC.,**
MERC-C., mez., nat-ar.,
nat-c., nat-m., **nat-p.,**
NAT-S., nux-v., oci-s.[9], oena.,
olnd., onos., op.[8, 13], paro-i.[14],
ph-ac., PHOS., pic-ac., plat.,
plb., podo., polyg-h.[3], psor.,
puls., rauw.[9], **rhus-t.,** ruta,
sabad., sabin.[3], sacch-l.[3], sars.,
sec., sel.[3], **sep.,** spig., spong.,
squil., stann.[14], sulph., **tarent.,**
tell.[14], **thuj.,** ven-m.[14], **VERAT.,**
vip., vip-a.[14], zinc.

afternoon[11]/après-midi/nach-
mittags
croc.

15 h[11]
caust.

evening[11]/soir/abends
oena.

night[11]/nuit/nachts
eup-per.

chill, during[1']
frissons, pendant les
Fieberfrost, während
bry., carb-v., tub.

fever, during[1']
fièvre, pendant la
Fieber, im
tub.

cold food agg.
ailments froids agg.
kalte Speisen agg.
acet-ac., acon.[3], agar., alum.,
alum-p.[1'], alum-sil.[1'], **alumn.**[2],
ant-c., arg-n., ARS., ars-s-f.[1'],
bar-c., **bell.**[3], bell-p.[9], **bov.,** brom.,

bry., calad., calc., calc-f., **calc-p.,**
calc-sil.[1]', canth., **carb-v.,**
carbn-s., caust., cham., chel.,
cocc., coloc., **con.,** crot-t.[3], cupr.[3],
dig., **DULC.,** elaps[2], ferr.[3], fl-ac.[3],
graph., hell., **hep., hyos.**[3], ign.,
ip.[3], kali-ar., **kali-bi.**[3]**, kali-c.,**
kali-i., kali-m.[1]', **kali-n.,**
kali-sil.[1]', **kreos., LACH.,** lept.[3],
LYC., mag-c., mag-m., mag-p.[3],
mang., merc., mez.[3], mur-ac.,
nat-ar., nat-c., nat-m., nat-p.,
nat-s., nat-sil.[1]'**, nit-ac., nux-m.,**
NUX-V., par., **ph-ac.,** plb., **puls.,**
rhod., RHUS-T., rumx., sabad.,
sep., SIL., spig., squil.[3],
staph.[3, 13]**,** stram.[3], sul-ac.[2, 3],
sulph., syph.[7]**,** thuj., **verat.**

frozen/glace/Gefrorenes

am.[2, 3]
acon., adlu.[14], agn.[3], alum.[3],
alumn.[2], am-c., **ambr.**[2, 3, 8, 13]**,**
anac., ang., ant-t., apis[3], arg-n.[3],
ars., **asar., bar-c., bell.,** bism.[3],
bor., brom.[3], **BRY.**[2, 3, 8, 13]**,**
calc., cann-s.[3], canth.,
carb-v., caust., cham., clem.,
coc-c.[3], **cupr.,** dros., **euph., ferr.,**
graph.[3], hell., **kali-c., lach.**[1'-3]**,**
laur., lyc.[8, 13], mag-c., mag-m.,
merc., mez., nat-m., nux-m.,
nux-v., op.[3], par., **ph-ac.,**
PHOS.[2, 3, 8, 13]**,** phyt.[3], **PULS.,**
pyrog.[3], rhod., rhus-t., sars.,
sep., sil.[2, 3, 8, 13], spig., squil.,
stann.[3], **sul-ac.,** sulph., tab.[3],
thuj.[3], verat., **zinc.**

aversion/Abneigung
acet-ac., alum-p.[1]', chel., cycl.,
kali-i.[13], phos.[13]

desire/désir/Verlangen
abel.[14], am-c., ang.[3], **ant-t.,**
arg-n.[1]', **ars.**[3]**,** asaf.[2], bell.[3],
bism.[3], **bry.**[3, 8, 13]**,** caust.[3],
cham.[3]**,** chin.[2], cina[3], cocc.[3],
croc.[3], cupr., cupr-ar., euph.[3],
ferr-p.[3], fl-ac.[7], **ign.**[1', 3]**,** kali-p.[3],
kali-s., lach.[1]', lept.[3], **lyc.,**

merc.[3, 11], merc-c., nat-m.,
nux-v.[2]**,** olnd.[3], **PHOS.,**
arg-n.[1]', asaf.[2], bell.[3], bism.[3],
bry.[3, 8, 13]**,** caust.[3], **cham.**[3]**,**
chin.[2], cina[3], cocc.[3], croc.[3],
cupr., cupr-ar., euph.[3], ferr-p.[3],
fl-ac.[7], **ign.**[1', 3]**,** kali-p.[3], **kali-s.,**
lach.[1]', **lyc.,** merc.[3, 11], merc-c.,
nat-m., **nux-v.**[2]**,** olnd.[3], **PHOS.,**
pic-ac.[13], pip-n.[3], plb.[3], **PULS.,**
rhus-t.[3], ruta[3], sabad.[3], sars.[1]',
sec.[3], **sil., thuj.,** ven-m.[14],
verat., zinc.

afternoon[11]/après-midi/nach-
mittags
nat-m.

menses, during
menstruation, pendant la
Menses, während der
am-c.

pregnancy, in[2]
grossesse, pendant la
Schwangerschaft, in der
verat.

cooked food agg.
ailments cuits agg.
gekochte Speisen agg.
ars.[14], podo.[1]'

warm f./a. chauds/warme Sp.

sensitive to the smell of
sensible à l'odeur des
empfindlich gegen den Geruch
von gekochten Sp.
ars.[1]', chin., **COLCH., dig.,**
eup-per., sep., stann.

aversion/Abneigung
am-c.[16], asar.[14], bell., bov., calc.,
chel., cupr., **graph.,** guare, ign.,
kreos.[2]**,** lach., **lyc.,** mag-c.,
merc., petr., phos., psor., **sil.,**
verat., zinc., zinc-p.[1]'

corn agg.[5]
maïs agg.
Mais agg.
 chin., kali-c., puls., sulph.

 meal/farine de/Maismehl
  calc-ar.

cucumbers agg.[6]
concombres agg.
Gurken agg.
 all-c., ars., puls.[6], sul-ac.[6, 16],
 verat.

 aversion[14]/Abneigung
  prot.

 desire/désir/Verlangen
  abies-n., **ant-c.,** verat.

delicacies, aversion to[13]
friandises, délicatesses, aversion des
Leckereien, Abneigung gegen
 caust.[1'], petr., sang.

 desire/désir/Verlangen
  acon-l.[11], aeth.[3], **aur.,** bufo, calc.,
  CHIN., cub., cupr., cupr-ar[13], **IP.,**
  kali-c., mag-c., mag-m.[3], nat-c.,
  paull.[11], petr., psor., rauw.[9],
  rhus-t., sabad., sang., **spong.,**
  TUB.

drinks, aversion to
boissons, aversion des
Getränke, Abneigung gegen
 agar., agn., aloe, ang., **apis,**
 arn., **bell.,** berb., bor.[3], bov.[3],
 bry.[3], bufo, calad.[3], calc.[7, 13],
 camph.[3], **canth.,** carb-an.,
 caust.[3], cham.[3], chin., chin-s.[3],
 chlor.[11], coc-c., cocc., coff.,
 colch.[3], coloc.[13], corn., cupr.,
 dros.[13], **FERR.,** graph.[1', 13],
 hell.[3], **HYOS.,** ign., kali-bi.[8, 13],
 lac-c., lach., lyc.[3, 13], **lyss.,**
 merc., nat-m.[3, 13], **nit-ac.,**
 NUX-V., phys., plb., plb-chr.[11],
 puls., rat., sabin.[3], samb., sec.,
 staph.[13], **stram.,** verat.[3]

 children, in[3]
 enfants, chez les
 Kindern, bei
  bor., bry.

 headache, during
 maux de tête, pendant les
 Kopfschmerzen, bei
  FERR.

 heat, during
 chaleur, fébrile, pendant la
 Fieberhitze, bei
  con.

 desire/désir/Verlangen
  cob-n.[9], lyc.[13]

 capricious, but refuses when
  offered[16]
 capricieux de boisson, qu'il
  refuse losqu'on lui en offre
 launisches Verlangen nach G.,
  die er ablehnt, wenn
  angeboten
  bell.

 without thirst[11]
 sans soif
 ohne Durst
  bell., camph., coloc., wies.

dry food agg.
nourriture sèche agg.
trockene Speisen agg.
 agar., bov.[3], **CALC.,** calad.[3], chin.,
 ferr.[3], ign.[3], ip., kali-i.[3], **lyc.,**
 nat-c., nit-ac., nux-v., ox-ac.[3],
 petr., ph-ac., **puls.,** raph.[3], sars.,
 sil., sulph.

 aversion[3]/Abneigung
  merc.

 desire/désir/Verlangen
  alum.

eel, desire for[13]
anguille, désir de
Aal, Verlangen nach
 med.

eggs agg.
œufs agg.
Eier agg.

anthraci.[7], **calc.**[3, 5, 7], calc-f.[6],
chin-ar., colch., **ferr.**, ferr-m.,
lyc.[3], merc-c.[3], **PULS.**[2, 3, 5, 6],
sulph.[3, 6]

smell of
odeur des
Geruch von Eiern
anthraci.[7], **colch.**

ailments, from bad[12]
troubles à la suite d'o. avariés
Beschwerden infolge von faulen
Eiern
carb-v.

aversion/Abneigung
bell.[3], calc-f.[9, 10, 14], carc.[7, 10],
colch.[5, 7, 13], **ferr.**, kali-s.,
nit-ac., prot.[14], puls.[5, 7],
saroth.[10, 14], sulph.

hard boiled/durs/hartgekochte
bry.[3, 6, 16], prot.[14]

smell of
odeur des
Geruch von Eiern
colch.

desire/désir/Verlangen
calc., calc-p.[3, 6], **carc.**[7, 10],
hydr., nat-p., ol-an., olnd.[13],
prot.[14]

fried/sur le plat/gebratenen
Eiern
nat-p.

hard boiled/durs/hartgekochten
CALC.

soft boiled/à la coque/weich-
kochten
calc., nat-p.[13], ol-an., olnd.[13]

farinaceous food agg.
farineux agg., ailments
Teigwaren agg.

alum.[3, 6], **bry.**[3], carb-v.[3, 13], **caust.**,
chin.[2], coloc.[3], iris[3], kali-bi.[2, 3, 6],
kali-c.[3], lyc., mag-c.[3, 6], **nat-c.**,
NAT-M., **NAT-S.**, nux-v.,
psor.[3, 13], **PULS.**[3], sulph., verat.[3]

starchy food/féculents/stärke-
haltige Speisen

aversion/Abneigung
ars., nat-m.[3, 6], ph-ac.[13], phos.,
plan.[13], ptel.[3, 6]

flour/farine/Mehl

desire/désir/Verlangen
calc-p.[8], lach., **nat-m.**, sabad.,
sumb.

fat agg.
graisse agg.
Fett agg.

acon., agn.[3], alet.[6], ant-c.,
ant-t., aran-ix.[10, 14], arg-n.[3],
ars., ars-s-f.[1'], **asaf.**, bell., bry.,
buni-o.[14], but-ac.[9], calc.[3, 8],
calc-f.[10], carb-an., **CARB-V.**,
carbn-s., **caust.**, chin., **colch.**,
convo-s.[9, 14], cupr.[13], **CYCL.**,
dros., erig.[10], euph., **FERR.**,
ferr-ar., **ferr-m.**, **GRAPH.**[3],
ham.[3], **hell.**, hep., hir.[14], **ip.**,
jug-r.[7], kali-ar., kali-c.,
kali-chl., **kali-m.**[1', 3, 8, 12],
kali-n., kali-sil.[1'], **lyc.**[3, 8],
mag-c., **mag-m.**, mag-s.[10],
mand.[9, 10, 14], meny., merc.,
merc-c., merc-cy.[13], **nat-ar.**,
nat-c., nat-m., **nat-p.**, nat-sil.[1'],
nit-ac., nux-v., phos., podo.[1'],
psor.[3], **ptel.**, **PULS.**, rob., ruta,
sep., sil., **spong.**, staph., **sulph.**,
TARAX., **TARENT.**[13], **thuj.**,
verat.

heavy food/lourde/schwere
Speisen
oil/huile/Öl
pork/porc/Schweinefleisch
rich/nourriture riche/reich-
haltige Speisen

infants, in[9]
petits enfants, chez les
Kleinkindern, bei
  but-ac.

rancid/rance/ranziges
  ars.[12], carb-v.[7, 12]

ailments from[12]
troubles à la suite de
Beschwerden infolge von
  ars., carb-v.

aversion to fats and rich food
aversion de graisse et de nourriture riche
Abneigung gegen fette und
  schwere Speisen
  acon-l.[7, 11], ang., **ars.**, ars-s-f.[1'],
  bell., **bry.**, calc., **calc-f.**[10],
  carb-an., carb-v., carbn-s.,
  carc.[7, 10], **CHIN.**, chin-ar., **colch.**,
  convo-s.[9], croc., **cycl.**, dros.,
  erig.[10], ferr.[3], grat., guare., hell.,
  hep., ip.[5, 7, 16], lyc.[13], lyss.,
  mag-s.[9, 10], mand.[10, 14], meny.,
  merc., nat-ar., nat-c., **nat-m.**,
  nit-ac.[13], nux-v.[13], **PETR.**, phos.,
  PTEL., PULS., rheum, rhus-t.,
  rib-ac.[14], sang., sec., **sep., sulph.**,
  tarent.[3], thyr.[14]

fat meat/gras/fettes Fleisch

desire/désir/Verlangen
  ars., calc.[7], **calc-p.**[3, 6], **carc.**[7, 10],
  hep., **mez.**[2-3, 6, 8], nat-c.[3], nat-m.[3],
  NIT-AC., nux-v., prot.[14],
  rad-br.[3], sanic.[3], **sulph., tub.**[3, 7]

bacon/lard/Speck
fat ham/jambon gras/fettem
  Schinken
lard/saindoux/Schweineschmalz
fried/rôti/Gebratenem

fat ham, desire for
jambon gras, désir de
fettem Schinken, Verlangen nach
  calc-p., **carc.**[7], **mez., sanic., tub.**

ham/jambon/Schinken

fat meat, aversion to
grase, aversion de viande
fettes Fleisch, Abneigung gegen
  carb-v., hell., phos.

fish agg.
poisson agg.
Fisch agg.
  ars.[3], calad., carb-an.,
  carb-v.[3-6, 8, 13], carb-ns.[1'],
  chin.[3, 6], chin-ar., fl-ac.[3], kali-c.,
  kali-s.[3, 6], lach.[6], lyc.[6], mag-m.[13],
  medus.[3, 6], nat-s.[8, 13],
  phenob.[13, 14], **plb., puls.**[3],
  sep.[3, 6], thuj.[3], urt-u.[3, 6, 8, 13]

pickled[2, 3]/salé/eingesalzener
  calad.

sensitive to smell of
sensible à l'odeur de
empfindlich gegen Fischgeruch
  colch.

shell-fish see shell-fish

spoiled/avarié/verdorbener
  all-c.[2, 7, 12], ars., bell.[3], **BERB.**[3],
  carb-an.[2, 12], **carb-v.**, chin.,
  COP.[3], euph.[3], kali-c.[2], lach.[3, 6],
  lyc.[3], **plb.**[2], puls., pyrog.[3, 6],
  rhus-t.[2, 3], ter.[6]

aversion/Abneigung
  carb-v.[13], **colch., GRAPH.**,
  grat.[7], guare., kali-i.[13], nat-m.,
  phos., sulph., **zinc.**

salt/salé/Salzfisch
  phos.

desire/désir/Verlangen
  calc-p.[10], mand.[9], **nat-m.**, nat-p.,
  phos., sul-ac.[8]

flatulent food agg.
flatulents agg., aliments
blähende Speisen agg.
  ars., **bry.**, calc., carb-v., **chin.**,
  cupr., hell., kali-c., **LYC.**, nat-m.,
  nat-p.[13], **PETR.**, puls., sep., sil.,
  verat.

beans and peas/fèves et pois/
  Bohnen und Erbsen
cabbage/chou/Kohl
sauerkraut/choucroute/Sauer-
  kraut

flour, aversion to
farine, aversion de
Mehl, Abneigung gegen
  ars., ph-ac., **phos.**

farinaceous/farineux/Teigwaren

desire/désir/Verlangen
  calc., lach., sabad.

food after eating a little, **aversion** to
nourriture à peine après avoir com-
  mencé à manger, **aversion** de toute
Speisen nach wenigem Essen, **Ab-**
neigung gegen
  bar-c., bry.[3], caust.[3], cham.[3],
  cina[3], **cycl.,** ign.[3], lyc.[3], **nux-v.,**
  prun.[3], **rheum,** rhus-t.[3], **ruta**[1, 7, 16],
  sil., **sulph.**

hunger, with
faim, avec
Hunger, mit
  act-sp., **agar.,** all-s.[2], **alum., ars.,**
  bar-c., bry., carb-v., **carbn-s.,**
  chin., chin-ar.[13], **chin-s., COCC.,**
  dulc., grat.[2], **hell., hydr., kali-n.,**
  lach., NAT-M., nicc., **NUX-V.,**
  olnd., op., **phos.,** psor., **rhus-t.,**
  ruta[13], sabad., **sil.,** stann.[2],
  sul-ac., sulph., tax., **tub.,** verb.

loathing of f. on attempting to eat
dégoût de n. en essayand de
  manger
Abscheu gegen Sp. beim Versuch
  zu essen
  ant-t.[1'], petros.[7], **sil.**

pregnancy, in [2, 7]
grossesse, pendant la
Schwangerschaft, in der
  ant-t., **laur., nat-m.**[2], sep.[16]

sudden, while eating
soudain en mangeant
plötzlich beim Essen
  bar-c., ruta

tastes it, until he, then he is
  ravenous
mais dès qu'il l'a goutée alors
  l'appétit devient vorace
aber nach dem Kosten Heißhunger
  LYC.

thinking of eating, when
rien qu'en pensant à manger
Denken an das Essen, beim
  arg-m.[16], **ars.**[2], **CHIN.**[2], colch.[7],
  mag-s., mosch.[2], sars.[2],
  sep.[2, 7, 16], **zinc.**[2]

pregnancy, in[7]
grossesse, dans la
Schwangerschaft, in der
  sep.

fried food, aversion to
rôtis, frits, aversion des aliments
Gebratenes, Abneigung gegen
  adel.[11], mag-s.[9]

desire/désir/Verlangen
  plb.

fried potatoes[9, 14]
pommes rissolées
Bratkartoffeln
  cob-n.

frozen, agg.
glacé agg.
Gefrorenes agg.
  arg-n., **ars.,** bry., **calc-p., carb-v.,**
  coloc.[3], dulc., **ip.**[1, 7], psor.[3],
  PULS., rumx.

am.[6]
  phos.

desire[6]/désir/Verlangen
  arg-m., eup-per., nat-s., phos.

fruit agg.
Obst agg.

acon., **aloe, ant-c.**, ant-t., **ARS.**,
ars-s-f.[1'], aster.[14], **bor., BRY.,**
calc., **calc-p., carb-v., caust.**[8],
CHIN., chin-ar., cist., colch.[3],
COLOC., crot-t., cub., elaps[2],
ferr., ign., iod.[3], **ip., iris,**
kali-bi.[8], kreos., lach., lith-c.,
lyc., mag-c., **mag-m.,** merc.[2, 3],
merc-c.[3], **mur-ac., nat-ar.,**
nat-c., nat-p., **NAT-S.,** olnd.,
ox-ac.[3], **ph-ac.,** phos., **podo.,**
psor., PULS., rheum, **rhod.,**
rumx.[8], ruta, samb.[2, 8, 13], **sel.,**
sep., sul-ac., sulph.[3], tarax.,
tarent.[13], trom., **VERAT.**

sour/acide/saures
ant-c., ant-t.[1'], cist.[6], ferr.[1', 2, 6],
ip., mag-c.[6], ox-ac.[1', 6], **ph-ac.,**
podo.[6], **psor., sul-ac.**[2], ther.[2]

spoiled[1]/avarié/verdorbenes
act-sp.

ailments from[12]
troubles à la suite de
Beschwerden infolge von
ars., rhod.

unripe[3, 12]/vert/unreifem
rheum

am.
lach.

sour[6]/acide/saures
lach.

aversion/Abneigung
aloe[13], **ant-t.**[13], **ars.**[5, 7, 13], bar-c.,
carb-v.[13], **carc.**[7, 10], **caust.**[13],
CHIN.[5, 7]. ferr-m.[13], ign.,
kali-bi[13], kali-br.[13], mag-c.[7],
phos.[13], **PULS.**[5, 7], **rumx.**[13],
sul-ac.[13]

green[7, 16]/vert/grünes
mag-c.

desire/désir/Verlangen
acon-l.[7, 11], aloe, **alum.,**
alum-p.[1'], alumn., **ant-t.,** ars.,
ars-s-f.[1'], asar.[14], calc-s.,
carb-v.[3, 6], **carc.**[7, 10], chin.,
cist., cub., gran., guaj.[3, 6], hep.,
ign., lach., lepi.[11], **mag-c.,**
mag-s.[9, 10, 14], med.[8], nat-m.,
paull.[11], **PH-AC.,** phos.[8], **puls.,**
staph.[3], **sul-ac., VERAT.**

green/vert/grünem
calc.[11], calc-s., lepi.[11], **med.**

sour/acide/saurem
adel.[11], ant-t.[1'], **ars.,** calc.,
calc-s., chin., **cist.,** cub., ign.,
lach.[6], **mag-c.**[6], thuj., **VERAT.**

garlic, agg. from the smell of[2, 3]
ail, agg. par l'odeur d'
Knoblauch-Geruch agg.
sabad.

aversion/Abneigung
prot.[14], **sabad.**

desire[3]/désir/Verlangen
nat-m.

grapes agg.[5]
raisins agg.
Weintrauben agg.
chin., verat.

gruel, agg.[5]
avoine agg., bouillie d'
Haferschleim agg.
chin., kali-c., kali-c., puls., sulph.

aversion/Abneigung
ars., **calc.**

desire[3]/désir/Verlangen
bel.

ham, aversion to[7]
jambon, aversion de
Schinken, Abneigung gegen
puls.

desire/désir/Verlangen
calc-p.[3, 7, 8], mez.[6], uran-n.[2, 7]

fat ham/jambon grass/fettem
Schinken

hearty food, desire for[11]
substantielle, désir de nourriture
herzhaften, kräftigen Speisen,
Verlangen nach
rhus-t., ust.

heavy food agg.
lourde agg., nourriture
schwere Speisen, agg.
bry., calc., **caust.,** cupr., **IOD.,** lyc.,
mag-c.[16], nat-c., **puls.,** sulph.

fat/graisse/Fett
rich/riche/reichhaltige

herring agg.[3, 7]
hareng agg.
Hering agg.
fl-ac., lyc., nat-m.[3]

sardines/Sardinen

aversion/Abneigung
phos.

desire/désir/Verlangen
cist., **NIT-AC., puls., verat.**

anchovies/anchois/Sardellen
sardines/Sardinen

highly seasoned food see spices

honey agg.
miel agg.
Honig agg.

nat-c., **nat-m.**[2, 13], phos.[3]

aversion[7]/Abneigung
nat-c.

desire/désir/Verlangen
sabad., verat.[3, 6]

hot drinks agg.[2]
très chaudes agg., boissons
heiße Getränke agg.
am-c., ambr., anac., ant-t., apis[6],
asar., **bar-c., bell., BRY.,**[2, 6, 8],

calc., **carbv-v.,** caust., **cham.,**
chion.[8, 13], cupr., euph., ferr.,
graph.[6, 8], hell., ign.[6,] kali-c.,
lach.[2, 6, 8], laur., **merc-i-f.,**
mez.[2, 6], oena.[11], **ph-ac.,**
PHOS.[2, 6, 8], **phyt.**[6], **PULS.**[2, 8],
pyrog.[6, 8], sep., sil.[1'], stann.[6, 8, 13],
sul-ac.

am.[3]: ars., chel.[6], lyc.[7], nux-v.,
sul-ac.

aversion/Abneigung
caust.[1', 13], cham.[6], chin.[1'], ferr.,
graph.[13], **kali-s., lyc.**[13], mang.[16],
oena.[11], ptel.[3], **puls.**[6, 13]

desire[2]/désir/Verlangen
ang., bell., **BRY.,** calad., casc.,
cast-v.[2, 13], cedr., chel., cupr.,
eup-pur., hyper., kali-i.[6], kreos.,
LAC-C., lyc., med.[8, 13], **puls.,**
spig.[8, 13]

hot food agg.
très chaude agg., nourriture
heiße Speisen, agg.
acon.[2], alum-sil.[1'], alumn.[2],
am-c.[2], **ambr.**[2], **anac.**[2], ang.[2],
ant-t.[2], apis[2], ars.[2], arum-t.,
asar.[2], **bar-c.**[2], **bell.**[2], bor.[2],
bry., calc.[2], canth.[2], caps.,
carb-v., **caust.**[2], **cham.**[2], chin.[13],
clem.[2], coff., **cupr.**[2], **euph.**[2], ferr.,
graph., **hell.**[2], kali-c.[2], **lach.**[2],
laur.[2], mag-c.[2], mag-m.[2], **merc.**[2],
mez.[2], nat-m.[2], **nat-s.,** nux-m.[2],
nux-v.[2], par.[2], **ph-ac.**[2], **PHOS.**[2],
phyt., **puls.,** rhod.[2], rhus-t.[2],
sars.[2], **sep.,** sil.[2], squil.[2], **sul-ac.**[2],
sulph.[2], thuj.[2], tub.[3], verat.[2],
zinc.[2]

am.[2]
agar., alumn., ant-c., **ARS.,**
bar-c., bell.[3], bov., bry., calc.,
canth., carb-v., caust., cham.,
chel.[3], **con., graph.,** hell, **ign.,**
kali-c., **kali-n., kreos., LYC.,**
mag-c., mag-m., **mang., mez.,**
mur-ac., nat-m., nit-ac., **nux-m.,**
NUX-V., par., ph-ac., **plb.,** puls.,

RHUS-T., sep., **sil.**, **spig.**, sul-ac.,
sulph., thuj., **verat.**

aversion/Abneigung
  calc.[7], **CHIN.**, ferr., kali-s.,
  merc-c., petr., pyrog.[13], sil.[1, 13],
  verat.[13]

desire[2]/désir/Verlangen
  ang., ars., chel., cupr.[2, 13], cycl.,
  ferr., **LYC.**, ph-ac., **sabad.**[2, 13]

ice agg.[3]
morceaux de glace agg.
Eisstücke agg.
  arg-n.[7], **ARS.**[3], bell., bell-p.[3],
  bry., calc-p., **CARB-V.**[3], hep.,
  ip., kali-bi[3], kali-c., **nux-v.**,
  puls.[3, 7], rhus-t.

ailments from ices[12]
troubles à la suite de
Beschwerden infolge von
  Eisstücken
    arg-n., ars., bell-p., carb-v.,
    puls.

ice-water[12]
d'eau de fusion
Eiswasser
  carb-v., rhus-t.

desire/désir/Verlangen
  arg-m.[3], arg-n.[1], **ars.**[3], **calc.**[7],
  elaps, eup-per.[3], lept.[3], **med.**,
  merc-c., merc-i-f.[13], nat-s.,
  paro-i.[14], phos.[13], sil.[1], **VERAT.**

ice-cream agg.[7]
glacée (crème) agg.
Speiseeis agg.
  arg-n., ars., kali-ar.[1], puls.[1]

ailments from[12]
troubles à la suite de
Beschwerden infolge von
  puls.

aversion[12]/Abneigung
  rad-br.

desire/désir/Verlangen
  arg-n.[1], **calc.**, **eup-per.**, **med.**[7],
  PHOS., puls.[1], rad-br.[12], **sil.**[1, 7],
  tub., verat.

indigestible things agg.[3]
indigestes agg., choses
Unverdauliches agg.
  bry., calc., **caust.**, cupr., **IOD.**,
  lyc., nat-c., **puls.**, sulph.

ailments from[12]
troubles à la suite de
Beschwerden infolge von
  ip.

desire/désir/Verlangen
  abies-c.[3, 6], **alum.**, alumn., **aur.**[7],
  bell, bry., **calc.**, **calc-p.**, cic.[3, 6, 7],
  con.[7], cycl., ferr.[6, 7], ign.[8], **LACH.**[7],
  nat-m.[7], **NIT-AC.**[3, 5-7], **nux-v.**[3, 6, 7],
  psor.[3], **SIL.**[3], **tarent.**[3]

ashes, charcoal, coal, lime,
* paper, rags, sand, strange,*
* tea grounds*
cendres, charbon, charbon de
* bois, chaux, chiffons, étranges,*
* marc de thé, papier*
Asche, Holzkohle, Kalk, Kohle,
* Lumpen, merkwürdigen,*
* Papier, Sand, Teesatz*

indistinct desire, knows not what
désire manger mais ne sait pas quoi
unbestimmtes Verlangen, weiß nicht
wonach
  arn.[3], **BRY.**, cham.[3], chin., cina[3],
  hep.[3], **IGN.**, ip., kreos.[3], **lach.**,
  mag-m., **PULS.**, sang., sil.,
  sulph.[3], **ther.**

capricious appetite (hunger, but
  knows not for what, or refuses
  things when offered)
appétit capricieux (a cependant
  faim, mais ne sait pas pour quoi
  ou refuse les choses qui lui sont
  offertes)
launenhafter Appetit (hat Hunger,
  aber weiß nicht worauf oder
  weist Angebotenes zurück)

ail., ang.[2], ars., aster., bell.,
BRY., bufo, carbn-s., **cham.**[3],
CHIN., CINA, coca, fago., ferr.[3],
hep., ign., ip., kali-bi., kreos.,
mag-c., **mag-m.,** merc.[3], merc-i-f.,
petr., **phos.,** phys.[3], **puls.,** rheum[3],
sang., staph.[3], sumb., symph.[7],
tep., **ther., tub.,** zinc.

juicy things, aversion to[13]
juteuses, aversion de choses
Saftiges, Abneigung gegen
    aloe

desire/désir/Verlangen
    aloe., **ant-t.**[8], chin.[8], gran.,
    graph.[3, 6], mag-c.[8], med.[8, 13],
    nat-ar., nux-v.[1', 7], **PH-AC.,**
    phos.[3, 8], puls., sabad.[3], **sabin.,**
    sars., staph.[3, 6], verat.

refreshing/rafraîchissantes/
    Erfrischendem

lard, desire for
saindoux, désir de
Schweineschmalz, Verlangen nach
    ars.

lemonade agg.
limonade agg.
Limonade agg.
    calc.[7], phyt., **sel.**

ailments form[12]
troubles à la suite de
Beschwerden infolge von
    sel.
    am.
        bell.[2, 3], cycl.[3, 8, 13], phyt.[3]

desire/désir/Verlangen
    am-m.[3, 6, 8, 13], **BELL.,** calc.,
    cycl., eup-per.[6], eup-pur.,
    fl-ac.[3, 6], jatr., lach.[3, 6], **nit-ac.,**
    puls., **sabin.,** sec., **sul-i.,** xan.[3]

    hot[2]/bien chaude/heißer
        puls.

lemons, desire for
citrons, désir de
Zitronen, Verlangen nach
    ars., **BELL.**[1', 2, 6, 7], ben-ac.[1], nabal.[1],
    puls.[7], verat.

lime, slate pencils, earth, chalk, clay,
    desire for
chaux, crayon, terre, craie, glaise,
    désir de
Kalk, Bleistift, Erde, Kreide, Lehm,
    Verlangen nach
    alum., alumn.[13], **calc.,** calc-p.[6],
    chel.[3], cic., con.[3], ferr., hep.[3],
    hyos.[3], ign.[3, 13], nat-m., **NIT-AC.,**
    nux-v., oci.[3], psor.[13], sil.[3], sulph.[3],
    tarent.[3, 7]

indigestible/indigestes/
    Unverdauliches

liqueur agg.[1, 3]
Likör agg.
    ant-**c.,** ars., bell., bov., **cann-i.,**
    carb-v., cimic., led., **ran-b.,**
    rhod., rhus-t., sel., sulph., verat.

desire[7]/désir/Verlangen
    med.

liquid food, desire for
liquide, désir de nourriture
flüssiger Nahrung, Verlangen nach
    ang., bell., bry., **calc-ar.,** caps.,
    ferr., merc., ph-ac., **staph., sulph.,**
    verat.

many things, desire for
beaucoup de choses, désire
vielerlei Verlangen nach
    CINA, kreos., phos.

indistinct desire/désir/
    unbestimmtes Verlangen

marinade, desire for[7]
marinade, désir de
Mariniertem, Verlangen nach
    ars., aster., **cist., fl-ac., hep., lac-c.,**
    nat-p., ph-ac., **sang.**

meat agg.
viande agg.
Fleisch agg.
  all-s.[8], arg-n.[3], **ars.**[3, 8], bor.[8],
  bry.[8], **calc.**[3], carb-an.,
  carb-v.[3, 8], caust., **chin.**[3, 8],
  colch., cupr., **ferr.**,
  ferr-ar.[13], ferr-i.[13], ferr-p.[13],
  graph.[3, 6], **kali-bi., kali-c.**[2],
  kreos.[3, 6], lyc.[5], lyss.[1], mag-c.,
  mag-m., med.[7], merc., nat-m.[8],
  nux-v.[1', 7], **ptel., puls.**, ruta,
  sel.[8], sep.[3], sil., staph., sulph.,
  ter., ther.[13], verat.[8]

bad, agg./avarié/verdorbenes
  absin.[8], acet-ac.[8], all-c.[8], **ARS.**,
  bell.[6], bry.[6], camph.[8], carb-an.[8],
  carb-v., chin., **crot-h.**,
  cupr.-ar.[8], gunp.[8], kreos.[8],
  lach., ph-ac.[6], **puls., pyrog.**,
  rhus-t.[6], urt-u.[8], **verat.**[8], vip.[6]

  sausages/saucisses/Wurst

fresh, agg./fraîche/frisches
  ars.[3, 13], **caust., chin.**[3], kali-c.[3]

smell of cooking, agg.
odeur de la v. cuisante
Geruch von kochendem
  ars., colch.

pickled, agg.[3, 7]
salée
Pökelfleisch
  carb-v.

am.
  lat.[13], **verat.**[2, 3, 6, 13]

aversion/Abneigung
  abies-c., adel.[11], agar., all-s.[13],
  aloe[2, 3, 8, 11], **alum.**, alum-p.[1'],
  alum-sil.[1'], alumn., am-c.,
  am-m.[13], **ang.**, aphis, **arn., ars.**,
  ars-s-f.[1'], asar.[14], aster., atro.[11],
  aur., aur-ar.[1', 12], aur-s.[1'], bell.,
  bor.[13], **bry., cact., CALC.**,
  calc-f.[10], **CALC-S.**, calc-sil.[1'],
  cann-s., carb-v., CARBN-S.,
  card-m.[8, 13], cary.[11], caust.,

cham., chel., chen-a.[2], **CHIN.**,
chin-ar., chin-b.[2], **coc-c.**,
colch.[8, 13], convo-s.[9], crot-c.,
crot-h.[8, 13], **cycl.**, der.[11], **elaps**,
ferr., ferr-ar., ferr-i., **ferr-m.**,
ferr-p., **GRAPH.**, hell., hydr.,
ign., kali-ar., kali-bi., kali-c.,
kali-m.[1'], kali-p., kali-s.,
kali-sil.[1'], kreos., lachn., lact.,
lap-a., lepi., **lyc.**, mag-c.,
mag-m.[13], mag-s., manc.,
meny.[13], **merc., mez.**,
morph.[7, 8], **MUR-AC.**, nat-ar.,
nat-c., **nat-m.**, nat-p., nat-s.,
nat-sil.[1'], nicc., **nit-ac.**,
NUX-V., ol-an., olnd.[13], op.,
PETR., phos., plan., **plat., ptel.**,
PULS., rad-br.[12], **rhus-t.**, ruta,
sabad., saroth.[10, 14], sec., sel.[13],
SEP., SIL., stront-c., **SULPH.**,
sumb., **syph., tarent.**, tep., ter.,
ther.[13], thuj., til., tril.[11], **tub.**,
upa., uran.[6], verat.[3], x-ray[9],
zinc., zinc-p.[1']

noon/midi/mittags
  ol-an., olnd.[13], sulph.

evening/soir/abends
  sulph.

boiled/bouillie/gekochtes
  ars., calc.[6], chel., nit-ac.

dinner, during
déjeuner, pendant le
Mittagessen, beim
  nat-c.

fresh/fraîche/frisches
  thuj.[1, 7]

men, in[9]
hommes, chez les
Männern, bei
  x-ray

menses, during
menstruation, pendant la
Menses, während der
  plat.

pickled[6]/salée/Pökelfleisch
  carb-v.

roast[3]/rôti/Braten
  ptel.

smell of[11]/odeur de/Fleischgeruch
  ars.

soup[3]/pot-au-feu/Suppenfleisch
  arn., cham., rhus-t.

spicy[7]/relevée/pikantes
  mag-c.

thinking of it, while
pensant, en y
Darandenken, beim
  GRAPH.

desire/désir/Verlangen
  abies-c., aloe, anth.[11], aur.,
  bell-p.[9], **calc.**[7], **calc-p.**[3, 8, 10, 13],
  canth., caust.[3], coca[3, 11], cocc.[3],
  cycl., erig.[10], ferr., **ferr-m.**,
  graph., hell., hydr.[13],
  iod., **kreos., lil-t., mag-c.,**
  mand.[9, 10, 14], med.[7], **meny.,**
  merc., morph.[11], nat-m.,
  nit-ac.[6], **nux-v.**[7], sabad., sanic.,
  staph.[7],**sulph.**[1, 7], thiop.[14], tub.,
  viol-o.[3]

boiled[3]/bouille/gekochtem
  caust.

children, in[7]
enfants, chez les
Kindern, bei
  mag-c.

lean[3]/maigre/magerem
  hell.

must have[7]
besoin impérieux de
unbedingtes
  calc., nux-v., staph., sulph.

pickled[3, 6]/salée/Pökelfleisch
  abies-c., ant-c., cori-r.[11],
  hyper., **mag-c.**[7]

smoked/fumée/Rauchfleisch
  calc-p., CAUST., kreos., **TUB.**

supper, at[11]
dîner, pendant le
Abendessen, beim
  graph.

melons agg.
Melonen agg.
  ars.[6, 7], fl-ac.[3], puls.[6], zing.[3, 6-8]

ailments from[12]
troubles à la suite de
Beschwerden infolge von
  zing.

aversion [5, 7]/Abneigung
  ars., chin., verat., zing.[13]

desire[6]/désir/Verlangen
  puls.

milk agg.
lait agg.
Milch agg.
  AETH., alum., alum-p.[1'],
  alum-sil.[1'], alumn.[2], **ambr.,**
  ang.[2, 3, 13], **ant-c.,** ant-t.,
  arg-m., ars., ars-s-f.[1'],
  brom., **bry., CALC.,**
  CALC-S., carb-an., **carb-v.,**
  carbn-s., **cham., chel., CHIN.,**
  cic., CON., crot-t., **cupr.,** ferr.[2],
  hell., hom.[1] (non: ham.), ign.,
  iris, kali-ar., kali-bi.[3], **kali-c.,**
  kali-i., kali-n.[3], kali-p.,
  kali-sil.[1'], lac-c.[10], **LAC-D.,**
  lach., lac-v.[12], lact.[8], levo.[14],
  lyc., mag-c., mag-f.[10], **MAG-M.,**
  merc.[1'], **nat-ar., nat-c., nat-m.,**
  nat-p., nat-s., nat-sil.[1'], **nicc.**[2, 8],
  NIT-AC., nux-m., **nux-v.,**
  ol-j., past.[12], **phos.,** podo.[8],
  psor., puls., rheum[8], rhus-t.,
  sabin., samb., **SEP.,** sil., spong.,
  STAPH.[5, 7], stram., sul-ac.,
  SULPH., valer., **zinc.,** zinc-p.[1']

cold[1']/froid/kalte: calc-sil.

hot[13]/très chaud/heiße
bry.

mother's[1, 3]/maternel/Mutter-
milch
cina[3], nat-c., **SIL.**

warm/chaud/warme
ambr.

ailments from[12]
troubles à la suite de
Beschwerden infolge von
hom., mag-c., nat-c., nat-p.,
nux-m.

boiled[12]/cuit/gekochter
sep.
cold/froid/kalter
calc-sil.[1'], kali-i.[12]

am.
acon.[3], **apis,** ant-c.[3], aran.[14],
arist-cl.[9], **ars., chel.**[2, 3, 6, 13],
cina[3], crot-t.[3], ferr.[3], graph.[3],
iod., lact.[13], merc.[3], mez.,
ph-ac.[3], rhus-t.[3], ruta, squil.[3],
staph.[3], verat.

hot[2]/bien chaud/heiße
crot-t.

warm/chaud/warme
chel., graph.[1']

aversion/Abneigung
acon.l.[11], **aeth.,** alum-p.[1'],
am-c., ammc.[11], **ant-t., arn.,**
ars.[3], bell., bov.[3], **bry., cact.**[13],
calad., **calc., calc-s.,** calc-sil.[1'],
carb-v., carbn-s., **carc.**[7, 10],
chin.[3], **cina,** con.[7], convo-s.[9],
elaps[13], esp-g.[13], ferr.[1'], ferr-p.,
guaj., guare., **ign.,** iod.[3, 6],
kali-i.[13], **LAC-D.,** lach.[3], **lec.,**
mag-c., **mag-m.**[13], merc.[3, 7],
NAT-C., nat-m.[3], nat-p., **nat-s.,**
nicot.[13], nit-ac.[3, 6, 13], nux-m.[3],
nux-v., ol-j.[11, 13], past.[8, 13],
pers.[14], **phos.,** podo.[13], **puls.,**
rheum, rhus-t.[3, 13], **sep., sil.,**
stann., **STAPH.**[5, 7], sul-ac.[3],
sulph.

morning/matin/morgens
puls.

boiled/bouilli/gekochte
phos.

cold[3]/froid/kalte
ph-ac., tub.

mother's/maternel/Muttermilch
ant-c., ant-t.[13], **cina,** lach.,
merc., nat-c.[13], rheum[3], **SIL.,**
stann., stram.

child refuses
enfant refuse
Kind verweigert
bor., calc., CALC-P., cina,
lach., **mag-c.**[7], **merc.,** sil.,
stann.[7]

smell of/odeur du/Milchgeruch
bell.

desire/désir/Verlangen
anac., **apis,** aran.[14], **ars., aur.,**
aur-ar.[1'], aur-s.[1'], bapt., bor.,
bov., **bry., calc.,** calc-sil.[1'],
carc.[7, 10], **chel., elaps,** kali-i.,
lac-c., lach.[3], lact.[13], **lycps.**[13],
mag-c., mang., **merc., nat-m.,**
nux-v., ph-ac., phel., **RHUS-T.,**
sabad., sabal[3, 8], sabin.,
sanic.[3], **sil., staph., stront-c.,**
sulph., **tub.**[7], **verat.**[13], **vip.**[3, 6]

boiled/cuit/gekochter
abrot., nat-s.

cold/froid/kalter
adlu.[14], **apis**[3, 6], ph-ac., phel.,
phos., rhus-t., sabad., staph.,
tub.

hot/bien chaud/heißer
calc., chel., graph., hyper.

sour/aigre/Sauermilch
ant-t.[3, 11], mand.[9], mang.

warm/chaud/warmer
bry.

mustard, desire for
moutarde, désir de
Senf, Verlangen nach
ars., cic.[14], **cocc.,** colch., hep.,
lac-c.[2], mez., mill., nicc.

mutton agg.
mouton agg.
Hammelfleisch agg.
bor.[16], lyss.[3], ov.

aversion/Abneigung
calc.[3], ov.

nuts, desire for
noix, désir de
Nüsse, Verlangen nach
cub.

oil agg.
huile agg.
Öl agg.
bry.[2, 3, 6, 13], **canth.**[2, 3, 6],
PULS.[1'-3, 6, 13]

onions agg.
oignons agg.
Zwiebeln agg.
acon-l.[12], alum.[3, 6], brom.[8],
kali-p.[3], **LYC.,** murx.[3, 6], nux-v.,
puls., sep.[3, 13], **thuj.**[1, 7]

ailments from[12]
troubles à la suite d'
Beschwerden infolge von
thuj.

aversion/Abneigung
brom.[13], lyc.[13], nit-ac.[5], **phos.**[13],
prot.[14], **sabad.,** sep.[13],
thuj.[5, 7, 13, 16]

desire for raw
désir d'o. crus
Verlangen nach rohen
all-c., all-s.[13], bell-p.[9, 10], cop.[3],
cub., med.[7], staph.[5], **thuj.**[3, 5, 7]

oranges, aversion to[13]
oranges, aversion d'
Apfelsinen, Abneigung gegen
elaps

desire/désir/Verlangen
cub., elaps, med., sol-t-ae., ther.

oysters agg.
huîtres agg.
Austern agg.
aloe, brom., bry., calc.[7],
carb-v.[3, 6, 8, 13], **coloc.**[3], **LYC.**[1, 7],
podo., puls.[3], **sul-ac.**

shell-fish/coquillage/Muschel-
tiere

am.[3]
lach.

aversion/Abneigung
calc.[7], lyc.[13], **phos.**

desire/désir/Verlangen
apis, brom., **bry., calc., LACH.,**
lyc., **LYCPS.**[13], nat-m., rhus-t.

pancakes agg.
crêpes agg.
Pfannkuchen agg.
ant-c.[3], **bry.,** ip., **kali-c., PULS.,**
verat.

paper, desire for[3]
papier, désir de
Papier, Verlangen nach
lac-f.

indigestible/indigestes/Unverdau-
liches

pastry agg.
pâtisserie agg.
Gebäck, agg., feines
ANT-C.[1, 7], arg-n., ars., **bry.**[2, 3],
carb-v., cycl.[3], ip., **kali-c.**[2, 3, 13],
kali-chl., kali-m.[3, 6, 8, 13], **lyc.,**
nat-s.[3, 6], **phos.,** ptel.[6], **PULS.,**
sulph.[3, 7], sumb.[11], **verat.**[2, 3]

sweets/sucreries/Süßigkeiten

ailments from[12]
troubles à la suite de
Beschwerden infolge von
puls.

aversion[2]/Abneigung
    ars., lyc.[13], **phos., ptel., puls.**[6, 13], sumb.[11]

desire/désir/Verlangen
    bufo, **calc.,** chin., mag-m.[14], merc-i-f.[7], plb., puls.[1'], sabad.[3], sulph.[7]

peaches, after
pêches, troubles après avoir mangé des
Pfirsichen, Beschwerden nach Genuß von
    all-c.[8], **fl-ac.**[3, 6], glon.[3, 7, 8], psor., verat.[5]

sensitive to the smell of
sensible à l'odeur de
empfindlich gegen den Geruch von
    all-c.

pears agg.
poires agg.
Birnen agg.
    bor., bry., merc-c.[3], nat-c.[3], puls-n.[7], **verat.**

pepper agg.
poivre agg.
Pfeffer agg.
    alum.[1'], ars., **chin.**[2, 3], **cina,** nat-c., **nux-v.**[2, 3, 7], sep., sil.

desire for black
désir de p. noir
Verlangen nach schwarzem
    lac-c., nux-v.[12]

cayenne (red)
Cayenne (rouge)
Cayenne-Pfeffer (rotem)
    merc-c.

pickles agg.[3]
cornichons au vinaigre agg.
Essiggurken agg.
    apis, ars., nat-m.[13], sul-ac., verat.

aversion/Abneigung
    abies-c., arund.[13]

desire/désir/Verlangen
    abies-c., alum.[13], am-m.[13], **ant-c.,** arn.[13], ars.[13], carb-an.[13], chel.[13], cod.[13], ham., hep., hyper., ign.[13], kali-bi.[13], **lach..** lact.[13], mag-c.[13], **myric.**[13], nat-ar., rib-ac.[14], sec.[13], **sep.**[13], **sul-i., sulph.,** verat.

plums agg.[3]
prunes agg.
Pflaumen agg.
    mag-c.[3, 16], **merc.,** puls.[5], rheum[3, 11]

ailments from[12]
troubles à la suite de
Beschwerden infolge von
    rheum

aversion/Abneigung
    bar-c., elaps[2], sul-ac.[13]

desire/désir/Verlangen
    sul-ac.

sauce/compote/Pflaumensoße
    arg-n.

pork agg.
porc agg.
Schweinefleisch agg.
    acon., acon-l.[12], **ant-c.,** ant-t., ars., asaf., bell., **CARB-V.,** caust., clem.[3], **colch., CYCL.,** dros.[2, 3], **GRAPH.**[3], ham., **ip., nat-ar., nat-c., nat-m., PULS., SEP.,** tarax., tarent.[13], thuj.

smell of p. agg.[2, 3]
odeur de p. agg.
Geruch von Sch. agg.
    colch.

ailments from[12]
troubles à la suite de
Beschwerden infolge von
    puls. sep.

am.[3, 6]
    mag-c.[2, 3, 6], nat-m., ran-b., ran-s.

aversion[7]/Abneigung
   ang., **colch., cycl., dros.,** prot.[14],
   psor., puls., sep.[3]

desire/désir/Verlangen
   calc-p.[3], **crot-h., mez.**[3], nit-ac.[3, 6],
   nux-v.[3, 6], rad.[7], rad-b.[3], **tub.**

potatoes agg.
pommes de terre agg.
Kartoffeln agg.
   alum., alum-p.[1'], **alumn.**[2], am-c.[3],
   am-m., **bry.**[2], calc., **coloc.,** gran.[3],
   mag-c.[7], mag-s., merc.[13], merc-c.,
   merc-cy.[13], **nat-s., puls.**[3], **sep.,**
   sil.[5], **sulph.**[3, 5], **verat.**

   aversion/Abneigung
      alum., alum-p.[1'], camph., sep.[13],
      thuj.

   desire/désir/Verlangen
      calc-p.[3, 6], hep.[13], med.[7], nat-c.,
      ol-an., olnd.[3, 6, 13]

   fried/rôties/Gebratenes
   raw/crues/rohen

poultry, ailments from[12]
volaille, troubles à la suite de
Geflügelfleisch, Beschwerden infolge
   von
   carb-v.

puddings agg.[2, 3, 6]
entremets agg.
Pudding agg.
   ptel.

sweets/sucreries/Süßigkeiten

aversion/Abneigung
   ars., **phos., ptel.**

desire/désir/Verlangen
   sabad.

pungent things, aversion to[13]
très assaisonné, aversion d'aliments
scharf gewürzte Speisen, Abneigung
   gegen
   fl-ac., sang.

spices/épices/Gewürze

desire/désir/Verlangen
   acon.[1'], ars., aster., caps.[3],
   caust.[1'], chin.[3], **cist., fl-ac., hep.,**
   lac-c., nat-p., nit-ac.[1'], **nux-v.**[1'],
   ph-ac., puls.[1'], **sang.,** sep.[1'],
   stry-p.[6], sulph.[1']

spices/épices/Gewürze

rags, desire for clean
chiffon propre, désir de
Lumpen, Verlangen nach sauberen
   alum., alumn.[13]

raw, agg.
crus agg., a.
rohe Sp. agg.

raw food, agg.
crus agg., aliments
rohe Speisen agg.
   ars., bry., chin., lyc., **puls.,**
   RUTA, Verat.

   am.[3]
      ign.

   desire/désir/Verlangen
      abies-c.[3, 8], ail., **all-c.**[3], alum.[3],
      ant-c.[3], calc.[3], cub.[3], ign.[3],
      lycps.[13], sil., **SULPH.,** tarent.

   onions/oignons/Zwiebeln

   ham/jambon/Schinken
      uran-n.

   potatoes/pommes de terre/Kar-
      toffeln
      calc., cic.[1']

   tomateos/tomates/Tomaten
      ferr.

refreshing things, aversion to[13]
refraîchissantes, aversion de
Erfrischendes, Abneigung gegen
   fl-ac., phos., rheum, sang.

desire/désir/Verlangen
  allox.[14], aloe, ant-t.[3], **ars., calc.,**
  calc-f.[10], **calc-p.**[13], calc-s.,
  carb-an., **caust., chin., cist.,**
  cocc., fl-ac., hep.[3], iod.[3], mag-s.[14],
  nat-ar., **PH-AC., phos., puls.,**
  rheum, **sabin.,** sang., sars., sel.[3],
  thuj., til., **tub.,** valer., **VERAT.**

rice agg.[5]
riz agg.
Reis agg.
  bry., puls., sulph., tell.[12]

desire for dry
désir de r. sec
Verlangen nach trockenem
  alum., mand.[9], ter., ther.[13]

rich, agg.
riche agg., nourriture
reichhaltige, gehaltvolle Speisen agg.
  ant-c., arg-n., ars.[3], **bry.,**
  buni-o.[14], calc.[7, 13], carb-an.,
  CARB-V., caust.[13], cupr.[13], cycl.,
  dros., ferr., iod.[13], **ip.,** kali-chl.,
  kali-m.[13], nat-c.[13], nat-m., **nat-s.,**
  nit-ac., phos., **PULS., sep.,** staph.,
  sulph.[13], tarax., thuj.

fat/graisse/Fett
heavy/lourde/schwere

ailments from[12]
troubles à la suite de
Beschwerden infolge von
  kali-m.

rolls, desire for **stale**[16]
petits pains rassis, désir de
Brötchen, Verlangen nach **altbackenen**
  aur.

salad agg.
salade agg.
Salat agg.
  all-c.[3], ars., bry., **calc.,** caps.[3],
  carb-v., ip.[3', 6], lach., lyc., nux-v.[5],
  puls.[3, 5, 6], sulph.[5]

aversion/Abneigung
  mag-c.[7], prot.[14]

desire/désir/Verlangen
  elaps, lepi.[11], lycps.[13],
  mag-s.[9, 10, 14]

salt agg.
sel agg.
Salz agg.
  alum., ars., bell.[3], calc., **carb-v.,**
  coca[2], **dros.,** lyc., mag-m.,
  NAT-M.[3, 8], **nit-s-d.**[2, 8], nux-v.,
  PHOS., puls.[3], **sel.,** sil.[3]

ailments from[12]
troubles à la suite de
Beschwerden infolge von
  carb-v., nat-m., nit-s-d., sel.

am.
  halo.[14], mag-c.[2, 3, 6, 13], nat-m.[3, 6]

aversion/Abneigung
  acet-ac., allox.[9, 14], bufo[3], **carb-v.,**
  carc.[7, 10], card-m., chin.[3, 6], **con.**[13],
  COR-R., cortico.[9], **GRAPH.,**
  lyc.[7, 16], lyss.[7], **nat-m.,** nit-ac.[13],
  phos.[13], puls.[3, 6], **sel., sep.,** sil.

desire/désir/Verlangen
  acet-ac.[13], **aloe, aq-mar.**[6],
  ARG-N., atro., calc.,
  calc-f.[9, 10, 14], **calc-p.,** calc-s.,
  CARB-V., carc.[7, 10], caste.[14],
  caust., cocc., **con., cor-r.,**
  galin.[14], halo.[14], **LAC-C.,**
  lycps.[13], **lyss., manc., med.,**
  meph., merc.[13], merc-i-f.,
  merc-i-r., **NAT-M., NIT-AC.**[1, 7],
  pers.[14], **PHOS.,** plb., prot.[14],
  sanic., sel., sulph., **tarent.,**
  tell.[14], teucr., **thuj.**[1, 7], **tub.**[1, 7],
  VERAT.

and dainties[7]
et friandises
und Leckereien
  ARG-N., calc., carb-v., caste.[14],
  med., plb.

pregnancy, during[2]
grossesse, pendant la
Schwangerschaft, in der
  nat-m., verat.

sand, desire for
sable, désir de
Sand, Verlangen nach
sil.[3], **TARENT.**

indigestible/indigestes/Unverdau-
liches

sardines agg.[7]
Sardinen agg.
fl-ac., **lyc.**

herring/hareng/Hering

desire/désir/Verlangen
cycl., verat.

anchovies/anchois/Sardellen
herring/hareng/Hering

sauces with f., desire for
sauces avec a., désir de
Soßen mit Sp., Verlangen nach
arg-n.[13], nux-v.[11]

sauerkraut agg.
choucroute agg.
Sauerkraut agg.
arist-cl.[9], ars., **BRY., calc.,**
carb-v., chin., cupr., hell., **lyc.,**
nat-m., **PETR., phos., puls.,** sep.,
verat.

aversion/Abneigung
hell., sulph.[6]

desire/désir/Verlangen
carb-an., cham., **lycps.**[13]

sausages agg.[8]
saucisses agg.
Würste agg.
acet-ac., **ars.**[3, 8], bell.[7, 12], bry.[3],
puls.

spoiled/avariées/ verdorbene
acet-ac.[12], **ARS., BELL., bry.,**
ph-ac., rhus-t., verat.[3]

ailments from[12]
troubles à la suite de
Beschwerden infolge von
bell.

aversion/Abneigung
ars.[13], puls.[7]

desire[13]/désir/Verlangen
acet-ac., calc-p.[6]

shell-fish agg.
coquillage agg.
Muscheltiere agg.
bell.[3, 4], carb-v., **coloc.**[3], cop.[4],
euph.[3], levo.[14], **lyc.,** phenob.[14],
rhus-t.[3], ter.[3, 6], **urt-u.**

sight of food agg.
vue de la nourriture agg.
Anblick von Speisen agg.
ant-t., **COLCH., kali-bi.,** kali-c.,
lyc., merc-i-f., mosch., ph-ac.,
sabad., **sil.**[3, 13], spig., squil.[3],
SULPH., xan.

aversion/Abneigung
ail.[2], **arn.**[2], **ARS.,** caust.[1'], chin.[1'],
colch.[13], dig.[8, 13], lyc.[13], **merc-i-f.**[2],
mang.[16], **mosch.**[2], nux-v.[13], ptel.[3],
sep.[3], **sil.,** squil., stann.[13]

smell of food agg.
odeur de la nourriture agg.
Speisengeruch agg.
ars., bell.[3], **cocc., COLCH.,**
dig., dros.[3], eup-per., **ip.,**
lach.[3], merc-i-f.[3, 6], nat-m.[3],
nux-m.[6], nux-v.[3], osm.[3], ph-ac.[3],
phos.[3], podo.[3, 6], ptel.[3], sang.[3],
sep., sil.[13], stann., sul-ac.[3],
sulph.[3], **thuj.,** xan.[3]

sensitive to the
sensible à l'
empfindlich gegen
arg-n., **ARS., cocc., COLCH.,**
eup-per., **ip.,** lach., **SEP.,**
stann.

aversion/Abneigung
  ars., bell.[13], caust.[1'], **COCC.,**
  COLCH., dig.[8, 13], **IP.,** lyc.[13],
  nux-v.[13], **podo., sep.,** stann.[8]

smoked food agg.
fumés agg., aliments
Geräuchertes agg.
  calc., sil.

  desire/désir/Verlangen
    calc-p., **CAUST., kreos.,** puls.[3, 6]

snow, desire for
neige, désir de
Schnee, Verlangen nach
  crot-c.

soft food, desire for[11]
tendre, désir de nourriture
weichen Speisen, Verlangen nach
  alumn., pyrus, sulph.

solid f., aversion to
solides, aversion d'a.
feste Sp., Abneigung gegen
  aether[11], ang., bell.[3], bry.[3], **ferr.,**
  lyc., merc., **staph.,** sulph.[3, 16]

soup agg.[8, 13]
soupe agg.
Suppe agg.
  alum., alumn.[2], chin.[5], kali-c.,
  staph.[5]

  aversion/Abneigung
    arn., ars., bell., carb-v.[5], cham.,
    chin.[5], **graph.,** kali-c.[13],
    kali-chl.[13], kali-i., merc-cy.[3],
    nat-m.[5], ol-an.[11], puls.[5], **rhus-t.,**
    staph.[5]

  desire/désir/Verlangen
    calc-ar., kali-chl.[13], ol-an.[11],
    staph.[2]

  liquid/liquide/flüssiger
  warm food/nourriture chaude/
    warme Speisen

sour, acids agg.
acides agg.
Saures agg.
  ACON.[3], aloe[2], **ANT-C.,** ant-t.,
  apis[2], **arg-n., ars.,** ars-s-f.[1'],
  aster.[14], **bell.,** bor., brom.,
  calad., calc.[3], **CARB-V.**[3, 8, 13],
  caust., chin., cimic.[3], cub.,
  dros., **ferr.,** ferr-ar., ferr-m.[13],
  ferr-p., fl-ac.[7], **HEP.**[3], ip.[13],
  kali-bi.[2], kreos., lach., mand.[10],
  merc-c., merc-cy.[13], merc-d.[3, 13],
  nat-c., nat-m., **nat-p.,** nux-v.,
  ph-ac., phos., **psor.**[13], **puls.**[3],
  ran-b., **rhus-t.**[3], sel., **sep.,**
  staph.[1], sul-ac.[3], **sulph.,**
  thuj.[1']

  sensitive to smell of
  sensible à l'odeur d'
  empfindlich gegen Geruch von
    Saurem
    dros.

  ailments from[12]
  troubles à la suite d'
  Beschwerden infolge von Saurem
    nat-m.

  am.[3, 6]
    arg-m., arg-n., lach.[3], ptel.[8, 13],
    sang.[8]

  aversion/Abneigung
    abies-c., arund.[13], **bell.,** chin.[13],
    clem.[3], **cocc., con.**[13], dros.[8, 13],
    elaps[13], **ferr.,** ferr-m., **fl-ac.**[13],
    ign., kali-bi.[3], lyc.[13], mand. [10],
    nat-m.[13], nat-p.[3], nux-v., ph-ac.,
    sabad., sulph.

  desire/désir/Verlangen
    abies-c.[8], **ACON.**[3], alum.,
    alum-p,[1'], alumn., am-c.,
    am-m., **ant-c., ant-t., apis,**
    arg-n., **arn., ars.,** ars-s-f.[1'],
    arund., bell., bism.[3], bol-la.,
    bor., brom., bry., calc., calc-s.,
    calc-sil.[1'], carb-an., **carb-v.,**
    carbn.[11], carbn-s., **cham.,** chel.,
    chin., chin-ar., **cist.,** cod.[8, 13],
    con., conv., **COR-R.,** corn.,

cub., cupr., cupr-a.[11], der.[11],
dig., dor.[2, 11], elaps, erig.[10,]
eup-per.[2], **ferr.**, ferr-ar.,
ferr-m., ferr-p., **fl-ac.**, gran.,
HEP., hipp., **ign.**, joan.[8],
kali-ar., kali-bi., **kali-c.**,
kali-p., kali-s., kreos., **lach.**,
lact.[8, 13], lyc.[13], **mag-c.**, mang.,
med., merc-i-f., **myric.**[6, 8, 11, 13],
nabal.[11], **nat-m.**, ph-ac.[8], phel.,
phos., plb., **podo.**, psor., ptel.,
puls., rauw.[9], rhus-t., **sabad.**,
sabin., sec., **sep.**, spirae.[11],
squil., staph.[2], **stram.**, stry-p.[6],
sul-i., **sulph.**, thea, ther., thuj.,
ust., **VERAT.**, ziz.

and salt[7]
et sel
und Salz
arg-n., **calc.**, **calc-s.**, **CARB-V.**,
con., **COR-R.**, **med.**, **merc-i-f.**,
NAT-M., **PHOS.**, **plb.**, **sulph.**,
thuj., **VERAT.**

and sweets[7]
et sucreries
und Süßigkeiten
bry., **calc.**, **carb-v.**, **kali-c.**,
med., **sabad.**, **sec.**, **sep.**,
SULPH.

pregnancy, during[2]
grossesse, pendant la
Schwangerschaft, in der
verat.

spices, condiments, highly seasoned food agg.
épices agg.
Gewürze agg.
bism.[3], ign.[3], kali-m.[3], naja[3],
NUX-V.[2, 3, 7, 8, 13], phos., sel.[3],
sep.[13], zinc.[3]

am.[3, 6]
hep., nux-m.

aversion[13]/Abneigung
mag-s.[12], phos., puls.[3, 6], **sang.,**
tarent.

*pungent/très assaisonné/scharf
gewürzte*

desire/désir/Verlangen
abies-c.[3], alum.[6, 8], ant-c.[3, 6],
arg-n.[3], **ars.**[3], aster.[2, 11], calc-f.[9],
calc-p.[3, 6, 10], caps.[3], **carc.**[7],
chel.[3, 6], **CHIN.**, cic.[14], **fl-ac.**[1, 7],
hep., hyper.[3, 6], **lac-c.,**
mand.[9, 10, 14], mag-s.[9], meph.[2],
nat-m.[3, 6], nux-m.[8], **nux-v.,**
PHOS., puls., **sang.**, sep.,
staph.[3, 8, 13], stry-p.[6], **SULPH.,**
tarent., **zing.**[7]

*pungent/très assaisonné/scharf
gewürzte*

starchy food agg.[8]
féculents agg. aliments
stärkehaltige Speisen agg.
alum.[1, 7], bry.[7], **carb-v.**, chin.,
coloc.[1'], lyc., **nat-c.**, nat-s.,
ox-ac.[1'], sulph.

*farinaceous food/farineux/
Teigwaren*

aversion[13]/Abneigung
chin., lyc., **nat-c.**, nat-s., **sulph.**

desire/désir/Verlangen
alum., atri.[7], calc., cic., **nat-m.**[13],
nit-ac., nux-v.

stimulants agg.[8]
Anregungsmittel agg.
agar.[1'], ant-c.[1', 8], cadm-s., chion.,
fl-ac., **glon.**, ign., lach., led., naja,
nat-sil.[1'], **nux-v.**[7, 8], op., thuj.[1'],
zinc.

tonics/toniques/Stärkungsmittel

am.[8]
gels., glon.

desire[11]/désir/Verlangen
alco., aloe[6, 11], ant-t., ars-s-f.[1'],
aster., aur., aur-s.[1'], calc-i.[1'],
caps.[7], caust.[3], chin.[6], crot-h.[9],
fl-ac.[6], gins., hep.[3], iber., iod.,

kali-i., naja, nat-p., nux-v.[7], **puls.,**
sol-t-ae., staph.[3, 6], sul-i.[1'],
sulph.[1', 6], sumb., tab., ziz.

strange things, desire for
étranges, désir de choses
Ausgefallenem, Verlangen nach
bry., calc., calc-p., chel., cycl.,
hep., lyss.[13]**, manc.,** ter.[2]

indigestible/indigestes/Unver-
dauliches

pregnancy, during
grossesse, pendant la
Schwangerschaft, in der
chel., LYSS., mag-c.

strawberries agg.
fraises agg.
Erdbeeren agg.
ant-c., ox-ac., sep., thlas.[3]

aversion[5, 7]/Abneigung
chin.[5, 7, 16], ox-ac.[13], **sulph.**

sugar agg.[6]
sucre agg.
Zucker agg.
arg-n.[1', 6, 7, 12], bell., **calc.**[2, 5, 7],
merc.[6, 8], nat-p.[8, 12], ox-ac.[1', 2, 6],
sang., **sel.**[1', 2, 6, 12], **SULPH.**[2, 5],
thuj. zinc.

aversion[6]/Abneigung
ars., caust., chloram.[14], graph.,
merc., phos., rauw.[9], sin-n.,
zinc.

desire/désir/Verlangen
am-c., am-m.[13], **ARG-N., calc.,**
kali-c., lyc.[2, 6], op.[11], prot.[14],
sec., sulph.[6]

evening/soir/abends
arg-n.

sugared water/eau sucrée/
Zuckerwasser
bufo[2, 7, 11], sulph.[11]

sweets agg.
sucreries agg.
Süßigkeiten agg.
acon., am-c., **ant-c., ARG-N.,**
ars.[3, 5], aster.[14], bad.[3], bell.[3],
calc., calc-f.[9, 10, 14], **cham.,**
cina[3], cycl.[6], ferr.[3], fl-ac.,
graph., hep.[5], **IGN., ip.**[2, 6, 8],
lach.[3], **lyc.**[6, 8, 13], mand.[9, 10, 14],
med.[7, 8, 13], **merc.,** nat-c.,
nat-p.[3], nux-v.[5], ox-ac., phos.,
puls.[5, 6], sang.[3, 8, 13], sel., spig.,
spong.[12], **sulph.,** thuj., zinc.,
zinc-p.[1']

delicacies/friandises/
Leckereien
pastry/pâtisserie/Gebäck
puddings/entrements/Pudding

sensitive to the smell of[3]
sensible à l'odeur de
empfindlich gegen den Geruch
von
aur., nit-ac., sil.

ailments from[12]
troubles à la suite de
Beschwerden infolge von
thuj.

am.
am-c.[14], bell.[3]

aversion/Abneigung
arg-n.[13]**, ars.,** bar-c., beryl.[9, 14],
caust., chloram.[14], erig.[14],
GRAPH., hipp., hippoz.[3'],
kali-c.[13], lac-c., lol.[6], **lyc.**[13],
med.[7, 15], **merc.,** nit-ac.,
nux-v.[5, 7, 16], petr.[13], **phos.,**
puls.[5, 7], rad.[13], rad-br.[3, 7, 8],
rauw.[9], rheum[13], senec.[3], **sin-n.,**
sul-ac.[13]**, sulph., zinc.,** zinc-p.[1']

desire/désir/Verlangen
alf.[8, 13], **am-c.,** aran-ix.[10, 14],
arg-m., **ARG-N., ARS.,**
ars-s-f.[1'], bar-c., bar-s.[1'], **bry.,**
bufo, cael.[14], **calc., calc-f.**[9, 10, 14],
calc-s., carb-v., caste.[14],
cere-b[11], **CHIN.,** chin-ar., **cina**[8, 13],

coca[8, 13], **cocain.**[8, 13], crot-h.[8, 13],
elaps, ferr.[3], **ip., joan.**[8], kali-ar.,
kali-c., kali-p., **kali-s.,** lil-t.[3],
LYC., mag-m., mand.[9, 10, 14],
med., meph.[14], **merc.**[1, 7],
merc-d.[3'], nat-ar., **nat-c.,**
nat-m., nux-v., onop.[14], op.,
petr., **plb.,** rad-br.[12], **rheum,**
rhus-t., rib-ac.[14], **sabad., sec.,**
sep., sil.[2], **SULPH., tub.,**
x-ray[9, 14]

dainties[7]/friandises/Leckereien
acon-l., arg-n., calc.

and salt[7]
et sel
und Salz
    ARG-N., calc., carb-v.,
    caste.[14], **med., plb.**

and sour[7]
et acides
und Saurem
    bry., calc., carb-v., kali-c.,
    med., sabad., sec., sep.,
    SULPH.

tea agg.
thé agg.
Tee agg.
    abies-c.[13], **abies-n.**[3, 8, 12], **aesc.,**
    agar.[3], ars.[3], aur-m.[1', 2], cham.[3, 6],
    chin., cocc.[3, 6], coff., dios., **ferr.,**
    fl-ac.[1'], hep.[3], kali-bi.[3], kali-hp.[8],
    lach., lob.[8, 12, 13], **nux-v.**[1', 7, 8, 12, 13],
    ph-ac.[3], puls.[3, 8, 13], **rhus-t.**[2, 12],
    rumx., **SEL., SEP.**[2, 3], **spig.**[3],
    thuj., verat.

ailments from[12]
troubles à la suite de
Beschwerden infolge von
    abies-n., **chin.,** cocc., dios., lob.,
    nux-v., sel., stroph-h., thuj.

am.
    carb-ac., dig., ferr., kali-bi.[3, 6],
    pyrus[13]

aversion/Abneigung
    carb-ac., carb-an.[13], chin.[13],
    dios.[13], ferr-m[13], kali-hp.[13], **phos.,**
    sel.[13], thea, thuj.[13]

desire/désir/Verlangen
    alum.[8], aster., calc-s., **chin.**[5, 7],
    hep., hydr., lepi.[11], nux-v.[5, 7],
    puls.[7], pyrus, sel.[,3 6], thuj.[7]

grounds/marc/Teesatz
    alum.

indigestible/indigestes/Unver-
*   daulichem*

thought of food agg.[3]
pensée des aliments agg.
Gedanke an Speisen agg.
    arg-n., bor., cann-s., carb-v., dros.,
    graph., lach., lil-t., nat-m., **puls.,**
    sars., **sep.,** thuj.

tomatoes agg.[3]
tomates agg.
Tomaten agg.
    lith-c., ox-ac.[1'], phos.

desire[7, 13]/désir/Verlangen
    ferr.

tonics agg.[13]
toniques agg.
Stärkungsmittel agg.
    carb-ac.

stimulants/Anregungsmittel

aversion[13]/Abneigung
    sul-ac.

desire/désir/Verlangen
    aloe, carb-ac., carb-an., caust.,
    cocc., nux-v., **rhus-t., ph-ac.,**
    puls., rheum, sul-ac., **valer.**

turnips agg.
navets agg.
weiße Rüben agg.
    bry., calc-ar., **lyc., puls.,** sulph.[5]

aversion/Abneigung
    bry.[7, 16], puls.[13], sulph.[5, 7, 16]

veal agg.
veau agg.
Kalbfleisch agg.
    ars., **calc.**, **caust.**, chin., **IP.**,
    KALI-N., nux-v., **sep.**, sulph.,
    verat., **zinc.**

ailments from[12]
troubles à la suite de
Beschwerden infolge von
    kali-n.

aversion/Abneigung
    merc.[3], phel., **zinc.**

vegetables agg.
légumes agg.
Gemüse agg.
    alum., ars., **bry.**, calc.[7], cupr.,
    hell., hydr.[2, 6, 8], **kali-c.**[2], lyc.,
    mag-c.[2], **nat-c.**, **NAT-S.**,
    petr.[3], verat.

decayed/pourris/verfaultes
    carb-an.[2, 12], **CARB-V.**

aversion/Abneigung
    bell., **hell.**, hydr., lyss.[13], **mag-c.**,
    mag-m.[2], ruta

desire/désir/Verlangen
    abies-c.[8], adel.[11], all-c.[3], **alum.**,
    alumn., ars., asar.[14], calc-s.,
    carb-an., cham., **lycps.**[13],
    mag-c.[1], **mag-m.**, onos.[13]

vinegar agg.
vinaigre agg.
Essig agg.
    acon.[3, 6], aloe, alum.[1'],
    ANT-C., **ars.**, **bell.**, bor.,
    calad., **carb-v.**[3, 8], caust., dros.,
    ferr., ferr-ar., **graph.**[3], hep.[3],
    kreos., lach., merc-c.[3], nat-ar.,
    nat-c., nat-m., **nat-p.**[3], nux-v.,
    ph-ac., phos., **puls.**[3], ran-b.,
    sep., staph., sul-ac.[3], **sulph.**

sensitive to the smell of
sensible à l'odeur de
empfindlich gegen Geruch von
    agar.

am.
    asar., bry., ign., meny., op., **puls.**,
    sang.[13], stram., tab.[6]

desire/désir/Verlangen
    apis, arn., ars., asar.[14], bell-p.[9, 10],
    chel., **HEP.**, kali-p., lepi., puls.[7],
    rib-ac.[14], **sep.**, sulph.

warm drinks agg.[13]
boissons chaudes agg.
warme Getränke agg.
    ambr.[2, 7, 8, 13], apis[1', 6], bry.[6, 8],
    CARBN-S., chel., fl-ac.[1'],
    graph.[6, 13], ign.[6], **lach.**[6, 8],
    phos.[6, 8, 13], **puls.**[8, 13], pyrog.[6],
    RHUS-T., sars.[1'], sep.[8], sil.[1'],
    stann.[8, 13, 14], **sulph.**, verat.,
    zinc-p.[1']

am.
    alum., apoc.[1'], arg-n., **ARS.**,
    bry., calc-f.[7], **carbn-s.**, **cedr.**,
    chel., cupr.[6], **graph.**, guare.,
    lyc., mang., nux-m., **NUX-V.**,
    pyrus, **RHUS-T.**, sabad.[6, 8, 13],
    spong., **sulph.**, verat.

aversion/Abneigung
    bry.[13], caust.[13], **cham.**, cupr.[13],
    graph.[13], kali-s.[8], **PHOS.**, **PULS.**,
    pyrog.[13], rib-ac.[14], zinc-p.[1']

desire/désir/Verlangen
    ang., **ARS.**, ars-s-f.[1'], bell.,
    BRY., **calad.**, carb-v., casc.,
    cast.[11], cast-v., cedr., **chel.**,
    chin-ar.[1'], cocc.[3], cupr.,
    eup-per., eup-pur., ferr.[3],
    ferr-p.[7, 8], graph., hep.[1'],
    hyper., kali-ar., kali-c.[14],
    kali-i.[3, 6], kreos., **LAC-C.**, lyc.,
    med.[7, 8], merc-c., pyrus, **sabad.**,
    spig.[3, 8], **sulph.**, tub.[7]

angina pectoris, in[7]
angine de poitrine, dans l'
Angina pectoris, bei
    spig.

chill, during
frissons, pendant les
Fieberfrost, während
   ARS., cedr., **eup-per.**

fever, during
fièvre, pendant la
Fieber, im
   casc., cedr., **eup-per.**, **lyc.**

warm food agg.
nourriture chaude agg.
warme Speisen agg.
   acon., agn., all-c., alum.,
   alum-p.[1'], alum-sil.[1'], am-c.,
   ambr., **anac.**, ang.[3], ant-t.,
   ars.[3], asar., **bar-c.**, **bell.**,
   bism., bor., **BRY.**, calc.,
   canth., **carb-v.**, carbn-s., caust.,
   cham., clem., **coc-c.**, **cupr.**, dros.,
   euph., ferr., gran., guat.[14], hell.,
   kali-c., **LACH.**, laur., **mag-c.**,
   mag-m., merc., **mez.**, nat-m.,
   nit-ac., nux-m., nux-v., par.,
   ph-ac., **PHOS.**, **PULS.**, rhod.,
   rhus-t., sars., sep., sil., spig.,
   squil., stann., sul-ac., sul-i.[1'],
   sulph., thiop.[14], thuj., verat.,
   zinc.

am.[13]
   asar., kreos.[8, 13], **laur.**, lyc.[3, 7, 8, 13],
   sabad.[1']

aversion/Abneigung
   alum-p.[1'], **bell.**, calc., chin., cupr.,
   GRAPH., guare., **ign.**, **lach.**, **lyc.**,
   mag-c., mag-s., merc., **merc-c.**,
   merc-cy[13], **nux-v.**[3], petr., **PHOS.**,
   psor., **PULS.**, **sil.**, **verat.**, zinc.

desire/désir/Verlangen
   ang., **ARS.**, ars-s-f.[1'], **bry.**[3], cast.[3],
   cedr.[3], **chel.**, china-ar.[1'], cocc.,
   cupr., cycl., **ferr.**, kali-i.[3], **lyc.**,
   med.[7], **ph-ac.**, sabad., sil.

soups/soupes/Suppen
   bry., **calc-ar.**, ferr., nat-m.,
   phel.

soup/soupe/Suppe

water agg.[13]
eau agg.
Wasser agg.
   arg-n.[6, 13], ars., bry., calc.,
   canth.[6, 13], chin-ar.[6], **cocc.**,
   crot-t., dros., ferr-m., lach.,
   lob., lyc., nux-m., puls.,
   sabad., sep., spong., stann.,
   sulph.

seeing or hearing of[13]
regardant ou en entendant l'e.,
   en
Sehen oder Hören von
   lyss.

am.[13]
   ars., **BRY.**

aversion/Abneigung
   apis, ars.[1', 13], **bell.**, berb.[1'], brom.,
   bry., **calad.**, cann-i., **canth.**, carl.,
   caust., cedr., chel.[13], **chin.**[1, 7],
   chin-ar.[13], coc-c., coloc., elaps,
   ham., hell., **HYOS.**, kali-bi.[1],
   lach.[5, 7], lyc., **lyss.**, manc.,
   merc.[13], merc-c., merc-cy.[13],
   nat-m., **NUX-V.**, onos., ox-ac.,
   phel., **phys.**, **puls.**, **STAPH.**[5, 7],
   STRAM., sul-ac.[5, 7], **tab.**[6], thea,
   zinc., zing.[13]

cold drinks-cold water/boissons
froides-eau froide/kalte
Getränke – kaltes Wasser

wine agg.*
vin agg.
Wein agg.
   acon., acon-l.[12], agar., alum.,
   am-m., **ant-c.**, **arn.**, **ARS.**, aur.,
   aur-m., bell., benz-ac.[3, 6, 8, 13],
   bor., bov., bry., cact., **calc.**,
   calc-sil.[1'], carb-an., carb-v.,
   carbn-s., **CHIN.**[1], chlol.,
   chlor.[13], cob-n.[10], coc-c.,
   COFF., coloc., **con.**, cor-r.,
   des-ac.[14], eup-per.[1'], **fl-ac.**,
   flav.[14], **gels.**, **glon.**, hyos.[4],
   ign., kali-chl., **lach.**, **led.**,
   LYC., mag-m.[14], **merc.**[2, 4], **naja**,
   nat-ar., **nat-c.**, **nat-m.**, nat-sil.[1'],

nux-m., NUX-V., OP., ox-ac.,
petr., phos.[16], prot.[14], puls.,
RAN-B., rhod., rhus-t., ruta,
sabad., sars.[1'], sel., SIL.,
staph.[3, 6], stront-c.,
sulph.[2, 3, 4, 5], thuj., verat.,
ZINC., zinc-p.[1']

champagne[7]
Champagner
calc.

red[3, 6, 7]
rouge
Rotwein
fl-ac.

sensitive to the smell of
sensible à l'odeur de
empfindlich gegen Weingeruch
tab.

sour/vert/saurer
ANT-C., ant-t., ars., ferr., sep.,
sulph.

sulphureted[2, 3, 7]
sulfuré
geschwefelter
ars., chin., merc., PULS., sep.

ailments from[12]
troubles à la suite de
Beschwerden infolge von
coff., lyc., nat-m.

bad[12]
mauvais
schlechter
carb-v.

am.
acon., agar., ars., bell., brom.,
bry., canth., carb-ac., chel.,
chen-v.[2], coca[8, 13], cocc., con.,
gels., glon., graph., lach., mez.,
nat-m.[3], nux-v., onos.[3, 6], op.,
osm., phos., ran-b.[13], sel.,
sul-ac., sulph., thea

sour[2, 7]/vert/saurer
ferr.

aversion/Abneigung
ACON.[13], agar., alum.[13], ars-m.,
carb-v.[13], carbn-s.[13], coff.[13], fl-ac.,
glon.[13], hyper.[13], ign., jatr.,
jug-r., lach., lact.[13], manc.,
mand.[9], merc., nat-m., nux-v.[13],
ph-ac., puls.[13], rhus-t.. SABAD.,
sil.[13], sulph., tub.[7], zinc., zinc-p.[1']

desire/désir/Verlangen
acon., aeth., arg-m., arg-mur.[11],
ars., asaf., bov., bry., calc.,
calc-ar., calc-s., CANTH.[13],
chel., chin., chin-ar., chlor.[3],
cic., colch., cub., eup-per.[1'],
fl-ac., hep., hyper., iod.[3, 6],
kali-bi., kali-br., kali-i., lach.,
lec., LYCPS.[13], merc., mez.,
nat-m., nux-v.[5, 12], op.[5, 13],
PHOS., puls., sec., sel., sep.,
spig., staph., sul-i.[3, 6], SULPH.,
sumb., ther., thiop.[14], vichy[11]

claret/rouge/Rotwein
calc-s., staph., sulph., ther.

FORCED through a narrow opening,
as if[3]
FORCÉ à travers une étroite ouverture,
comme
GEZWUNGEN WIRD, als ob etwas
durch eine enge Öffnung
BAR-C., bell., bufo, carb-an., card-m.,
coc-c., cocc., dig., glon., lach., op.,
plb., puls., sulph., tab., thuj., tub.,
valer.

FOREIGN BODIES or grains of sand
were under the skin, sensation as if
small
CORPS ÉTRANGERS ou de grains de
sable sous la peau, sensation de petits
FREMDKÖRPERN oder Sandkörnern
unter der Haut, Gefühl von kleinen
COCAIN.

FORMICATION, external parts
FORMICATION externe
AMEISENLAUFEN, Kribbeln, äußerliches
  abrot.[3], **ACON.,** acon-c.[11], acon-f.[11], aconin.[11], aesc., aether[11], agar., agn.[1',3], alco.[11], all-s., aloe[3,11], **alum.,** alum-p.[1'], alum-sil.[1'], **alumn.**[2], am-c., am-m., ambr., anac., ang.[3], ant-c., ant-t., apis[3], **aran.**[2,6], arg-m. **ARG-N.**[3,6], **ARN.,** ars., ars-i., ars-s-f.[1'], arum-t.[7], arund., asaf., asar., aur., aur-ar.[1'], aur-s.[1'], **bar-c.,** bar-i.[1'], bar-m., bar-s.[1'], bell., bor., bov., bry., bruc.[11], bufo[3], cadm-s.[1'], calad., calc., calc-p., camph., cann-i., cann-s., canth.[2,4], caps., carb-an., carb-v., carbn-s.[1'], card-b.[11], **carl.**[11], **cast.**[3,6], **caust.,** cedr.[2,3,11], cham., **chel.,** chin., cic., cina, cist., clem., **cocc., COLCH.,** coloc., con., conin.[11], **croc.,** cupr-s.[2], cur.[7], dros., dulc., euon.[4,11], euphr., fago.[11], ferr., ferr-ma.[4], fl-ac.[3], **gran.,** graph., guaj., guare.[11], halo.[14], ham.[11], hep., hist.[10], hydr-ac.[2], hyos., **hyper.**[3,6], ign., iod., ip., kali-ar., **kali-br.**[3,6], **kali-c.,** kali-m.[1'], kali-n., **kalm.**[3,6], kreos., kres.[13], lach., lath.[6], laur., led., **lyc., m-arct.**[4], m-aust.[3,4], mag-c., **mag-m.,** mang., **med.**[1'], **merc.,** merc-c., merc-i-r.[11], **mez.,** morph.[11], mosch., mur-ac., nat-ar., **nat-c., nat-m.,** nat-p., nat-sil.[1'], nit-ac., nit-s-d.[11], nux-m., **NUX-V.,** ol-an.[3], ol-j.[11], olnd., onos., op., pall., par., petr.[3,6], **ph-ac., phos.,** phys.[6], **pic-ac., PLAT.,** plb., **puls., ran-b.,** ran-s., rheum, **rhod., RHUS-T.,** rumx.[3,11], **sabad.,** sabin., samb., sars., **SEC.,** sel., seneg., **SEP.,** sil., **SPIG.,** spong., **squil.**[4], stann., staph., stram., stront-c., sul-ac., sul-i.[1'], **sulph.,** tab.[3,6,11], tarax., **tarent.,** teucr., thuj., tub.[1'], urt-u., valer., verat., verb., viol-t., **visc.**[3,6], **zinc.,** zinc-p.[1']

internally
interne
innerliches
  acon., acon-f., agar., agn., aloe[3], alum., alum-sil.[1'], am-c., am-m., ambr., ant-t., apis[3], arg-m., **arn.,** ars., asaf., bar-c., bell., bor.[3], bov.[3], brom.[3], **bry.,** cadm-s.[1'], calc., **canth.,** caps.[3], carb-an.[3], carb-v., caust., **cham.**[3], chel., **chin.,** cic., cina[3], cocc., **COLCH.,** coloc., con.[3], cupr., dig.[3], dros., dulc., euphr., ferr.[3], graph., guaj., hep., hyos., ign., iod., **ip.**[3], kali-ar.[1'], kali-c.[3], kali-n.[3], kres.[13], **lach.**[3], laur., led., mag-c.[3], mag-m.[3], meny., merc., mez., mur-ac.[3], nat-ar., nat-c., **nat-m.**[3], nat-p., nat-sil.[1'], nux-m., nux-v., olnd.[3], ph-ac., phos., **PLAT.,** plb., prun.[3], **puls.,** rheum, rhod., **RHUS-T., sabad.,** sabin., **SANG., sec.,** sel., seneg., sep., sil., spig., spong., stann., staph., sul-i.[1'], **SULPH.,** tarax., teucr.[3], thuj., **verat.**[3], viol-o., **zinc.,** zinc-p.[1']

bones
os, dans les
Knochen, in den
  acon., arn., cham., colch., ign.[2,11], kali-bi.[3], merc., mez.[3], nat-c., nat-m., nux-v., ph-ac., plat., **plb.,** puls., rhod., **rhus-t.,** sabad., sec., **sep.,** spig., sulph., zinc.

emissions, after seminal[16]
pertes séminales, après
Samenverlusten, nach
  mez.

glands
glandes, dans les
Drüsen, in den
  acon., **arn.,** bell., calc., cann-s., canth., **CON.,** ign., m-aust.[4], laur., merc., nat-c., ph-ac., **plat.,** puls., rhod., **rhus-t.,** sabin., **sep., spong.,** sulph., zinc.

painful sensation of crawling through
  whole body if he knocks against
  any part
douloureuse de fourmis rampant à
  travers tout le corps s'il se heurte
  quelque part, sensation
schmerzhaftes Kribbeln durch den
  ganzen Körper, wenn er sich
  anstößt
  spig.

suffering parts, of[16]
souffrantes, des parties
leidenden Teile, der
  con.

FROSTBITE, ailments from[12]
GELURE, troubles à la suite de
ERFRIERUNG, Beschwerden
  infolge von
  zinc.

FULL feeling **externally**
PLÉNITUDE, sensation **externe** de
VÖLLEGEFÜHL, äußerliches
  aesc., aloe[1'], ars., aur., aur-m.,
  caust., kali-n., laur., nux-m., par.,
  phos., sul-i.[1'], verat.

blood-vessels, of[3]
vaisseaux sanguins, des
Blutgefäße, der
  ham., sang.

internally
interne
innerliches
  ACON., AESC., agar., aloe[3],
  alum., alum-sil.[1'], am-c., am-m.,
  aml-ns., anac., ant-c., **ant-t., apis,**
  arg-n.[3], **arn.**, ars., **asaf., asar.,**
  aur., aur-m.[1'], aur-s.[1'], **bar-c.,**
  bar-i.[1'], bar-m., bar-s.[1'], **bell.,** bor.,
  bov., **bry.,** cact., calc., calc-i.,
  calc-s.[1'], calc-sil.[1'], camph.,
  cann-i., cann-s., **canth., caps.,**
  carb-an., carb-v., carbn-s., caust.,
  cench.[1'], **cham.,** chel., **CHIN.,** cic.,
  CIMIC., coc-c.[11], cocc., coff.,

colch., coloc., com., **con.,**
conv.[3], croc., **crot-t., cycl., dig.,**
dirc.[11], **ferr.,** ferr-ar.[1'], gels.[3],
GLON., graph., guaj., halo.[14],
ham., hell., hyos., ign., iod., **iris,**
kali-c., kali-m.[1'], **kali-n.,** kreos.,
lach., laur., led., **lil-t.**[3], lob.[3], **lyc.,**
mag-c., mag-m., mang., **MELI.,**
meny., merc., mez., **MOSCH.,**
mur-ac., **nat-ar.,** nat-c., nat-m.,
nat-s.[1', 3], **nit-ac., nux-m.,**
nux-v., olnd., op., par., petr.,
ph-ac., **PHOS.,** phys.[11], **phyt.,**
plat., plb., **psor., puls., ran-s.,**
rheum, rhod., **RHUS-T.,** ruta,
sabad., **sabin.,** sars., **sep.,** sil.,
spig., spong., stann., staph., stict.,
stront-c., sul-ac., sul-i.[1'], **SULPH.,**
thuj., **valer.,** verat., verat-v.,
verb., vip.[6], zinc.

playing piano, after[1]
piano, par jouer du
Klavierspiel, durch
  anac.

GAIT REELING, staggering, tottering
  and wavering[3]
DÉMARCHE CHANCELANTE,
  titubante, mal assurée, vacilante
GANG SCHWANKEND, stolpernd,
  wackelig und taumelnd
  acet-ac.[11], acon.[3, 6, 8], **AGAR.**[3, 4, 6, 8, 11],
  agro.[8], ail., **alum.**[3, 6], am-c.[4], anan.[2],
  ang.[8], ant-c., **arg-m.**[3, 8], arn., ars.[3, 11],
  ars-s-f.[2], **asar.**[3, 8, 11], aster.[8], astra-m.[8],
  aur., aur-s.[2], **BELL.**[3, 4, 6, 8, 11], bov.,
  BRY.[2, 3, 11], calc., calc-p.[8, 11], **camph.,**
  cann-s.[3, 4], canth., **caps.,** carb-an.,
  carb-v.[3, 11], **carbn-s.**[8], **CAUST.**[3, 4, 6, 8],
  cham., chel., chin.[2, 3], cic.[3, 11],
  COCC.[3, 4, 6, 8], **coff.,** colch.[3, 8],
  con.[3, 6, 8, 11], croc., crot-h.[2], cupr.[3, 4],
  cupr-ar.[6], cycl., dig.[6], dros.[3, 11],
  dub-m.[8], dulc., euph., ferr., **gels.**[3, 8],
  glon.[2, 3], graph., hell.[3, 4], helo.[8],
  hydr-ac.[2, 4], hydrc.[6], **hyos.**[3, 6],
  ign.[3, 4, 6, 8], ip., kali-br.[3, 6], kali-c.,
  kali-n., lac-c.[8], lach.[4], lact.[11], **lath.**[8],
  laur., led., lil-t.[8, 11], lol.[3, 6, 8], lyc.[11],
  mag-c., **mag-m.**[3, 4], mag-s.[6], mang.[3, 8],

merc.[3, 8, 11], **mez.,** morph.[11], mosch.,
mur-ac.[3, 8], **mygal.**[8], naja[11],
nat-c.[3, 6, 8, 11], nat-m.[3, 4, 6], nit-ac.,
nux-m.[3, 8], **NUX-V.**[3, 8], **olnd.,** onos.[3, 8],
OP.[3, 4, 6], **oxyt.**[8], paeon.[8], par.,
petr.[3, 4, 6], **ph-ac.**[3, 4, 6, 11] **phos.**[3, 11],
phys.[11], phyt.[2], pic-ac., plat.[4], plb.,
prun.[4, 6], puls., rheum, **rhod.**[3, 4, 6],
RHUS-T.[3, 4, 6, 11], ruta[3, 4, 6], sabad.[3, 4, 6],
samb., sars., **sec.**[3, 4], seneg., sep., **sil.,**
spig., spong., **STRAM.**[2-4, 6, 11],
stront-c., sulph.[3, 11], tab., tanac.[11],
tarax.[3, 11], teucr.[3, 4, 6], **thuj.**[3, 4, 11],
valer., **VERAT.**[3, 4], **verat-v.,** verb.[3, 4],
viol-o., viol-t.[3, 11], vip.[3, 4], visc., zinc.

gangrene see blackness

GLANDERS
MORVE
ROTZKRANKHEIT
    acon.[8], **ars.,** calc., chin-s.[8], **crot-h.**[8],
    hep.[8], hippoz.[8, 12], **kali-bi.**[8, 12], **lach.**[8, 12],
    merc.[8], ph-ac., phos.[8], sep.[8], sil.[8],
    sulph., thuj.[8]

GONORRHOEA, suppressed
GONORRHÉE supprimée
GONORRHOE, unterdrückte
    acon.[3], agn., ant-t.[8], aur., benz-ac.,
    brom., **calc., CANTH.**[2], **chel.**[2], **clem.,**
    coca[2], crot-h., daph., graph.[8], kali-i.[8],
    kalm., **MED.,** merc., mez.,
    NAT-S.[1', 2, 7, 8, 12], **nit-ac.,** phyt.[3],
    psor.[8], **puls.,** sars., sel.[3], sep.[1'], sil.[1'],
    staph., SULPH.[2, 3, 7], **THUJ.,** verat.,
    viol-t.[2, 12], x-ray[8], zinc.

sycosis/sycotique/sykotische

GOOD HEALTH before paroxysmes[7]
BONNE SANTÉ avant les paroxymes
WOHLBEFINDEN vor Anfällen
    bry., carc., helon., nat-m.[3], phos.[3],
    psor., sep.[3]

GROWTH in length too fast[8]*
CROISSANCE en longueur trop rapide
LÄNGENWACHSTUM, zu schnelles
    calc.[7, 8], **calc-p.,** ferr.[3], ferr-a., iod.[3],
    irid., kreos., **ph-ac.**[3, 8], **phos.**[3, 8]

    children-growing/enfants-
      croissance/Kindern – wachsen
    pains-growing/douleurs-crois-
      sance/Schmerzen – Wachstums-
      schmerzen
    weakness-growing/faiblesse-
      croissance/Schwäche – Wachstum

    young people, in[2]
    jeunes, chez les
    Jugendlichen, bei
      hippoz., kreos.[12], **ph-ac.**[2, 12], **PHOS.**

HAEMORRHAGE
HÉMORRHAGIE
BLUTUNG
    abies-n.[12], acal.[8], acet-ac., **acon.,**
    adren.[6, 8], **agar.**[3, 4, 6], alet.[1'], aln.[12],
    aloe, **alum.,** alumn.[8, 12], am-c.,
    am-caust.[10], am-m.[4], ambr., **ammc.**[2],
    anac.[3, 4], **ant-c.,** ant-t.[3, 4], anthraci.[8],
    apis, apoc.[1', 6], **aran.,** arg-m.[4],
    arg-n., ARN., ars., ars-h.[8], ars-i.,
    arum-t.[6], asaf.[1', 4, 11], asar.[3, 4], aur.[12],
    aur-m.[12], bapt.[6], **bar-c.,** bar-i.[1'],
    bar-m., **BELL.,** bell-p.[6, 10], bism.[3, 4],
    bor.[3, 4], **BOTH., bov.,** brom.[6], **bry.,**
    bufo[2], **cact., CALC.,** calc-f.[6],
    CALC-S., calc-sil.[1'], cann-s.[3, 4],
    CANTH., caps., carb-an., **CARB-V.,**
    carbn-s., card-m.[1', 12], casc.[2, 12],
    caust.[3], **cham., CHIN.,** chin-ar.,
    chin-s.[4, 8, 12], cina[3, 4], cinnb., **cinnm.,**
    cit-l.[12], clem.[3, 4], cob.[12], coc-c.[6, 12],
    cocc.[3, 4, 11], **coff.,** coff-t.[7], colch.[3, 4],
    coll.[12], **coloc.,** con.[3, 4], **croc.,** crot-c.[7],
    CROT-H., cupr., des-ac.[14], dig.,
    dor.[6, 7], **dros., dulc.,** elaps, equis.[10],
    erech.[7, 8, 12], ergot.[8, 12], **ERIG.,**
    erod.[12], euphr.[3, 4], eupi.[12], **FERR.,**
    ferr-ar., ferr-i., ferr-m.[2, 12], **ferr-p.,**
    ferr-s.[12], fic.[8, 10, 12], gal-ac.[8, 12],
    ger.[8, 10, 12], glon.[10], **graph., HAM.,**
    HELL.[2], hep.[3, 4], hir.[7, 8, 10, 12, 14], hydr.[6],
    hydrin-s.[8], **hyos.,** ign.[3, 4], **iod., IP.,**

jug-c.[6], juni-c.[12], kali-c., **kali-chl.**,
kali-i., kali-m.[1'], kali-n., **kali-p.**,
kreos.[1], **LACH.**, lachn.[2], **led.**, leon.[12],
lyc., lycps.[3, 6], m-arct.[4], m-aust.[4],
mag-c.[3, 4], mag-m.[3, 4], **MELI.**,
MERC., MERC-C., merc-cy.[8, 12],
mez., MILL., mosch., mur-ac.,
MURX.[2], nat-c., **NAT-M., nat-n.**[6, 10],
nat-s.[6, 10], nat-sil.[8], **NIT-AC.**,
nux-m., **NUX-V.**, op.[4, 8], par.[3, 4],
petr.[4], **ph-ac., PHOS., plat.**, plb.[3, 4],
psor., PULS., pyrog.[6], rat.[4, 6, 12],
rhod., rhus-a.[12], rhus-g.[12], **rhus-t.**,
ruta[3, 4, 12], sabad.[3, 4], **SABIN.**,
sal-ac.[6], sang., **sanguiso.**[6], sars.,
scir.[12], **SEC.**, sel.[3, 4], **senec., SEP.**,
sil., squil., stann., staph.[3, 4], **stram.**,
SUL-AC., sulfa.[14], **SULPH.**, syph.[7],
tarax.[3, 4], **ter.**, thlas.[6, 8, 12], thuj.,
til.[8], **tril.**, urt-u.[12], ust.[6, 8], valer.[3, 4],
verat.[3, 4, 8], vib.[3], vinc.[4, 6], vip.[4, 6, 12],
vip-a.[14], wies.[12], x-ray[9, 14], xan.[8],
zinc.[3, 4, 6]

agg., slight h.[3]
agg. par la moindre h.
agg., geringe B.
   bufo, **carb-an.**, chin., ham.,
   HYDR., sec.

after h.[3]/après/nach
   CHIN., ferr., nat-m., ph-ac., sep.[1'],
   sul-ac.[3]

ailments from[12]
troubles à la suite de
Beschwerden infolge von
   senec., squil., stict., stront-c.

am.
   ars.[3], bov., brom.[3], bufo[3], calad.[3],
   card-m.[3], coloc.[3], ferr.[3], ferr-p.[3],
   ham.[3], kali-n.[3], **lach.**[3], mag-c.[3],
   meli.[3], sars., sel., tarent.[3], thiop.[14]

blood, acrid[4]
sang âcre
Blut, scharfes
   am-c., ars., bar-c., bov., canth.,
   carb-v., graph., hep., **kali-c.**[3, 4, 6],
   kali-n.[3, 4, 6], rhus-t., sars., **sil.**[3, 4, 6],
   sul-ac.[3, 4, 6], sulph.[3, 4, 6], zinc.

black[4]/noir/schwarzes
   am-c.[1', 4], arn., ars.[1'], asar.,
   bapt.[1'], ben-n.[11], both.[7, 11], canth.,
   carb-v.[1', 4], **chin., croc.**,
   crot-h.[1', 3], elaps[1', 3], **ferr.**[4, 11]
   fl-ac.[3], ham.[1'], kali-n., kreos.,
   lach.[1'], led.[1'], **mag-c.**, mag-m.,
   mag-s., nat-c., **nat-m.**[4, 11], nat-s.,
   nit-ac., ol-an., op.[11], **puls.**,
   sec.[1', 4, 12], stram., sulph.

bright red[4]/rutilant/hellrotes
   abrot.[3, 6], **ACON.**[2, 3, 6, 8], am-c.,
   ant-t.[2, 4], **arn.**[3, 4], **ars.**[1', 2, 4], bar-c.,
   bell.[3, 4, 6, 8], bor., bov., bry., calc.[4, 7],
   canth., carb-an., carb-v.[3, 4],
   chin., cinnm.[6], **crot-h.**[6], dig.,
   dros.[2, 4], **dulc.**[2-4], erech.[7, 8],
   erig.[3, 6-8, 10], **ferr.**[3, 4, 8], **ferr-p.**[2, 8],
   graph.[2, 4], **ham.**[2], **hyos.**[2, 3, 4, 6],
   IP.[2, 3, 4, 6, 8], kali-n.[3, 4, 6], **kali-p.**[2],
   kreos., laur., led.[3, 4, 8], **m-aust.**,
   mag-m., meli.[3, 6], **MILL.**[1'-3, 6-8, 10],
   nat-c., **nat-m.**[2], nit-ac.[3, 4, 6, 8],
   nux-m., **phos.**[1'-4, 6, 8, 10], plb.[3],
   puls., rhus-t., sabad.,
   sabin.[1', 3, 4, 6, 8, 10], **sec., sep.**,
   sil., stram., stront-c., **sulph.**[3, 4],
   tril.[2, 3, 6, 8], ust.[8], zinc.

with dark clots[3]
avec caillots foncés
mit dunkelroten Blutgerinnseln
   ferr., sabin., sang.

brownish[3, 4, 6]/brunâtre/bräunliches
   ben-n.[11], bry., calc.[4], **carb-v.**,
   con., ferr.[1'], puls.[4], rhus-t.[4],
   sul-h.[11]

clots[4]/caillots/Blutgerinnsel
   am-m., arn.[3, 4], ars.[1'], **bell.**[3, 4, 6],
   bry., calc.[3], canth.[3, 4], carb-an.,
   caust., **CHAM.**[3, 4, 6], **chin.**[3, 4, 6],
   con., croc.[3, 4, 6], erig.[8],
   ferr.[1'-4, 8], ferr-p.[2], **hyos.**[3, 4],
   ign.[3, 4], **ip.**[3, 4], **kali-m.**[1'-3, 6],
   kali-n., **kali-p.**[2], lach.[1', 3],
   mag-m., **merc.**[2, 3, 4, 6], **nat-m.**[2, 11],
   nat-s., nit-ac.[3, 4, 6], nux-v.[3, 4],
   ph-ac., phos.[1'], **PLAT.**[2, 3, 4, 8],
   puls.[3, 4, 8], rat.[8], **RHUS-T.**[3, 4, 6],

rhus-v., **sabin.**[1', 3, 4, 8], sec.,
sep., **stram.**[3, 4], stront-c.,
sul-ac.[3, 6], sulph.[3, 11], **thlas.**[2],
ust.[3, 8], zinc.

dark[8]/foncés/dunkelrote
alum., anthraci., chin.,
CROC.[2, 8], crot-h., **elaps,** ham.,
kali-m.[1'], lach., mangi., merc.,
merc-cy., mur-ac., plat., **puls.**[2],
sec.[2], **sul-ac.,** ter., **thlas.,** tril.

dark[4]/foncé/dunkelrotes
acon.[3, 4], agar.[3, 6], **am-c.**[1'-3, 4, 6],
ant-c., anthraci.[7], arn., **asar.**[3, 4],
bell.[4, 12], **bism.,** bov.[3, 6], bry.,
canth.[3, 4], **carb-v.**[3, 4, 6], carbn-h.[11],
carbn-o.[11], card-m.[3, 6], caust.[3],
cham.[3, 4], **chin.**[3, 4], cocc., con.,
croc.[3, 4], **crot-h.**[3, 6], cupr., cycl.[3],
dig., dros., **ferr.**[1', 2, 4, 11], graph.,
ham.[1', 3, 6], kali-m.[1'], kali-n.,
kreos.[3, 4], **lach.**[3, 4, 6], led., lyc.,
mag-c., merc.[3, 6], nit-ac.[1', 3, 4, 6],
nux-m.[3, 4, 6], **NUX-V.**[2-4],
ph-ac.[3, 4], phos., plat., **puls.**[3, 4],
sec.[3, 4, 6, 12], sel., **sep.**[3, 4], **stram.**[3, 4],
sul-ac.[1', 3, 6], sulph.[4, 11], **thlas.**[2],
ust.[3, 6], verat.[3]

decomposed[3, 4]/décomposé/
zersetztes
cic., **crot-h., lach., vip.**[4]

hot[3, 6]/chaud/heißes
acon., anac.[11], **bell.,** dulc.[3], sabin.

non-coagulable, hemophilia
non-coagulable, hémophilie
nicht gerinnbar, Hämophilie
adren.[6, 8], ail.[8], am-c., anthraci.,
apis, aran.[2], **arn.**[3, 6], ars.,
BOTH.[1, 7], bov.[6, 8], calc.[3, 6],
calc-lac.[6], calc-p.[6], carb-an.[3, 6],
carb-v., chin., chlol., chloram.[14],
cortico.[9], croc.[6], **CROT-C., crot-h.,**
dig., dor., **elaps, erig.**[1],
FERR.[2, 6, 8], ferr-m.[6], **ham.**[2, 3, 6, 8],
HIR.[7], ip.[6], **kali-p.,** kreos.[3, 6-8],
LACH., LAT-M.[1, 7], led.[6],
merc.[6, 8], mill.[6, 8], nat-m., nat-n.[6],
nat-s.[3, 6, 10], **nat-sil.**[6, 8], **NIT-AC.,**

op.[11], ph-ac.[6, 10], **PHOS.,** puls.[6],
rad-br.[7], **sec.,** sil.[3, 6], **sul-ac.,**
sulph.[6, 11], ter.[2, 6, 8], vip.[3, 11], x-ray[7]

offensive[4]/fétide/übelriechendes
ars.[1', 4], bapt.[1'], **bell., bry.,**
carb-an., carb-v., caust., **cham.,**
chin., **croc.,** ign., kali-c., **kali-p.**[1'],
merc., mur-ac.[3], phos., plat.,
rheum, sabin., sec.[1', 3, 4], sil.,
sulph.

pale[3]/pâle/blasses
apis[11], carb-ac., carb-an., carb-v.,
ferr., graph.[1', 3], kreos., **phos.**[3, 11],
sabad., sulph., tarent.[11]

ropy, tenacious[3, 4, 6]
visqueux, collant
fadenziehendes, zähes
anthraci.[2], apis[2], **CROC.**[2-4, 6],
cupr., kali-chl.[4], **kali-m.**[2], kreos.[3],
lach.[3], mag-c., **merc.**[3, 6], naja[3],
sec., ust.[3], verat.[3]

thick[4]/épais/dickflüssiges
agar.[3], bov.[3], carb-v., cham.[3],
chin.[3], **croc.**[3], cupr.[3], **ferr-m.**[11],
kali-n., kreos., lach., laur.[3],
mag-c., mag-s., **nux-m.**[3, 4],
plat.[3, 4], **puls.,** rhus-t.[3], sep.[3],
sulph.

thin[3]/fluide/dünnflüssiges
ant-t.[11], ben-n.[11], both.[11], carb-v.,
crot-h., ferr.[1'], ham., lach., laur.[3],
nit-ac., phos.[3, 11], **sec.**[3, 12], sul-ac.,
tab.[11], ust.

watery[4]/aqueux/wässriges
alum., am-c., ant-t., **berb.,** bor.,
bov., carb-v.[3, 4], crot-h., dulc.,
ferr.[1', 4], **graph.,** hir.[12], kali-c.,
kreos., lat-m.[12], laur., mang.[1'],
nat-m.[1'], nat-s., nit-ac.[3, 4], phos.,
prun., **puls.,** rhus-t., sabin.[3, 4],
sec.[4, 12], stram., sulph.

mixed with clots[3]
mêlé de caillots
mit Blutgerinnseln
arn., bell., caust., puls., sabin.

climacteric period, in[7]
ménopause, pendant la
Klimakterium, im
phos.

exertion, after
exercices physiques, suite d'
Anstrengung, nach
bell-p.[10], mill., NIT-AC.[2]

exudates, hemorrhagic[2]
exsudats hémorrhagiques
Exsudate, hämorrhagische
anthraci.

internally[3]
interne
innerliche
acon.[15], alumn.[2], bell.[3, 15], bry.,
cham., chin.[3, 15], cic., con., dulc.,
euph., ferr., ferr-p.[15], hep., hyper.,
iod., lach., laur., mill.[15], nux-v.,
par., petr., phos., plb., puls., rhus-t.,
ruta, sabin.[15], sec., sul-i.[1'], sulph.,
thlas.

mucous membranes, from[1']
muqueuses, des membranes
Schleimhäute, der
calc-sil.

orifices of the body, from
orifices du corps, des
Körperöffnungen, aus allen
anthraci.[7], aran., BOTH., chin.,
CROT-H., elaps, ip.[1, 7], lach.,
PHOS., sul-ac.

passive, oozing[3]
passive, suintante
passive, sickernde
ars-h.[11], bov., bufo, carb-v., chin.,
crot-h., ferr-p., ham., ph-ac., sec.,
tarent.[11], ter., ust.

vicarious[1']
vicariante
vikariierende

abrot.[6], bry., ham., ip.[6], kali-c.[6],
phos., sec.

HAIR brushing back agg.[3]
CHEVEUX, agg. en se brossant en
arrière les
HAARE agg., Zurückbürsten der
carbn-s.[2, 3], puls., rhus-t.

combing agg.[3]
peignant, agg. en se
Kämmen der, agg.
asar.[2], bell.[1'], bry., chin., ign.,
kreos., nat-s., sel.

cutting agg.[3]
coupant les, agg. en se
Schneiden der, agg.
acon.[8], BELL.[2, 3, 6, 8], glon.[2, 3, 6, 8],
kali-i.[3, 6], lappa, led.[3], phos.[2, 3, 6],
puls., sep.

ailments from[12]
troubles à la suite de couper
Beschwerden infolge vom
bell., glon.[6], kali-i.[6], led., phos.

distribution masculine in women[9]
hirsutisme chez la femme, dans l'
männliche Behaarung bei Frauen,
Hirsutismus
cortico.

sensation of a
sensation d'un cheveu quelque part
Gefühl eines Haares
all-c.[3], arg-n., ars., bell.[3], caps.[3],
carbn-s., caust.[3], coc-c., croc.[3],
kali-bi., lac-c.[3], laur.[3], lyc., mosch.[3],
nat-m., nat-p., nux-v.[3], ptel.[3], puls.,
ran-b., rhus-t.[3], sabad.[3], SIL., sulph.,
ther.[3], thuj.

touching agg.[3]
toucher agg.
Berühren agg.
ambr., APIS[2, 3, 6], ARS.[2, 3], bell.[3, 6],
carb-v.[2, 3], chin.[3, 6], ferr.[3, 6], ferr-p.[2],
hep., ign.[3, 6], mez., nit-ac.[6],
nux-v.[3, 6], ph-ac., phos., puls.[3, 6],
rhus-t., SEL.[3, 6], sep.[3], stann.,
verat.[3], zinc.[2, 3, 6]

HAND on part **am.**, lying
MAIN sur la partie malade **am.**,
   application de la
AUFLEGEN DER HAND auf die kranke
   Stelle **am.**
      bell., calc., canth., carb-an.[3],
      croc., dros., **mang.**[1, 16], meny.,
      mur-ac., nat-c., olnd., par., **phos.**,
      rhus-t., sabad., sep., sil.[16], spig.,
      sulph., thuj.

    magnetism/magnétisme/
    Magnetismus

   hand near part am.[16]
   la main près de la partie malade
   am.
   Annähern der Hand am.
      sul-ac.

  agg.[16]
      kali-n.

HANG DOWN, letting limbs, agg.
PENDRE le membre agg., laisser
HERUNTERHÄNGENLASSEN der
   Glieder agg.
      alum., **am-c.**, ang.[3], bar-c.[3], **BELL.**[3],
      berb., **CALC.**, **carb-v.**, **caust.**, cina,
      con.[3], dig., hep., ign., lyc., m-aust.[3],
      nat-m., nux-v., ox-ac., par., ph-ac.,
      phos., phyt., plat., plb., **puls.**, ran-s.,
      ruta, **sabin.**, sil.[3], stann., stront-c.[3, 6],
      sul-ac., sulph., thuj., valer., **vip.**,
      vip-a.[14]

  am.
      acon., am-m., anac., ant-c., arg-m.,
      arg-n., **arn.**, asar., **bar-c.**, **bell.**,
      berb.[3], bor., **bry.**, calc.[3], camph.,
      caps., caust., chin., cic., cina, **cocc.**,
      coff., colch., coloc., **CON.**, cupr.,
      dros., euph., ferr., graph., hep., ign.,
      iris, **kali-c.**, kreos., **lach.**, **led.**, lyc.,
      mag-c., **mag-m.**, mang.[3], merc.,
      mez., nat-c., nat-m., nit-ac., nux-v.,
      olnd., **petr.**, phos., plb., puls.,
      ran-b., rat.[3], **rhus-t.**, ruta, **sil.**,
      stann., sul-ac., sulph., teucr.,
      thuj., verat., verb.

HARD bed, sensation of
DUR, le lit paraît
HARTEN Bettes, Gefühl eines
   acon., agar., alum.[3], **ARN.**, ars.,
   BAPT.[1, 7], bar-c., bry., caust., cham.[6],
   con., dros., eup-per.[6], euphr.[3, 11],
   fago.[11], **ferr.**, **ferr-p.**, graph., hep.[4], ip.,
   kali-c., lach.[3], lyc., mag-c., mag-m.,
   manc., merc., **nat-s.**[3, 6], nux-m., nux-v.,
   op.[1, 7], petr.[3, 7, 11], phos., plat., podo.[3],
   psor.[3, 6], puls., **PYROG.**[1, 7], **rhus-t.**,
   RUTA[1, 7], sabad., **SIL.**, spong., stann.,
   sulph., tarax., thuj., til.[3], verat.

HEAT, flushes of
CHALEUR, bouffées de
HITZEWALLUNGEN
   acet-ac., **acon.**[1, 7], aesc., agar.[6, 11],
   agn., ail., **all-c.**[11], aloe[6], alum.,
   alum-sil.[1'], **alumn.**, am-c., am-m.,
   ambr., **AML-NS.**[1, 7], ang., ant-t., apis,
   apoc.[11], aran-ix.[10, 14], **arg-n.**[6, 7],
   arist-cl.[10], **arn.**, ars., **ars-i.**, arum-t.,
   asar., aur., bapt., bar-a.[11], bar-c.,
   bell.[1, 7], berb., bism., bol-la.[11], bor.,
   bor-ac.[8, 12], bov., brom., bruc.[4], bry.,
   bufo, buth-a.[9], **cact.**, **CALC.**, **calc-s.**,
   calc-sil.[1'], camph.[1'], cann-s.[4, 11],
   carb-an., **carb-v.**, **carbn-s.**, carl.[11],
   CAUST., cedr.[11], cench.[1'], **cham.**[1, 7],
   chel., chim.[11], **chin.**, chin-s., cic.[6],
   cimic.[6, 8, 10], cimx., **cina**[2, 7], clem.[11],
   COCC., coff., **colch.**, coll.[3], coloc.,
   corn., croc., **crot-h.**[1, 7], **crot-t.**[1, 7],
   cupr., cupr-am-s.[11], cyt-l.[10], dig.,
   dros.[11, 16], dulc.[4], **elaps**, ery-a.[2, 7, 11],
   eucal.[7], eup-per., euphr.[11], fago.[11],
   ferr., ferr-ar., ferr-i., ferr-p.,
   fl-ac.[3, 6, 7], flav.[14], flor-p.[10, 14],
   frax.[7, 11], galin.[14], **gamb.**[1, 7],
   GELS.[3], **GLON.**, **graph.**, guaj.[6],
   hep., helon., hura, hydr-ac.[7],
   hyos., **IGN.**[1, 7], **iod.**, ip.[1], **jab.**[6-8, 12],
   jug-r.[11], kali-ar.[1], **kali-bi.**[1],
   kali-br.[3, 6, 8], **KALI-C.**[1], **kali-i.**[1],
   kali-n.[4, 11], **kali-p.**[1], **kali-s.**, kiss.[11],
   kreos., kres.[13], lac-ac., **LACH.**,
   lachn.[11], lat-m.[14], laur.[11], lil-s.[11],
   lipp.[11], lob., **LYC.**, lyss., m-aust.[4],
   mag-c.[4], mag-m., **MANG.**, med.[2, 7],

MELI.[3], meny., meph.[6], **merc.,**
merc-i-r.[11], methys.[14], mit.[11],
morph.[11], mosch.[11], nat-ar., nat-c.,
nat-m., nat-p., **NAT-S.,** nep.[13, 14],
nicc-s.[8], nid.[14], **NIT-AC.,** nit-s-d.[2, 7, 11],
nux-v., ol-an.[6, 11], ol-j.[11], olnd., op.,
ov.[6, 8], **ox-ac., petr.,** ph-ac., **PHOS.,**
pilo.[8], pip-m.[11], **PLAT.**[1, 7], plb.[11],
podo., **PSOR.,** ptel.[2, 7], **PULS.**[1, 7],
raph., rauw.[14], rumx., **rhus-t.,** ruta,
sabad., sabin., sal-ac.[6], samb.[4],
sang., saroth.[14], sec.[6], sed-ac.[8],
sel.[6, 14], seneg, **SEP., sil.,** sol-a.[1],
spig., **spong.,** squil.[6], stann.,
stront-c.[3, 6, 8], **SUL-AC., SUL-I.**[1'],
SULPH., SUMB., tab.[6, 11], tanac.[11],
ter.[7], teuer., thala.[14], **THUJ.,**
thyr.[3, 14], til.[11], trom.[2, 7], **TUB.,**
uran-n.[6], **ust.**[6-8], valer., verat-v.[8],
vesp.[8], vinc.[6, 8], vip.[11], visc.[14],
voes.[11], **xan.,** zinc., zinc-val.[6, 8]

weakness–heat/faiblesse–chaleur/
Schwäche–Hitzewallungen
Vol. I: *anxiety–flushes/anxiété–*
bouffées/Angst–Hitzewallungen

daytime[11]
journée, pendant la
tagsüber
bar-c.[2], bism., bor., bry., **lach.**[2],
nit-ac., **petr.**[2, 12], senec.[2]

morning/matin/morgens
bism., bor., ox-ac.[2]

eating, after
mangé, après avoir
Essen, nach dem
thuj.

forenoon agg.[11]/matinée agg./vor-
mittags agg.
sabad.

11 h with hunger[2]
11 h avec faim
11 h mit Hunger
SULPH.

afternoon/après-midi/nachmittags
ambr., bell., bor.[2], colch., con.,
fago.[11], laur., meny., **nat-p.**[1], plb.,
samb., **SEP.**

14 h[11]
ptel.

16–21 h[2, 7, 11]
arum-t.

evening/soir/abends
acon., all-c., arum-t., bor.,
carb-an., carb-v., **elaps**[1, 7], **lyc.,**
merc-c., nat-p., **nat-s.,** nit-ac.,
phos., **psor., SEP., stann.**[2, 7],
sulph.

19 h[11]
gins.

20 h with nausea
20 h avec nausée
20 h mit Übelkeit
ferr.

20.30 h
arum-t., cimic.[11], cina, sep.

eating, after
mangé, après avoir
Essen, nach dem
carb-v., upa.[11]

falling asleep, before
s'endormir, avant de
Einschlafen, vor dem
carb-v.

night/nuit/nachts
arum-t.[2], bar-c., flav.[14], **kali-i.**[2, 7],
rhod.[2], **sep.**[2], spig., **sulph.**[2]

orgasme of blood–night/orgasme
sanguin–nuit/Blutwallungen–
nachts
Vol. III: *sleeplessness–*
climacteric period/insomnie–
ménopause/Schlaflosigkeit–
Klimakterium

3 h[11]
fago.

feeling as if sweat would break
out
sensation que la sueur va sortir
Gefühl eines bevorstehenden
Schweißausbruches
bapt.

air, am. in open[11]
air, am. en plein
Freien, am. im
mosch.

alternating with anxiety[2, 7]
alternant avec anxiété
abwechselnd mit Angst
calc., dros., plat.

chills/frissons/Frösteln
acon., ang.[11], ars., asar., **calc.**[1, 7],
chin-s.[1, 7], corn., iod., jug-c.[11],
kali-bi., kalm.[11], med., morph.[11],
pin-s.[11], **sep.,** spig.

headache[2, 7]/maux de tête/Kopf-
schmerzen
lyss.

anger, after
colère, par
Zorn, durch
petr.[2], **phos.**

back or stomach, from[1']
dos ou de l'estomac, partant du
Rücken oder Magen ausgehend, vom
phos.

bed, in[11]
lit, au
Bett, im
eupi.

chill, before
frissons, avant les
Fieberfrost, vor
CAUST., sang.

after[2]/après les/nach
ail., cimx.,

chilliness, with
frissonnement, avec
Frösteln, mit
agar., am-br.[11], apis, **ars., carb-v.,**
colch., corn., eup-per., kali-bi.,
lach., lob., **merc., petr.**[2, 7], plat.,
puls., sang.[2], sep., sulph., ter.,
thuj.

after[11]/après/nach
corn., gast., gels., nat-p.[2, 11],
nit-ac., **puls.**[2], rhus-t., sang.

climacteric[2, 6]
climactériques
klimakterische
acon.[6, 8], **aml-ns.**[2, 6, 8, 12], **arg-n.**[2],
aur.[6], **bell.,** bor-ac.[12], calc.[6, 8], con.[2],
croc.[6], **crot-h.**[2], **dig.,** eucal.[2], ferr.[6],
glon.[2, 6, 8], hydr-ac.[2], jab.[2, 6, 12],
kali-bi.[2, 6, 12], **kali-br.,** kali-c.[6],
LACH.[2, 6, 8], lyc.[2], **MANG.**[2, 12],
nux-v.[6], ol-an.[6], ov.[6], ph-ac.[6], **plat.**[2],
sang.[2, 6, 8, 12], **sep.**[2, 6, 8], **stront-c.**[6],
SUL-AC., SULPH.[2, 6, 8], sumb.,
ter.[2], **ust.**[2, 6, 8], valer., vinc.[6], xan.[2],
zinc-val.[6]

coitus, after[2, 7]
coït, après le
Koitus, nach
dig.

dinner, during
déjeuner, pendant le
Mittagessen, beim
calc-s., nux-v.

after[11]/après le/nach dem
par., sumb.

downward
vers le bas
von oben nach unten
aesc.[2, 7], glon., sang., xan.[2]

down back[2, 7]
dans le dos
den Rücken herunter
nat-c., sumb.

head to stomach
de la tête à l'estomac
vom Kopf zum Magen
   sang.

eating, while
mangeant, en
Essen, beim
   bov.[2], **calc-s.,** nux-v., psor.

   after
   après avoir mangé
   nach dem
      alum., arg-n., carb-v., card-b[11],
      cinnb.[2], **lach.**[2], par., sumb., upa.[11]

   am.[16]: chin.

emotions, from
émotions, par
Gemütsbewegungen, durch
   lach., **phos.**

exertion, from least
exercice physique, par le moindre
Anstrengung, durch die geringste
   alum., **merc.**[2], olnd.[2], sep., **sumb.**

fainting, with[2]
évanouissement, avec
Ohnmacht, mit
   crot-t., **SULPH.**

headache, during[16]
maux de tête, pendant les
Kopfschmerzen, bei
   agar.

leucorrhoea, with[2]
leucorrhée, avec
Fluor, mit
   lach., lyc., **sulph.**

lying down am.
couché am., étant
Liegen am.
   nux-v.[2, 11], thuj.[11]

menses, before
menstruation, avant la
Menses, vor den
   alum., ferr.[8], glon.[8], iod., kali-c.[15],
   lach.[8], **sang.**[8], sulph.[8]

during/pendant la/während der
   nat-p.

mental exertion, from
travail intellectuel, par
geistige Anstrengung, durch
   lach.[2], olnd.

motion, from
mouvement, par
Bewegung, durch
   helon.[1, 7], nux-v.[11], **sep.**[2, 7]

nausea, with[2]
nausée, avec
Übelkeit, mit
   merc.[2, 7], **nux-v.,** sang.

palpitation, with
palpitations, avec
Herzklopfen, mit
   calc.[2, 7, 15], iod.[2], **KALI-C.,** lach.[15],
   sep.[15], sul-i.[1']

perspiration, with
transpiration, avec
Schweiß, mit
   acet-ac., am-m., ant-c.,
   aran-ix.[10, 14], aur., bell.,
   camph.[1', 7], **carb-v., chin.**[7], cob.[2, 7],
   CON.[2, 7], **hep.,** hipp.[7], **ign.**[2, 7],
   ipom.[2], jab.[6], kali-bi., **kali-i.**[7],
   kres.[14], **lach.,** lyss.[7], nux-v.[6], op.,
   ox-ac.[2, 7], petr.[15, 16], **PSOR.**[2, 7],
   sep., SUL-AC.[1, 7], sulph., **ter.**[2, 7],
   TUB., valer.[6], **xan.**

   face and hands[16]
   de la face et des mains
   im Gesicht und an den Händen
      calc.

and anxiety/et anxiété/und Angst
   ang., kali-bi.

without[7]/sans/ohne
   LACH.

pregnancy, during[2, 7]
grossesse, pendant la
Schwangerschaft, in der
   glon.[6], **sulph., verat.**

room, in[11]
chambre, dans une
Zimmer, im
  helon.

running[1']
courir
Laufen, beim
  sul-i.

sleep, before[2, 7]
sommeil, avant le
Schlaf, vor dem
  carb-v.

  during/pendant le/im
    cham., nat-m., **phos.**, ran-b.[11], sil.,
    zinc.

  preventing the[2, 7]
  empêchant de s'endormir
  verhindert den
    psor., puls.

sexual excess, after[2]
excès sexuel, après un
sexueller Ausschweifung, nach
  dig.

sitting, on[16]
assis, étant
Sitzen, beim
  sep.

stool am., after[11]
selle, am. après
Stuhlgang am., nach
  agar.

upwards
ascendantes
von unten nach oben
    alum., alumn., ars., ars-h.[2], asaf.,
    calc., carb-an., carb-v., chin.,
    cinnb., **ferr.,** ferr-ar., **GLON.,**
    graph., indg., iris, kali-bi., **kali-c.,**
    laur., **lyc.,** mag-m., mang., nat-s.,
    nit-ac., **phos.,** plb., **psor., SEP.,**
    spong., sulph., sumb., tarent.,
    valer.

  from back[2, 7]
  depuis le dos
  vom Rücken aus
    sumb.

  from the hips
  depuis les hanches
  von den Hüften aus
    alumn.

vomiting, after[11]
vomissement, après
Erbrechen, nach
  tab.

walking am.[11]
marchant, am. en
Gehen am., beim
  fago.

walking in open air
marchant en plein air, en
Gehen im Freien, beim
  caust., tarax.[11]

warm water were poured over one,
  as if
eau chaude par dessus,
  comme si on lui versait de l'
warmem Wasser übergossen, wie mit
  ARS., bry., ph-ac., phos., **PSOR.,**
  puls., rhus-t., SEP.

  dashed over one
  l'aspergeait d'
  bespritzt
    calc., cann-s., nat-m., phos.,
    puls., rhus-t., sep.

  water/eau/Wasser

  when an idea occurs vividly
  à l'occasion d'une pensée très
    vive
  wenn ein Gedanke lebhaft ein-
    fällt
  phos.

weakness, with[2]
faiblesse, avec
Schwäche, mit
  phos.

after fl. of h.
après b. de ch.
nach H.
  dig.[12], **SEP.**[2, 7], **SULPH.**[2], **xan.**[7]

HEAT, sensation of
CHALEUR, sensation de
HITZEGEFÜHL
  acet-ac.[1'], achy.[14], agar., agn.,
  allox.[9], **alum., alumn.**[2], am-c.,
  anh.[9, 10], ant-t., **APIS**, aran-ix.[10],
  arg-n., ars., ars-i., asaf., **asar.**[2, 3, 6],
  aur., aur-i., aur-m., bar-c., bov.,
  bry., **calc., calc-i., CALC-S.,**
  camph., CANN-S., canth., caps.,
  carb-an.[3], caust., chel., chin., cina,
  cob-n.[9], **COC-C.**, cocc., **COFF.**,
  colch., com., **croc.**, cycl., cyt-l.[14],
  dros., euph., **FL-AC.**, flor-p.[10],
  graph., hed.[10], hell., hist.[10, 14],
  hyos.[5], hypoth.[14], ign., **IOD., ip.,**
  kali-c., **kali-i.**, kali-n., **KALI-S.,**
  kreos., **lach.**, laur., **LIL-T., LYC.,**
  lyss.[10], mag-c., **mag-m.**, mand.[9],
  mang., meph.[3, 6], **merc.**, nat-c.,
  NAT-M., NAT-S., nit-ac.[3, 16],
  nux-m., nux-v., oci-s.[9], ph-ac.,
  phos., plat., psor., ptel., PULS.,
  ran-b., rauw.[9], rheum, rhod.,
  rhus-t., sabad., sabin., samb.,
  sars., **SEC., seneg.**, sep.[3], **spong.,**
  staph., **SUL-AC., SUL-I., SULPH.,**
  tab.[3, 6], teucr., thuj., **tub.**[1], valer.,
  verat., zinc.

evening, in bed
soir au lit, le
abends im Bett
  bry., fl-ac.[1']

night/nuit/nachts
  bar-c.[16], cham., con.[16], fl-ac.[1'],
  nat-m., **phos.**, puls.[6, 16], rhus-t.[16],
  sil., zinc.

alternating with sensation of cold[14]
alternant avec sensation de froid
abwechselnd mit Kältegefühl
  hist.

ascending[9]/ascendante/aufstei-
  gendes
  cob-n.

beer, after[7]
bière, après avoir bu de la
Bier, nach
  bell.

eating, after[1']
mangé, après avoir
Essen, nach dem
  cycl.

eating warm food
mangeant des aliments chauds, en
Essen warmer Speisen, beim
  carb-v., ferr., **kali-c.**, lach.,
  mag-c., PHOS., PULS., sep.,
  sul-ac.

coughing, on[16]
toussant, en
Husten, beim
  squil., sep.

exertion, on
exercice physique, par l'
Anstrengung, bei
  alum., squil.

hand has lain, where[16]
main repose, à l'endroit où la
Hand gelegen hat, wo die
  hyos.

nausea, with[7]
nausée, avec
Übelkeit, mit
  chel.

motion, at least[16]
mouvement, au moindre
Bewegung, bei der leichtesten
  squil.

rest agg.[14]
repos agg.
Ruhe agg.
  achy.

single parts, in[3]
certaines parties, de
einzelnen Teilen, in
  apis, bor., par., ph-ac.

talking, on[16]
parlant, en
Sprechen, beim
  squil.

waking, on
réveil, au
Erwachen, beim
  BAR-C., fl-ac., **graph.**, nat-m.,
  sil., zinc.

walking, on[16]
marchant, en
Gehen, beim
  samb.

bloodvessels, in
vaisseaux sanguins, dans les
Blutgefäßen, in den
  agar., am-m.[1'], **ARS.**, **aur.**,
  benz-ac.[7], **bry.**, calc., **hyos.**, med.,
  nat-m., nit-ac., op., **RHUS-T.**,
  sulph., syph.[1', 3, 7], **verat.**

vital, lack of
vitale, manque de ch.
Lebenswärme, Mangel an
  aesc., **agar.**, allox.[9, 14], **alum.**,
  alum-p.[1'], **ALUMN.**[1], am-br.[6],
  am-c., am-m.[1], anac.[7], ang.[4, 6],
  anh.[9, 10, 14], **ant-c.**, **ARAN.**,
  aran-ix.[9, 10, 14], **arg-m.**, **arg-n.**,
  arist-cl.[9, 10], **ARS.**, ars-h.[2], **ars-i.**,
  asar., **aur.**, aur-s.[1'], **BAR-C.**,
  bar-m., bar-s.[1'], **bor.**, **brom.**, bufo[1],
  buth-a.[9, 10], cact., cadm-s., **CALC.**,
  CALC-AR., calc-f., **CALC-P.**,
  calc-s., calc-sil.[1'], calen.[7],
  CAMPH., caps.[1], **CARB-AN.**,
  carb-v., carbn-s., **caul.**, **CAUST.**,
  chel., chin., chlor.[2], chloram.[14],
  chlorpr.[14], cic.[14], **cimic.**, **cinnb.**,
  CIST., cob-n.[10], **cocc.**, colch.[6],
  con., **CROT-C.**, cupr-a.[2], cycl.,
  cyt-l.[9, 10], dicha.[10, 14], **dig.**, **DULC.**,
  elaps, esp-g.[10, 13], eucal.[2],
  euph.[4, 6, 16], **FERR.**, **ferr-ar.**,
  ferr-p.[1'], **GRAPH.**, **guaj.**, hed.[14],
  HELO., **HEP.**, hir.[14], hydr-ac.[4, 6],
  ip., **KALI-AR.**, **KALI-BI.**, kali-br.[2],
  KALI-C., **KALI-P.**, **kalm.**, **kreos.**,
  lac-ac., **lac-d.**, **lach.**, lat-m.[9, 14],

  laur.[1], **LED.**, lyc., lycps.[2], **mag-c.**,
  mag-m., **MAG-P.**, mag-s.[10],
  mang., **med.**, **merc.**, **mez.**, **mosch.**,
  naja, **nat-ar.**, nat-c., **nat-m.**,
  nat-p., **nat-sil.**[1'], nep.[10], **NIT-AC.**,
  nux-m., **NUX-V.**, ol-j., penic.[13, 14],
  perh.[14], **petr.**, **PH-AC.**, **PHOS.**,
  plb., **PSOR.**, **PYROG.**, ran-b.,
  rhod., **RHUS-T.**, rumx., **sabad.**,
  sarcol-ac.[14], saroth.[10, 14], sars.,
  senec., **sep.**, **SIL.**, spig., **stann.**,
  staph., **stront-c.**, **sul-ac.**, **sulph.**,
  sumb., **tarent.**, thal.[14], **ther.**, **thuj.**,
  tub., v-a-b.[13, 14], verat.[1', 12],
  vip-a.[14], x-ray[9], zinc., zinc-p.[1']

afternoon after siesta[16]
après-midi après le sieste
nach dem Mittagsschlaf
  con.

and warmth agg.[7]
et agg. par la chaleur
und Wärme agg.
  agar., **ALUM.**, ant-c., **APIS,**
  arg-n., **ars-i.**, aur., **bar-c.**, bor.,
  BRY., **CAMPH.**, **CARB-AN.**,
  carb-v., **CARBN-S.**, caust., cocc.,
  dig., **dros.**, **dulc.**, **GRAPH.**, guaj.,
  ip., **kali-s.**, lach., laur., <u>**LED.**</u>,
  LYC., merc., **MEZ.**, nat-c., **nat-m.**,
  nat-s., **ph-ac.**, **phos.**, <u>**PULS.**</u>,
  sabad., spig. staph., <u>**sulph.**</u>, **thuj.**,
  zinc.

climacteric period, during[7]
ménopause, pendant la
Klimakterium, im
  chin.

exercise, during
exercices physiques, pendant les
Körperübungen, bei
  plb., **sil.**

nausea, with[9]
nausée, avec
Übelkeit, mit
  arist-cl.

walking, after
marche, après la
Gehen, nach
  gins.

warm covering does not am.
se couvrir chaudement n'améliore
  pas
warmes Zudecken bessert nicht
  asar.

HEATED, becoming
S'ÉCHAUFFE, agg. lorsqu'on
ERHITZUNG agg.
  acon., am-c., **ANT-C., arg-n., arn.,**
  bell., bor.[3], **brom., BRY.,** calc.[3],
  calc-s., calc-sil.[1]′, **camph.,** caps.,
  carb-v., coff., **cycl., dig.,** dros.,
  dulc.[1]′, **ferr.,** fl-ac.[3], gels.[1]′, **glon.,**
  graph.[7, 10], hep., ign., **IOD.,** ip.,
  kali-ar.[1]′, **KALI-C., KALI-S.,** lach.[3],
  lyc.[1]′, [3], merc., mez., **nat-m.,** nux-m.,
  nux-v., olnd., **op., phos., PULS.,**
  ran-b., sep., SIL., staph., **thuj.,**
  zinc.

old drunkards
ivrognes vieux, chez les
alten Trinkern, bei
  bar-c.

HEAVINESS externally
LOURDEUR externe
SCHWEREGEFÜHL, äußerliches
  acon., **AESC.,** agar., agn., aloe,
  alum., alum-p.[1]′, alum-sil.[1]′, am-c.,
  ambr., ammc.[4], anac., ang.[3], ant-c.,
  an-t., arg-n.[3], arn., **ars., ars-i.,** asaf.,
  asar., aur., aur-ar.[1]′, **bar-c.,** bar-m.,
  bar-s.[1]′, **BELL.,** berb.[4], bor., bov.,
  BRY., cact., calc., camph., cann-i.,
  cann-s., canth., caps., carb-ac.,
  carb-an.[4], **carb-v., carbn-s.,** caust.,
  cham., chel., **chin.,** cic., cimic.[3],
  cina[4], clem., cocc., coff., colch.,
  coloc., **CON.,** croc., crot-h., crot-t.,
  cupr., cur., dig., dulc., euph., euphr.,
  ferr., ferr-ar.[1]′, **GELS.,** graph., grat.[4],
  hell., hep., ign., iod., **ip.,** kali-c.,

kali-m.[1]′, kali-n., kali-s., **kreos.,**
lach.[4], laur., **led.,** lyc., m-arct.[4],
m-aust.[4], mag-c., mag-m., **meli.,**
meny., **merc., mez.,** mosch., mur-ac.,
nat-c., nat-m., nat-sil.[1]′, nit-ac.,
nux-m., **NUX-V.,** ol-an.[4], **onos.,** op.,
par., **petr., ph-ac., PHOS.,** pic-ac.,
plat., plb., **psor., PULS.,** ran-b.,
rheum, **rhod., RHUS-T., ruta,**
sabad., sabin., samb., sars., sec.,
SEP., sil., SPIG., spong., squil.,
STANN., staph., stram., stront-c.,
sul-ac., sul-i.[1]′, **SULPH.,** teucr.[3],
ther.[4], **thuj.,** valer., **verat.,** verb.,
viol-o., **zinc., zinc-p.**[1]′

internally
interne
innerliches
  ACON., agar., agn., **ALOE,** alum.,
  am-c., am-m., ambr., anac., ang.[3],
  ant-t., arg-n., arn., ars., ars-s-f.[1]′,
  asaf., asar., aur., **bar-c.,** bar-m.,
  bell., BISM., bor., bov., bry., calad.,
  CALC., calc-sil.[1]′, camph., **cann-i.,**
  cann-s., canth., carb-ac., **carb-an.,**
  carb-v., carbn-s., caust., cham.,
  CHEL., chin., cic., clem., **cocc.,**
  coff., colch., **coloc., con., croc.,**
  cupr., dig., dros., dulc.[1], euphr.,
  ferr., ferr-ar.[1]′, **GELS.,** graph., **hell.,**
  hep., hyos., ign., iod., ip.[1], **iris,**
  kali-bi.[3], **kali-c.,** kali-m.[1]′, kali-n.,
  kreos., **lach.,** laur., lob., lyc., **mag-c.,**
  mag-m., mang., **meny., merc.,** mez.,
  mosch., **mur-ac.,** nat-c., **NAT-M.,**
  nat-sil.[1]′, nit-ac., **nux-m., NUX-V.,**
  olnd., onos., op., par., **PETR.,** ph-ac.,
  PHOS., plat., **plb., prun.,** psor.[3],
  PULS., ran-b., ran-s., rheum, rhod.,
  RHUS-T., ruta, **sabad.,** sabin.,
  samb., **sang.,** sars., sec., sel.,
  senec., seneg., SEP., SIL., spig.,
  spong., squil., **STANN., staph.,**
  stram., stront-c., sul-ac., sul-i.[1]′,
  SULPH., tarax., thuj., valer., verat.,
  verb., viol-o., viol-t., zinc.,
  zinc-p.[1]′

morning[16]/matin/morgens
  kali-c., lyc., nat-c., zinc.

night[16]/nuit/nachts
  mag-c.

menses, during[16]
menstruation, pendant la
Menses, während der
  kali-c.

sleep, after[16]
sommeil, après le
Schlaf, nach dem
  rheum

storm, before and during[16]
tempête, avant et pendant la
Sturm, vor und bei einem
  sil.

walking in open air, on[16]
marchant en plein air, en
Gehen im Freien, beim
  nit-ac.

bones, of[3]
os, des
Knochen, der
  sulph.

muscles, of[9, 10]
muscles, des
Muskeln, der
  mand.

high see ascending–high

HODGKIN'S disease, lymphogranulo-
  matosis[8]
LYMPHOGRANULOMATOSE maligne
HODGKIN, Morbus
  acon.[8, 12], acon-l.[8, 12], **ars.**[8, 12], **ars-i.,**
  bar-i., buni-o.[14], **calc-f.**[8, 9, 12], ferr-pic.,
  iod., kali-m.[8, 12], **nat-m.**[8, 12], phos.,
  saroth.[14], scroph-n., syph.[1', 7]

HUNGER agg.[6*]
FAIM agg.
HUNGER agg.
  anac., ars-i.[1'], chel., cina, graph.,
  iod., kali-c., lyc., olnd., phos., sil.,
  staph.

ailments from
troubles à la suite de
Beschwerden infolge von
  alum., aur., **cact.,** calc-f.[10, 14], canth.,
  caust., CROT-H.[1], ferr., **GRAPH.,**
  hell., **IOD., KALI-C.,** olnd., **phos.,**
  plat., **psor.,** rhus-t., **SIL., spig.,**
  stann., **SULPH.,** valer., verat.,
  zinc.

HYPERTENSION[7]
HYPERTONIE
  acon.[6], adon.[6], **adren.**[6, 7], agar.[6],
  aml-ns.[6], anh.[14], ant-ar., aran.[10, 14],
  aran-ix.[10], arg-n., arn.[7, 10], ars., asar.[6],
  aster.[14], **aur.**[6-8, 10], aur-br., aur-i.[6, 7],
  aur-m., aur-m-n., **bar-c.**[6, 7, 10],
  bar-m.[6, 8], cal-ren., calc., calc-f.[6],
  calc-p., caust., chin-s., chlor.[11],
  chloram.[14], chlorpr.[14], coff.[6, 7, 11],
  convo-s.[9], cortico.[9, 10], cortiso.[14],
  cupr., cupr-a., cupr-ar., cyna.[14],
  cyt-l.[9, 10, 14], dig., ergot.[14], esp-g.[14],
  fl-ac.[6], gels.[11], glon.[6-8, 10], **grat.,** ign.,
  iod.[6, 7, 10], iris[6], kali-c., kali-m., kali-p.,
  kali-sal., kres.[10, 13, 14], lach.[7, 10],
  lat-m.[9, 14], lyc., mag-c., mand.[14],
  methys.[14], naja[10], nit-ac., nux-v.[6, 7],
  onop.[14], ph-ac., phos., pic-ac.,
  pitu.[9, 14], **plb.**[6, 10], plb-i.[6, 7], psor.,
  pulm-a.[13], puls., rad-br., reser.[14],
  rauw.[9, 10, 14], rhust.[15], sang., **sec.**[6, 7, 10],
  sep., sil., squil.[6], **stront-c.**[6, 7], **stront-i.**[6],
  sulph., **sumb.,** tab., thal.[14], thlas.,
  thuj., valer.[6], vanad., **VERAT.,**
  verat-v.[7, 8], **visc.**[6-8, 10, 14]

HYPOTENSION[10]
HYPOTONIE
  acon., adlu.[14], agar., aran., chlorpr.[14],
  cortico.[14], cur.[7], gels.[8], halo.[14], hist.[9],
  lach., lat-m.[9, 14], levo.[14], lyc.[1'],
  meph.[14], naja, nat-f.[9], rad-br.,
  rauw.[9, 14], reser.[14], rib-ac.[14], staph.,
  sulfa.[14], thiop.[14], thymol.[9], v-a-b.[13, 14],
  verat.

INDOLENCE and luxury, ailments
from[7]
PARESSE et vie dans le luxe, troubles
à la suite de
FAULHEIT und Wohlleben, Beschwerden infolge von
carb-v., helon., nux-v.

INDURATIONS
VERHÄRTUNGEN
ambr., **ant-c.**[3], **anthraci., apis**[2, 3],
arg-m., arg-n., arn., **ars.**, ars-i.,
ars-s-f.[1], asaf., **aur.**, aur-ar.[1],
aur-i.[1], **aur-m.**, AUR-M-N.[2],
aur-s.[1], **BAD., bar-c.**, bar-i.[1],
bar-m.[4], **BELL.**, bov.[4], **bry., calc.,**
CALC-F., calc-i.[1], camph.,
cann-i.[2], cann-s., caps.,
CARB-AN., CARB-V., carbn-s.,
caust., cham., chel., **CHIN.**, cina,
cist.[3, 6], **CLEM.**, cocc.[4], coloc.,
CON., cupr., cycl., dulc., ferr.,
ferr-ar., fl-ac.[3, 6], **graph., hep.,**
hydrc.[2], hyos., ign., **iod.**, kali-c.,
kali-chl., kali-i., kali-m.[1, 3],
LACH., lap-a.[6], led., **lyc.**, mag-c.,
MAG-M., mang.[1, 3], **merc.,**
merc-i-r.[3], mez., nat-c., nux-v.,
op., **petr.**[4], **PHOS., phyt.**[3], **plb.,**
plb-i.[8], **psor., puls.**, ran-b.[3, 6],
ran-s., rhod., **RHUS-T.**, sec., **SEL.,**
SEP., SIL., spig., spong., squil.[4],
STAPH., stram., sul-i.[3], **sulph.,**
syph.[7], tarent.[3], thuj., valer.,
verat.

painful[16]
douloureuses
schmerzhafte
bell.

pressure, from[1]
pression, par
Druck, durch
sulph.

glands, of
glandes, des
Drüsen, der
aethi-a.[6], agar., agn., **alum.,**
alumn.[1, 8], am-c., **am-m.**[3, 6],

ambr., ant-c., **anthraci.**[2], **apis**[2],
arg-n.[2], arn., ars., ars-br.[8], ars-i.,
asaf.[2, 3, 6], astac.[2], **aster**[8], **aur.,**
aur-ar.[1], aur-i.[1], **aur-m.,**
aur-m-n.[2], aur-s.[1], **BAD., bar-c.,**
bar-i.[1, 8], **BAR-M.**, bar-s.[1], **BELL.,**
berb-a.[8], bov., **BROM., bry.,**
bufo[3], **CALC.**, calc-chl.[8],
CALC-F., calc-i.[6], **calc-s.**[1, 2],
calc-sil.[1], camph., cann-s., canth.,
caps., **CARB-AN., carb-v.,**
carbn-s., caust., cham., **chin.,**
cinnb.[2], cist., **CLEM., cocc.,**
coloc., **CON.**, cupr., cycl., **dig.,**
dulc., ferr., **ferr-i., graph.,**
hecla[2, 8], hep., hydr.[1], hyos., ign.,
IOD., kali-c., **kali-chl., kali-i.,**
kali-m.[1], kali-n.[2], kali-sil.[1],
lap-a.[6, 8], **lyc., mag-m.**, mang.,
merc., merc-aur.[6], **merc-c.**[2],
merc-d.[3, 6], **merc-i-f.**[2, 6, 8],
merc-i-r.[3, 6, 8], merc-sul.[2], nat-ar.,
nat-c., nat-m.[3, 6], nat-sil.[1], nit-ac.,
nux-v., oper.[8], petr., phos.,
PHYT., plb., **psor., puls.**, raph.[4],
rhod., **rhus-t., sars.**, sep., **sil.,**
spig., **SPONG.**, squil., staph.,
SUL-I.[1, 3, 6], **SULPH.**, syph.[7],
thuj., thyr.[8], trif-r.[8], tub.[6], verat.,
viol-t.[2]

injuries, after
traumatismes, par
Verletzungen, durch
CON.

knotty like ropes
noueux, comme des cordons
perlschnurartige
aeth.[3], **BAR-M.**, berb.[3], **calc.,**
cist., con., **dulc.**, hep., **iod.**, lyc.,
nit-ac.[3], rhus-t., **sil.**, sul-i.[1, 3],
tub.

nodes under the skin, like
nodules sous la peau, comme des
Knoten unter der Haut, wie
bry., **calc.**, caust., mag-c., nit-ac.

sensation of small foreign bodies
sensation des petits corps
   étrangers
Gefühl kleiner Fremdkörper
   cocain.

muscles, of
muscles, des
Muskeln, der
   alum., **anthraci., bad.,** bar-c., **bry.,**
   CALC-F.[1], carb-an., carb-v., **caust.,**
   con., dulc., hep., hyos., iod., kali-c.,
   kali-chl., kali-m.[1]', kali-sil.[1]', lach.,
   lyc., nat.-c., nux-v., ph-ac., puls.,
   ran-b., rhod., rhus-t., sars., sep.,
   sil., spong., sul-i.[1]', sulph., thuj.

INFLAMMATION externally
INFLAMMATIONS externes
ENTZÜNDUNGEN, äußerliche
   acon., agar., agn.[4], alum.[7], alumn.[1]',
   am-c., ambr., ant-c., **apis**[2, 3], arn.,
   ARS., ars-i., asaf., asar., aur.
   aur-ar.[1]', bar-c., **BELL.,** bor.[1] (non:
   brom.), bov., **bry., cact., calc.,**
   calc-i.[1]', calc-sil.[1]', camph., cann-s.,
   canth., caps., carb-an., carb-v.,
   caust., **cham.,** chel., chin., chin-s.[4],
   cina[4], clem., cocc., coff., colch.[4],
   coloc., **con.,** cortiso.[9], croc.[4],
   crot-h., crot-t.[4], cupr., cupr-a.[4], dig.,
   dulc., **ECHI.,** euph., **euphr., ferr.,**
   ferr-ar.[1]', **FERR-P.**[2], **fl-ac., gels.**[2],
   gran.[4], graph., **gunp.**[7], hell., **hep.,**
   hyos., ign., iod., ip., **kali-ar.,**
   kali-c., kali-m.[1]', kali-n., kreos.,
   LACH., lact.[4], led., **lyc., m-arct.**[4],
   mag-c., mag-m., mang., **merc.,**
   merc-d.[4], mez., mur-ac., myris.[3],
   nat-ar., nat-c., nat-m., nat-sil[1]',
   nit-ac., nux-v., op., **petr.,** ph-ac.,
   phos., plb., **PULS.,** ran-b., **rhus-t.,**
   sabad., sabin., samb., sars., sep.,
   SIL., spig., spong., squil.[2], stann.,
   STAPH., stram., sul-ac., sul-i.[3],
   sulph.[2, 3, 4], tarax., teucr., thuj.,
   valer., verat., **VERAT-V.**[2], zinc.

internally
internes
innerliche
   ACON., agar., aloe[3], alum., ang.[3],
   ant-c., ant-t., **apis,** arg-m.,
   arg-n.[3], arn., **ARS.,** ars-i.,
   ars-s-f.[1]', **arum-t.,** asaf., **aur.,**
   aur-ar.[1]', aur-i.[1]', aur-s.[1]', bar-c.,
   bar-i.[1]', **BELL.,** bell-p.[9], **berb.,**
   bism., **BRY., cact.,** calad., calc.,
   calc-sil.[1]', camph., **cann-s.,**
   CANTH., caps., carb-ac., carb-v.,
   cham., chin., cic., cina, clem.,
   coc-c., cocc., coff., colch., coloc.,
   con., cortiso.[9], crot-h., **cub.,**
   cupr., dig., dros., dulc., **ECHI.,**
   equis., euph., **ferr.,** ferr-ar.[1]',
   FERR-P.[2], **GELS.,** graph., guaj.,
   ham., hell., hep., hydr-ac.[6], **hyos.,**
   ign., **IOD.,** ip., **kali-ar., kali-c.,**
   kali-chl., kali-i., kali-n., LACH.,
   laur., lil-t., **lyc.,** mag-m., mang.,
   MERC., MERC-C.[3], mez., nat-ar.,
   nat-c., nat-m., nat-s.[6], nit-ac.,
   nux-m.[2], **NUX-V.,** op., par.,
   pareir., petr., ph-ac., **PHOS.,**
   phyt., **PLB.,** podo.[6], **PULS.,** ran-b.,
   ran-s., rheum, rhus-t., ruta,
   sabad., sabin., samb., sang.,
   sang-n., **SEC.,** senec., seneg., sep.
   sil., spig., spong., **squil.,** stann.,
   stram., stront-c., sul-ac., sul-i.[1]',
   sulph., tab.[6], tarent.[6], **TER.,** thuj.,
   uva, **verat., verat-v.**[6], vip.[6]

blood vessels, of
vaisseaux sanguins, des
Blutgefäße, der
   acon., **ant-t., ARN'., ARN., ARS.,**
   ars-i., **BAR-C.,** calc., cham., **cupr.,**
   ham., kali-c., kreos., lach., lyc.,
   puls., sil., spig., **SULPH.,** thuj.,
   zinc.

   arteriitis[8]/artérite/Arteriitis
   ars., **calc.**[2], echi., hist.[14], **kali-i.,**
   lach., **nat-i.,** sec., sulfa.[14]

phlebitis, milk leg
phlébite, phlegmasia alba dolens
Phlebitis, Phlegmasia alba dolens
  ACON.[3, 8], agar.[8], all-c., ant-c.,
  ant-t.[2, 3, 12], apis, arist-cl.[10, 14],
  arn., ars., bell., both.[7], BRY.,
  bufo, CALC., calc-ar.[6], calc-f.[6],
  carb-v.[3, 6, 10], carbn-s., cham.,
  chin., chlorpr.[14], crot-h., ferr-p.[2],
  graph., ham., hecla[14], hir.[14], hep.,
  iod., kali-c., kali-m.[6], kreos.,
  LACH., led., lyc., lycps., mag-c.[10],
  mag-f.[14], merc., merc-cy.[12],
  merc-i-r.[10]. nat-s., nux-v., phos.[8],
  puls., rhod., RHUS-T., ruta[8],
  sep., sil., spig., stront-br.[12],
  stront-c.[8, 12], sulfa.[14], sulph.,
  thiop.[14], thuj.[3, 4], verat.,
  VIP.[3, 6-8, 10, 12], vip-a.[14], zinc.

injuries, after[6]
traumatismes, après
Verletzungen, nach
  rhus-t.

bones, of; osteitis
os, des; ostéite
Knochen, der; Ostitis
  acon., ang.[3, 6], ars., ars-i., asaf.,
  aur., aur-ar.[1'], aur-i.[1', 7, 8], aur-m.,
  aur-s.[1'], bell., bry., calc., calc-f.[3, 6],
  calc-sil.[1'], chin., clem., coloc.,
  con., conch.[7, 8, 11, 12], cupr., dig.,
  euph., FL-AC., guaj., hecla[2, 7, 8],
  hep., iod., kali-i.[7, 8, 11], kreos.,
  lac-ac., lach., lyc., mag-m., mang.,
  MERC., merc-c.[3], merc-sul.[7],
  MEZ., nat-c., nat-sil.[1'], nit-ac.,
  PH-AC., phos., phyt.[2], plb., psor.,
  PULS., rhus-t., sep., SIL., spig.,
  STAPH., still.[7, 8], stront-c.[7, 8],
  sulph., symph.[2], thuj., verat.,

osteomyelitis[7, 8]/ostéomyélite/
Osteomyelitis
  achy.[14], acon., arg-m.[14], bell.[6],
  chin-s., conch.[11], des-ac.[14], gunp.,
  ph-ac.[12], phos., sil.[6]

periosteum, of; periostitis
périoste, du; périostite
Periost, des; Periostitis
  acon.[2, 3, 7], ant-c., apis, aran.[8],
  ars., asaf., aur., aur-ac.[1'], aur-m.,
  bell.[1, 7], calc.[1', 3, 8], calc-p.[3, 6],
  calc-sil.[10], chin., clem.[8], colch.[8],
  con.[3, 7, 8], conch.[11], ferr-i.[2, 7, 8, 12],
  ferr-p.[2, 7], FL-AC., graph.[8], guaj.[8],
  hecla[2, 7, 8, 12], hep.[3], iod.[8, 10],
  kali-bi.[3, 7, 8], kali-l., lach.[3], led.,
  mang., merc., merc-c., MEZ.,
  nat-sal.[12], nit-ac., PH-AC.,
  phyt.[2, 7, 8, 10], plat-m.[8], psor.,
  puls., rhod.[8], rhus-t., RUTA[1, 7],
  SABIN.[3], sars.[8], sep.[3], sil., staph.,
  still.[7, 8, 10, 12], sulph.[3], symph.[2, 7, 8],
  tell.[3]

bursae, of; bursitis[2]
bourses, des; bursite
Schleimbeutel, der; Bursitis
  ant-c., apis, ars., bell., bell-p.[7],
  graph., hep., iod., lycpr.[7], puls.,
  ruta[7, 12], SIL., stict., sulph.

cartilages, of; chondritis, perichon-
  dritis
cartilages, des; chondrite, périchon-
  drite

Knorpel, der; Chondritis, Perichon-
  dritis
  asaf[1], ARG-M., bell.[8, 12], cham[8, 12],
  cimic.[8, 12], lob-s.[12], nat-m., olnd.[8, 12],
  plb.[8, 12], Ruta[8, 12]

cellulitis[8]
cellulite
Zellgewebsentzündung
  apis[3, 8], arn., ars.[3, 8], bapt., bell.[3],
  crot-h., graph[3], hep.[3], lach., mang.,
  merc-i-r., myris.[3], rhus-t[1', 3, 8],
  sil.[3, 8, 12], sul-i.[3], sulph.[3], vesp.

chronic appendicitis[6]
chronique, appendicite
chronische Appendizitis
  bell-p.[14], but-ac.[14], coloc.,
  iris-t.[6, 8], kali-c.[14], merc-d., plb.,
  pyrog.[7], sil., sul-i.[6, 10], sulph.,
  tub-k.[10]

hepatitis
hépatite
Hepatitis
  adlu.[14], **arn., aur.**[2], **bell.**[2], cael.[14],
  calc-f.[10, 14], **card-m., corn.,**
  crot-h., flor-p.[10], **iod.**[6], kali-c.[6, 14],
  lach., LYC., mag-m., mand.[10],
  nat-c., **nat-m., NAT-S., nit-ac.,**
  nux-v., phos., phyt.[2], **podo.**[2],
  psor., ptel.[2], ran-s., sel., **sil.**[2],
  stann.[10, 14], **sulph.,** vip-a.[14]

ovaries, of[2]
ovarite
Ovarien, der
  ars., bry., chin., cod., coloc.,
  con.[8], graph.[8], **guaj.,** ign., **iod.**[2, 8],
  lach.[2, 8], **lil-t., lyc.,** nux-v., **pall.**[2, 8],
  ph-ac., **plat.**[2, 8], pyrog.[7], rhus-t.,
  sabal[8], sabin., sep.[8], staph.,
  thuj.[8]

prostatitis[8]
prostatite
Prostatitis
  alum., anac.[14], arg-m.[14], **aur.**[6, 8],
  bar-c., brach., calad., carbn-s.,
  caust.[2, 8], cic.[14], clem., **con.,**
  ferr-pic., graph., hep., hydrc.,
  iod.[6, 8], **kali-bi.**[2], kali-c.[14], **lyc.**[6, 8],
  merc., merc-c., nit-ac., nux-v.[2, 8],
  phyt., **puls.,** pyrog.[7], sabad.,
  sabal, sel., senec.[2], **sep.**[8, 10], sil.,
  solid., **staph.**[2, 8], sulph., **thuj.,**
  trib.

sinusitis[6, 8]
sinusite
Sinusitis
  ant-c.[8, 10], ars-i., aur.[8], **calc.**[2, 3, 6, 8],
  calc-f.[8, 10], calc-s.[7], cinnb.[6, 10],
  eucal.[8], fl-ac.[10], hecla[14], **hep.**[6, 8, 10],
  hydr., kali-bi., kali-c.[8, 10],
  kali-i.[2, 6, 8], kali-s.[7], lyc.[3, 6],
  mag-c.[10], mag-f.[10], mag-m.[10],
  med.[10], **merc.,** nat-m.[3, 6],
  nit-ac.[3, 6, 10], penic.[14], **phos.,**
  puls.[3, 6], pyrog.[7], spig.[8],
  SIL.[2, 3, 6, 8, 10], stann.[10, 14],
  stict.[8, 10], **sulph.**[6, 8, 10], teucr.,
  thuj.[8]

tonsillitis
amygdalite
Tonsillitis
  alum.[6], **alumn., BAR-C.,**
  bar-i.[6, 10], **bar-m.,** bar-s.[1'],
  brom.[3, 10], calc.[6, 10], calc-i.[6, 10],
  calc-p.[7, 8], con.[6], fuc.[6, 8], guaj.[7],
  hep., ign.[2, 6], iod.[6, 10], kali-bi.[6],
  kali-i.[3, 6], lach., lyc., mag-f.[10, 14],
  nat-m.[3, 6], **NIT-AC.**[2, 6], **PSOR.**[1, 7],
  sang., sep., sil., staph.[2, 6],
  sul-i.[3, 6, 10], sulph., teucr.[6],
  thuj.[3, 6, 10], **TUB.**[6, 7], v-a-b.[14]

gangrenous
gangreneuse
gangränöse
  ARS., bell., CANTH., carb-an.,
  carb-v., chin., colch., crot-h.,
  euph.[16], hep., **iod.,** kali-n.[16],
  kali-p., LACH., merc., **phos.,**
  plb., rhus-t., SEC., SIL.

glands, of; adenitis
glandes, des; adénite
Drüsen, der; Adenositis
  acon., ail.[8], **alumn., anan.,**
  apis[2, 3, 8, 10], arn., ars., ars-i.,
  ars-s-f.[1'], **aur.,** aur-ar.[1'], aur-i[1'],
  aur-m., aur-s[1'], **bad., bar-c.,**
  bar-i.[1', 8, 10], **BAR-M.,** bar-s.[1'], **BELL.,**
  berb.[4], **brom., bry.,** bufo, **CALC.,**
  calc-f.[10], calc-hp.[10], calc-i.[10],
  calc-sil[1', 10], **camph.,** canth.,
  caps.[3], **carb-an.,** carb-v., **cham.,**
  cist., clem., **con.,** cor-r.[12],
  crot-h.[2, 3], dros.[7], dulc., echi.[3],
  ferr-ar., fl-ac.[10], **graph.**[3, 4, 8], **hep.,**
  hippoz.[2, 12], iod.[8, 10], **iodof.**[8], kali-ar.,
  kali-c., kali-i., kali-m.[2], kali-p.,
  lach., laur., **lyc.,** m-aust.[4], mag-m.[4],
  MERC., merc-c.[11], **merc-i-r.**[8, 10],
  nat-s.[3], **nit-ac., nux-v.,** oper.[8], petr.,
  ph-ac., **PHOS., phyt.,** plb., **psor.,**
  puls., pyrog.[3], raph.[4], rhus-t., samb.,
  sanic.[10], sars., scroph-n.[10], sieg.[10],
  sil., sil-mar.[8], spig., spong.[1', 10],
  squil., staph., still.[10], sul-ac.,
  sul-i.[1', 10], **SULPH.,** tarent-c.[3], thuj.,
  tub.[10], verat., zinc.

joints, of; arthritis
articulations, des; arthrite
Gelenke, der; Arthritis
abrot.[3, 6, 8], **ACON.,** am-be.[6], am-c.[6],
am-caust.[6], am-m.[6], am-p.[6], **ang.,**
ant-c.[6], **ant-t.**[2, 6], **APIS,** aran.[10, 14],
aran-ix.[10], arb.[8, 11, 12], arist-cl.[9], **arn.,**
ars.[6], asar.[6], **aur.,** bar-c.[6], **BELL.,**
benz-ac.[3, 6, 8], berb.[6, 8], **BRY., calc.,**
calc-p.[6], caul.[6], **caust.,** cham.[6, 12],
chin.[6, 8], chin-s.[6], cimic.[8], clem.[6],
colch.[6, 8], coloc.[8], conch.[11],
cortiso.[9], crot-h.[6], cycl.[6], **dulc.**[1′, 3, 6],
elat.[8], eup-per.[6], euphr.[10], ferr.[6],
ferr-p., fl-ac.[3], form.[3, 6], **form-ac.**[6, 10],
gaul.[6], gins.[6], gnaph.[8], **guaj.,** hed.[10],
hep.[6], hyper., ichth.[12], **iod.,** kali-ar.[1′],
kali-bi.[8], **kali-c., kali-i.,** kali-m.[6],
kalm., kreos., lac-ac., lach., **LED.,**
lil-t.[8], **lith-be.**[6], lith-c., **lyc.,**
mand.[10, 14], **mang.,** meny., **merc.,**
mez.[6], **nat-m., nat-s.,** nat-sil.[8],
nit-ac.[8], ph-ac.[6], phos.[6], **phyt., psor.,**
puls., pyrog.[6], rad-br.[6, 8], ran-b.[6],
rhod., rhus-t., ruta, sabad.[6], sabin.,
sal-ac.[6, 8], sang.[6], **sars., sep., SIL.,**
solid.[8], spong.[6], **stel.**[6, 8], stict.[6],
stront-c.[6], sul-i.[10], sul-ter.[8], **sulph.,**
syph.[1′], tarax.[6], thuj.[6], tub.[6],
ven-m.[14], verat.[6], verat-v., viol-t.[8],
visc.[10]

arthritis deformans[6, 8]
arthrite déformante
Arthritis deformans
abrot.[6], **am-p.,** ant-c., aran.[10],
aran-ix.[10], arb.[8], arn.[8], **ars.**[3, 8],
aur.[3], **benz-ac.,** cal-ren.[8],
calc.[6, 8, 10], calc-caust.[6], calc-f.[10],
calc-p.[6], caul., **caust.**[3, 6, 8, 10],
chin.[8], **cimic.**[8], clem.[6], colch.,
colchin.[8], cupr.[3], euphr.[10], ferr-i.[8],
ferr-pic.[8], fl-ac.[10], form-ac.[6, 10],
graph.[6], **guaj.**[3, 6, 8], hed.[10], hep.[3, 6],
ichth.[6], **iod.,** kali-br.[8], **kali-i.,**
kalm.[10], lac-ac.[8], **led.,** lith-be.[6],
lith-c.[6], lith-sal.[6], lyc., mand.[10],
mang.[6], merc.[3], merc-c.[8], nat-br.[8],
nat-p.[8], nat-s., nit-ac.[6], onop.[14],
pipe.[8], **puls.**[3, 8], rad.[8], rad-br.[3, 6, 10],
rhod.[6], **sabin.**[3, 6, 8], sal-ac.[8], sars.[6],
sep., **sil.**[6], staph.[6], sul-i.[10],

sul-ter.[8], **sulph.**[6, 8, 10], symph.[10],
thuj.[6], thyr.[8], urt-u.[6], visc.[10]

lymphangitis[6]
lympgangite
Lymphangitis
aethi-a., all-c., **anthraci.**[6-8], **apis**[6, 8],
arn., **ars.,** ars-i.[6, 8], **bell.**[6, 8], both.[6, 8],
BUFO[6-8], **buth-a.**[9], carb-v., **chin-ar.,**
croth-h.[6, 8], cupr.[7], **echi.**[6, 8], euph.,
graph., hep., hippoz.[8], iod.[7], **lach.**[6-8],
lat-k.[8], **merc.**[6, 8], merc-i-r.[8],
mygal.[7, 8], **myris.,** nat-s., **pyrog.**[6, 8],
rhus-t.[6, 8], sil., sulph., **tarent-c.**

muscles, of; myositis[8]
muscles, des; myosite
Muskeln, der; Myositis
arn., bell., **bry.,** ham[1′], hep., kali-i.,
merc., **mez., rhus-t.**

nerves, of; neuritis
nerfs, des; névrite
Nerven, der; Neuritis
ACON., aesc.[8], **all-c.**[8], **alum-sil.,**
anan.[8], **ant-c.,** arg-n.[8], **arn.**[8], **ars.,**
BELL., bell-p.[8, 9], ben-d.[8], berb.[8],
cact., carbn-s.[8], caust., **cedr.**[8, 12],
cic., cimic.[8], **coca,** con.[8], ferr-p.[8],
gels., hep., hyper., iod., **ip.,** kali-i.,
kalm., lac-c., **lec., led., merc., nat-m.,**
nit-ac.[1′], **nux-v.,** pareir.[8], ph-ac.[8],
PHOS., plb-p.[8], **puls., rhus-t.,**
sang.[8], **sil., stann.**[8], stront-c.[8],
stram., stry.[8], sulph., **thal.**[8, 12],
urt-u.[8], zinc., zinc-p.[8]

serous membranes, of
membranes séreuses, des
serösen Häute, der
acon.[1], am-c., **APIS, apoc.**[1], arg-m.,
ARS., ars-i., asaf., **aur.,** aur-ar.[1′],
aur-i.[1′], **aur-m.,** aur-s.[1′], bell., **BRY.,**
CALC., calc-p., **carb-v.,** colch., ferr.,
fl-ac., **HELL.,** indg., **iod., kali-c.,**
lach., **led., LYC.,** mag-m., **merc.,**
nat-m., ph-ac., phos., plat., **psor.,**
puls., samb., seneg., **SIL., squil.,**
stram., sulph., ter., zinc.

sudden[16]
soudaine
plötzliche
   bell.

synovitis
synovite
Synovitis
   acon.[8], **am-p.**[8], ant-t.[12], apis, arn.[8],
   bell., **benz-ac.**[8], **berb.**[8], bry., calc.,
   calc-f.[8], calc-p.[8], canth.[8], caust.,
   ferr-p., fl-ac.[8], **hep.**[8], iod., kali-c.,
   kali-i., led., lyc., merc., phyt., puls.,
   rhus-t., ruta[8], **sabin.**[8], sep., sil.,
   slag[8], staph.[8], **stel.**[8], stict.[8], sulph.,
   tub.[8], verat-v.

tendency to[16]
tendance à
Tendenz zu
   camph.

tendons, of; tendinitis
tendons, des; tendinite
Sehnen, der
   anac.[7], ant-c.[12], **rhod., rhus-t.**

wounds, of[4]
plaies, des
Wunden, der
   acon., arist-cl.[9], arn., calc-f.[2],
   calen.[2, 11], **cham., con.**[2], hyper.[1'],
   kali-bi.[11], lach., led.[1'], mez.[4, 16],
   nat-m., plb., **puls., rhus-t.**[4, 11],
   sul-ac., sulph., vip.[11]

INJURIES (including blows, bruises,
   falls)
TRAUMATISMES (coups, meurtrissu-
   res, suites de chutes)
VERLETZUNGEN (einschließlich Folgen
   von Schlag, Quetschung, Fall)
   absin.[2], acet-ac.[7, 8], **acon.**[2, 3, 4, 7, 8, 12].
   agn.[2], all-c.[3, 8, 12], aloe.[3], alum.[3, 4],
   am-c.[3, 4], am-m.[3], ang.[3, 6-8, 12],
   ant-c.[2, 3], apis[12], **arg-m.**[2, 3], arg-n.[3],
   ARN., aur-m.[2], **bad.,** bell.[3, 4],
   bell-p.[1, 7], bor.[3, 4], bry., bufo[3, 7, 8],
   calc., calc-p.[3], calc-s.[12],
   CALEN.[1'-3, 6-8, 10], **CAMPH.**[7],
   CANN-I.[7] **cann-s.**[3], canth.,

carb-v., caust.[2, 3, 4], cham., chin.,
chion.[3], chin-s.[4], **cic., CON.,**
croc., crot-t.[7, 8], dig.[3],
dros.[2, 3], **dulc.,** echi.[3, 7, 8], erig.[12],
eug.[4], euph.[3], euph-pi.[12], euphr.,
ferr-p.[12], **form.**[2, 12], gamb.[12],
glon.[2, 3, 6-8, 12], **ham.**[2, 3, 6-8, 12], hell.[12],
HEP., hyos., **HYPER., iod.,** ip.[12],
kali-c., kali-i.[3], kali-m.[12], kali-p.[12],
kali-s.[12], kalm.[3], kreos., lac-c.[12],
lac-d.[12], **lach.,** laur., **led., lith-c.**[2, 3, 12],
lyc., mag-c.[7, 8, 12], merc., mez.,
mill.[2, 3, 7, 12], mosch.[2], **naja**[3], nat-c.,
nat-m., **nat-s., nit-ac.,** nux-m.[3],
nux-v., oena.[12], **olnd.**[2, 3], par.,
pareir.[2], **petr.**[2, 3, 4], ph-ac., **phos.,**
phys.[3, 7, 8, 12], **plan.**[2, 12], plat., plb.,
polyg-h.[2], psor.[12], **PULS.,** pyrog.[3],
ran-b.[12], **rhod.**[2, 3], **RHUS-T., ruta,**
samb., sec., seneg., sep.[2, 3, 4, 12],
sil., spig.[3], **staph.,** stict.[12],
stront-c.[3, 7, 8], **SUL-AC.,** sul-i.[1'],
sulph., symph., tab.[3], tarent.[3, 12],
tell.[12], ter.[12], teucr.[2, 3], urt-u.[12],
valer.[3], vario.[12], verat., **verb.**[2, 3, 7, 8],
zinc.

lifting/soulever/Heben
shocks/choc/Schock

ailments from[12]
troubles à la suite de
Beschwerden infolge von
   acon., all-c., arn., bell-p., con.,
   dulc., ferr-p., glon., ham., hell.,
   hep., ip., kali-m., kali-p., kali-s.,
   lac-c., lac-d., lach., led., lith-c.,
   mag-c., mill., nat-s., nux-v., oena.,
   paeon., par., ph-ac., phys., plan.,
   psor., ran-b., ruta, sec., sep., sil.,
   staph., stict., sul-ac., sulph.,
   symph., tarent., tell., ter., teucr.,
   urt-u., valer., vario.,

wounds-constitutional effects/
   blessures-effets constitutionnels/
   Wunden – konstitutionelle
   Folgen

concussion[2, 3]
commotion
Erschütterung
    acon., **anac., ARN.**[2, 3, 6], aur.,
    BAD.[2], **bell.**[2, 3, 7], bry.[3, 4], **calc.,**
    calen.[2], camph., cann-s., caust.,
    chin.[2, 3], cic.[2, 3, 6, 8, 12], cina, **cocc.,**
    con.[2], cupr., euphr.[2], **glon.**[3],
    hell.[2, 12], **hyos., HYPER.**[2, 7], **iod.**[2],
    kali-p.[2], kreos., **lach.**[2], laur., **led.,**
    lyc., m-arct.[3], mag-m., **mang.,**
    mez., nat-m., **NAT-S.**[2], nux-m.,
    nux-v.[2, 3, 6], ph-ac., **puls.**[2-4],
    rhus-t.[2, 3], seneg., **sep.**[2, 3, 12], **sil.,**
    spig., staph., stry.[6], sul-ac.[2],
    sulph.[3], **valer., verat.,** viol-t.

ailments from[6]
troubles à la suite de
Beschwerden infolge von
    am-c., **arn., hyper.,** valer.

am.[3]
    hell.

commotion of the brain, ailments
    from[12] *
commotion du cerveau, troubles
    à la suite de
Commotio cerebri, Beschwerden
    infolge von
    sul-ac., teucr.

    convulsions–c./Konvulsionen–C.
    faintness–injury–c./évanouisse-
    ment–choc–c./Ohnmacht–
    Verletzungsschock–G.

dislocation, luxation[3]
dislocation, luxation
Luxation
    acon., agar., **AGN.**[2, 3, 12], alum.,
    am-c.[2, 3, 12], am-m., **ambr.**[2, 3],
    anac., ang.[2, 3], ant-c., ant-t.,
    ARN.[2-4, 7], ars., asar., aur.,
    bar-c.[2, 3], **bell.**[2, 3], bov.[2, 3], **bry.**[2-4],
    calad., **CALC.**[2, 3], **calc-f.,** calc-p.,
    camph., cann-s.[2, 3], caps.[3, 4],
    carb-an.[2-4], **carb-v.**[2-4],
    carl.[11], **caust.**[2, 3], cham.,
    chel., chin., cina, cocc., **coloc.,**
    con.[2-4], croc., cycl., dig., dros.,

dulc., euph., **ferr-s.**[2], **form.**[2, 12],
graph.[2, 3], hell., hep.[2, 3], **IGN.**[2-4],
ip., kali-c., **kali-n.**[2, 3], kreos.[2, 3],
lach.[4], led., **LYC.**[2, 3], m-arct.[4],
m-aust.[12], mag-c.[3, 4], mag-m.,
mang., meny., **merc.**[2-4], mez.[2],
mosch.[2-4], mur-ac., **NAT-C.**[2-4],
NAT-M.[2-4], **nit-ac.**[2, 3], nux-m.,
nux-v.[2, 3], par.[4], **PETR.**[2-4],
ph-ac., **PHOS.**[2-4], plat., plb.,
prun., psor.[3, 12], **PULS.**[2, 3], ran-b.,
rhod.[2, 3], **RHUS-T.**[2-4, 7], **ruta**[2, 3, 12],
sabin.[2, 3], sars., seneg., sep.[2, 3, 4],
sil., **spig.**[2-4], spong., stann.[2, 3],
staph.[2, 3], **stront-c., sulph.**[2-4],
thuj., valer., verat., verb.,
zinc.[2, 3]

ailments from[12]
troubles à la suite de
Beschwerden infolge von
    psor., rheum

extravasations, with
extravasations, avec
Blutaustritt, mit
    acet-ac.[2], agar.[2, 7], **ARN., bad.,**
    bell-p.[7], both.[7], bry., calen.[2, 7],
    cham., chin., cic., **con.,** crot-h.[4, 7],
    dulc., euphr., ferr., **ham.**[2], **hep.,**
    hyper.[7], iod., **lach.,** laur., **led.**[2, 3, 7, 8],
    mill.[2], nux-v., par., plb., **puls.,**
    rhus-t., **ruta,** sec., staph.[7], **SUL-AC.,**
    sul-i.[1], **sulph.,** symph.[7]

operation, disorders from[8] *
opération, troubles par
Operation, Störungen durch
    acet-ac., **acon.**[2, 3, 7, 12], all-c.[12],
    apis[8, 12], **arn.**[3, 6-12], **bell-p.**[7-9],
    berb.[6, 8], calc-f., calc-p.[12],
    calen.[1'-3, 8], camph., carb-v.[1'],
    chin.[6], croc.[8, 12], ferr-p.,
    hyper.[3, 6, 8, 12], kali-s., led.[1'],
    merc.[12], mill., naja, nit-ac.,
    nux-v.[6], op.[6], ph-ac.[12], pop.[6],
    raph., rhus-t., ruta[1'],
    STAPH.[1', 7, 8, 12], **stront-c.**[1', 3, 7, 8],
    sul-ac.[12], verat., zinc.[12]

    fistulae–operation/fistules–
    opération/Fisteloperation

weakness-operation/faiblesse-
opération/Schwäche –
Operation

ailments from[12]
troubles à la suite d'
Beschwerden infolge von
   acon., all-c., calc-p., ph-ac.,
   staph., stront-c., sul-ac., zinc.

stretching, with[1']
extension, avec
Überdehnung, mit
   staph.

overexertion, strain, from[12]
effort, suite d'
Überanstrengung, durch
   arn.[2, 7], **ars.**[2, 12], **CALC.**[2, 12], calc-f.,
   carb-an., carb-v., cocc., **con.**[2],
   ham.[2], lyc., **mill.**[2], nat-c., ovi-p.,
   rhus-t.[2, 12], sanic., sil., ter.

prophylaxis of tetanus[7]
prophylaxie du tétanos
Tetanus-Prophylaxe
   ARN., HYPER., LED., tetox., thuj.

convulsions–tetanic/convulsions–
tétaniques/Konvulsionen–
tetanische

rupture of bloodvessel[2]
rupture des vaisseaux sanguins
Gefäßruptur
   mill.

muscles, of[2]
muscles, des
Muskelriß
   calen.

tendons, of[7]
arrachement ligamentaire
Bänderriß
   rhus-t.

sprains, distorsions[3]
distorsions, foulures
Verstauchungen, Zerrungen
   acet-ac.[8], **acon.**[8], agar.,
   AGN.[2-4, 8, 12], all-s.[12], **am-c.**[2-4, 6, 12],
   am-m.[6, 12], am-p., ambr.,
   amgd-p.[12], ang.[3, 4],
   ARN.[1'-3, 4, 6-8, 10, 12], ars.[12],
   asaf.[2], asar.[6], bar-c., bell.[2-4, 8, 11],
   bell-p.[6-8, 10], benz-ac., bov.[3, 6],
   bry.[2-4, 6, 7], **CALC.**[2, 3, 4, 7, 8],
   calc-f.[8, 12], calc-p.[3, 6], calc-sil.[1'],
   calen.[8], cann-s., canth.[4], caps.,
   carb-an.[2-4, 6, 8], carb-v.[2-4], carl.[12],
   caust.[3, 4, 6], chin.[4], **cic.**[3, 4, 11, 12],
   coloc., con., cupr.[4], ferr-p.[1', 2, 12],
   ferr-s.[2], form.[8], graph.[3, 4, 6],
   guaj., hep., hyos.[3, 4], **hyper.**[8],
   ign.[2-4], kali-i., **kali-n.,** kreos.[3],
   led.[3, 6, 7], lith-c., **LYC.**[2-4, 6, 12],
   m-aust.[3, 4], mag-c.[6], **merc.,**
   mez.[3, 6], **MILL.**[2, 7, 8, 12], mosch.,
   NAT-C.[2-4, 6], **NAT-M.**[2-4, 6],
   nit-ac.[2-4, 6], **nux-v.**[2-4, 6, 8],
   onos., **PETR.**[2-4, 6, 8, 12],
   PHOS.[1'-4, 6, 12], plat., polyg-h.[2],
   polyg-pe.[12], **prun.**[6, 12], psor.[12],
   puls.[2-4, 6], rad., rhod.[3, 6, 8, 12],
   RHUS-T.[1'-3, 6-8, 10, 12],
   RUTA[1'-4, 6-8, 10, 12], sabin.,
   sep.[2-4, 6], sil.[3, 6, 12], sol-n.[4],
   spig.[3, 4], stann., staph.[3, 6], stram.,
   stront-c.[2, 3, 6-8, 12], **sulph.**[2-4, 6],
   sumb.[11], **symph.**[2, 8, 10, 12],
   tarent.[11], thuj., zinc.

ailments from[12]
troubles à la suite de
Beschwerden infolge von
   agn., kali-m., kreos., lach., petr.,
   phos., polyg-h., prun., psor.,
   rhod., rhus-v., ruta, seneg.,
   stront-c., sul-ac., sulph.

traumatic fever[3]
fièvre traumatique
traumatisches Fieber
   acon.[2, 3, 7, 8, 12], **apis.**[3, 7],
   ARN.[2, 3, 7, 8, 12], **ars.**[7, 8, 12], bry.,
   cact.[12], **calen.**[2, 7], carb-v., **chin.**[7, 8, 12],

coff.[2, 7], croc., euphr., hep., **iod.**[7],
lach.[3, 7, 8, 12], **lyss.**[7], merc.[3, 7], nat-c.,
nit-ac., ph-ac., phos., **puls., rhus-t.,**
staph., sul-ac., **sulph.**[1, 3]

bones, of; fractures ✶
os, des; fractures
Knochen, der; Frakturen
  acon.[7], ang.[3, 6], **arn.**[1, 3, 4, 6-8],
  asaf.[2], bell-p.[9, 10], calc., **calc-f.**[2, 3, 6],
  calc-p., **calen**[2, 3, 4, 6, 7],
  CARB-AC.[2], con.[3], cortico.[9],
  cortiso.[9], croc.[3], **eup-per.**[3, 12],
  ferr.[3, 6], hep.[3], iod.[3, 6],
  kali-i.[3, 6], lyc.[2], nit-ac.[2], petr.[3],
  ph-ac.[3, 4, 6], phos.[3, 4], **puls.**[3, 4],
  rhus-t.[1, 3, 4], **RUTA, sil.**[2, 3, 4, 6, 7, 12],
  staph.[3, 4], stront-c.[7], **sul-ac.,**
  sulph.[2, 3, 6], **symph.**, valer.[3]

shock–injury/choc–
  traumatismes/Schock–
  Verletzungen

ailments from[12]
troubles à la suite de
Beschwerden infolge von
  hecla, ruta, symph.

compound fracture[3]
fracture compliquée
komplizierter Bruch
  ang., **ARN.**[2, 3, 7, 8], calc., **calen.**[3, 6-8],
  con., crot-h.[2], hep., hyper.[12],
  iod., **lach.**[2], **petr.**, ph-ac., phos.,
  puls., rhus-t., **RUTA**, sil., staph.,
  symph.

slow repair of broken bones
retard de calcification dans les
  fractures
langsame Frakturheilung
  asaf., **CALC.**, calc-f.[3, 7],
  CALC-P., calen.[7, 8], des-ac.[14],
  ferr.[1, 7], fl-ac.[1], iod.[7, 8], lyc.,
  mang.[7, 8], merc., **mez.**[1, 7],
  nit-ac., **ph-ac.**, phos., puls.,
  RUTA[1, 7], sep., sil., staph.,
  sulph., **SYMPH.**[1, 7], **thyr.**[7, 8, 12]

children, in[7]
enfants, chez les
Kindern, bei
  calc., calc-f., calc-p., sil.

glands, of
glandes, des
Drüsen, der
  arn., aster.[8], cann-s.[3], cic., **CON.,**
  dulc., hep., **iod.**, kali-c.[3], kalm.[2],
  merc., **petr.**[2, 3, 4], **phos.**, puls.,
  rhus-t., **sil., sul-ac., sulph.**[3, 4]

muscles, of[3]
muscles, des
Muskeln, der
  arn.[1, 3], calc.[1], nat-c., nat-m.,
  phos., **RHUS-T.**[1, 3]

nerves with great pain, of
névritiques, avec fortes douleurs
Nerven mit heftigen Schmerzen, der
  bell-p.[7-9], **cur.**[2], glon.[3, 6], **HYPER.,**
  led.[1], mag-p.[2], meny.[2, 12], **phos.,**
  tarent.[2], ther.[2], xan.[12]

ailments from[12]
troubles à la suite de
Beschwerden infolge von
  hyper., meny., xan.

periosteum, of
périoste, du
Periost, des
  calc.[1], **ruta**, symph.[12]

ailments from[12]
troubles à la suite de
Beschwerden infolge von
  symph.

soft parts, of
parties molles, des
Weichteile, der
  ARN., bell-p.[7], cham., **CON.**, dulc.,
  euphr., ham.[7], hyper.[7], lach.,
  nat-c.[4], nat-m.[4], phos.[4], **puls.,**
  rhus-t.[4, 7], samb., **sul-ac.**, sulph.,
  symph.[7]

stump neuralgia[2, 6, 7]
névralgie des moignons
Amputationsneuralgie
   all-c., am-m., arn.[2, 6], **hyper.**[2, 7],
   kalm.[2, 6], ph-ac.[2, 6], symph.

   pain-amputation/douleurs-
   amputation/Schmerzen-
   Amputation

tendons, of
tendons, des
Sehnen, der
   anac., calen.[7], rhus-t.[7], ruta[1']

INTOXICATION, after
IVRESSE, suite d'
RAUSCH, Folgen von
   abies-c.[11], absin.[11], acet-ac.[11], acon.,
   aether[11], agar., agn.[11], **am-m.,**
   aml-ns.[11], amyg.[11], arg-m., ars.[11],
   atro.[11], bart.[11], bell., bov., **bry.,**
   camph.[11], cann-s.[11], **caps.**[3, 11],
   carb-an.[11], **carb-v.,** chel.[11], chin.,
   cic.[11], cinch.[11], coca[11], **cocc., coff.,**
   con.[3, 11], conin.[11], cori-r.[11], dat-m.[11],
   eucal.[11], fagu.[11], ferr.[11], **gels.**[3, 11],
   grat.[11], hyos.[11], ign.[11], ip., kali-bi.[11],
   kali-c., kali-i.[11], kali-n., kiss.[11],
   kreos., lach.[3], lact.[11] **laur.,** led.[11, 12],
   lol.[11], merc.[11], mez.[11], mill.[11],
   morph.[11], nabal.[11], naja[11], nat-m.,
   nux-m., **NUX-V, OP.,** ph-ac., phel.[11],
   pip-m.[11], **puls.,** ran-b.[3], rheum, rhod.[11],
   sabad.[11], samb., sec.[11], **spong.,** squil.,
   stram., tab.[11], tax.[11], ter.[11], teucr.,
   thea.[11], til.[11], tus-fr.[11], valer.,
   verat.[11], vip.[11], zinc.[3, 11]

   index: *alcohol/alcool/Alkohol*
   index Vol. I: *drunkenness/ivresse/*
   Trunkenheit

IODINE, after abuse of[6]
IODE, abus de
JOD, Mißbrauch von
   ant-c., ant-t.[2], **ars.**[2, 4, 6, 12], bell.,
   camph., chin., chin-s.[2], coff., **conv.,**
   hep., lycps., merc.[2], **op., phos.**[2, 4, 6]
   sec., spong.[2], sulph.[4, 6]

IRON, after abuse of
FER, après abus de; sidérose
EISENPRÄPARATEN, nach Mißbrauch
von
   ars., calc-p.[6], **chin.**[2, 3, 6, 8], chin-ar.[6],
   cupr.[3, 6], **hep.**[2, 3, 6, 8], iod.[2], ip.[2, 3],
   merc.[2], nat-m.[6], **puls., sulph.,** thea[3],
   verat.[3], **zinc.**

IRRITABILITY, excessive physical
IRRITABILITÉ physique excessive
REIZBARKEIT, außerordentliche
physische
   absin., acon., agar., alum.[12],
   ambr., anac., ant-c., ant-t.[1],
   APIS, arg-n.[8]**, ARN., ars., asaf.,**
   ASAR., AUR., aur-ar.[1']**, aur-m.**[2],
   bar-c., bar-m.[2], **BELL., bell-p.**[8],
   berb.[12], bor., bov., bry., **calad.**[12],
   calc.[3], camph., cann-i., **CANTH.,**
   carb-ac.[12], **carb-v.**[3, 12], carbn-s.,
   caust., **cham., CHIN.,** chin-ar.[8],
   chin-s., chlol.[2], cina[3], cob.[8],
   coc-c.[12], coca[2], **cocc., COFF.,**
   coll.[12], con.[3], croc., cupr., dig.[3],
   dulc.[12], ery-a.[2], **ferr.,** ferr-ar.[1'],
   ferr-i.[11] **gels.,** graph., gua.[8], hell.,
   hep., hyos., **hyper.**[8]**, ign.,** indg.[2],
   kali-c.[3, 8], kali-p.[8], kreos., **lach.,**
   laur., **lil-t., lyc.**[3, 12], mag-c.,
   mag-m., mang., **MED.,** meny.[3],
   MERC., mez., **morph.**[12]**, mosch.,**
   naja[8], nat-ar., nat-c., **nat-m.,**
   nat-p., nat-sil.[1']**, NIT-AC.,**
   nux-m.[3]**, NUX-V.,** ox-ac.[8], par.,
   ped.[12], petr., **ph-ac., phos.,**
   phys.[8]**, pic-ac.**[8], plat., podo.[2],
   puls., ran-b.[8], rhus-t., **rhus-v.**[12],
   rumx.[12], sabin., sars.[3], sec., sel.,
   sep., **SIL.,** spig., spong.[2, 3], squil.,
   STAPH., stram., stry-p.[8], sulph.,
   TARENT., tell.[8]**, TEUCR.,** ther.[8],
   tub.[8], **valer., verat., vib.**[2]**, zinc.**[8],
   zinc-val.[8], ziz.[2]

   sexual excesses, from[8]
   sexuels, par excès
   sexuelle Exzesse, durch
     agar., kali-p., nat-m.

when too much medicine has produced an over-sensitive state and remedies fail to act

quand l'abus de médicament a crée un état d'hypersensibilité et que les remèdes restent sans effet

nach Medikamenten-Mißbrauch Überempfindlichkeit und Mittelunwirksamkeit

ph-ac., **TEUCR.**

medicaments/médicaments/ Medikamenten

lack of
manque d'
Unempfindlichkeit
acon.³, agn., **alum.**, alum-p.¹′, **am-c.**, am-m.³, **ambr.**, **anac.**, ang.³, ant-c., ant-t., arn., **ars.**, asaf., asar.³, bar-c., bell.³, bism., bor.³, brom., bry., **CALC., CALC-I., camph.**, cann-s., canth.³, **CAPS., carb-an., CARB-V.**, caust., cham.³, chel.³, chin.³, cic., clem.³, **cocc.**, colch., coloc., **CON.**, croc., cupr., dig.³, **dulc.**, euph., ferr., ferr-i.¹′, **GELS.**, graph., **guaj., HELL.**, hep.³, hyos., ign.³, **iod., ip., kali-br.¹** (non: kali-bi.), kali-c., kali-s.¹′, lach., **LAUR.**, led., **lyc.**, mag-c., mag-m., merc.³, mez., **mosch.**, mur-ac., nat-c.³, nat-m.³, **nit-ac.³**, nux-m., nux-v.³, **OLND., OP.**, petr., **PH-AC.**, phos., plb., **PSOR.**, puls.³, **rhod.**, rhus-t., sec., seneg., **sep.**, sil.³, spong., stann., staph.³, **stram.**, stront-c., **sulph., TEUCR.⁷**, thuj., valer., verat.⁴′⁶, verb., **zinc.**

*anaesthesia/anesthésie/Anästhesie
analgesia/analgésie/Analgesie
painlessness/insensibilité/
Schmerzlosigkeit
reaction/réaction/Reaktionsmangel*

ITCHING of **glands**
PRURIT glandulaire
JUCKEN von **Drüsen**
am-c., **anac.**, ant-c., canth., carb-an., carb-v., **caust.**, cocc., **CON., kali-c.**, mag-c., merc., nit-ac.¹⁶, **phos.**, ran-s., rheum, rhus-t., sabin., sep., **sil., spong.**, sulph.³

affected parts, of¹⁶
souffrantes, des parties
leidenden Teile, der
dig.

bones, of¹⁶
os, des
Knochen, der
verat.

internal¹⁶
interne
innerliches
phos.

ITCHING and **TICKLING** internally³
PRURIT et **CHATOUILLEMENT** interne
JUCKEN und **KITZELN,** innerliches
acon., agar., alum., am-c., am-m., **AMBR.**, anac., ang., ant-t., apis, arn., asar., bar-c., bell., bor., bov., brom., bry., calc., caps., carb-v., caust., cham., chin., cic., cina, cocc., colch., **con.**, croc., dig., euph., **ferr.**, fl-ac., graph., hep., ign. **IOD.**, ip., **kali-bi.**, kali-c., lach., **laur.**, led., mag-c., mag-m., meny., merc., mosch., nat-c., nit-ac., nux-m., **NUX-V.**, olnd., petr., ph-ac., **PHOS.**, plb., puls., rhod., rhus-t., ruta, sabad., sabin., sang., seneg., sep., sil., spig., spong., squil., **stann.**, sulph., tarax., teucr., thuj. verat., zinc.

JAR, stepping **agg.**
SECOUSSES en marchant **agg.**
STÖSSE beim Auftreten **agg.**
acon., aloe³, alum., alum-p.¹′, alum-sil.¹′, am-c., ambr., **anac.**, ang.³, **ant-c.**, arg-m., **arg-n.**,

ARN., ars., **asar.**, bapt.[3],
bar-c., **BELL.**, berb.[3, 7, 8], bor.,
BRY., **cact.**, calad., **calc.**, calc-p[1]',
calc-sil.[1]', camph., canth., carb-ac.[3],
carbn-s., **caust.**, cham., chel., **chin.**,
CIC., cina[3], **cocc.**, coff., **CON.**,
crot-h.[8], dros., dulc., euphr., **ferr.**,
ferr-ar., ferr-p.[1]', form.[3], glon.,
graph., **ham.**, **hell.**, **hep.**,
ign., kali-c., **kali-i.**, kali-n.,
kali-sil.[1]', **lac-c.**[6, 7], **LACH.**, led.,
lil-t., **lyc.**, mag-c., **mag-m.**, meny.,
merc., nat-ar., **nat-c.**, **nat-m.**,
nat-p., nat-s.[3], nat-sil[1]', **NIT-AC.**,
nux-m., **nux-v.**, **onos.**, par., petr.,
ph-ac., **phos.**, plat., plb., podo.[3],
puls., rhod., **RHUS-T.**, ruta, **sabad.**,
sabin., **sanic.**, seneg., **sep.**, **SIL.**,
spig., spong., stann., staph., **sulph.**,
tab.[3], tarax.[3], **THER.**, **thuj.**, valer.[6],
verb., viol-t.

am.
caps., gels.[3], hell.[3], nit-ac.[3]

JERKING internally
SECOUSSES, saccades internes
RUCKE, innerliche
acon., agar., ambr., anac., ang.[3],
aran-ix.[10], arn., ars.,**bell.**, bov., bry.,
calad., **CALC.**, **CANN-I.**, cann-s.[1],
caust., cic., clem., coca, colch.,
con., **croc.**, dig., dulc., **GLON.**,
kreos., **lyc.**, mag-c., mang., mez.,
mur-ac., nat.-c., nat-m., **nux-m.**,
nux-v., petr., phos., **PLAT.**, **PULS.**,
ran-s., rhod., rhus-t., ruta, samb.,
sep., **sil.**, **SPIG.**, **spong.**, **STANN.**,
stront-c., sul-ac., sulph.[3], teucr.,
thuj., **valer.**

shocks, electric-like/chocs-électri-
que/Schock – elektrischer Schlag
twitching/soubresaut/Zucken

bones, in[3]
os, dans les
Knochen, in den
chin., sil.

convulsions, as in
convulsions, comme dans
Konvulsionen, wie bei
acon., agar., **alum.**, am-c.[4], am-m.[4],
AMBR., ant-c., ant-t.[4], arg-m., arn.,
ars., asaf.[4], bar-c.[4], bar-m.[4], bell.,
bry., **calc.**, camph., cann-s., canth.[4],
caps., carb-v., **CAUST.**, **cham.**,
chin., chin-s.[4], chlol.[7], **cic.**, cina[4],
cocc.[4], coff.[4], colch.[4], coloc.,
crot-h.[4], **cupr.**, cupr-a.[4], cupr-c.[4],
dig., dros., dulc., graph.[4], hep.,
hyos., **ign.**, ip., kali-c., kali-chl.[4],
kreos.[4], lach., lact.[4], laur., led.[4],
lil-t., lob.[4], lyc., m-arct.[4], mag-c.,
mag-m.[4], mang.[4], **meny**, **merc.**,
mez., mosch.[4], mur-ac., nat-c.,
NAT-M., nat-s.[4], nit-ac., nux-v., op.,
petr., ph-ac.[4], phel.[4], **phos.**, plat.,
PLB., puls.[4], **ran-b.**, ran-s.[4], rat.[4],
rhod., rhus-t.[4], sabad., **sec.**, sep.,
sil., sol-n.[4], squil., staph., **stram.**,
stront-c., sul-ac., **sulph.**, tarent.[1]',
teucr.[4], thuj., valer.[4], verat., viol-t.,
vip.[4], **zinc.**

night[16]/nuit/nachts
staph.

joints, in[3]
articulations, dans les
Gelenken, in den
alum., bell., bry., bufo, **coloc.**,
graph., nat-m., puls., sil., spig.[3, 6],
spong., **sul-ac.**, sulph.[3, 6], **verat.**

muscles, of
muscles, des
Muskeln, der
acon, aesc., **agar.**, alum.,
alum-p.[1]', alum-sil.[1]', am-c.,
ambr.[6], **anac.**, ant-c., **ant-t.**, apis,
aran-ix.[10], **arg-m.**, **arg-n.**, arn.,
ars., asaf.[1], asar., **bar-c.**, bar-s.[1]',
bell., berb.[4], bor.[3], **bry.**, bufo[1]',
cadm-s., calc., calc-f.[10, 14],
CALC-P., **cann-i.**, caps.,
carbn-s., caust.[4, 6], cham.,
chin., **chion.**, **CIC.**, **cimic.**,
clem.[4], cocc., **colch.**, coloc.[3, 4],
con., **croc.**, **cupr.**, cyt-l.[10], dulc.,
eucal.[6], euph., euphr., **ferr.**,

ferr-ar., **gels., glon., graph.,**
hist.[9, 10, 14] **HYOS.,** hyper.[1'],
ign.[4, 6] ind.[14] iod.[6] ip., kali-i.,
kali-n.[4] kali-p.[1'], kali-s., **lach.,**
lil-t., lyc.[3, 6] lyss.[10] mag-c.,
mag-m.[1'] **meny, merc.,** merc-c.,
MEZ., mosch., **nat-c.,** nat-f.[10]
nat-m., nit-ac., **nux-m., nux-v.,**
olnd., **op.,** petr., ph-ac., **phos.,**
phyt.[1'] **plat., plb., puls.,**
ran-b.[4] rat.[3] **rhus-t.,** ruta,
sabad., sabin., sal-ac.[6] sec.[4, 6]
SEP., sil., **spig., stann.,** staph.,
STRAM., stront-c., SUL-AC.,
sul-i.[1'] **SULPH.,** tab.[3] tarax.[14]
tarent., ter., teucr.[4] **valer.,**
viol-t., **visc., ZINC.,** zinc-i.[3]
ZINC-P.[1']

paralyzed parts, of
parties paralysées, de
gelähmter Teile
arg-n., merc., **nux-v.,** phos.,
sec.[1'], stram.[1'], **stry.**

side lain on, in
côté sur lequel on est appuyé,
    sur le
Seite, auf der man liegt
cimic.

sleep, on going to
s'endormant, en
Einschlafen, vor dem
acon., **agar.,** all-s.[2] **aloe**[2]
alum., arg-m., **ARS.,** bell.[3]
cob., **colch**[1] hyper., **ign.,**
iodof.[2] **KALI-C.,** kali-cy.[7]
nit-ac.[3] nux-v.[1'] op.[3] phys.,
puls.[16] ran-b., **sel.,** sep.[3] sil.,
stront-c., stry., sul-ac., sulph.,
tub.[1', 7] **zinc.**

shocks, electric-like sleep/
chocs-électrique-s'endormir/
Schock – elektrischer – Ein-
schlafen

during
sommeil, pendant le
Schlaf, im
agar., aloe, **alum.,** ambr.,
anac., ant-t., arg-m., **ars., bell.,**
bry., calc.[4] carb-v.[3] cast.,
cham., cimic., cob., colch.[1]
con., cor-r., **cupr.,** cupr-ar.[6]
daph., dig.[3] dulc., hep.,
ign., ip., **kali-c.,** lyc., merc.,
nat-c., **nat-m.,** nat-s., nit-ac.,
nux-v.[1', 6, 7] op., phos., puls.,
ran-s., rheum, rhus-t., sel., sep.,
sil., stann., staph., stront-c.,
sul-ac., **sulph.,** thuj., tub.[1', 7]
viol-t., zinc.

KNEE in[7]
GENU valgum
bar-c., lach., nux-v.

out[7]
varum
calc., nux-v., sulph.

KNEELING, ailments on
S'AGENOUILLANT, troubles en
KNIEN, Beschwerden beim
calc.[3] **cocc.,** mag-c., puls.[3] sep.,
spig.[3] tarent.[3]

am.[3]
euph.

KNOTTED sensation internally
« NOUÉ » intérieurement, sensation
d'être
KNOTEN, Gefühl eines inneren
ambr., ant-t., arn., **ars.,** asaf.[3] bell.[3]
bry., carb-an., carb-v.[6] cham., cic.,
cina[3] con., cupr., gels., graph.[3]
hydr.[3] hydr-ac., ign.[3] kali-p.[3, 6]
kreos., **LACH.,** lob.[3] mag-m.,
mag-p.[3, 6] **merc-i-r.,** nux-v., petr.,
phyt., puls., **rhus-t., sabad.,** sec., sep.,
SPIG., staph., stict., **SULPH.,** valer.[3]
zinc.[3, 6]

ball/boule/Kugel

LABOR agg., manual[3]
TRAVAIL manuel agg.
HANDARBEIT agg.
   am-m., bov., ferr., kali-c., **lach.**,
   mag-c., merc., **NAT-M.**[3, 6], nit-ac.,
   phos., **sil.**, **verat.**

LASSITUDE
MATTIGKEIT
   abies-n.[2], **ACON.**, **aesc.**, aeth.,
   agar.[1], ail., **alet.**[2], aloe[2], **ALUM.**,
   alumn.[1'], **ALUM-P.**[1'], alum-sil.[1'],
   AM-C., **am-m.**[2], **ambr.**, aml-ns.[2],
   ammc.[2], anac.[2], ang.[2], anh.[9], ant-c.,
   ant-t., **APIS**, apoc., **ARAN.**,
   aran-ix.[10], arg-m., arg-n.[2], **arn.**[2],
   ars., ars-h.[2], **ars-i.**, ars-met.[2],
   ars-s-f.[1'], arum-d.[2], arum-m.[2],
   arum-t.[2], asaf., asar., asc-t.[2],
   aspar.[2], astac.[2], aster., atro.[2],
   aur., aur-m-n., bar-c., bar-i.[1'],
   bar-m., bar-s.[1'], **bapt.**, **bell.**, bell-p.[7],
   benz-ac., **berb.**, bism., **bol-la.**[2], bor.,
   bov., brach.[2], bry., cact.,
   cadm-met.[9], cain.[7], **CALAD.**,
   CALC., calc-ar.[1', 2], calc-i.[1'],
   CALC-P.[2], calc-s.[2], calc-sil.[1'],
   calen.[2], **camph.**, cann-s., canth.,
   caps., **carb-ac.**, **carb-v.**, **CARBN-S.**,
   card-m.[2], **casc.**, **caust.**, cedr.[2],
   cham., **chel.**, chen-v.[2], **CHIN.**,
   chin-ar.[2], **chin-s.**, chlf.[2], chlol.[2, 7],
   chr-ac.[2], **cic.**, cina, cinnb.[2], cist.[2],
   cob-n.[9, 14], coc-c.[2], **coca**[2], **cocc.**,
   coff., **colch.**, **coloc.**, **CON.**, conv.[7],
   cop., croc., **CROT-C.**, crot-t.[2],
   CUPR., cupr-ar[2], cupr-s.[2], cyn-d.[14],
   daph.[2], dicha.[14], **dig.**, dios.[2], **dulc.**[2],
   ery-a.[2], eucal., eup-pur.[2], euph.[2],
   euphr., **FERR.**, ferr-ar., ferr-p.,
   fl-ac[2], **form.**, gamb.[2], **GELS.**,
   GRAPH., grat.[1', 2], guaj., **guar.**[2],
   halo.[14], **ham.**[2], harp.[14], **hell.**[2],
   hep., hippoz.[2], **hydr.**, **hydrc.**[2], hyos.,
   ign., iod., ip., **kali-bi.**[2, 3], **kali-br.**[2],
   kali-c., **kali-m.**[1', 2], kali-n., **kali-p.**,
   kali-sil.[1'], lac-ac.[2], **lac-d.**[1', 2, 7],
   LACH., **laur.**, led., **lept.**[2], levo.[14],
   lob., luf-o.[14], **lyc.**, lyss.[2], mag-c.,
   mag-m., manc.[2], **mang.**, **med.**[2],
   meny., **merc.**, methys.[14], **mez.**,

mosch., mur-ac., myric.[2], naja[14],
nat-ar., **nat-c.**, **nat-m.**, **nat-p.**,
nat-s.[2], **nat-sil.**[1'], nep.[13, 14], nit-ac.,
nuph.[2], **nux-m.**, **NUX-V.**, ol-an.[2],
olnd., onop.[14], **op.**, **ox-ac.**, oxyt.,
pall.[2], petr., **PH-AC.**, phel.[2], **phos.**,
phyt., **PIC-AC.**, plat., **plb.**, **psor.**,
ptel.[2], puls., **ran-b.**, **raph.**[2], **rat.**[2],
rhod., **rhust-t.**, **rhus-v.**[2], rib-ac.[14],
RUTA, sabad., sabin., **SANG.**,
sarr.[2], sec., sel., **senec.**[1', 2], **seneg.**,
sep., **SIL.**, spig., **spong.**, **stann.**,
staph., **stram.**, stront-c., **SUL-AC.**,
sul-i.[1'], sulfa.[14], sulfonam.[14], **sulph.**,
sumb., **tab.**[2], tarax., **TARENT.**,
tell.[2], **ter.**[2], **teucr.**, ther., thiop.[14],
thuj., **tub.**[2], uran-n.[2], ust.[2], vac.[2],
valer., verat., viol-t., x-ray[9], **ZINC.**,
ZINC-P.[1'], zing.[2]

weakness/faiblesse/Schwäche

daytime[2]
journée, pendant la
tagsüber
   am-m., asc-t., **calc.**, calc-f., cob-n.[9],
   ferr., **kali-bi.**, **senec.**

morning/matin/morgens
   am-c., ant-c., calad.[2], **kali-m.**[2],
   lyc., **mag-m.**[2], nat-c., nat-p.,
   nux-v., staph.[2], **sulph.**[2], sumb.

and afternoon[2]
et après-midi
und nachmittags
   bry.

bed, in[4]
lit, au
Bett, im
   acon., alum., **ambr.**[2, 4], **aur.**, **bell.**,
   bor., **bry.**, **carb-v.**[2, 4], **caust.**,
   cham.[2], clem., con., crot-t., dros.,
   hell. iod., kali-c., **lach.**, mag-c.,
   mag-s., mang., nat-m., **op.**,
   petr.[2, 4], phos., plb., **puls.**, ran-s.,
   sep., sil., spig., **squil.**, thuj.,
   verat., zinc.[2, 4]

rising, on[4]
levant, en se
Aufstehen, beim
   dig., **ferr.**[2], kreos., **nux-v.**[2],
   osm.[2], petr., ph-ac., plb., **sep.**[2],
   sil., stann., vib.[2]

   am.[4]
      acon., mag-c.

forenoon/matinée/vormittags
   alum., ran-b.

noon[2]/midi/mittags
   cic.

afternoon/après-midi/nachmittags
   arg-n., **calc-s.**[2], **card-m.**[2], gels.,
   hyos.[16], lil-t.[7], lyc., petr.[16], thuj.

siesta, after[16]
sieste, après le
Mittagsschlaf, nach dem
   kali-c.

16 h[14]
   trios.

evening/soir/abends
   am-c., ars., calc-sil.[1'], carb-v.,
   CAUST., graph., ign.[2], **myrt-c.**[2],
   naja, nat-m., pall.[2], sang.[7], spig.,
   sulfonam.[14], thuj.

night[1']/nuit/nachts
   calc-sil.

2 h[14]
   trios.

and morning[2]
et matin
und morgens
   nat-s.

Addison's disease, in[2]
maladie bronzée, dans la
Addison' Syndrom, bei
   calc.

air agg., in open[2]
air agg., en plein
Freien agg., im
   petr.

alternating with activity
alternant avec activité
abwechselnd mit Aktivität
   aloe, aur.

coldness, objective or subjective[2]
frissonnement objectif ou subjectif
Kälte, objektiver oder subjektiver
   spig.

chilliness, with[2]
frilosité, avec
Frösteln, mit
   cimic., corn.

coition, after
coït, après le
Koitus, nach
   agar.[2, 4, 6, 15], **CALC.,** con.[4], graph.[4],
   led.[4], lyc.[4], nat-m.[4], **phos.**[6], plb.[4],
   sep.[4], staph.[4], tax.[4], **ziz.**[2]

conversation, from
conversation, par la
Unterhaltung, durch
   sil.

eating, after
mangé, après avoir
Essen, nach dem
   act-sp.[2], ant-c.[2], bar-c.[2, 16], bov.[2],
   calc-p.[2], **carb-an.**[2], **card-m.**[2], chin.[2],
   lach.[2], **lyc.,** lyss.[2], mur-ac., **nat-m.**[2],
   nux-m.[2], ol-an.[7], **PH-AC., rhus-t.**[2],
   sel., sep.[16]

emissions, from seminal[2]
pertes séminales, par
Samenverluste, durch
   bar-c.[4], **ery-a.,** ham.

lie down before dinner, must
s'étendre avant le déjeuner, doit
hinlegen, muß sich vor dem Mittagessen
      mez.

if he does not eat frequently[2]
s'il ne mange pas souvent
wenn er nicht häufig ißt
  sulph.

menses, before
menstruation, avant la
Menses, vor den
  alum.[4, 6], **bell.**[2, 6], calc., lyc.,
  nux-m.[4, 6]

during[4]/pendant la/während der
  alum.[4, 6], **am-c.**[2], bell.[6], bor.[2, 4],
  bov., calc-p.[2], carb-an.[4, 6], cast.,
  caust.[2, 4], ign., iod.[2, 4], **kali-c.**[2, 4],
  kali-n., lyc., **mag-c.**, mag-m.,
  nit-ac.[2], **nux-m.**[2], **petr.**[2, 4], phel.,
  phos., thuj.[2]

after[2, 4]/après la/nach den
  berb., nux-v., thuj.[2]

mental exertion, from[2]
travail intellectuel, par
geistige Anstrengung, durch
  AUR., podo., **puls.**

motion, on
mouvement, par
Bewegung, durch
  phos.

  am.[16]: nat-c.

pregnancy, during[2]
grossesse, pendant la
Schwangerschaft, während der
  calc-p.

restlessness, with[2]
agitation, avec
Unruhe, mit
  dios., tell.

sexual excesses, after[6]
sexuels, après excès
sexuellen Ausschweifungen, nach
  agn.

sitting, on
assis, étant
Sitzen, im
  merc.[2], phos.

sleep, after
sommeil, après le
Schlaf, nach dem
  ant-t.[2], kali-c.[16], **PULS.**[2], sil.

spring, in[2]
printemps, en
Frühling, im
  apis, **bry., gels.**

stool, before[2]
selle, avant la
Stuhlgang, vor
  mez.

during[2]/pendant la/während
  bor., ip.

after/après la/nach
  ip.[2], **lyc.**[2], mag-m.

stormy weather
temps orageux, pendant
stürmischem Wetter, bei
  psor., **sang., tub.**

talking, after
parlé, après avoir
Reden, nach
  alum., dor.[2]

waking, on[4]
réveil, au
Erwachen, beim
  acon., alum., ambr., **arg-m.**[2], aur.,
  bell., bor., **bry., carb-v.,** card-m.[2],
  caust., chin.[2], clem., crot-t., dios.[2],
  dros., hell., hyper.[2], kreos., lac-ac.[2],
  lach., mang., **op.,** petr., **ph-ac.**[2, 4],
  phos., plb., **podo.**[2], **ptel.**[2], puls.,
  ran-s., sep., sil., spig., **squil.,** stann.,
  thuj., verat., xan.[2], zinc.

walking in open air am.
marchant en plein air am.
Gehen im Freien am.
  alum., am-c., graph.[16]

warm room, in
chambre chaude, dans une
warmen Zimmer, im
  iod.

weather, during warm
temps chaud, par
Wetter, durch warmes
  nat-p.

wet[2]/humide/feuchtes
  SANG.

LEAD, chronic effects of
SATURNISME, effets chroniques du
BLEIVERGIFTUNG, chronische
  alum., alum-sil.[12], **alumn.,** ant-c.[2],
  ars., **bell.,** carbn-s.[8], **CAUST.,** chin.,
  cocc.[2, 6], **coloc.**[6, 8, 12], crot-t.[6], cupr.[6],
  gels.[6], hep.[2, 10], iod.[8, 10], kali-br.[8],
  kali-i.[6, 8], kreos.[2], lyc.[2], mang.[6],
  merc.[8], **nat-s.**[6], nux-v., **op.,** petr.[2, 8],
  pipe.[12], **plat.,** plb.[3, 10], sul-ac., **sulph.,**
  zinc.[2]

paralysis-poisoning/paralysie-
empoisonnement/Paralysis-
Vergiftung

LEAN people
MAIGRE, personne
MAGERE Personen
  acet-ac.[12], alum.[3, 5-7], **AMBR.,**
  arg-m.[1', 3, 6, 14], **arg-n.,** ars.[12], ars-i.[7],
  bar-c.[3, 6], beryl.[9], bry., cadm-met.[9],
  calc-f.[9], **CALC-P.,** caust., chin.[12],
  coff.[7, 12], cupr.[7], ferr.[3, 6], fl-ac.[7],
  flor-p.[14], graph.[5, 12], ign., **iod.,** ip.[3, 6],
  kreos.[3, 6, 12], lach., **lyc.,** mag-c.[3, 5, 6],
  mang.[3, 6], merc.[12], nat-c.[6], nat-m.[5, 12],
  nit-ac., nux-m.[3, 6], **nux-v.,** perh.[14],
  petr.[1', 3, 6, 12], ph-ac.[7], **phos.,** plb.[12],
  saroth.[14], **SEC.,** sep., **sil.,** stann.[12],
  SULPH., tub., v-a-b.[14], verat.[12]

LEANING against anything **agg.**[3]
S'APPUYER contre n'importe quoi **agg.**
SICHANLEHNEN agg.
  arg-m., arn., bell., cann-s.,
  canth., cimic., coloc.[6], con.,
  cycl., graph., **hell.,** hep., mag-m.,
  nit-ac., phos., plat., samb., sil.,
  stann., staph.[3, 6], sulph., ther.,
  thuj.

after[3]/après/nach
  coloc.

am.[3]
  bell., **carb-v.,** dros., **FERR.,**
  kali-c., mang., merc., **nat-m.,**
  nux-v., rhod., rhus-t., sabad., sabin.,
  seneg., spig., staph.

backward agg.[3]
en arrière agg.
rückwärts agg.
  nit-ac., staph.

desire for[11]
désire
Verlangen, sich anzulehnen
  gymne., op., tub.[7]

hard am.[3]
dur am.
hartes A. am.
  bell., **rhus-t.**

pressure/pression/Druck

sharp edge agg., a[3]
bord saillant agg., un
scharfe Kante agg., eine
  agar.[3, 6], caust., chin-s., lyc.,
  ran-b., ruta, **samb.**[3, 6], stann.,
  valer.

am.[3]
  nat-c., stann.

sideward agg.[3]
à côté agg.
seitwärts agg.
  meny.

LEUCORRHEA am.[3]
LEUCORRHÉE am.
FLUOR am.
  arist-cl.[9], cimic., lach., puls.

mucous secretions/muqueuses,
sécrétions/Schleimabsonderungen

LEUKAEMIA
LEUCÉMIE
LEUKÄMIE
acet-ac., acon.[2], aran.[2, 8], ars., **ars-i.**[8],
bar-i.[8], benzol.[8], bry.[8], **calc., calc-p.,**
carb-v., **carbn-s.,** cean.[8], chin., chin-s.[8],
con.[8], cortiso.[9], crot-h., **ferr-pic.**[8], ip.,
kali-p., merc.[8], **NAT-AR., nat-m.,**
nat-p., NAT-S., nux-v., op.[11], phos.[8],
pic-ac., sulfa.[14], sulph., thuj., tub.[7],
x-ray[9, 14]

LIE DOWN, desire to[11]
S'ÉTENDRE, désir de
SICH HINZULEGEN, Verlangen
abrot., absin., acon., adlu.[14], aether,
alet.[1'], alum-p.[1'], **alumn.,** aur-ar.[1'],
aur-s.[1'], bar-s.[1'], bell., caj., carbn-o.,
cench.[1'], chlor., cocc., coloc., dor.,
dros., ferr., ferr-m., gels., grat.,
ham., hell., hipp., hydr., iber.,
kali-m.[1'], **kali-sil.**[1'], lach., lyc.,
manc., merc., merc-i-f., mez., nat-c.,
nat-sil.[1'], nux-v., op., ox-ac., paull.,
phos., polyp-p., **rhus-t.,** sal-n.,
sang., sel., sumb., tab., tarent.,
thea, wildb., zinc., zinc-p.[1']

inclination to
inclination pour
Neigung
ACON., ALUM., am-c., ambr.,
amor-r.[14], **anac., ant-c.,** ant-t.,
apis, ARAN., arn., **ARS.,**
ars-s-f.[1'], asar., **aur., bapt., bar-c.,**
bar-m., bell.[1], bism., bor., bry.,
buni-o.[14], **CALAD., calc.,** calc-s.[2],
cann-s.[3, 4], canth., **caps., carb-an.,**
carb-v., CARBN-S., casc., **caust.,**
CHAM., chel., chin., chin-ar.,
chlol.[3], cic.[4], cina, clem.[4], **cocc.,**
coff., colch.[1', 3], **con.,** croc.,
crot-h.[4], crot-t.[4], cupr., **cycl.,**
daph.[4], dig., dros., dulc., euonin.[4],
FERR., ferr-ar.[1'], ferr-p., **form.**[3, 16],
gels., gran.[4], **graph.,** grat.[4], **guaj.,**
hell.[4], hep.[4, 16], hipp., hyos.[4, 16],
iber.[14], **ign.,** ip., **KALI-AR.,**
kali-bi., kali-br.[3], KALI-C.[1, 7],
kali-n.[3, 4, 6], kali-s., lach., laur.[4],
led., lil-t.[3], **lyc.,** m-arct.[4], mag-c.,

mag-m., mang.[16], merc., merc-c.[3],
mez.[3], mosch.[2], mur-ac., nat-ar.,
nat-c., **nat-m.,** nat-p., nat-s.[3, 4],
nit-ac.[1], nux-m.[3, 4], **NUX-V.,**
olnd.[3, 4], op., ox-ac.[4, 6], par.[4],
petr., ph-ac., phos., phyt., pic-ac.,
plan.[3], plb.[4], **psor.**[1', 6], **puls.,**
ran-b., raph.[4], **rhus-t.,** ruta,
sabad., sabin.[4], **SEL.,** senec.[6],
seneg.[2], **sep., SIL., spong., stann.,**
staph., **stram.,** stront-c.,
sulfonam.[14], **sulph., sumb.,**
tarax., **tarent.,** teucr., thea[4],
ther.[4], thuj., verat., vip.[4], visc.[9],
zinc., zing.[2]

abdomen in pregnancy, on[7]
ventre dans la grossesse, sur le
Bauch in der Schwangerschaft,
    auf den
    podo.

but agg. thereby[3]
mais en agg.
aber dadurch agg.
    alum.

eating, after
mangé, après avoir
Essen, nach dem
    ant-c.[3, 16], caust.[3], chel.[16],
    chin.[3, 16], clem.[16], **lach.,** nat-m.[3, 16],
    nit-ac.[16], **sel.**

will not lie down, sits up in bed
refuse de s'étendre, s'assied dans
    son lit
will sich **nicht** hinlegen, sitzt aufrecht
    im Bett
    kali-br.

LIFTING, straining of muscles and
    tendons, from
SOULEVER qc., suites d'effort
    musculaire et tendineux
HEBEN, Überanstrengen der Muskeln
    und Sehnen durch
    acet-ac.[7], **acon.**[7], **agn.**[2, 7, 12], alum.,
    alum-sil.[1'], alumn.[2], **ambr.,**
    arist-cl.[9], **ARN.,** ars.[3], bar-c., bell.[7],
    bell.-p.[7], **bor., bov.**[2], **bry., CALC.,**

calc-f.[7, 9], calc-p.[12], **calc-s.,**
calc-sil.[1'], calen.[7], **CARB-AN.,**
carb-v., carbn-s., caust., chin., **cocc.,**
coloc., **CON.,** croc., cur., **dulc.**[1, 7],
ferr., ferr-p., **form.**[2, 7, 12], **GRAPH.,**
hyper.[1', 7], **ign.**[3], iod., **kali-c.,**
kali-m.[1'], kali-sil.[1'], **kalm.**[2], lach.,
lyc., mag-c.[4], merc., **mill.,** mur-ac.,
nat-c. nat-m., nit-ac., nux-v., olnd.,
ph-ac., phos., plat., podo.[2, 12],
prun.[12], psor.[12], rhod., **RHUS-T.,**
RUTA[1, 7], **sec.,** sep., **SIL.,** spig.,
stann., staph., stront-c.[7], sul-ac.,
sulph., thuj., valer.

ailments from[12]
troubles à la suite de
Beschwerden infolge von
   agn., alum., calc., calc-p.,
   carb-an., carb-v., graph., lyc.,
   mill., ph-ac., phos., podo., prun.,
   psor., rhus-t., ruta, sec., sep.

arms, of[12]
bras, lever les
Arme, der
   rhus-t., sul-ac.

reaching high[12]
tendre en haut
Hochgreifen
   sulph.

tendency to strain o.s. in lifting[6]
tendance de se donner un tour de
   reins en soulevant q.q.c.
Neigung sich zu verheben
   arn., bry., **calc.,** carb-v., con.,
   graph., lyc., **nat-c.**[6, 7], nat-m.[7],
   psor.[7], **rhus-t., SIL.**[6, 7], **symph.**[7]

LIGHT agg.[3]
LUMIÈRE agg.
LICHT agg.
   achy.[14], **acon.**[3, 8], agar., agn., alum.,
   am-c., am-m., anac., anh.[10, 14],
   ant-c., arg-n.[3, 7], arn., **ars.,** asar.,
   bar-c., BELL.[3, 7, 8], bor., bry.,
   buth-a.[10], **CALC.**[3, 8], camph.,
   carb-an., caust., cham., **chin.,**
   cic., cina, clem., coca[8], cocc.,

coff., **colch.**[3, 8, 14], **CON.**[3, 8], **croc.,**
culx.[1'], cupr., dig., **dros., EUPHR.,**
glon.[3, 12], **GRAPH.**[3, 8], hell., **hep.,**
hyos., **ign.**[3, 8], kali-c., kali-n., lach.,
laur., levo.[14], **lyc., lyss.**[8], mag-c.,
mag-m., mang., **merc.,** mez.,
mim-p.[14], mur-ac., **nat-c.,** nat-m.,
nat-s., nit-ac., nux-m., **nux-v.**[3, 7, 8],
op.[7], petr., **ph-ac., PHOS.**[3, 8], plat.,
puls., rhod., **rhus-t.,** ruta, samb.,
sang.[3], sars., sel., seneg., **SEP., sil.,**
spig.[3, 8], stann., staph., **stram.**[3, 8],
sul-ac., **sulph.,** tarax., thuj., **valer.,**
verat., zinc.

ailments from bright[12]
troubles à la suite de l. claire
Beschwerden infolge von hellem
   glon.

snow/neige/Schnee

am.[2, 3]
   am-m., anac., ars., bar-c., **calc.,**
   carb-an.[2, 3, 6], **carb-v.**[2, 3, 6], **caust.,**
   coff.[3], **plat.**[2, 3, 6], **staph.,**
   stram.[2, 3, 6, 8], **STRONT-C.**[2, 3, 6],
   valer.

artificial l. agg.[3]
artificielle agg.
künstliches L. agg.
   agn., am-m., anac., **apis, bar-c.**[3, 6],
   bell.[3, 6], bor., **CALC-C.**[3, 6], carb-an.,
   caust., chin-s., cina, **CON.**[3, 6],
   croc.[3, 6], **DROS., GLON.**[3, 6],
   graph.[3, 6], **hep.**[3, 6], **ign.,** kali-c., laur.,
   LYC., manc., mang., **MERC.**[3, 6],
   mez., nat-c., nat-m., **nat-s.,** nit-ac.,
   nux-m., petr., **ph-ac., PHOS.**[3, 6],
   plat., **PULS.,** ruta[3, 6], sars., seneg.,
   sep.[3, 6], **sil.**[3, 6], staph., stram.[3, 6],
   sulph.

daylight agg.[3]
lumière du jour agg.
Tageslicht agg.
   acon., am-m., **ant-c.,** bell., **calc.,**
   CON., dros., EUPHR.[3, 6], **GRAPH.,**
   hell., **HEP.,** hyos., mag-c., mang.,
   merc., nit-ac., **NUX-V.,** petr.,
   ph-ac., **PHOS.,** rhod., samb., sang.,
   sars., **sep., SIL., stram.,** sulph., thuj.

fire agg., of[3]
lueur du feu agg.
Feuerschein agg.
    ant-c., bry., **euph.**, **glon.**, mag-m.,
    merc., puls., **zinc.**

sunlight agg.[3]
soleil agg.
Sonnenschein agg.
    acon., agar., anh.[9, 10], **ant-c.**[3, 6],
    ars., asar., bar-c.[3, 6], bell.[3, 10],
    bry., **CALC.**[3, 6], camph., **chin.**[3, 6],
    con.[3, 6], **euphr.**[3, 6], **GLON.**,
    GRAPH.[3, 6], **ign.**[3, 6], lach.,
    mag-m., merc-c., **nat-c.**[3, 6],
    nux-v.[3, 6], **PH-AC.**[3, 6], phos.[3, 6],
    puls.[3, 6], sang.[6], sel., seneg., sil.[6],
    stann., stram., **sulph.**[3, 6], valer.,
    verat., zinc.

sun/soleil/Sonne

am.[2, 3]
    anac., con., **plat.**, **stram.**,
    STRONT-C., thuj.[3]

LIGHTNESS, sensation of[16]
LÉGÈRETÉ, sensation de
LEICHTIGKEIT, Gefühl von
    mez.

LIGHTNING, ailments from[12]
ÉCLAIR, troubles à la suite d'
BLITZ, Beschwerden infolge von
    crot-h., morph., phos.

weather–storm/temps–tempête/
* Wetter–Sturm*

LOSS of **blood**[6] ✱
PERTE de **sang,** troubles à la suite de
BLUTVERLUST, Folgen von
    abrot., arn., carb-an., **chin.**[1', 6],
    chin-ar., **ferr.**[1', 6], ferr-pic.[12], ham.,
    helon., hydr., ip.[12], **nat-m.,**
    ph-ac.[1', 6], phos., sep.[1'], staph.[1']

fluids, of ✱
fluides vitaux, de
Säfteverlust, von
    abrot.[3], acon.[3], agar., alet.[6],
    alum., anac., ant-c., ant-t.,
    arg-m., arn., **ars.**, ars-i., **aven.**[6],
    bell., bism.[3], bor., bov.,
    brom.[3], bry., bufo[3], **calad.,**
    CALC., **CALC-P.**, cann-s., canth.,
    caps., carb-ac.[3], **carb-an.,**
    CARB-V., **carbn-s.**, caust., cham.,
    CHIN., **chin-ar.**, **CHIN-S.**, cimic.[3],
    cina, coff., **con.**, **crot-h.**, **cupr.**[3, 6],
    dig., dulc., **ferr.**, ferr-ar., **GRAPH.**,
    ham.[3, 6, 8], helon.[3, 6], hep., ign.,
    iod., ip., **kali-c.**, **kali-p.**, lach.[3],
    led., lyc., mag-m., **merc.**, mez.,
    mosch., nat-c., nat-m., **nat-p.,**
    nit-ac., nux-m.[1], **nux-v.**, petr.,
    PH-AC., **phos.**, plat.[3], plb., psor.[8],
    PULS., ran-b., rhod., rhus-t., ruta,
    sabad., samb., sec., **SEL.**, **SEP.**,
    sil., spig., **squil.**, stann., **STAPH.**,
    stram.[3], sul-ac.[7], **sulph.**, thuj.,
    valer., verat., zinc.

emissions/pertes séminales/
* Samenverluste*
nursing/allaiter/Stillen

ailments from[12]
troubles à la suite de
Beschwerden infolge von
    calc., carb-an., chin., nat-m.,
    ph-ac., phos., sel., sil.

LYING agg.
COUCHÉ agg., étant
LIEGEN agg.
    abies-n., **acon.**, aesc.[3, 6], **agar.,**
    agn.[3], alum., alum-p.[1'], **alumn.**[2],
    am-c., **am-m.**, ambr., anac.,
    ang.[2, 3], ant-c., **ant-t.**, **APIS,**
    apoc., aral., aran.[3], **arg-m.**, arn.,
    ARS., ars-i., ars-s-f.[1'], arum-t.[8],
    asaf., asar., **AUR.**, aur-ar.[1'], **aur-i.**[1'],
    aur-s.[1'], **bapt.**, bar-c.[2, 3], **bell.,**
    bism., bor., bov., **bry.**, cact., calad.,
    calc., calc-p., camph., cann-i.,
    cann-s., canth., **CAPS.**, carb-an.,
    carb-v., carbn-s., caust., cench.[7, 8],
    CHAM., chel., chin., cic., cina,
    clem., cocc., coff., colch., coloc.,

CON., croc., crot-h.[3], crot-t., cupr.,
cycl., dig., dios., DROS., dulc.,
EUPH., euphr., FERR., ferr-ar.,
ferr-i., ferr-p., fl-ac., gels., glon.,
gnaph.[7], graph., grin., guaj., hell.,
hep., HYOS., iber.[8], ign., iod., ip.,
kali-bi., kali-br., KALI-C., kali-i.,
kali-m.[1'], kali-n., kali-s.[1'], kalm.[3, 6],
kreos., lach., lact., laur., led., lil-t.[3],
LYC., mag-c., mag-m., mang.,
MENY., meph.[3], merc., mez.,
mosch., mur-ac., murx., naja,
nat-ar., nat-c., nat-m., NAT-S.,
nit-ac., nux-m., nux-v., olnd., op.,
ox-ac.[3], par., petr., ph-ac., phel.,
PHOS., PLAT., plb., prot.[14], PULS.,
ran-b., ran-s.[3], raph., rheum, rhod.,
RHUS-T., RUMX., ruta, sabad.,
sabin., sal-ac., SAMB., SANG.,
sars., sec., sel., seneg., sep.,
sil.[2, 3, 6, 8], spig., spong., squil.,
stann., staph., stict., stram.,
stront-c., sul-ac., sul-i.[1'], sulph.,
TARAX., tarent.[3], teucr., thuj.,
trif-r.[8], valer., verat., verb., viol-o.,
viol-t., x-ray[8], zinc., zing.

am.
acon., agar., agn., alum., alum-sil.[1'],
alumn.[2], am-c., AM-M., ambr.,
anac., ang.[2, 3], anh.[8, 10], ant-c.,
ant-t., arg-m., arn., ars., asaf.[3],
ASAR., aur.[3], bar-c., bar-i.[1'], BELL.,
bell-p.[8], bor., bov.[3], brom.[8], BRY.,
calad., CALC., calc-i.[1'], calc-p.,
calc-sil.[1'], camph., cann-s., canth.,
caps., carb-ac., carb-an., carb-v.,
carbn-s., caust., cham.[2, 3], chel.,
chin., cic., cimic., cina, clem.,
coc-c.[2], cocc., coff., colch., coloc.,
con., conv., croc., cupr., cycl.[3, 6],
dicha.[10], dig., dios., dros., dulc.,
equis.[8], euph., euphr.[3], FERR.,
fl-ac.[3], form.[3], gels.[3], glon.,
graph., guaj., hell., hep., hyos.,
ign., iod., ip., kali-c., kali-n.,
kalm., kreos., lach., laur., led., lyc.,
mag-c., mag-m., mag-s.[4], MANG.,
merc., merc-c.[3], methys.[14], mez.,
mur-ac., nat-c., NAT-M., nat-sil.[1'],
nit-ac., nux-m., NUX-V., olnd.,
onos.[8], op., par., petr., ph-ac., phos.,

PIC-AC., plat.[3, 6], plb., psor., pulx.[8],
puls.[3, 8], rad-br.[8], ran-b., rheum,
rhod.[3], rhus-t., ruta, sabad., sabin.,
samb.[3], sang.[3], sars., sec., sel.,
seneg., sep., sieg.[10], sil.[2, 3], spig.,
spong., SQUIL., stann.[2, 3, 6, 8],
staph.[2, 3, 6], stram.[2, 3], stroph-s.[14],
stry.[8], sul-ac.[2, 3], sulph., sym-r.[8],
tarax.[3], teucr.[2, 3], thuj.[2, 3], valer.[3],
verat.[2, 3, 4, 6], verb.[3], zinc.[2, 3, 16]

after l. agg.
après être c. agg.
nach dem L. agg.
acon., agar., agn., alum., am-c.,
am-m., AMBR., ant-c., ant-t.,
arg-m., arn., ARS., asaf., asar.,
AUR., bar-c., bell., bism., bor.,
bov., bry., calad., calc., canth.,
caps., carb-an., carb-v., caust.,
cham., chel., chin., clem., cocc.,
coff., colch., coloc., con., croc.,
cupr., cycl., dros., DULC., euph.,
euphr., ferr., graph., guaj., hell.,
hep., hyos., ign., ip., kali-c.,
kali-m.[1'], kali-n., lach., laur., led.,
LYC., mag-c., mag-m., mang.,
meny., merc., mez., mosch.,
mur-ac., nat-ar., nat-c., nit-ac.,
nux-m., nux-v., olnd., op., par.,
petr., ph-ac., phos., PLAT., plb.,
PULS., ran-b., ran-s., rhod.,
RHUS-T., ruta, sabad., sabin.,
SAMB., sars., sel., seneg., sep.,
sil., spig., stann., staph.,
STRONT-C., sul-ac., sulph.,
tarax., teucr., thuj., valer., verat.,
verb., viol-o., viol-t., zinc.

am.
acon., agar., agn., am-m., ambr.,
anac., ant-c., ant-t., arg-m., arn.,
ARS., asaf., aur., bar-c., bell.,
bov., BRY., caj., calad., CALC.,
calc-f., camph., cann-s., canth.,
caps., carb-an., carb-v., carbn-s.,
caust., chel., chin., cic., cina,
cocc., coff., colch., coloc., con.,
croc., crot-h., cupr., dig., dios.,
dros., dulc., euphr., fl-ac., graph.,
guaj., hell., hep., hyos., ign., iod.,
ip., kali-c., kali-n., kreos., lach.,

laur., led., lyc., mag-c., mag-m.,
meli., **merc.**, nat-c., **NAT-M.,**
NIT-AC., nux-m., **NUX-V.**, olnd.,
pall., par., petr., ph-ac., phos.,
PULS., ran-b., rheum, rhod.,
rhus-t., sabin., samb., sars., sec.,
sel., **sep.**, sil., sin-n., **spig.**, spong.,
SQUIL., stann., **staph.**, **stram.**,
sul-ac., sul-i.[1]', **sulph.**, tarax.,
thuj., valer., verat., verb.

abdomen agg., on[3]
ventre agg., sur le
Bauchlage agg.
  ambr.

  am.
    acet-ac., adlu.[14], aloe, am-c.,
    ambr., ant-t.[8], ars., bar-c., **BELL.,**
    bell-p.[3], bry., calc., calc-p.[3, 7],
    chel., chion.[3], **cina, coloc.**, crot-t.,
    cupr.[3, 6], **elaps, eup-per.**[3, 6], ind.[3],
    lach., lept.[3, 7], mag-c., **MED.**[3, 7, 8],
    nit-ac., par.[3, 7], pareir.[3], **phos.**,
    phyt., plb., **podo.**[3, 7, 8], psil.[14],
    psor.[3], rhus-t., rib-ac.[14], sel., sep.,
    stann., stram.[3], **tab.**[8], thyr.[3]

    pregnancy, in[15]
    grossesse, pendant la
    Schwangerschaft, in der
      podo.

back agg., on
dos agg., sur le
Rückenlage agg.
    acet-ac., acon., agar.[3], aloe,
    alum., alum-p.[1]', alum-sil.[1]',
    alumn.[2], am-c., **am-m.**, ang.[2, 3],
    arg-m., arg-n.[3, 6], arn., **ars.**,
    ars-s-f.[1]', aur-m., bar-c., bar-i.[1]',
    bell., bor., bry., bufo, calc., canth.,
    carb-v.[16], **caust., cham.**, chin.,
    cimic.[3, 6], cina, clem., **colch.**[2, 3],
    coloc., cupr., cycl.[3], dulc.,
    eup-per., euph., hyper., **IGN.**[2-4],
    iod., kali-c., **kali-n.**[2, 3, 6], kreos.[3, 6],
    lach., lob.[3], mag-m.[2, 3], mag-p.[3, 6],
    merc., merc-i-f.[3], nat-c., nat-m.,
    nat-s., NUX-V., op., par., **PHOS.,**
    plat., **plb.**[3], **puls.**[2-4, 8], ran-b.,
    rhus-t., rib-ac.[14], sang.[3, 6], **sep.,**
    sil., spig., spong., stront-c.,
    sul-i., **sulph.**, thuj.

am.
  acon., aeth., am-c., **AM-M., anac.,**
  ang.[2, 3], **apis**, arn., bar-c., bell.,
  bor., **BRY., cact.**[1], calad., **CALC.,**
  calc-sil.[1]', **camph.**[7], **canth.,**
  carb-an., caust., chin., cimjc.,
  cina, clem., **colch.**, con., conv.,
  crot-h.[3, 6], **cycl.**[3, 6], **dig.**[3, 6, 8], ferr.,
  grat., hell., **ign.**, ip., **kali-c., kalm.,**
  kreos., lach., **lyc.**, mag-m.[3], merc.,
  MERC-C., mosch., nat-c., **nat-m.,**
  nat-s., nux-v., ox-ac., par., **phos.,**
  plat., **PULS.**, ran-b., **RHUS-T.,**
  sabad., sabin.[3, 6], **sang.**, senec.,
  seneg., sep., sil., spig., **spong.,**
  stann., sulph., sym-r.[8], tell.[14],
  thuj., verat., viol-t.

unable to turn from the back
incapable de se retourner étant
  couché sur le dos
unfähig, sich aus der Rückenlage
  umzudrehen
  cic., elaps

bed agg., in
lit agg., au
Bett agg., im
    acon., **agar.**, agn.[1], aloe, alum.,
    am-c., am-m., **AMBR.**, anac.,
    ang.[3], ant-c., **ant-t., arg-m.**, arn.,
    ars., ars-i., asaf., asar., **aur.**,
    aur-i.[1]', aur-s.[1]', bar-c., bar-i.[1]',
    bell., bism., **bor.**, bov., **bry.**,
    bufo[3], calad., calc., calc-i.[1]',
    camph., cann-s., canth., caps.,
    carb-an., carb-v., caust., cham.,
    chel., chin., cic., cina, **clem.,**
    cocc., coff., colch., **coloc.**, con.,
    croc., cycl., dig., dios., **dros.,**
    dulc., **euph.**, euphr., **FERR.,**
    FERR-I., ferr-p.[1]', fl-ac.[3], graph.,
    guaj., hell., hep., hyos., ign., **IOD.,**
    kali-c., kali-i., kali-m.[1]', kali-n.,
    kali-p., kali-s., **kalm.**, kreos.,
    LACH., laur., **led., lil-t., lith-c.,**
    LYC., mag-c., mag-m.[3], **mang.,**
    meny., **MERC.**, merc-c.[3],
    merc-i-f., mez., mosch., mur-ac.,
    nat-c., **nat-m.**, nit-ac., nux-m.,
    nux-v., olnd., op., **ox-ac.**, par.,
    petr., **ph-ac., PHOS.**, phyt., **plat.**

plb., **PULS.**, ran-b., rheum, **rhod.,**
rhus-t., RUMX., ruta, sabad.,
sabin., samb., **SANG., sars.,** sec.,
sel., seneg., **SEP., SIL., spig.,**
spong., squil., stann., staph.,
stict., stram., **stront-c.,** sul-ac.,
sul-i.[1'], **SULPH.,** tarax., **tell.,**
teucr., thuj., valer., **verat.,** verb.,
viol-o., viol-t., **zinc.,** zinc-p.[1']

am.

   acon., agar., **am-m.,** ambr., anac.,
   ang.[3], ant-c., ant-t., arg-m., arn.,
   ars., asar., aur., aur-ar.[1'], **bar-c.,**
   bell., bov., **BRY.,** calad., calc.,
   calc-sil.[1'], camph., cann-s., **canth.,**
   caps., carb-an., carb-v., **caust.,**
   cham., chel., chin., **CIC.,** cina,
   clem., **coc-c., COCC.,** coff., colch.,
   coloc., **con.,** croc., cupr., dig.,
   dulc., ferr., graph., guaj., hell.,
   HEP., hyos., ign., iod., ip., kali-c.,
   kali-n., kreos., **lach.,** laur., led.,
   lyc., mag-c., mag-m.[3], merc.,
   mez., mur-ac., nat-c., **nat-m.,**
   nit-ac., nux-m., **NUX-V.,** olnd.,
   par., petr., ph-ac., phos., puls.,
   ran-b., rheum, rhod., **rhus-t.,**
   sabad., sabin., samb., sars., sec.,
   sel., sep., **sil.,** spig., spong.,
   SQUIL., STANN., staph., stram.,
   stront-c., sul-ac., sulfonam.[14],
   sulph., tarax., thuj., valer., verat.,
   verb., viol-t.

doubled up agg.[3]
jambes repliées agg.
zusammengekrümmtes L. agg.
   hyos., lyc., spong., teucr., valer.

   am.[2, 3, 6]

      bell.[3], cham.[3], cocc.[3], **colch.,**
      COLOC., mag-m.[3, 6], mag-p.[3, 6],
      merc-c.[3], plat.[3], **puls., rheum,**
      rhus-t.[6], staph.[3], stram.[3], **sulph.**[2],
      verat.[3]

down, immediatly after[1']
étendu, immédiatement après s'être
Hinlegen, sofort nach dem
   cench., ferr-i.

face am., on the [3, 6]
face am., sur la
Gesicht am., auf dem
   led., **psor.,**

half reclining posture am.[3]
à moitié c. am., en position
halb zurückgelehnte Lage am.
   acon., gels., sang.

hand knee position am.[3]
mains et les **genoux** am., position
   sur les
Hand-Knie-Lage am.
   con., eup-per., euph., **lach.,** med.,
   pareir., sep., tarent.

hard bed agg., on a[6]
dur, agg. sur un lit
hartes L. agg.
     arn., bapt., bar-c., graph., kali-c.,
     lach., puls., **rhus-t.,** sil.

   am.[3, 6]

      acon.[3], bell., mag-m.[3], nat-m.[3],
      rhus-t.[3], **sep.**[3]

head high am., with[8]
tête surélevée am., avec
erhöhtem Kopf am., mit
   petr., puls., spig., spong.[6]

head low agg., with[2, 3]
tête basse agg., avec
tiefliegendem Kopf agg., mit
     ant-t., apis[3], **arg-m.**[3], arn.,
     ARS.[2, 3, 8], bell.[3], cact.[3], **cann-s.,**
     caps., carb-v.[3], **chin., clem.,**
     colch., con.[3], gels.[3], glon.[1'], **hep.,**
     KALI-N., lach., nux-v., petr.,
     phos., **PULS.,** sang.[3], **spig.,**
     spong.[3], stront-c., **sulph.**

   am.[3]

      apis, **arn.**[2, 3, 8], bell., calc.[3, 6],
      caust.[3, 6], cycl., lach., laur.[3],
      nat-m.[3, 6], sang.[3], **spong.**[2, 3, 8],
      tab., **verat., verat-v.**[7]

knee chest position am.[3]
génu-pectorale am., en position
Knie-Brust-Lage am.
   sep.

knee elbow position am.[3]
coudes et **genoux** am., position sur
Knie-Ellbogen-Lage am.
   con.[3, 6], eup-per., euph.[3, 6], **lyc.**[3, 6],
   med., pareir., petr., sep.

legs drawn up am.[6]
jambes relevées am.
Beine angezogen am.
   bell., cocc., coloc., **mag-p.**, stram.,
   verat.

moist ground or floor agg., on a[3]
sol humide agg.
feuchtem Boden agg., auf
   ars., calc., calc-p.[3, 6], caust., **dulc.**[3, 6],
   rhus-t.[3, 6], **sil., sulph.**[3, 6]

side agg., on
côté, agg. sur le
Seite agg., auf der
   ACON., am-c., am-m., **ANAC.,**
   ang.[2, 3], **arg-n.,** arn., ars.[16], aur.,
   bar-c., bell., bor., **BRY., calad.,**
   CALC., canth., **CARB-AN.,** caust.,
   chin., **cina,** clem., colch., **con.,**
   ferr., ign., ip., **KALI-C.,** kali-n.[16],
   kreos., lach., lil-t.[1', 3], **LYC.,**
   mag-m.[2, 3], **merc., merc-c.,** mosch.,
   nat-c.[2, 3], nat-m., **nat-s.,** nux-v.,
   par., ph-ac., phos., plat., **puls.,**
   ran-b., **RHUS-T.,** sabad., **seneg.,**
   sep., **sil.,** spig., spong., **STANN.,**
   sulph., thuj., verat., viol-t.

  am.
   acon., alum., am-c., am-m.,
   ang.[2, 3], arn., ars., bar-c., bell.,
   bor., bry., calc-p., canth., caust.,
   cham., chin., cina, clem., **COCC.,**
   colch., **coloc.**[2, 3], cupr., dulc.,
   euph., ign., iod., kali-c., **kali-n.**[2, 3],
   lach., mag-m.[2, 3], merc.[2, 3],
   nat-c.[2, 3], nat-m., **NUX-V.,** par.,
   phos., plat., puls.[2, 3], ran-b.,
   rhus-t., **sep., sil.**[2, 3], spig., spong.,
   stront-c., sulph., thuj.

left s. agg.
gauche agg.
linken S. agg.
   acon., ail., **am-c.**[2, 3, 6], anac.,
   ang.[2, 3], ant-t., apis[3], **arg-n.,**
   arn., **bar-c.,** bell., brom.[6], bry.,
   cact., calad.[8], calc.[2, 3], canth.,
   carb-an., chin., coc-c.[8], **colch.,**
   con., cycl.[3], dig.[3], eup-per.,
   glon.[3], hydroph.[14], iber.[3, 8],
   ind.[3], ip., kali-ar., kali-c., kalm.,
   kreos., lil-t.[3], lyc., mag-m.,
   magn-gr.[8], merc., **naja, nat-c.,**
   nat-m., nat-p., **nat-s.,** op., **par.,**
   petr., **PHOS.,** plat., **ptel.**[3, 8],
   PULS., rhus-t., rumx.[3], seneg.,
   sep., sil., **spig.**[2, 3, 8], **stann.**[2, 3],
   sulph., tab., **thuj.,** tub.[3], vib.[3],
   visc.[8], zinc-i.[3]

  am.[2]
   acon., **am-m.,** anac., arg-n.[3, 6],
   bor., bry., calc., carb-an.,
   caust., cina, clem., con., ign.[8],
   ip., kali-c., lach., lyc., **mag-m.,**
   merc., mur-ac.[8], nat-c., nat-m.[8],
   nux-v., puls., ran-b., seneg.,
   spig., **spong.,** stann., sulph.,
   thuj.

pain goes to side on which he is
  not lying[3]
douleur va au côté sur lequel il
  n'est pas couché, la
Schmerz geht in die Seite, auf der
  er nicht liegt
   arn., **bry.,** calc-ar., cupr., cur.,
   fl-ac., graph., **ign.,** kali-c.,
   kali-bi., merc., ph-ac., puls.,
   rhus-t., sil.

  lain on[3]
  il est couché
  auf der er liegt
   arn., **ars., bry.,** calc., cimic.,
   graph., **kali-c.,** merc., mosch.,
   nat-m., ph-ac., phos., phys.,
   PULS., sep., sil.

painful s. agg.
douloureux agg.
schmerzhaften S. agg.
  acon., agar., am-c., am-m.,
  ambr., anac., ang.[2, 3], **ant-c.**,
  arg-m., arn., **ars.**, ars-i., **bapt.**,
  BAR-C., bell., bry., **CALAD.**,
  calc., calc-f., cann-s., caps.,
  carb-an., carb-v., caust., **chin.**,
  cina, clem., croc., cupr.,
  CYCL.[3, 16], dios., **dros., graph.**,
  guaj., **HEP.**, hyos., ign., **IOD.**,
  kali-c., kali-i., kali-m.[1', 2],
  kali-n., **LACH.**[2, 3, 6], **laur.**[3], led.,
  lyc., mag-c., MAG-M.[2, 3],
  mang., **merc.**, mez., **mosch.**,
  mur-ac., nat-m., **nit-ac.**,
  NUX-M., nux-v., olnd., **par.**,
  petr., **ph-ac., phos.**, plat., puls.,
  pyrog.[3, 6], ran-b., ran-s., **rheum**,
  rhod., **rhus-t., rumx., RUTA**,
  sabad., sabin., samb., sars.,
  sel., sep., **SIL., spong.**, staph.,
  stram., sulph.[2, 3], tarax.,
  tell.[3, 8], teucr., thiop.[14], thuj.,
  valer., verat., verb., vib.[8]

am.
  am-c.[8, 15], ambr., arn., bell.,
  bor.[8], **BRY., calc.**, cann-s.,
  carb-v., caust., **cham.**, chel.[3],
  coloc., cupr-a.[8], esp-g.[13], fl-ac.[3],
  ign., kali-c., lyc., mag-p.[3, 6],
  nux-v., plb.[3, 6], **puls.**, rhus-t.,
  sec.[3], **sep.**, stram., sul-ac.[8],
  sulph., viol-o., viol-t.

painless s. agg.
sans douleur agg.
schmerzlosen S. agg.
  ambr., arg-m., arn., bell., **BRY.**,
  calc., cann-s., carb-v., **caust.**,
  CHAM., chel., chin.[3, 16],
  COLOC., con.[3], cupr., **FL-AC.**[3],
  graph.[3], hyper., **ign., kali-c.**,
  lyc., merc-i-r., naja, nat-c.[1],
  nat-m.[3], nat-s.[3], nux-v., phos.,
  plan., ptel.[8], **PULS., rhus-t.**,
  SEC.[3], **sep.**, stann., sul-ac.,
  ter.[3], viol-o., viol-t.

am.
  acon., agar., am-c., am-m.,
  ambr., anac., ang.[2], ant-c.,
  arg-m., arn., ars., **bapt., bar-c.**,
  bell., bry., **calad.**, calc.[2], calc-f.,
  cann-s., caps., carb-an.,
  carb-v., caust., chin., cina,
  clem., croc., cupr., dios., dros.,
  graph., guaj., **hep.**, hyos., ign.,
  iod., kali-c., kali-m.[1'], kali-n.,
  lach., led., lyc., mag-c.,
  mag-m.[2], mang., merc., mez.,
  mosch., mur-ac., naja[14], nat-m.,
  nit-ac., **nux-m., nux-v.**, olnd.,
  par., petr., ph-ac., **phos.**[2], plat.,
  puls., ran-b., ran-s., rheum,
  rhod., rhus-t., **ruta,** sabad.,
  sabin., samb., sars., sel., sep.,
  sil., spong., staph., stram.,
  sulph.[2], tarax., teucr.[2], thuj.,
  valer., verat., verb.

part on which he is lying, agg.[3]
partie où il est couché, agg. sur la
Körperteils, auf dem man liegt,
  agg. des
  aloe, am-c., ars., **arn.**, bar-c., **bry.**,
  calc., caust., **chin., graph.**, hep.,
  hyper., mag-m., merc., mosch.,
  nat-s., nit-ac., ph-ac., **PULS.**,
  rhus-t., sep., sil., thuj.

right s. agg.
droit agg.
rechten S. agg.
  acon., **alum.**, am-c., **am-m.**,
  anac., bad.[3], bell.[3], **benz-ac.**,
  bor., bry., bufo, calc.[2, 3, 16],
  cann-i.[8], carb-an., caust.[1],
  cimic.[14], cina, clem., con.,
  hydr.[3], ip., iris[3], **kali-c.**, kali-i.,
  kali-m.[1'], kreos., lach.[2, 3], lyc.,
  lycps.[3, 6], mag-c.[3'], **mag-m.**,
  MERC., mur-ac., nat-c.[2, 3],
  nux-v., phos., prun-s., psor.,
  puls.[2, 3], ran-b., **rhus-t.**[3, 8],
  rumx.[3, 6], sang.[3'], scroph-n.[8],
  sec.[3], seneg., spig.[2, 3], **spong.**,
  stann.[2, 3, 8], sul-ac., sulph.,
  thuj.

am.[2, 3]
>
> acon., am-c., anac., ang.,
> ant-t.[8], arn., bar-c., bar-m.[3],
> bell., brom.[3], bry.[2, 3, 6], cact.[3],
> calc., canth., carb-an., chin.,
> colch., con., crot-h.[3], ip.,
> kali-c., kreos.[3], lyc.,
> mang.[3, 6], merc., nat-c.,
> nat-m.[2, 3, 8], par., PHOS.[2, 3, 8],
> plat., ptel.[3, 6], PULS., seneg.,
> sep., sil., spig.[2, 3, 6], stann.,
> sulph.[2, 3, 8], tab.[8], thuj.

with head high[8]
avec tête surélevée
mit erhöhtem Kopf
>
> ars., cact., spig., spong.

stretched out l. agg.[3]
étendus agg., membres
ausgestreckstes L. agg.
>
> cham., colch., coloc., plat., puls.,
> rheum, rhus-t., staph.

MAGNETISM am.
MAGNÉTISME am.
MAGNETISMUS am.
>
> acon., bar-c., bell., calc., calc-p., chin.,
> con., CUPR., graph., ign., iod., nat-c.,
> nux-v., PHOS., sabin., sep., sil.,
> sulph., teucr., viol-o.

hand-laying/main-application/Hand-auflegen

MANY SYMPTOMS[3]
NOMBREUX SYMPTOMES
SYMPTOMFULLE
>
> agar., tub.

contradictory/contradictoires/ widerspruchsvolle

MASTURBATION, onanism, from*
MASTURBATION, onanisme, troubles
à la suite de
MASTURBATION, Onanie,
Beschwerden durch
>
> abrot.[8], agar., agn.[3, 8], aloe[12],
> alum., ambr., anac., anan.[11], ant-c.,

apis[8, 12], arg-m., arg-n.[7, 12], ars.,
aur.[3], aven.[6], bar-c.[3, 6], bell.[2],
bell-p.[7, 8, 12], bov., bufo, calad.,
CALC., calc-p.[3, 6, 8, 12], calc-s.,
calc-sil.[1'], cann-i.[6], cann-s.[3], carb-v.,
carc.[7], caust.[5, 7], CHIN., cina[3], cob.[12],
COCC., coff.[5, 7], CON., dig.,
dios.[3, 6, 8, 12], dulc.[3], ferr., GELS.,
graph.[8], grat.[7, 8, 12], hyos., ign.[3], iod.,
kali-br.[3, 6, 8, 12], kali-c., kali-p.,
lach.[3, 12], lyc., mag-p.[1], med.[12], merc.,
merc-c.[1], mosch., nat-c., nat-m.,
NAT-P., nux-m., nux-v., op.[11], ORIG.,
petr., PH-AC., phos., pic-ac.[3, 6, 8],
plat.[3, 8, 12], plb., puls., sal-n.[8, 12],
sars.[12], SEL., SEP., sil., spig., squil.,
stann.[3, 12], STAPH., stict.[3, 6], still.[8],
stram.[3, 6], SULPH., tab.[8, 12], thuj.[3, 8],
trib.[8], ust.[3, 8], zinc.[8, 12], zinc-o.[8]

MEASLES, after
ROUGEOLE, après
MASERN, Folgekrankheiten nach
>
> acon.[3], am-c.[3], ant-c., ant-t.[3],
> arg-m.[2], ars.[2-4], bell., bry., calc.[2],
> CAMPH., CARB-V., carbn-s.,
> caust.[2], cham., chin., cina[3], coff.[3, 6],
> cupr-a.[3], dros.[2, 3], dulc.[2, 4], euphr.[2],
> hell.[3], hyos., ign., iod.[4], ip.[7],
> kali-c.[3, 6], kali-m.[2, 6], lob.[7], MORB.[7],
> mosch., nux-m.[2], nux-v., oxyd.[7],
> phos.[4], PULS., rhus-t., sep.[2, 3],
> stict.[2], stram.[2], sulph., zinc.[3]

exanthema repelled[3, 4]
exanthème supprimé
Exanthem, unterdrücktes
>
> bry.[3], phos., puls., rhus-t.

MEDICAMENTS, abuse of[7]
MÉDICAMENTS, abus des
MEDIKAMENTEN, Mißbrauch von
>
> aloe[8], ars.[3], bapt., camph.[3, 6],
> carb-v., cham.[3, 4, 6], coff.[4], hep.[3],
> hydr.[3, 8], kali-i.[3], lob.[7], mag-s.[9],
> nat-m.[3], nit-ac.[3], NUX-V.[2-4, 6-8, 12],
> puls.[3, 6], sulph.[3], teucr.[2, 8, 12],
> thuj.[12]

arsenical poisoning/arsenic,
empoisonnement/Arsen-
Vergiftung
china/quinique/Chinarinde
iodine, abuse/iode, abus/Jod,
Mißbrauch
iron, abuse/fer, abus/Eisen-
präparaten, Mißbrauch
mercury, abuse/mercure, abus/
Quecksilber, Mißbrauch
narcotics/narcotiques/Narkotika
paralysis-poisoning/paralysie-
empoisonnement/Paralysis-
Vergiftung
purgatives/Abführmitteln
quinine, abuse/quinine, abus/
Chinin, Mißbrauch
sulphur, abuse/sulphur, abus/
Schwefel, Mißbrauch

vegetable[8]/végétaux/pflanzlichen
camph., **nux-v.**

addiction
asservissement à l'usage d'une
drogue
Arzneimittelsucht
buth-a.[9], tab.[12]

Vol. I: *morphinism/morphino-*
manie/Morphinismus
narcotics-desire/narcotiques-désir/
Narkotika-Verlangen

oversensitive to[5, 7]
hypersensible aux
überempfindlich gegen Medikamente
acon., arn., asar.[3], cham.[3, 5, 7],
chin.[3], coff., **ign.**[3], lyc., nit-ac.[1'],
NUX-V.[1', 3, 5, 7], **PULS.**[3, 5, 7], sep.[5],
sil.[5], **SULPH.**, teucr.[3, 12], **valer.**[3]

high potencies, to[1']
hautes dynamisations, aux
Hochpotenzen, gegen
ars-i., caust.[5], hep.[5], lyc.[5],
NIT-AC.[1', 4, 5, 7], nux-v.[1', 5],
sep.[5]

quick reaction[1']
réaction rapide
schnelle Reaktion auf Medikamente
bell., cupr., nux-v., zinc.

reaction, lack-remedies/réaction,
manque-remèdes/Reaktions-
mangel – Arzneimittel

MENSES, before
MENSTRUATION, avant la
MENSES, vor den
alum., alum-p.[1'], **am-c.**, am-m.,
arg-n., arist-cl.[9, 10, 14], asaf., asar.,
bar-c., bar-i.[1'], bar-m., bar-s.[1'],
bell., berb.[4], bor., **BOV.**, brom.[3],
bry., **CALC., CALC-P.**, calc-sil.[1'],
canth., carb-an., **carb-v.**, carbn-s.,
caul.[3, 6], **caust.**[1, 7], cham., chin.,
cimic.[3, 14], cina, cocc., coff., **coloc.**[3],
con., croc., **CUPR.**, dig.[3], dulc.,
ferr.[1], ferr-i., foll.[14], gels., graph.,
hep., **hyos.**, ign., iod., ip., **kali-c.**,
kali-m.[1'], kali-n., **kreos., LACH.**,
LYC., mag-c.[1, 7], mag-f.[9, 10, 14],
mag-m., mag-s.[9, 10], **mang., merc.**,
mez., mosch., mur-ac., nat-c.,
NAT-M., **nat-p.**, **nit-ac.**[3, 4], nux-m.,
nux-v., ol-an.[4], petr., **ph-ac., phos.**,
plat., psor.[3, 6], **PULS.**, rhus-t., rob.[7],
ruta, sabad., sars., **SEP.**, sil., spig.,
spong., stann., staph., sul-ac.,
SULPH., thuj.[7], valer., **VERAT.**,
vib., vip-a.[14], **ZINC.**, zinc-p.[1']

at beginning of
au début de la
am Anfang der
acon., arg-n.[3], asar., bell., bry.,
cact., **CALC-P., caust.**, cham.,
cimic.[3], cocc., coff., graph.,
HYOS., ign., iod., ip., **KALI-C.**,
LACH.[3, 8], lac-c.[7], **lyc.**, mag-c.,
mag-m., mag-p.[3, 6], merc., mosch.,
nat-m., nit-ac., **phos., plat.**, plb.[3],
puls., ruta, sars., **sep., sil.**, staph.,
zinc.[3]

am.[6]
lach., mag-p., plb., zinc.

during
pendant la
während der

acon., agar., aloe, alum., alum-p.[1]',
AM-C., am-m., ambr., **ant-c.,**
ARG-N., ars., ars-i., ars-s-f.[1]',
asar., aur.[3], bar-c., bar-i.[1]',
bar-m., bars-s.[1]', bell., berb.[4],
bor., **BOV.,** bry., **bufo,** but-ac.[14],
calc.[1], calc-p., calc-sil.[1]', cann-s.,
canth., caps., carb-an., carb-v.,
CARBN-S., cast.[3, 4, 6], caust.,
CHAM., chel., chin., chin-s.[4],
cimic., cocc., coff., con., croc.,
crot-h., crot-t.[4], cupr., ferr.,
ferr-i., ferr-p., gels., gran.[4],
GRAPH., ham.[3, 8], hep. **HYOS.,**
ign., iod., **KALI-C.,** kali-i.[4],
kali-m.[1]', kali-n., **kreos.,** lach.,
laur., **lyc., MAG-C., mag-m.,**
mag-s.[4, 9, 10], merc., mosch.,
mur-ac., nat-c., **nat-m.,** nat-p.,
nat-s.[3, 4], nicc.[4], nit-ac., **nux-m.**[1],
NUX-V., oena., ol-an.[3, 4, 6], op.,
petr., ph-ac., phel.[4], **phos.,** plat.,
prun.[4], psor.[3, 6], **PULS.,** rat.[4,]
rhod., rhus-t., sabin., sars., sec.,
sel., **SEP., sil.,** spong., stann.,
staph.[3, 4], stram., stront-c., sul-ac.,
SULPH., thea, thyr.[14], **verat.,**
vib., vinc.[4], **ZINC., ZINC-P.**[1]'

am.
all-s.[3], alum., am-c.[8], apis, aran.,
arg-n.[3], arist-cl.[9, 10, 14], bell.,
calc., calc-f.⌀cimic., cortiso.[9, 14],
cycl., dicha.[10, 14], ferr-p.[3], foll.[14],
gels.[3], ign.[3], iod.[3], kali-bi., **kali-c.,**
kali-p., lac-c., **LACH.,** lycps.[2],
mand.[14], **mosch.,** phenob.[13, 14],
phos., plb.[6], puls., rhus-t., senec.,
sep., **stann.,** sulph., ust., verat.,
vip-a.[14], **zinc.**

retarded[2]
retardée
verspätete
   lach.

after
après la
nach den

alum., alum-p.[1]', am-c.,
arist-cl.[9, 10, 14], ars.[4], berb.[4], **BOR.,**
bov., bry., calc., calc-sil.[1]',
canth., carb-an., carb-v.,
carbn-s., chel., chin., **cocc.**[6], **con.,**
cupr., **ferr.,** ferr-i., **GRAPH.,** iod.,
kali-c., KREOS., LACH., lil-t.,
lyc., mag-c., merc., **nat-m.,**
nat-p., **NUX-V., nit-ac., ph-ac.**[1],
phos., plat., puls., rhus-t., ruta,
sabin., **SEP.,** sil., **stram.,** sul-ac.,
sulph., tarent.[6], verat., **zinc.,**
zinc-p.[1]'

am.[3, 6]
aran.., arist-cl.[9], calc., cimic.,
lycps.[3], thyr.[14], **zinc-p.**[1]'

MERCURY, abuse of*
MERCURE, abus de
QUECKSILBER, Mißbrauch von

acon.[3], agn.[3], alumn.[7], anan.[7], ang.[3, 6, 8],
ant-c., ant-t.[8], **arg-m.,** arn.[3], ars.[3, 6],
asaf., AUR., aur-m.[1]', aur-s.[1]', **bell.,**
bor.[7], bry.[3], calad.[2, 3], **calc.,** camph.[2, 3],
CARB-V., caust.[3, 8], **chel., chin.,** cic.,
cina[3], **clem.,** cocc.[1, 3, 16], coff.[3], **colch.,**
con., **cupr.,** dig.[3, 7], dulc., **euph.,**
euphr.[3], ferr.[2, 3], fl-ac.[3, 6, 8], graph.,
guaj., HEP., hydr.[3, 6, 7], **iod.,** iris[6],
kali-bi., **kali-chl.**[2, 3, 6, 12], **KALI-I.,**
LACH., laur.[3], **led., lyc.**[3, 4, 16], merc.[2],
merc-i-r.[12], **mez., mur-ac., nat-m.**[3, 7],
NAT-S., NIT-AC., nux-v.[3], op.[2, 3, 8],
ph-ac., PHYT., plat.[3], plat-m.[8, 12],
podo., **puls.,** rheum, rhod., rhus-t.[3],
sabad.[3], **sars.,** sel., sep., **sil.,** spong.,
STAPH., still.[2, 3, 6], stram., stront-c.,
sul-i.[1]', **SULPH.,** thuj., valer., verat.[3],
viol-t., zinc.

paralysis-poisoning/paralysie-empoi-
sonnement/Paralysis-Vergiftung

METASTASIS
MÉTASTASES
METASTASIERUNG, Verlagerung von
Krankheitsprozessen
ABROT., agar.$^{1', 7}$, apis^3, ant-c.$^{1', 3, 6}$,
ars.$^{1', 3, 6}$, asaf.^{6}, cact.^{6}, calc.^{3}, carb-v.,
caul.^{6}, cimic.$^{6, 7}$, colch., crot-t.^{6}, cupr.,
dig.^{6}, dulc.^{6}, graph.^{6}, hep.^{3}, kali-bi.^{6},
kalm.^{6}, kreos.^{3}, lac-c., lach.$^{3, 6}$, lith-c.^{6},
lyc.^{3}, mag-c.^{10}, merc.^{3}, mez.^{6}, nat-m.^{6},
nat-p.^{15}, nux-v.^{6}, plat.^{6}, puls., sang.,
senec.^{6}, sep.$^{3, 6}$, sil.^{3}, sulph., zinc.^{6}

MINING, ill effects of^8
MINEURS, maladies des
BERGLEUTEN, Krankheiten bei
card-m., nat-ar., sulph.$^{1'}$

stone-cutters/tailleurs de pierre/
   Steinstaub

moistening affected part am. see
bathing–affectet am.

MOON agg., **full** (Kent's Rep.1897) ✱
LUNE agg., **pleine**
MOND, Vollmond agg.
alum., apis^7, arn.$^{3, 6}$, ARS.$^{3, 7}$,
bar-c.^{7}, bell.$^{3, 7}$, brom.^{3}, bry.^{7}, calc.,
calc-p.^{7}, canth.^{7}, caust.$^{3, 6, 7}$, cina^3,
croc.$^{3, 6}$, cupr.^{7}, cycl., fl-ac.^{3}, gels.^{7},
graph., hep.^{7}, ign.^{7}, kali-bi.$^{6, 7}$,
kali-n., lach.^{2}, led.^{7}, LYC.$^{3, 7}$, merc.^{7},
nat-c., nat-m., nit-ac.^{7}, nux-v.^{7},
ph-ac., PHOS.$^{3, 7}$, psor.$^{3, 7}$, PULS.^{7},
rhus-t.^{7}, sabad., sang.^{7}, sep., sil.,
sol-m.^{7}, sol-t-ae.^{7}, spong., sul-i.^{7},
sulph., teucr., thuj.^{7}, thuj.^{7},
verat-v.^{7}

convulsions–moon/convulsions–
   lune/Konvulsionen–Vollmond

decreasing m. agg.
dernier quartier agg.
abnehmender M. agg.
alum.^{15}, apis^7, ars.^{7}, bry.^{7}, calc.^{7},
clem.^{3}, daph.$^{2-4}$, dulc., gels.^{7},
kali-bi.^{7}, kali-c.^{7}, lach.^{7}, lyc.$^{3, 7}$,
merc.^{7}, merc-i-r.^{7}, nat-m.^{7}, nux-v.^{7},
ph-ac.^{7}, phel.$^{2, 3}$, PHOS.^{7}, phyt.^{7},
plat.^{7}, PULS.^{7}, RHUS-T.^{7}, SEP.$^{3, 7}$,

---

sil.^{7}, sul-i.^{7}, SULPH.$^{3, 7}$, tab.^{7}, thuj.^{7},
tub.^{7}, verat.^{7}

new m. agg. ✱
nouvelle l. agg.
Neumond agg.
agar.^{7}, alum., am-c., apis^7, arg-n.^{7},
arn.$^{3, 6, 7}$, ARS.$^{3, 7}$, ars-i.^{7}, bell.^{7},
bry.^{7}, bufo, calc., calc-p.^{7}, canth.^{7},
caust., chin.^{7}, cina^3, clem., croc.$^{3, 6}$,
cupr., daph., graph.^{7}, hep.^{7},
kali-bi.$^{6, 7}$, lach.^{7}, lyc., merc.^{7},
merc-c.^{7}, merc-i-f.^{7}, nat-m.^{7},
NUX-V.$^{3, 7}$, PHOS.^{7}, phyt.^{7},
PULS.^{7}, RHUS-T.$^{3, 7}$, sabad., sep.,
sil., SULPH.^{7}, thuj.$^{3, 7}$

chorea–moon/chorée–lune/
   Chorea–Neumond
convulsions–moon/convulsions–
   lune/Konvulsionen–Neumond

increasing m. agg.
premier quartier agg.
zunehmender M. agg.
alum.$^{3, 6, 7}$, apis^7, arn., ARS.$^{3, 7}$,
arum-t.^{7}, bell.^{7}, bry.$^{3, 7}$, CALC.^{7},
calc-p.^{7}, caust.^{7}, chin.^{2}, cimic.^{7},
clem., cupr.$^{3, 7}$, graph.^{7}, ign.^{7},
kali-bi.^{7}, kali-c.^{7}, lach.^{7}, lyc.$^{3, 7}$,
med.^{7}, merc-i-f.^{7}, nat-m.$^{3, 7}$, nit-ac.^{7},
nux-v.^{7}, phel.$^{2, 3, 7}$, PHOS.^{7},
PULS.^{7}, rhus-t.^{7}, sang.^{7}, SEP.^{7}, sil.^{7},
staph.^{3}, sul-i.^{7}, SULPH.^{7},
thuj.$^{3, 4, 6, 7}$

MOONLIGHT agg.
CLAIR DE LUNE agg.
MONDSCHEIN agg.
ant-c., bell., calc.$^{3, 6}$, ovi-p.^{7}, sep.^{3},
sulph.^{3}, thuj.

morphinism/morphinomanie/
   Morphinismus see Vol. I

MOTION agg.
MOUVEMENT agg.
BEWEGUNG agg.
abrot., achy.^{14}, acon., adlu.^{14},
aesc.^{8}, agar., agav-t.^{14}, agn., aloe,

aml-ns.[8], anac., **ang.**[2, 3], ange-s.[14],
anh.[8, 10, 14], ant-c., ant-t., **apis,** apoc.,
aq-mar.[14], arg-m.[2, 3], arg-n.[7], **arn.,**
ars., ars-h., **ars-i.,** asaf., **asar.,**
aspar., aster.[14], **aur.,** aur-ar.[1'],
aur-i.[1'], aur-s.[1'], bapt., **bar-c.,**
bar-i.[1'], bar-s.[1'], **BELL., berb.,**
beryl[14], **BISM.,** bor., bov.,
BRY., bufo, **but-ac.**[8], **cact.,**
cadm-met.[10, 14], cadm-s., **calad.,**
calc., calc-ar.[8], **calc-p., calc-s.,**
calc-sil.[1'], **camph.,** cann-i., **cann-s.,**
canth., caps., carb-an., carb-v.,
carbn-s., card-m., caust., cean.[8],
cham., **CHEL., CHIN.,** chin-ar.,
chion., cic., **cimic., cimx.,** cina,
cinnb., clem., coc-c., **COCC., coff.,**
coff-t.[7], **COLCH., COLOC., con.,**
cortico.[9], **croc., crot-h.,** crot-t.,
cupr., cupr-ar., cur.[7], **cycl.**[2, 3],
des-ac.[14], **dig.,** dros., dulc.[2, 3], elaps[3],
eup-per., euph., equis.[8], **ferr.,** ferr-i.,
ferr-p.[1', 3, 8], **fl-ac., foll.**[14], form.,
gels., get.[8], **glon., graph., GUAJ.,**
guat.[14], hed.[9], **hell.,** helon.[8], **hep.,**
hip-ac.[9, 14], hist.[10, 14], hoit.[14], hyos.,
iber.[8], ign., **iod., ip., iris,** jac.,
jug-c.[8], jug-r.[7], **kali-bi., kali-c.**[2, 3, 6],
kali-m.[1', 8], **kali-n.,** kali-p., kali-sil.[1'],
kalm., kreos.[2, 3], lac-c.[1', 8], **lac-d.**[1', 7],
lach., lat-m.[14], laur., **LED.,** lina.[8],
lob.[8], **lyc.**[2, 3], lycpr.[8], lycps., mag-c.,
mag-m., **mag-p., mang.,** med.[1],
meli., meny., meph.[4], **MERC.,**
merc-c., mez., mim-p.[14], mosch.,
mur-ac.[2, 3], naja[3, 14], **nat-ar.,**
nat-c.[2, 3, 4, 16], **nat-m., nat-p., nat-s.,**
nat-sil.[1'], nit-ac., nux-m., **NUX-V.,**
ol-an., olnd., onop.[14], **onos.,** op.,
osm., ovi-p.[7], **ox-ac.,** pall., par.,
paro.[14], penic.[13, 14], **petr.,** ph-ac.,
phos., phyt., pic-ac.[8], plan.[12],
plat., **plb.,** psil.[14], **psor.,** ptel.,
puls., puls-n.[8], pulx.[8], pyrog.[3],
RAN-B., ran-s., **rheum,** rhod.[2, 3],
rhus-t.[2, 3], rumx., ruta[2, 3, 8], sabad.,
SABIN., samb., sal-ac.[6], **sang.,**
sanic., sarcol-ac.[9, 14], **sars.**[2, 3], **sec.,**
sel., senec., seneg., **sep.,** sieg.[10],
SIL., spig., spong., **squil., stann.,**
staph., still.[8], stram., stront-c.,
stroph-s.[9, 14], stry.[8], sul-ac., sul-i.[1'],

SULPH., syph.[7], tab.[3, 8], tarax.,
tarent.[3, 6, 8], teucr., thea[8], **ther.,**
thuj., thymol.[8], tril., trios.[14], tub.[3, 7],
valer.[2, 3], **verat.,** verb., vib.[3],
viol-o., viol-t., **visc.,** x-ray[14], **zinc.,**
zinc-p.[1], zinc-val.[3]

am.
abrot.[8], **acon.,** aesc.[3, 8], **agar.,**
agn.[3], **aloe, alum., alumn.**[2], **am-c.,**
am-m., ambr., **anac., ang.**[2, 3],
ant-c.[2, 3], ant-t., apis[6], aran-ix.[10, 14],
arg-m., arg-n., arist-cl.[10, 14], arn.,
ars., ars-s-f.[1'], asaf., asar., **atro,**
AUR., AUR-M., aur-m-n., bar-c.,
bar-m., bell.[2, 3, 6, 8], bell-p.[8, 10, 14],
benz-ac., **bism.,** bor., bov., **brom.,**
bry.[2, 3], cact.[6], calc., calc-p., cann-s.[3],
canth., **CAPS.,** carb-ac., carb-an.,
carb-v., **caust.,** cham., chel.[3], chin.,
chin-ar., cic., cina, coc-c.[2, 8],
coca, **cocc., coloc., com., CON.,**
cupr., **CYCL.,** dig.[3], **dios.,** dros.,
DULC., erig.[10], **EUPH.,** euphr.,
FERR., ferr-ar., ferr-p., **fl-ac.**[3, 6-8],
gamb., gels., glon.[3], graph.[3], guaj.,
hed.[10, 14], hell.[3], **helon.**[3, 8], hep., hom.[8],
hyos., ign., **indg., iod.**[3], iris[8],
kali-br.[6], **kali-c., kali-i., kali-n.,**
kali-p., **KALI-S., kreos.,** lach., laur.,
led.[3], **lil-t.,** lith-c., lith-lac.[8], lob.,
LYC., mag-c., mag-m., magn-gr.[8],
mand.[9], mang., **meny., med.,**
merc.[2, 3], **merc-c., merc-i-f.,** mez.[2, 3],
mosch., mur-ac., **nat-c.,** nat-m.[2, 3],
nat-s., nit-ac., nux-m., olnd., op.,
par., parth.[8], petr., **ph-ac.,** phel.[4],
phos.[2, 3], pip-m.[8], **plat.,** plb.[2, 3],
pneu.[14], **PULS., PYROG.,** rad-br.[8],
raja-s.[14], **rat., RHOD., RHUS-T.,**
ruta, SABAD., sabin.[2, 3], **SAMB.,**
sars.[2, 3], **sel.,** seneg., **sep.,** sel.[2, 3],
spig., spong.[2, 3], **stann.,** staph.[2, 3],
stel.[8], **stront-c.,** sul-ac., **SULPH.,**
syph.[8], **TARAX., TARENT.,** teucr.,
thala.[14], thiop.[14], thuj., **tub.,**
VALER., ven-m.[14], verat., **verb.,**
vib., viol-o.[3], **viol-t.,** visc.[14], xero.[8],
zinc., zinc-p.[1']

affected part agg., of
affectées agg., des parties
leidender Teile agg.

    acon., **AESC.**, agar., am-c., anac.,
    ang.[3], **ant-t., ARN., ars.**, asaf.,
    asar., bar-c., **bell., BRY.**, bufo[3],
    camph., **cann-s., caps.**, caust.,
    CHAM., chel., **chin.**, cic., cimic.,
    clem., **cocc.**, coff., **COLCH.,**
    coloc., com., con., croc., cupr.,
    dig., ferr-ar., form., **gels., glon.**,
    guaj., hep., ign., iod., kali-bi.[3],
    kali-c., **kalm., lach., LED.**, mag-c.,
    mang., meny., **merc., mez.**, nat-c.,
    nat-m., nux-m., nux-v., olnd.,
    petr., **phos.**, phyt., plat., plan.[12],
    puls., ran-b., rheum, **RHUS-T.,**
    rhod., rumx., ruta, sabad., **sabin.**,
    samb., **sang., sars.**, sel., sep.,
    sil., SPIG., stann., staph., **sulph.**,
    thuj., zinc.

am.

    abrot., acon., **agar.**, agn., **am-m.**,
    ang.[3], apis[3], arn., **ars.**, ars-i.,
    asaf., asar., **aur.**, bell.[3], calc.,
    CAPS., cham., **chin.**, cina, **con.**,
    croc., **DULC., euph., FERR.**,
    hyos.[3], **kali-bi.**, kali-c., lith-c.[3],
    lyc., mag-c., **mag-m.**, meny.,
    mosch., mur-ac., nat-c., **ph-ac.**,
    PULS., rhod., RHUS-T., sabad.,
    samb., sep., squil., stann.,
    stront-c., **SULPH.** tarax., thuj.,
    valer., verb., viol-t.

after m. agg.
après le m. agg.
nach B. agg.

    AGAR., am-c., anac., arn., **ARS.**,
    aspar., calad., camph., **CANN-S.**,
    carb-v., caust., cocc., coff., **croc.**,
    dros., hydr.[3], **hyos.**, iod., **kali-c.**,
    laur., merc., **nit-ac.**, nux-v., olnd.,
    phos., plb., **PULS., RHUS-T., ruta,**
    sabin., sep., spig., **SPONG.,**
    STANN., staph., **stram.**, sul-ac.,
    VALER., zinc.

aversion to
aversion pour
Abneigung gegen

abrot.[7], **ACON.**, agar.[11], alco.[11],
aloe[1',11], alum., alum-p.[1'], alum-sil.[1'],
am-c., ambr., anac., ant-c., ant-t.,
arn., **ARS.**, ars-s-f.[1'], asar., atro.[11],
bapt.[3,11], **bar-c., BELL.**, bol-la.[11],
bor., **BRY.**, cadm-s., **CALAD.,**
CALC., CALC-S., cann-i.[11], canth.,
caps., carb-an., carb-v., carbn-s.,
caust., cham., **chel., chin.**,
chin-ar., cina, coc-c.[11], **cocc.**, coff.,
colch.[1'], **con.**, croc., cupr., **cycl.**,
dig., dios.[11], dros., dulc., eryt-j.[11],
ferr., ferr-i., **gels.**, gins.[11], **graph.**,
GUAJ., ham.[11], hell.[4], hydr-ac.[11],
hyos., hyper.[2], **ign.**, iod.[4], ip.,
kali-ar., **kali-bi., kali-c.**, kali-p.,
kali-sil.[1'], **LACH.**, led., lob.[11], **lyc.**,
mag-c., mag-m., merc., **mez.**,
mur-ac., myric.[11], **nat-ar.**, nat-c.,
nat-m., nit-ac., nux-m.[11], **NUX-V.**,
oena.[11], op., peti.[11], petr., **ph-ac.**,
phos., phys.[11], psor., ptel.[11], puls.,
RUTA, sang., sapin.[11], sep., **SIL.**,
stann., stront-c., **SULPH.**, tarax.,
tarent.[11], teucr., **thuj.**, zinc.,
zinc-p.[1']

at beginning of m. agg.
au début de m. agg.
am Beginn der B. agg.

    agar., am-c.[7], ant-t., asar., bry.[3],
    cact., calc., **CAPS., carb-v., caust.**,
    chin., cina, cocc., **CON.**, cupr.,
    dig.[16], dros., **EUPH., FERR.**, fl-ac.,
    graph., hecla[14], hed.[10], **kali-p.**,
    lach., led., **LYC.**, mag-c., mand.[14],
    med.[7], nit-ac., petr., **ph-ac., phos.**,
    plat., plb., **psor., PULS.**, rhod.,
    RHUS-T., ruta, **sabad.**, sabin.,
    samb., sanic.[3,7], sars., sep.[1'], **sil.**,
    stront-c.[8], **ther.**, thuj., tub.[7], valer.,
    verat., **zinc.**, zinc-p.[1']

walking – beginning / marcher –
début/Gehen – Beginn

continued m. am.
continu am.
fortgesetzte B. am.
    agar., **am-m., ambr.,** anac.[3],
    aran-ix.[10], bell-p.[10], bry., **cact.,**
    CAPS., carb-v., caust., chin., **cina,**
    cob.[3], com., **CON., cycl., dros.,**
    EUPH., FERR., FL-AC.[3], gels.,
    graph.[3], hecla[14], hed.[10], ind., iod.[10],
    iris, kali-c., **lyc.,** mag-c.[10],
    mand.[10, 14], med.[1'], plat., plb., **ptel.,**
    PULS., rauw.[14], **rhod., RHUS-T.,**
    ruta, **sabad.,** sabin., **SAMB.,** sep.,
    sil., SYPH.[7], tarax., thuj., **valer.,**
    verat., zinc.[3]

desire for[3]
désir de
Verlangen nach
    acon., agar., alum.[3, 4], am-c., **ambr.,**
    arg-m., arg-n., **arn.**[3, 4], ars.,
    ars-i.[1'], asar., aur., aur-ar.[1'], **bell.**[3, 4],
    bell-p.[10, 14], bism., bor., bry.[3, 4],
    calc.[3, 4], con., canth., cench.[1'],
    CHAM.[3, 4], **CHIN.**[3, 4], coff., coloc.,
    con., **cupr.,** euphr., **FERR.**[3, 4],
    ferr-ar.[1'], ferr-i.[1'], hyos., ign., iod.,
    ip., kali-i.[1'], kreos., lyc.[3, 4, 11],
    macro.[11], mag-c., mag-m., mang.,
    merc.[3, 4], mosch., mur-ac., nat-c.,
    nit-ac., nux-m., nux-v., op., petr.[11],
    ph-ac., phos., puls., ran-b., rhod.,
    RHUS-T., ruta, samb., sec., sep.,
    sil., squil.[3, 4], stann., staph.,
    stront-c., sul-i.[1'], sulph.[1', 3], **teucr.**
    tub.[1'], valer., verat.

open air agg., in[3]
plein air agg., en
Freien agg., im
    bell., bry., **calc.,** cocc., colch.,
    led., nux-v.

    am.[3]
        dios., **iod.,** kali-i., **lil-t.,** mag-c.,
        mag-m., **PULS.**

rapid m. am.[3]
rapide am.
schnelle B. am
    ars., aur-m., **bry., ferr.**[1'], fl-ac., sep.,
    sil., stann., sulph.

slow m. agg.[3]
lent agg.
langsame B. agg.
    sep.

    am.[3]
        agar.[3, 8], alum., ambr.[3, 8], asaf.[1'],
        aur., bell., calc.[15], coloc.,
        FERR.[1', 3, 6-8, 15], ferr-a.[8], ferr-ar.[1'],
        ferr-p.[1'], glon., kali-bi., **kali-p.,**
        mag-m., plat.[8], **PULS.**[1', 3, 7, 15],
        stann.[8], **sulph.**[15], sumb.,
        SYPH.[3, 7, 15], tarent., zinc.[8]

violent m. agg.[3]
violent agg.
heftige B. agg.
    acon., arn., ars., bry., calc.,
    camph., lyc., mag-c., nux-v.,
    rhus-t., ruta, sep., sil., sul-ac.,
    sulph.

    am.[3]
        aesc.[3, 6], **ARS., BROM.,** dulc.,
        phys., **SEP.**[3, 6], sil., **sul-ac.**[3, 6]

MOUNTAIN sickness[7]
MAL DE MONTAGNE, mal d'altitude
HÖHENKRANKHEIT
    acon.[2, 8], **ars.**[6-8, 12], aur., bell.,
    CALC., carb-v., caust.,
    COCA[2, 6-8, 12], con., conv., cupr.,
    gels., kola[6], **lach.,** lyc., nat-m.,
    olnd., puls., spig., verat.[12]

ascending–high/monter–haut/
Steigen–Hochsteigen

am. in mountains
am. en montagne
am. im Gebirge
    prot.[14], **syph.**[7, 8]

climbing m., ailments from[12]
alpinisme, troubles à la suite d'
Bergsteigen, Beschwerden infolge von
ars.

MUCOUS SECRETIONS increased
MUQUEUSE, hypersécrétion
SCHLEIMHAUTABSONDERUNGEN,
  vermehrte
  acet-ac., acon., agar., agn.[4],
  ALL-C., alum., alum-sil.[1'], am-c.,
  am-m., ambr., **ammc.,** ang.[3, 4],
  ant-c., ant-t., aphis[4], **arg-m., arg-n.,**
  arn., **ars.,** ars-i., arum-m.[4], asaf.[4],
  asar.; aur., aur-s.[1'], **bar-c., bar-m.,**
  bell., benz-ac., bism., bond.[11], **bor.,**
  bov., bry., **CALC.,** calc-s.[3],
  calc-sil.[1'], camph., **cann-s.,** canth.,
  caps., carb-an., **CARB-V., carbn-s.,**
  caust., cham., chel., **chin.,** chlor.[11],
  chr-ac.[11], cina, cinnb.[11], **coc-c.,**
  cocc., coff., colch., coloc., **con.,**
  cop., croc., cupr., dig., dros.,
  DULC., euph., **euphr., ferr.,** ferr-i.,
  graph., grat.[4], guaj., hell., **hep.,**
  HYDR., hyos., ign., **IOD.,** ip., iris[3],
  jab.[3], kali-ar., **KALI-BI., kali-c.,**
  kali-chl.[4], **kali-i.,** kali-m.[1'], kali-n.,
  kali-sil.[1'], kreos., **LACH.,** lact.[4],
  laur., **LYC.,** m-arct.[4], m-aust.[4],
  mag-c., mag-m., mec.[11], med.[3, 7],
  MERC., mez., mur-ac.[4, 11], myric.[2],
  nat-ar., **nat-c., nat-m., nat-s.**[3, 4],
  nicc.[4], **nit-ac., nux-m., NUX-V.,**
  olnd.[1], op.[3], **par., PETR.,** ph-ac.,
  phel.[4]**, PHOS.,** plat., plb., podo.,
  PULS., ran-b., raph.[4], rat.[4], rheum,
  rhod., **rhus-t., rumx.,** ruta, sabad.,
  sabin., **samb.,** sars., sec., sel.,
  seneg., sep., sil., sin-n.[2], spig.,
  spong.[3, 4], **squil., stann.,** staph.,
  stroph-h.[3], sul-ac., sul-i.[1'], **SULPH.,**
  TAB., tax.[11], teucr., thal.[11], thuj.,
  tong.[4], valer., verat., zinc.

  am.[3]
  apis, arg-m., arist-cl.[9, 10], ars.,
  bry.[3, 6]**,** calc., camph., cimic.[3, 6],
  cupr.[3, 6], dulc.[6], graph.[6], ip.,
  kali-bi.[6], **LACH.**[1', 3, 6, 8], lyc.,
  mosch.[6, 8], nux-v.[3, 6], ph-ac., psor.,

puls.[3, 6, 10]**,** rhus-t., senec.[6], sep.[3, 6],
sil., squil., stann.[8], stict., stram.,
SULPH.[3, 6]**,** thuj.[6], verat., **zinc.**[3, 6, 8]

leucorrhea/leucorrhée/Fluor

  acrid[4]
  âcre
  scharfe
  aesc.[7], all-s.[3], **alum., am-c.**[1', 4, 7]**,**
  am-m., anac., ant-c., arum-t.[1', 3],
  ars.[1', 3, 4]**,** ars-i.[3], **bor.,** bov., **brom.**[3]**,**
  calc., cann-s., canth., carb-an.,
  carb-v.[1', 4]**, caust.**[3]**, cham.**[3, 4]**,** chin.,
  con., euph., **ferr.,** fl-ac.[1', 7], **graph.**[3]**,**
  hep.[3, 4], **ign., iod.**[3, 4]**,** kali-c.,
  kali-i.[3, 4], **kreos.**[1', 3, 4, 7]**, lach.,**
  lyc.[3, 4]**,** m-arct., mag-c., **mag-m.,**
  mang., **merc.**[3, 4]**,** merc-c.[3], **mez.,**
  mur-ac., **nat-m.**[2, 4]**, nit-ac.**[2-4]**, nux-v.,**
  ph-ac., **phos.**[3, 4]**,** prun., **puls.,**
  rhus-t.[3], **ran-b.,** ruta, sang.[1'], **sep.**[3, 4]**,**
  sil.[3, 4]**,** spig., squil., **sul-ac.,**
  sulph.[1', 3, 4]**,** thuj.

  albuminoid[3, 4]
  albuminoïde
  eiweißähnliche
  alum.[3], am-m., berb.[3], bor., bov.[4],
  coc-c.[3], graph.[1'], grat.[1'], jatr.[4],
  kali-m.[2]**,** mez., **NAT-M.**[3]**,** pall.[3],
  petr., plat., sep.[3], stann.[3]

  bitter taste[8]
  amer, goût
  bitterer Geschmack
  aloe, cocc., **kali-bi.,** nat-m., nux-v.,
  puls.

  bland[6]
  douce
  milde
  alumn.[1'], arg-n., cycl., euphr.[3],
  hep.[3]**,** kali-i.[3], kali-m.[3], kali-s.,
  merc.[3, 6]**, PULS.**[1'-3, 6, 7]**,** sil.[3],
  sulph.[3]

  bloody[4]
  sanguinolante
  blutige
  acon.[3, 4, 6], ail.[3], aloe[3], alum.[3, 4],
  alum-sil.[1'], am-c., am-m., aphis,

arg-n.[3, 6, 7], arn.[3, 6], ars.[1', 3, 4],
ars-s-f.[1'], **asar., bar-c.**[3, 4], bar-m.[1'],
bell.[1', 3, 4], bor., brom.[3], bry.[3],
calc-s.[1', 2], **canth.**[3, 4, 6], caps.,
carb-an.[6], **carb-v.**[1', 3, 4], caust.[3, 4],
chin.[3, 4], cocc.[3, 4], cop., **crot-h.**[3, 6],
daph., dros.[3], euon., ferr.[3, 4], form.[6],
graph., ham.[1', 2], hep., iod.[3, 4],
kali-ar.[1'], kali-c., kali-chl., kali-n.,
kreos.[1', 3], **lach.**[3, 4, 6], led., lyc.[3, 4],
mag-c., mag-m., mang.[6], **merc.**[3, 4, 6],
mez., mur-ac.[3], murx., nat-m.[3, 4],
nit-ac.[1', 3, 6], nux-m., **nux-v.**[3, 4], op.,
par., petr., **phos.**[3, 4, 6], **puls.**[1', 3, 4],
sabin.[3, 4], sang.[3], **sep.**[3, 4], **sil.**[3, 4, 6],
sul-ac.[1', 3, 4], sul-i.[1'], sulph.[3, 4],
ter.[2, 6], thuj.[3, 4], verat.[3, 4], vip.,
zinc.[3, 4, 6], zinc-p.[1']

bluish[3, 4]
bleuâtre
bläuliche
ambr., ars., cupr.[3], cupr-a.[4], lach.[6]

brownish[3, 4]
brunâtre
bräunliche
am-m.[4], ambr.[3], ars., **bell.**, bism.[4],
bor., carb-v., grat.[4], nit-ac., sulph.

burning[6]
brûlante
brennende
acon., aesc., **ail.**[3, 6], all-c.[3, 6], alum.[4],
alum-p.[1'], am-c.[4, 6, 7], am-m.[4],
ars.[1', 3, 4, 6], ars-i.[6, 7], ars-s-f.[1'],
arum-t., bad., brom.[3, 6], calad.[4],
calc.[3, 4], canth., caps., carb-ac.,
carb-an.[4, 6], carb-v., cast.[4], chin.[4, 6],
chlor., cina[4], **con.**[4], crot-h., fl-ac.[1', 6],
gels.[3, 6], graph., guaj., hep., hydr.,
iod.[6], kali-c., **kali-i.**[3, 4, 6], kreos.[3, 6],
lach., lyc.[6], mag-s.[4], **merc.**[3, 6],
merc-c.[3], mez.[4], mur-ac., nat-m.,
nit-ac.[6, 7], petr., phos., phyt.,
puls.[3, 4], ran-s., **sabad.**[3, 6], sang.,
sep., sil., sin-n.[3], sul-ac.[4, 6],
sulph.[3, 4, 6, 7]

cold[1']
froide
kalte
verat.

corrosive[3]
corrosive, excoriante
ätzende
ALUM., am-c.[1', 3, 7], **am-m.,** ant-c.[4],
ARS.[1'-4, 6], ars-i.[7], **ars-s-f.**[1'], arum-t[1'],
bor., **bov.,** carb-v., **CAUST.,**
cham.[3, 4], **con.**[4], ferr.[3, 4], **HYDR.,**
ign., **iod.**[6], ip.[4], kali-ar.[1'], **kali-bi.,**
kali-i.[2, 3, 6], **kreos.**[1', 3], **lach.**[3, 4], lyc.[6],
MERC.[3, 4, 6], mez., nat-m.[3, 4, 6],
NIT-AC.[1', 3], **nux-v., phos.**[3, 4], **puls.,**
rhus-t., ruta, sep.[3, 6], **SIL.**[3, 4, 6],
staph., sul-ac.[1', 3], **sulph.**[1', 3, 4, 7],
thuj.

flocculent[3]
floconneuse
flockige
agar., ambr., kali-bi., kali-c.,
kreos., mag-c., merc., phos.,
sabad., sep., sil., sulph., thuj.

frothy[4]
spumeuse
schaumige
aphis, ars., ferr., **NAT-M.**[2], op.,
sec., sul-ac.

gelatinous[3, 4]
gélatineuse
gallertartige
aloe[2, 3], arg-m., **arg-n.**[3], bell.[3], berb.,
caust.[3], chin-s.[4], cocc.[1'], **colch.**[3],
coloc.[3], dig.[3], **hell., kali-bi.**[1', 3],
laur., podo.[3], **rhus-t.,** sabin.[3], sel.,
sep.[3]

gray[3, 4]
grise
graue
ambr., anac., **arg-m.**[1', 3, 4], ars.,
carb-an., caust., chin., cop.[4],
kali-m.[6], kreos., lach., **lyc.**[3],
mag-m., merc., sep., **sil.,** thuj.

greenish[3, 4]
verdâtre
grünliche
acon.[3], **ars.**, asaf.[4], aur.[4], bor.[4, 6],
carb-v., caust.[4], cham.[3], colch.[4],
con.[3], **dros.**, ferr., hyos.[4], ip.[3],
kali-bi.[3, 4, 7], kali-c.[4], **kali-i.**[1'-3],
kali-s.[1', 2], kreos., lach.[4], led., **lyc.**,
m-aust.[4], **mag-c.**, mang.[4], med.[3, 7],
merc., murx.[4], nat-c., nat-m.[4],
nat-s.[1', 3], nit-ac.[4], nux-v.[4], **par.**[4],
phos., **PULS.**[1', 3, 4, 6], rhus-t.,
sabad.[4], sec.[3], **sep.**, sil.[4], **stann.**,
sul-ac.[3], **sulph.**, thuj., **verat.**[3]

hard[3]
dure
harte
agar., bry., con., **KALI-BI.**, **mosch.**,
nat-c., **phos.**, **sep.**, **sil.**, stict.[6],
sulph., **thuj.**

honey-like[1']
comme du miel
honigartige
ars-i.

hot[3]
chaude
heiße
acon., **ars.**, **bell.**, bor., euphr., **iod.**,
kreos., op., **puls.**, sabin., **sulph.**

lumpy[4]
grumeleuse
klumpige
calc-s.[2], **hep.**[2], kali-c., kreos., phos.,
sabad., sabin., sin-n.[2], stann.

metallic taste[4]
métallique, goût
metallischer Geschmack
calc., cupr., ip., nux-v., rhus-t.

milky[4]
laiteuse
milchige
calc.[3, 4], carb-v., con., ferr.,
kali-m.[1', 3], kali-p.[3], lyc., nat-s.[3],
ph-ac.[3], phos., **puls.**[3, 4], sabin.,
sep.[3, 4], **sil.**, sul-ac.

musty smell[3]
moisie, odeur
schimmliger Geruch
bor.[3, 4], **carb-v.**[3, 4], **coloc.**, crot-h.,
merc., nux-v., **phos.**, **puls.**, **rhus-t.**,
stann.

offensive, fetid[6]
fétide
übelriechende, stinkende
ail., arg-n., arn., arum-t.[3],
ars.[1'-3, 4, 6], **ars-s-f.**[1'], asaf.[1', 6],
aur-s.[1'], bals-p., **BAPT.**[1'-3, 6], bell.[4],
calc.[3, 4], calc-f., calc-sil.[1'], caps.[4],
carb-ac., carb-an., **carb-v.**[1'-3, 6],
chel.[4], chin., chlor., cist.[1'], con.[4],
cop., crot-h., cupr.[4], cur.[7], echi.,
ferr.[4], fl-ac.[1', 6, 7], **graph.**[1', 2, 4, 6],
guaj.[1', 2, 6], helon., hep.[1', 3, 4, 6],
kali-ar.[1'], kali-bi., kali-br.[6], kali-i.,
kali-p.[1'], kali-perm., kali-s.,
KREOS.[1', 2, 4, 6], **LACH.**[2, 3, 6],
lyc., mag-c.[4, 10], **merc.**[2, 4, 6],
mur-ac.[4, 6], **NAT-C.**[1', 3, 4],
NIT-AC.[1'-3, 4, 6], **nux-v.**[4], petr.,
psor.[1', 3, 6, 7], puls.[1', 4], **pyrog.**[1', 3, 6],
rob.[2], sabin.[4], sang., sec.[3], **sep.**[3, 4, 6],
sil.[4, 6], stann.[4], **sulph.**[1', 3, 4], ther.,
tril.[2], vip.

purulent[3]
purulente
eitrige
aur., **CALC.**, **CON.**, cop.[4], **graph.**,
ign.[4], lyc.[6], **merc.**[3, 4, 6], nat-c.[6], **puls.**,
sep.[4], **sil.**, sulph.[7]

ropy, tenacious[4]
tenace, visqueuse
fadenziehende, zähe
acon., agn., **alum.**[4, 6], alum-p.[1'],
am-m., anac., **ant-c.**, ant-s-aur.[11],
ant-t.[3, 4], arg-m.[1', 3, 6], arg-n.[3], **ars.**,
asaf., bar-a.[6], bar-c.[4, 6], bar-m.[6],
bell., bor.[3, 6], **bov.**[2-4], bry.[3, 4, 6],
calc.[3, 4], cann-s.[4], canth.[4, 6], carb-an.,
carb-v.[4, 6], carbn-s.[1'], caust.[1', 3, 4, 6],
cham., chin., **chin-s.**, **cist.**,
coc-c.[1', 3, 6, 15], cocc., colch., con.,
croc.[3], culx.[1'], dulc.[4, 6], euphr.,
form.[6], graph.[1', 3, 4, 6], hep.,
hydr.[1'-3, 6, 15], iod., **KALI-BI.**[1'-3, 6, 7, 15],

kali-c.³, ⁴, ⁶, **kali-m.**¹', ³, kali-s.¹',
lach.³, ⁴, ⁶, lact., lap-a.³, laur., lob.,
lyc.³, m-arct., m-aust., **mag-c.,**
mag-m., **merc.**³, ⁴, **mez.**³, ⁴, myrt-c.³,
nat-c., nat-m.³, nux-v., ol-an., osm.³,
par., ph-ac., phos.³, ⁴, phyt.³, ⁶,
plat., plb.⁴, ⁶, puls.¹', ³, ⁴, **ran-b.,**
raph., rhus-t., sabad., sabin., **samb.,**
scroph-n., **seneg.,** sep., sin-n.²,
spig., spong., squil., **STANN.**³, ⁴,
staph., sul-ac.³, **sulph.,** sumb.¹²,
tab., thuj.⁶, tong., ust.³, verat.³, ⁴,
zinc.

salty taste⁴
salé, goût
salziger Geschmack
alum., **ambr., ars., bar-c.,** calc.,
chin., dros., fl-ac.⁷, **graph., iod.⁶,**
kali-i.⁶, lyc.⁴, ⁶, mag-c., mag-m.,
merc., nat-m.⁶, **nat-c.,** nux-v., **petr.,**
phos., puls., samb., **sep., sil.,** stann.,
staph., sulph., zinc.

sour taste⁴
acide, goût
saurer Geschmack
calc., graph., **hep.**¹', ², ⁴, kali-c.,
kali-n., lam., mag-m., merc., nat-c.,
nat-p.⁷, nit-ac.⁷, nux-v., **plb.,** sep.,
sulph.⁴, ⁷, tarax.

suppressed
supprimée
unterdrückte
abrot.⁷, ⁸, agar.¹¹, **ant-c.²,** arist-cl.¹⁴,
ars.¹', asaf.⁶, ⁸, **ASAR.,** aur-m.⁸,
bar-c.⁸, bell.¹', **bry.**³, ⁸, ¹², bufo¹',
calc.¹', carb-v.¹', ⁸, **dulc.**³, ⁶,
graph.¹', ⁸, **lach.**³, ⁶, ⁸, led.¹², **lob.⁸,**
med.⁸, merc.⁶, ⁸, mill.⁶, **mosch.²,**
nux-v.³, ⁶, plb.⁶, **psor.⁸, puls.**³, ⁶, ⁷,
sanic.⁸, senec.⁶, **sil.**¹', ³, ⁸,
STRAM.², ³, ⁶, ⁸,¹¹, **sulph.**¹', ³, ⁶, ⁸,
verat.³, viol-o.¹², zinc.⁶⁻⁸

sweetish taste⁴
douceâtre, goût
süßlicher Geschmack
asar., **calc.**¹', cham.¹¹, lach.⁴, ¹¹,
mag-c., merc-c., phos.¹', stann.¹'

thick, slimy⁴
épaisse
dicke, schleimige
acon., agar., **alum.,** alum-sil.¹',
am-m., ant-c., arg-m.¹', ³, ⁴, **arg-n.⁶,**
ars.³, ⁴, ars-i.¹', ars-s-f.¹', **aur-s.**¹',
bals-p.⁶, **bar-c.,** berb., bor.³, ⁴, ⁶,
calc.³, ⁴, calc-s.¹', ³, carb-an.,
carb-v.³, ⁴, carbn-s.¹', cast., caust.¹',
chin.³, cist.¹', coc-c.¹', con.³, ⁴, cop.,
croc.³, cycl.⁶, graph., helon.³, **hep.⁶,**
hydr.¹', ³, ⁶, iod., ip., **kali-bi.**¹', ³,
kali-br.⁶, **kali-i.**¹', ⁴, **kali-m.**¹', ²,
kali-s.¹', ⁶, kali-sil.¹', kreos., lac-ac.⁶,
lam., lith-c.⁶, lyc.³, ⁴, m-arct.,
mag-c.³, **mag-m.,** mag-s., mang.⁶,
merc.¹', ³, ⁶, merc-d.³, mur-ac.,
murx., **nat-c.**⁴, ⁶, nat-m.¹', ³, ⁴,
nat-s.¹', nat-sil.¹', nicc., nit-ac.,
ol-an., op., par.³, ⁴, phos.³,
PULS.¹'⁻⁴, ⁶, ruta, sabad., samb.,
sars., scroph-n., sec., sel., seneg.,
sil.¹', ³, ⁴, staph., **sulph.**¹', ³, ⁴, tong.,
tub.⁷, zinc., zing.

thin⁴
fluide
dünnflüssige
ambr., ant-t., **ars.**¹', ⁶, **ars-s-f.**¹',
asaf.⁶, asar., **bell.**¹', ⁴, bor., bov.,
calc., canth., caps., **carb-v.**¹', ⁴,
caust., colch., **con.,** ferr., **fl-ac.**¹', ⁶,
gels.⁶, **graph., kali-i.**², ⁴, kali-n.,
kali-s.¹', laur., lyc., **mag-c.,** mez.,
mur-ac.⁶, nat-m.⁴, ⁶, **NIT-AC.**¹', ², ⁶,
nux-v., ol-an., **puls.**¹, ⁴, rhus-t.,
seneg., **sil.⁶,** stann., staph.,
sul-ac.¹', ⁴, ter.⁴, ⁶, thuj.⁶

transparent⁴
transparente
durchsichtige
aesc.⁷, alum., cast., crot-h., ferr-m.,
fl-ac.⁷, graph., kali-i., mag-s., mang.,
NAT-M.², ⁴, phos., puls., sabad.,
sep., sil., stann., sul-ac.

urinous odor³
urine, odeur d'
Uringeruch, mit
benz-ac., canth., **coloc.,** nat-m.,
nit-ac., ol-an., sec., urt-u.

vicarious[3]
vicariante
vikariierende
    bry., con., dig., ferr., ham., **lach.**,
    lycps., mill., nux-v., **PHOS.**, **puls.**,
    sec., senec., **sep.**, sulph.

watery[4]
aqueuse
wäßrige
    acon.[6], aesc.[7], **agar.**, alum., **am-c.**,
    am-m., ambr., ant-c., arg-m.,
    ars.[3, 4, 6], **asaf.**[1', 3], asar., bell.,
    bov., brom.[6], calc., cann-s.,
    carb-an., **carb-v.**, cast., **caust.**[3],
    cham.[3, 4], **chin.**, chlor[6], clem., coff.,
    con., crot-h.[3], cupr.[3], elat.[2], fl-ac.[1'],
    gamb.[3], **gels.**[2], **graph.**[3, 4], grat.[3],
    guaj., ign., iod., iris[3], kali-i.[3, 4, 6],
    kali-n., **kali-s.**[1'], kreos.[1', 4], **lach.**,
    m-arct., **mag-c.**, **mag-m.**, meny.,
    merc.[3, 4], **mez.**, murx., **mur-ac.**,
    NAT-M.[1', 2, 6], nat-s.[3], nicc., **nux-v.**,
    par., phos.[3, 4], **plb.**, **podo.**[3], puls.[1', 4],
    ran-b., rhus-t.[3, 4], sabin.[3], sec.[3],
    seneg., **sep.**, **sil.**, **squil.**, stann.,
    staph., sul-ac., **sulph.**, thuj.,
    verat.[1', 3]

white[4]
blanche
weiße
    bell.[1'], ferr., graph., grat., hell.,
    kali-m.[1', 2, 6] kali-n., kreos., lyc.,
    m-arct., mag-c., **merc.**,
    NAT-M.[1', 2, 4], nat-s.[1'], nux-v.,
    ol-an., **phos.**, prun., **puls.**, raph.,
    rat., sabin., **sep.**[1', 4], **sil.**, sul-ac.,
    tab.

yellow[4]
jaune
gelbe
    acon., agar.[2], agn., **alum.**, alum-p.[1'],
    alum-sil.[1'], alumn.[1'], am-c., am-m.,
    ambr., anac., ang., **ant-c.**, arg-m.[1', 4],
    arg-n.[6, 7], **ars.**, ars-i.', **ars-s-f.**[1'],
    aur., aur-ar.[1'], **aur-i.**[1'], **aur-s.**[1'],
    bar-c., bar-i.[1'], bar-s.[1'], **bell.**, **berb.**,
    bov., **bry.**, **calc.**, calc-s.[1'], calc-sil.[1'],
    cann-s., **canth.**, caps., **carb-an.**[3, 4],

carb-v., cast., caust., cench.[1'],
cham., **cic.**, cist.[1'], clem., con.,
cor-r., croc., cycl.[6], **daph.**, **dros.**,
dulc., **eug.**, form.[6], gran., **graph.**,
hep., **hydr.**[1', 3, 6], **iod.**, kali-ar.[1'],
kali-bi.[3, 7], **kali-c.**, **kali-m.**[1', 2], kali-n.,
kali-s.[1'-3, 6], kali-sil.[1'], **kreos.**,
lac-ac.[6], lach., **lyc.**, mag-c., mag-m.,
mag-s., mang., merc., merc-i-f.[3],
mez., mur-ac., nat-ar.[11], **nat-c.**,
nat-m., nat-p.[2], nat-s.[2, 3], **nat-sil.**[1'],
nit-ac., **nux-v.**, ol-j.[3], ph-ac., **phos.**,
prun., **puls.**[1', 4, 6], rhus-t., ruta,
sabad., sabin., sec., **sel.**, seneg.,
sep., **sil.**[1', 4], **spig.**, **stann.**, staph.,
sul-ac.[1, 4], **sul-i.**[1'], **sulph.**, sumb.[3, 12],
thuj., verat., viol-t., zinc-p.[1']

yellowish-green[1']
jaunâtre-verte
gelblich-grüne
    ars-i.[1', 3], **calc-sil.**, kali-bi.[7],
    mang.[3, 6], **merc.**[1', 3], nat-s.[1'],
    NIT-AC.[1', 2], **PULS.**[1'-3], sulph.

MUSHROOMS POISONING[7, 8]
CHAMPIGNONS, intoxication
PILZVERGIFTUNG
    absin., agar.[2, 8], ars.[7], atro., **bell.**,
    camph., pyrog.

MYATROPHY, progresse spinal[8]
AMYOTROPHIE spinale progressive
MUSKELATROPHIE, progressive
    spinale
    ars., carbn-s.[8, 12], hyper., kali-hp.,
    PHOS.[2, 8, 12], phys.[8, 12], **plb.**[1', 2, 8, 12],
    sec.

MYXEDEMA[14]
MYXOEDÈME
MYXÖDEM
    ars.[2, 7], cortico., dor.[12], penic., sulfa.,
    thyr.[7, 8, 12]

NARCOTICS agg.
NARCOTIQUES, agg. par les
NARKOTIKA agg.

acet-ac.[8, 12], acon., agar., am-c.[3], apom.[8], ars., aur., **aven.**[6, 8], **BELL.,** bry., calc., **camph.**[6, 8], cann-i.[8], canth., carb-v., caust., **CHAM.,** chin., cic.[3, 6], cimic.[8], **COFF.,** colch., croc., cupr., **dig.,** dulc., euph., **ferr., graph.,** hep., **hyos.,** ign., **ip.,** kali-perm.[6], **LACH.,** lob.[7], **lyc.,** macro.[8], mag-s.[9], merc., mosch., mur-ac.[3, 6, 8], nat-c., nat-m., nat-p.[3, 6, 7], nit-ac., nux-m., **NUX-V., op.,** ox-ac.[7], oxyg.[12], passi.[6], ph-ac., phenob.[14], phos., plat., plb., **puls.,** rhus-t., seneg., **sep.,** staph., sulph., thuj.[8], **valer.,** verat., zinc.

ailments from[12]
troubles à la suite de
Beschwerden infolge von
ip., oxyg., verat.

desire for[11]
désir de
Verlangen nach
buth-a.[9], op., tab.

Vol. I: *morphinism/morphino-
manie/Morphinismus*

NECROSIS bones
NÉCROSE des os
KNOCHENNEKROSE

ang.[6, 8], aran.[6], **arg-m.**[6, 8], **ARS.,** asaf., **aur.**[3, 6], aur-i.[8], **aur-m.**[2, 8], bac.[12], bell., both.[11, 12], **calc.**[2, 6, 8], **calc-f.**[2, 6, 8], calc-i.[3, 6], calc-hp.[6, 8], calc-p.[6, 8], calc-sil.[8], caps.[6], carb-ac., carb-an.[6], chin.[6, 8], **cist.**[6], con., euph., **FL-AC.**[1', 2, 6-8], graph.[6, 8], hecla[6, 8], **hep.**[1', 6, 8], **iod.**[3, 6, 8], kali-bi.[6, 8], kali-c.[6], kali-i.[6, 8], kreos., lach.[6, 8], lap-a.[6], lyc.[6], mang.[1'], med.[8], **merc., merc-c.,** mez.[1', 6, 8], **nat-sil-f.**[8], **nit-ac.**[3, 6, 8], ph-ac., **phos.,** plat.[6], plat-m.[8], plb., psor.[6], puls.[3], rad-br.[3], **sabin.,** sal-ac.[2], sec., sil., staph.[8], stront-c.[6], sul-ac.[8, 12],

sulph., symph.[8], syph.[8], teucr.[6], thea[8], ther., thuj., **tub.**[6, 8], vitr.[8]

*caries/carie/Knochenkaries
softening/ostéomalacie/Knochen-
erweichung*

NOISES am.[1']
BRUITS am.
GERÄUSCHE am.

apoc., aur-ar., calad.[2], calc.[3], graph.[3], hell.[3], kali-ar., mag-p., med., puls.[3], pyrog., stram.[3], tarent.

Vol. I: *sensitive – noise/sensible –
bruits/empfindlich – Geräusche*

NUMBNESS externally
ENGOURDISSEMENT externe
TAUBHEIT, äußerliche

abrot., absin., acet-ac.[11], **acon.,** acon-f.[11, 12], aesc.[3, 6], ail., agar., aloe[3, 6], alum., alum-p.[1'], alum-sil.[1', 8], alumn.[1'], am-c., am-m., **ambr., ANAC.,** ang.[3, 4], anh.[9], ant-c., **ant-t., apis,** aran.[6], aran-ix.[9], **arg-m.**[1'-3, 6], **arg-n.,** arn., ars., ars-i., asaf., asar., aur., **bapt., bar-c.,** bar-m., **bell., BERB.,** bism., bov., brom., bry., bufo, cact., caj., calc., **calc-p.**[8], calc-sil.[1'], camph., cann-i., cann-s., canth., caps.[3], carb-ac., **carb-an., carb-v., CARBN-S., caust.,** cedr., **cham., chel.,** chin., chlor., **cic.,** cimic., cinnb., cob-n.[9], coca, **cocain.**[8], **COCC.,** cod.[8, 11, 12], coff.[3], colch., coloc., **CON.,** conin.[12], croc., **crot-c., crot-h.,** crot-t.[4], cupr., cur., cycl.[3, 4], dig., dios., dulc., euph.[3], euphr., elaps, ferr., fl-ac., form.[6], gast.[11], **gels., glon., gnaph., GRAPH., guaj.**[2, 3, 4], **hell., helo.**[8, 12], hep.[3], hydr-ac., **HYOS., hyper., ign.,** iod., ip., irid.[8, 12], iris, kali-ar.[1'], kali-bi.[3], kali-br., **KALI-C., kali-fcy., kali-n.,** kali-p., kalm., keroso.[11], kreos.[3], lach., lath.[6], laur., **led.,** lepi.[11], **LYC.,** mag-m., mag-s.[9], mand.[10],

mang.[3, 6], **merc., mez.**[3, 4, 6],
mosch., mur-ac.[3], naja[3],
nat-m.[2, 3, 4], nit-ac.[3], **nux-m.,**
nux-v., OLND., onos., **OP., ox-ac.,**
oxyt., par., petr., **PH-AC., PHOS.,**
phys., phyt.[6], **pic-ac., plat., PLB.,**
puls., raph.[8, 11, 12], rheum[3, 4],
rhod., **rhus-t.,** samb.[3, 6], sang.[3],
SEC., sep., sil., spig., spong.,
stann.[3, 8], staph., **STRAM.,**
stront-c.[3, 6], sul-ac.[3], sulph., tab.,
tanac.[11], tang.[11], teucr.[3, 4], thal.[8],
thea, thuj.[3, 4, 6], thymol.[9], **urt-u.,**
valer., verat., verat-v., verb.,
vip.[11], **zinc.,** zinc-p.[1']

night[16]/nuit/nachts
　sil.

　on waking[16]
　au réveil
　beim Erwachen
　　mez.

alternating
　with hypersensitiveness[3]
alternant avec hypersensibilité
abwechselnd mit Überempfindlich-
　keit
　　plat.

bruised part, in the
contuse, dans la partie
geprellten Teil, im
　　arn.

climacteric period, during
ménopause, pendant la
Klimakterium, im
　　cimic.

epilepsy, before
épileptiques, avant les attaques
epileptischen Anfällen, vor
　　bufo

feels neither heat nor cold[3']
sent ni le chaud ni le froid, ne
fühlt weder Wärme noch Kälte
　　berb.

left half of body
moitié gauche du corps, de la
linken Körperhälfte, der
　caust.[1], mez.[16], xan.[12]

right half of body[3]
moitié droite du corps, de la
rechten Körperhälfte, der
　ars., lyc.[16]

whole body
corps entier, du
ganzen Körpers, des
　acon.[11], apis[11], arg-n., asc-t.[11],
　bar-m.[1], bell.[11], caj.[11], caps.[16],
　cedr., chel.[16], crot-c.[11], gels.[11],
　gymno.[11], kali-bi.[11], **KALI-BR.,**
　kreos.[11], lyss., merc.[11], nitro-o.[11],
　nux-v.[16], OLND.[1], **ox-ac.,**
　pic-ac.[11], tarent.[11], tab.[11]

glands, in
glandes, des
Drüsen, der
　anac., asaf., bell., cocc., con., lyc.,
　plat., puls., rhus-t., sep., sil., spong.

internally
interne
innerliche
　acon.[3], aloe[3], alum.[3], am-c., ambr.,
　ang.[3], ant-c.[3], **ant-t.**[3], arg-n.[3], **ars.,**
　asaf., asar.[3], aur.[3], bar-c., **bell.,**
　bism.[3], bor.[3], **bov., bry.**[3], bufo[3],
　calad.[3], calc., camph.[3], cann-s.[3],
　CANTH.[3], caps.[3], carb-an., carb-v.[3],
　carbn-s.[3], caust., cham., chel.[3], chin.,
　cic.[3], cina, cocc.[3], coff., colch.,
　coloc.[3], con., croc.[3], crot-t., cupr.,
　dig., dulc.[3], euph.[3], ferr., **GELS.,**
　glon.[3], graph., **hell.**[3], hep.[3], **hyos.,**
　ign., iod.[3], ip.[3], **kali-br.,** kali-c.,
　kali-n.[3], kreos.[3], lach.[3], laur., lyc.,
　mag-c., mag-m., mang.[3], meny.[3],
　merc., merc-c.[3], mez.[3], mosch.[3],
　mur-ac., nat-c.[3], nat-m., nit-ac.,
　nux-m., **NUX-V.**[3], olnd., **op.,** par.[3],
　petr., ph-ac.[3], phos., **PLAT.,** plb.,
　podo.[3], puls., ran-b., ran-s.[3], rheum,
　rhod.[3], rhus-t.[3], ruta[3], sabad.[3],
　sabin.[3], sars., sec.[3], seneg., sep.[3],
　sil., **spig.,** spong.[3], squil.[3], stann.,

staph.[3], stram., stront-c., sul-ac.[3],
sulph.[3], tarax.[3], teucr.[3], thuj., valer.,
verat., verb.[3], viol-o.[3], zinc.[3]

lower half of body, of[3]
moitié inférieure du corps, de la
unteren Körperhälfte, der
  spong.

pains, after[3]
douleurs, après des
Schmerzen, nach
  acon., agar., graph., mez., plat.

  from[3]/par/durch
    cham., **coloc.,** kalm., plat., puls.,
    rhus-t.

parts, lain on
couché, sur la partie sur laquelle
  on est
Teile, auf denen man liegt
  ambr., am-c., **arn.**[3], ars., **bar-c.,**
  bufo[3], **calc.,** calc-sil.[1'], carb-an.[3],
  carb-v., carbn-s., chin.[3, 15], cop.,
  graph., ign., kali-c., **lach.,** mag-c.[3],
  nat-m., pall.[7], **phos., PULS.,**
  RHUS-T., sep.[7], sil., sumb., zinc.

single parts, in
certaines parties, de
einzelner Teile
  acon., agar., alum., alum-p.[1'],
  alum-sil.[1'], am-c., am-m., **ambr.,**
  anac., ang.[3], anh.[9], ant-c., **ant-t.,**
  aran-ix.[9], **arg-m., arg-n.,** arn., ars.,
  ars-i., asaf., asar., aur., aur-ar.[1'],
  aur-i.[1'], aur-s.[1'], **bar-c.,** bar-s.[1'],
  bell., bor., bov., bry., cadm-s.[1', 7],
  calc., calc-i.[1'], **calc-p.,** calc-sil.[1'],
  camph., cann-s., canth., caps.,
  CARB-AN., carb-v., CARBN-S.,
  caust., **cham.,** chel., **chin.,** cic., cina,
  COCC., colch., **coloc.,** con., **CROC.,**
  dig., dros., dulc., euph., euphr.,
  ferr., ferr-ar.[1'], ferr-p., **GRAPH.,**
  guaj., hep., hyos., **ign.,** iod., ip.,
  kali-ar., **KALI-C., kali-fcy.,**
  kali-m.[1'], **kali-n.**[1], kali-p., kali-s.[1'],
  kreos., laur., led., **LYC.,** mag-c.,
  mag-m., mang., **MERC.,** mez.,
  mosch., **mur-ac.,** nat-c., **nat-m.,**

nat-p., nit-ac., **nux-v.,** olnd., op.,
par., petr., ph-ac.[7], **phos.,** plat., plb.,
PULS., rheum, rhod., RHUS-T.,
sabad., sabin., samb., **sars., sec.,**
sep., SIL., spig., spong., squil.,
stann., staph., **stram.,** sul-ac.,
sul-i.[1'], **sulph.,** teucr., thuj., valer.,
verat., zinc., ZINC-P.[1']

spots, in
localisé
Stellen, an kleinen
  cadm-s.[7], caust.[7], **lyc., plat.**

suffering parts, of
parties souffrantes, des
leidender Teile
  acon., alum., alum-sil.[1'], **agar.**[3],
  ambr., **anac.,** ang.[3], ant-t., aran.[3],
  arn., **ars.,** ars-i., **asaf.,** aur., aur-ar.[1'],
  aur-i.[1'], bell., bor., bov., bry., calc.,
  calc-sil.[1'], cann-s., carb-an., carb-v.,
  caust., **CHAM.,** chel., chin., cic.,
  cina, **cocc.,** coff., colch., coloc.,
  CON., croc., cupr., cycl., dig., dulc.,
  elaps, euphr., ferr., ferr-ar., ferr-p.,
  gnaph., graph., hell., hep., hyos.,
  ign., iod., kali-c., **kali-n.**[1], **KALM.**[3],
  kreos., **lyc.,** mag-m., mang.[3], merc.,
  mez., mur-ac., nat-m., nux-m.,
  nux-v., **olnd.,** petr., ph-ac., phos.,
  PLAT., PLB., PULS., rheum, rhod.,
  rhus-t., ruta, samb., sec., sep., sil.,
  spong., stann., staph., stram.,
  stront-c., sul-ac., sul-i.[1'], sulph.,
  thuj., verat., verb., viol-o., zinc.

  bruised parts
  contuses, des parties
  geprellten, gequetschten Teilen,
    in den
    arn.

unilateral[3]
unilatéral
einseitige
  ars., caust., chel., **COCC.,** nat-m.,
  phos., puls.

upper half of body, of
moitié supérieure du corps, de la
oberen Körperhälfte, der
  bar-c.

NURSING, suckling agg.[3, 13]*
ALLAITER agg.
STILLEN agg.
abrot.[6], acon., agn., ant-t.[13], ars.[3],
bell., bor.[3, 6, 13], **BRY.**[3, 6, 13],
CALC.[3, 6, 13], **calc-p.**[3, 6, 13], carb-an.,
carb-v.[3, 6, 13], cast-eq.[13], caust.[13],
cham., chel., **chin.**[3, 6, 13], chin-ar.[6],
chion.[12], cina, **cocc.**[2], con., crot-h.[2],
crot-t.[13], **dulc.**, ferr., graph., ign.,
iod., ip., **kali-c.**[3, 6, 13], lac-c.[13],
lach., lyc., **merc.**, mill.[13], nat-c.,
nat-m., **nit-ac.**[13], nux-v., olnd.[3, 6, 13],
ph-ac.[3, 6, 7, 13], phel.[3, 6, 13], phos.,
PHYT.[3, 6, 13], **PULS.**[3, 6, 13], rheum,
rhus-t., samb., sec., sel.[3], **SEP.**[3, 6, 13],
SIL., spig., squil.[3], stann., **staph.**[3, 6],
stram., **sulph.**[3, 6, 13], zinc.[3, 6, 13]

loss – fluids / perte – fluides vitaux /
Blutverlust – Säfteverlust
trembling–nursing/tremblement–
allaitement/Zittern–Stillen
weakness – lactation / faiblesse –
lactation / Schwäche – Stillen

NURSLINGS[13]
NOURRISSONS, enfants au sein,
  maladies des
SÄUGLINGEN, Krankheiten bei
acon., aeth., ant-c., ant-t., **arn., ars.,**
bell., BOR., BRY., CALC., calc-p.,
camph., carb-v., CHAM., chin., cina,
coloc., crot-t., dulc., ferr., graph.,
hep., ign., **ip.**, kali-bi.[3], kali-c., lach.,
lyc., mag-c., merc., nat-c., nat-m.,
NAT-P., nux-v., OP., ph-ac., phos.,
podo., psor., PULS., rheum, rhus-t.,
samb., sec., sil., stann., staph., stram.,
verat., sulph., zinc.

OBESITY
OBÉSITÉ
FETTLEIBIGKEIT
acon.[3], adon.[6], agar., ail.[12], alco.[11],
all-s.[7, 8], **am-br.**[2, 8, 12], **am-c.**[3, 6–8, 12, 16],
am-m., ambr., **ang.**[2, 3], **ant-c.**,
ant-t.[2, 3], apis[3], aran-ix.[10],
arist-cl.[9, 10, 14], arn.[2, 3], **ars.**[2, 5, 8],

asaf.[1], **aur.**, bac.[12], bar-c., **bell.**[2, 3],
blatta[6, 8, 12], bor., brom.[3, 11], bry.,
bufo[3], calad.[6], **CALC.**, calc-a.[6],
calc-ar., calc-caust.[6], **calo.**[8].
camph., canth., **CAPS.**, carb-v.[3, 8],
caust.[3], cham.[2, 3], chin., chlorpr.[12],
cic.[3], cimic.[10, 14], clem.[2, 3], **coc-c.**[2],
coca[12], cocc., coloc.[2, 3, 8], con.,
cortiso.[14], **croc.**[2, 3, 8, 12],
crot-h.[4, 6], **cupr.**, cyna.[14], dig.[2, 3],
elaps[7, 8], euph., euphr.[2], **FERR.**,
fuc.[6, 8, 10, 12], **GRAPH.**, guaj.,
hell.[2, 3], **hura**[7], **hyos.**[2, 3], iod., ip.,
kali-bi., kali-br.[8, 12], **kali-c., lac-d.,**
lach., laur., lith-c.[12], lob.[8], **lyc.,**
lycpr.[12], mag-c., mag-p.[12], mang.[8],
med.[7], merc., merc-d.[6], mur-ac.,
nat-ar.[11], nat-c., **nat-m.**[5, 16], nux-m.,
nux-v.[5], olnd., op., **phos.**[3, 8, 12],
PHYT.[2, 3, 6, 8, 10, 12], plat., plb., **puls.,**
rauw.[9], rheum[2], rhus-t.[3], sabad.,
sabal[8, 12], sars., sel.[3], seneg., sep.,
sil., spig., spong., stram.[2, 3],
stront-c.[3], **sulph.**, thuj.,
thyr.[8, 11, 12, 14], tus-fr.[7, 8, 11, 12],
valer.[3], verat., viol-o.[2, 3]

weakness–reaction/faiblesse–
réaction/Schwäche–Reaktions–
mangel

body fat, but **legs thin**
jambes maigres, avec
Beine dünn, aber
  am-m., ant-c.[3]

children, in
enfants, chez les
Kindern, bei
  ant-c.[2, 8], **bad.**[2], bar-c.[6, 8],
  CALC.[1'-3, 7, 8, 12], **caps.**[1', 8], **ferr.**[8],
  kali-bi.[2, 8, 12], sacch.[8, 12], seneg.[12]

climacteric period, during
ménopause, pendant la
Klimakterium, im
  calc-ar.[12], **GRAPH.**[6, 7], sep.[6]

old people, in
vieillesse, dans la
Alter, im
    am-c.[7], **AUR.**[7], bar-c.[6], fl-ac.[7],
    KALI-C.[1, 7], op.[7], sec.[7]

young people, in
jeunes, chez les
Jugendlicher
    ant-c.[2, 4, 6, 7], calc.[4], calc-a.[6], lach.[6]

OLD AGE, premature
VIEILLESSE prématurée
ALTERN, vorzeitiges
    agn.[1, 7], alco.[11], alum.[6], **ambr.,**
    arg-m.[14], arg-n.[7], **bar-c.,** berb.[1'],
    bufo, carb-v.[1'], chin-s.[1], coca[11],
    con.[3, 6, 10], cortico.[14], **cupr.**[1'],
    des-ac.[14], esp-g.[14], **fl-ac.**[3, 6, 7, 12],
    kali-c., kres.[14], lyc., mag-f.[10],
    nux-v.[1'], op.[11], prot.[14], psor.[6],
    reser.[14], sars.[1'], **SEL.,** sep.[1'], staph.[6],
    stram.[7, 12], sulph.[6], **vip.**[7, 11, 12]

old people*
personnes âgées
alte Menschen
    acet-ac.[7, 12], **acon.,** agar., agn.[7],
    all-s.[7], **aloe, alum.**[3, 7, 8, 12], alumn.,
    am-c., am-m.[7], **AMBR., ammc.,**
    anac., ant-c., ant-t., apis[12], **arg-n.**[7],
    arn.[3, 6], **ars.,** ars-s-f.[1'], **AUR.,** bapt.[12],
    BAR-C., bar-m.[8], **bry.**[1, 7], calc.[3, 7],
    calc-p., camph., cann-i.[7], caps.[8],
    carb-an., carb-v., caust., cham.[7, 12],
    chin.[3, 12], chin-s.[4, 6], cic., cit-v.[8],
    COCA, cocc.[3], **colch., con.,** crot-h.[8],
    cupr.[1'], dig.[7], **fl-ac.,** gamb.[7], gins.[3],
    graph.[7, 12], **hydr.**[2, 3, 7, 8, 12], hyos.[3],
    iod., irid.[7, 12], **iris**[7], kali-ar.[7], kali-bi.[7],
    KALI-C., kreos.[3, 12], **LACH.**[3, 7, 12],
    LYC., mag-f.[14], merc.[5, 7],
    mill.[2, 7, 8, 12], nat-c.[7], **nat-m.,** nat-s.[12],
    nit-ac., nux-m.[8, 12], nux-v.[3], **OP.,**
    orch.[7, 12], **ov.**[7, 8], perh.[14], ph-ac.[3],
    phos.[3, 7, 8], puls.[7], rhus-t.[3], ruta[3, 7],
    sabad., sanic.[3], sarcol-ac.[14], sars.[3],
    SEC., SEL., seneg., sep.[7], **sil.**[5, 7],
    sul-ac., **sulph.**[1, 7], sumb.[3], syph.[3],

ter.[6, 12], **TEUCR.**[1, 7], thiosin.[7], thuj.[7],
tub.[3], **verat.**[3, 7, 8, 12], zinc.[7]

senile decay[8]
déchéance sénile
Altersverfall
    agn., arg-n., ars., bar-c., cann-i.,
    con., fl-ac., iod., **lyc., ov.,** phos.,
    thiosin.

onanism see masturbation

ORGASME of BLOOD
ORGASME SANGUIN
BLUTWALLUNGEN
    ACON., aloe, alum., alum-p.[1'],
    alum-sil.[1'], alumn., **am-c., am-m.,**
    ambr., aml-ns., ant-c., ant-t.,
    anthraco.[2], arg-m., **ARG-N., arn.,**
    ars.[3, 16], **ars-i., asar.**[1], **AUR.,** aur-ar.[1'],
    aur-i.[1'], aur-s.[1'], bar-c., bar-s.[1'],
    BELL., berb., bor.[2, 3], **bov., bry.,**
    CALC., calc-ar., calc-i.[1'], calc-s.,
    cann-i., cann-s., carb-an., **carb-v.,**
    CARBN-S., caust., cench.[1'], **cham.,**
    chin., cina, cocc., coff., **con.,** corn.[3],
    croc., cupr., dig., dulc., erig.[10],
    FERR., ferr-ar., **ferr-i.,** ferr-p., **gels.,**
    GLON., graph., guaj., **hep.,** hyos.,
    ign., **iod.,** jab.[3], kali-bi.[3], kali-br.[3],
    kali-c., kali-p., kali-s., kali-sil.[1'],
    kiss., **KREOS., LACH.,** lil-t., **LYC.,**
    mag-c.[3], mag-m., mang., **meli.,**
    merc., merl., **mill.**[1'], mosch., nat-c.,
    nat-m., nat-p., nit-ac., **nux-m.,**
    nux-v., op., ox-ac.[1'], **petr.,**
    PH-AC.[2, 3], **PHOS.,** plb., rhod.,
    puls., rhus-t., sabad., sabin., **samb.,**
    sang., **sars., sel.**[3], seneg., **sep., sil.,**
    SPONG., stann., staph., **STRAM.,**
    stront-c.[3], **sul-ac.**[3], sul-i.[1'], **SULPH.,**
    tab., tell., ter.[3], **thuj.,** ust.[3], valer.[3],
    verat.

heat–flushes/ chaleur–bouffées/
Hitzewallungen

morning in sleep
matin en dormant
morgens im Schlaf
    ang.

after restless sleep
après sommeil agité
nach ruhelosem Schlaf
   calc.

on waking
au réveil
beim Erwachen
   calc.[16], graph., kali-c.[16], lyc.,
   nux-v.

rising am.
en se levant am.
Aufstehen am.
   nux-v.

evening/soir/abends
   arn., **asar.**[1], **caust.**, dig., kali-c.[16],
   lyc., **merc.**[2], petr., phos., rhus-t.,
   sars.[2], thuj.

after lying down
après s'être couché
nach dem Hinlegen
   ign., samb., sars.[16], sil.

during sexual excitement
pendant l'excitation sexuelle
bei sexueller Erregung
   clem.

sitting am.
étant assis am.
Sitzen am.
   thuj.

night/nuit/nachts
   am-c., arg-n., **calc.**, **carb-an.**,
   carb-v., hep., ign., mag-c., **merc.**,
   mur-ac., **nat-c.**, nat-m., **phos.**,
   puls., ran-b., raph.[2], senn.[7], **sep.**,
   sil., **sulph.**

   heat–flushes–night/
     chaleur–bouffées–nuit/
     Hitzewallungen–nachts
   Vol. III: *sleeplessness–*
     climacteric period/insomnie–
     ménopause/Schlaflosigkeit–
     Klimakterium

bed, drives him out of
lit, le poussant hors du
Bett, treiben ihn aus dem
   iod.

beer, after
bière, après avoir bu de·la
Bier, nach
   sulph.

anxiety with[2]
anxiété avec
Angst mit
   acon., aloe, am-m., **bar-c.**, chel.

ascending stairs, on[16]
montant des escaliers, en
Treppensteigen, beim
   thuj.

burning in hands, with[2]
brûlantes, avec mains
Brennen in Händen, mit
   SULPH.

   skin, of[2]
   peau brûlante, avec
   Haut, der
     sang.

coition, after
coït, après le
Koitus, nach
   am-c., **sep.**

disagreeable news, from
désagréables nouvelles, par
unangenehme Nachrichten, durch
   lach.

eating am.
manger am.
Essen am.
   alum., chin.

warm food, while
chauds, en mangeant des aliments
warmer Speisen, beim
   mag-c.

emotions, after
émotions, après
Gefühlserregungen, nach
   acon., apis, **aur., bell.,** bry., calc.,
   CHAM., coff., colch., **coloc., con.,**
   cupr., **HYOS., IGN.,** kali-c., **kali-p.,**
   lach., lyc., mag-c., nat-m., **nat-p.,**
   nit-ac., nux-v., op., **petr., ph-ac.,**
   phos., plat., **PULS., sep., staph.,**
   stram., teucr., thuj., verat.

everything were moving in body,
   as if
tout bougeait dans le corps,
   comme si
alles im Körper bewegt, als ob sich
   croc.

faintness, with[7]
évanouissement, avec
Ohnmacht, mit
   petr.

falling asleep, on
s'endormant, en
Einschlafen, beim
   petr., sep.[16]

lying on left side
couché sur le côté gauche, étant
Liegen auf der linken Seite, beim
   bar-c.

menses, before
menstruations, avant la
Menses, vor den
   alum., **cupr.,** merc.

   during/pendant la/während der
   calc., merl.

motion, on[16]
mouvement, au
Bewegung, bei
   nat-m.

motion or speaking agg.
mouvement ou parler agg.
Bewegung oder Sprechen agg.
   iod., nat-c., thuj.[16]

nervousness, from
nervosité, par
Nervosität, durch
   ambr., **bell.,** calc., ferr., kali-n.,
   merc., **nit-ac., ph-ac., phos.,** sep.

palpitation, with[16]
palpitations, avec
Herzklopfen, mit
   kali-c., phos., sul-i.[1']

restlessness, with[2]
agitation, avec
Ruhelosigkeit, mit
   aloe, ph-ac.

sensual impressions, from
sensorielles, par impressions
Sinneseindrücke, durch
   phos.

sitting, while
assis, en étant
Sitzen, im
   mag-m.

smoking tobacco, on[16]
fumant du tabac, en
Rauchen, beim
   phos.

vertigo, during
vertige, pendant le
Schwindel, bei
   nat-c.

vexation, after
vexations, après
Ärger, nach
   acon., **CHAM.,** coloc., ign., merc.,
   petr., SEP., staph.

vomiting, after[16]
vomissement, après
Erbrechen, nach
   verat.

walk, after a long
marche, après une longue
Spaziergang, nach einem langen
   arg-n.

walking, after
marche, après une
Gehen, nach
    arg-n., berb., **petr.**[2], sul-i.[1']

am.
    mag-m.

wine, after[16]
vin, après injestion de
Wein, nach
    sil.

OVULATION, at
OVULATION, à l'
OVULATION, bei der
    foll.[14]

PAIN, ailments from[12]
DOULEURS, troubles à la suite de
SCHMERZEN, Beschwerden infolge von
    cham., scut.

sensitiveness–pain/sensibilité–
douleur/Empfindlichkeit–
Schmerzempfindlichkeit

  Vol. I: *sensitive – pain/sensible –*
douleurs/empfindlich –
Schmerzen

morning[16]/matin/morgens
    sil.

evening[16]/soir/abends
    ars.

night[16]/nuit/nachts
    con., kali-c.

en dormant
in sleep[4]
im Schlaf
    alum., aur., bell., kali-n., lach.,
    lyc., **merc.,** mosch., **nit-ac.,** vip.

appear gradually
apparaissent graduellement
beginnen allmählich
    acon., bry., calc-sil.[8], carbn-o.,
    caust., chin.[8], con., ign., lact.,
    lob., rad-br.[8], sars., sul-ac., tell.[8]

and disappear gradually
et disparaissent graduellement
und hören allmählich auf
    acon., **arg-n.**[2, 6, 8], arn., ars.,
    bar-c., bufo, cact.[3], cast.[3],
    chel.[3], coloc.[3], crot-h., epiph.[3],
    euphr.[3], form.[3], **gels.**[3, 6], glon.,
    ign.[3], jab., kali-bi.[6], **kalm.,**
    lach.[3, 6], lol.[3], mez., **nat-m.,**
    op., **phos.,** pic-ac., **PLAT.,**
    psor., **puls.**[3, 6], sabin.,
    SANG.[3, 6], sars., sel.[3], sep.[3],
    spig., STANN., staph.,
    stront-c., **sul-ac.,** sulph.,
    SYPH.[1', 6-8], verb.

suddenly
soudainement
plötzlich
    arg-m., arg-n.[2], bell.[3], caust.,
    ign.[3, 8], **puls.,** rhus-t.[3], rad.[3],
    sul-ac.

appear suddenly
apparaissent soudainement
beginnen plötzlich
    acon.[3, 6], agar., am-c.[3, 6], anh.[9],
    arg-m., ars.[6], aster., atro.[6],
    bar-a.[3, 6], **BELL.,** berb., camph.,
    canth.[3, 6], carb-ac.[3, 6], caust.[6],
    cimic., cob-n.[10], **coloc.**[3, 6], croc.,
    crot-h.[3, 6], **cupr.**[3, 6], cupr-ar.[6],
    daph.[7], **dios.**[6], eup-per.[3], ferr.,
    form.[3, 6], **glon.**[3, 6], kali-bi[3, 6], lyc.,
    mag-c.[3, 6], mag-p.[3, 6], med.[7], mez.,
    morph., **nat-s.**[3, 6], **NIT-AC.,**
    nux-v.[6], ox-ac.[3, 6], phys., plb.[3, 6],
    podo.[3, 6], **puls.,** ran-b.[3, 6], **sabin.,**
    sep., sil.[6], spig.[3], stann.[3, 6],
    stry-p.[6], sul-ac.[3, 6], **tab.,**
    tarent.[3, 6], thala.[14], thuj.[3, 6],
    valer., verb.[6], vip.[3, 6], zinc.[6],
    zinc-val.[6]

and disappear gradually
et disparaissent graduellement
und hören allmählich auf
    asaf., **bell.**[3], buni-o.[14], calc.,
    coloc.[3], fl-ac., **hyper.**[3], ign.[6],
    lach.[3], **med.**[3], **puls.,** rad.[3],
    rad-br.[3], ran-s., sabin.[1], sep.[1],
    sul-ac.[8]

pain

suddenly
soudainement
plötzlich
 arg-n., asaf., aster., **BELL.,**
 bor.[3], cact.[8], canth.,
 carb-ac.[3, 6, 8], carbn-s.,
 cham.[7], coff.[7], crot-h.[3], cupr.[3],
 dios.[3], eup-per.[8], eup-pur.,
 fl-ac., ictod.[8], ign., **KALI-BI.,**
 kalm., lyc., mag-p., merc-c.,
 nat-f.[10], **NIT-AC.,** nux-m.[3],
 ovi-p.[3, 7], oxyt.[3], petr.[7, 8],
 phyt., puls.[8], rhus-t.[3, 8], sabin.,
 spig., **stry.**[8], thal.[14], thuj.[3],
 tub.[8,] valer.[3]

disappear suddenly[3]
disparaissent soudainement
hören plötzlich auf
 arum-t.[2], **BELL.**[2, 3, 6], carb-ac.[2, 6],
 caust., cimic.[2], **dios.**[6], mag-p.[6], puls.,
 sul-ac., stry-p.[6], sulph., thuj.[6]

direction of pain backward[3]
direction des douleurs vers l'arrière
Schmerzverlauf rückwärts
 bar-c., bell., **bry.,** chel., con.,
 crot-t., cupr., gels., **kali-bi.,**
 kali-c., kali-i., lil-t., merc.,
 nat-m., par., phos., phyt., prun.,
 puls., **sep.,** spig., **SULPH.**

crosswise[3]
croisée
kreuzweise

 acon., ambr., anac., arg-m., **bell.,**
 berb., bov., bry., calc., canth.,
 caust., cham., **chel., chin.,** cocc.,
 ferr., hell., kali-bi., kali-c.,
 kali-m., **lac-c.**[3, 6], laur., lyc.,
 mang.[6], merc., mur-ac., phos.,
 rhus-t., seneg., **sep., sil.,** spig.,
 stront-c., sul-ac., **sulph.,** tarax.,
 valer., **verat.,** zinc.

downward[3]
vers le bas
abwärts
 acon., agar., agn., aloe[3], alum.,
 alumn.[2], ant-t., apis[7], arn., asaf.[6],
 aur., bar-c., bell., benz-ac.[3, 6],

berb., bor.[8], bry., cact.[8], canth.,
caps., carb-v., caust., chel., chin.,
cic., cina, coff., **FERR.,** goss.[11],
graph., hyper., kali-c.,
kalm.[1', 3, 6-8], lach., led.[7], **LYC.,**
merc., mez.[1'], nat-c., nat-m.,
nux-v., ph-ac., **puls.,** rheum[2, 7],
rhod., rhus-t., **sanic.**[8], sars.,
sel.[2, 3], seneg., sep., sil., sulph.,
verat., verb., zinc.

forward[3]
vers l'avant
nach vorn
 berb., bry., carb-v., **gels., lac-c.,**
 sabin., sang., sep., sil., **SPIG.**

inward[3]
vers le dedans
nach innen
 alum., arg-n., **ARN.**[3, 6], bell.,
 bov., **calc.,** cann-s., **CANTH.**[3, 6],
 carb.-v., caust., chin., cina, con.,
 hyos., **ign., laur.,** meny., merc.,
 mez., petr., phel., phyt.[6], **plb.**[3, 6],
 ran-b.[3, 6], rhus-t., **sabin.**[3, 6], sep.,
 spig., spong., squil., stann.,
 staph., sul-ac., sulph., valer.,
 verb.

left side, on[11]
gauche, le côté
linken Seite, auf der
 benz-ac., brom., chel., cinnb.,
 crot-c., crot-h., daph., ind., kalm.,
 lepi., lil-t., lycps., merc.,
 merc-i-f., oena., ol-j., op., ox-ac.,
 phys., pic-ac., plan., puls-n.

outward[3]
vers le dehors
nach außen
 alum.[3, 6], am-m., anh.[9, 14], **arg-m.,**
 arg-n.[3, 6], arn., **ASAF.**[1', 3, 6], bell.,
 berb., bry., calc., canth., carb-v.,
 chel.[3, 6], **chin.**[3, 6], cimic.[3], cocc.,
 CON.[3, 6], dros., dulc., hyos.,
 kali-c.[3], kali-bi., kali-m., kalm.,
 led.[1'], lith-c., lyc.[1', 3], mang.,
 merc.[3, 6], mez., mur-ac., nat-c.,
 nit-ac., phel.[6], phos., phyt.[3, 6],
 plat., plb., prun.[3], ran-b.[3, 6],

rhod., rhus-t., sabad., sabin.,
sep.[3], sil.[3, 6], spig.[3, 6], spong.[3, 6],
stann.[3, 6], stann-i.[6], staph.,
SULPH.[3, 6], tarax., **valer.**[3, 6],
viol-t., zinc.

radiating[3]
irradiante
ausstrahlend
agar.[3, 6], apis[6], arg-n.[3, 6], ars.[3, 6],
bapt., berb., caust., cham., cimic.,
coloc., cupr.[3, 6], **dios.**[3, 6], hyper.,
kali-bi., kali-c.[3, 6], kalm., lil-t.[6],
mag-m., mag-p., **merc.**, mez.,
nux-v., phyt., plat., plb., sec.,
sil., spig.[3, 6], xan.

right side, on[11]
droit, le côté
rechten Seite, auf der
arist-m., brach., bry., cedr., oena.,
pic-ac., sulph., tarent., wye., yuc.

upward[3]
vers le haut
aufwärts
acon., aloe, alum-sil.[1'], anac.,
arn., ars., **asaf.**[3, 6], aur., **BELL.**,
calc., canth., caust., cham., chin.,
cimic., colch., con., croc.,
cupr.[3, 6], dulc., eup-pur.[3, 6],
euphr., gels., **glon.**, hyper.[6],
IGN., kali-bi., kalm.[1', 3], kreos.,
LACH.[1', 3], **led.**[1', 3, 6, 8], mag-c.,
mang., meny., naja, nat-c.,
nat-m., nit-ac., nux-v., op.,
PHOS., puls., rhus-t., sabad.,
samb., **SANG., SEP., SIL.**, spong.,
stront-c., stroph-h., sulph., thuj.,
valer., zinc.

amputation, after
amputation, après
Amputation, nach
acon.[7], **all-c.**[2, 7], am-m.[2, 7], arn.[2],
asaf., bell.[7], cupr.[7], hell.[7], **hyper.**[7],
ign.[7], kalm.[2], **ph-ac.**[2, 7], rauw.[10],
spig.[7], **staph.**[7], symph.[2, 7], verat.[7]

bones, of
os, des
Knochen, der
abies-n., acon., **agar.**, agn.,
all-c.[11], alum.[4], am-c., am-m.,
ambr.[4], anac., ang.[3, 4, 8, 12],
ant-c.[3, 4], aran.[2], **arg-m.**, arn.,
ars., ars-i., **ASAF., aur.**, aur-ar.[1'],
aur-i.[1'], aur-m.[1', 8], aur-s.[1'],
bar-c., bar-i.[1'], bar-s.[1'], bell.,
berb.[1], bism., bry., **calc., calc-p.**,
calc-s., camph.[4], cann-s., canth.,
caps., carb-an., carb-v., carbn-s.,
cast-eq.[8], caust., **cham.**, chel.,
chin., chin-m.[2, 12], chin-s., cic.,
cinnb., cinnm.[2, 12], clem., cob-n.[14],
cocc., colch., coloc., **con.**,
conch.[11], crot-c.[8, 11], **crot-h.**[4, 8, 11],
cupr., cycl., **daph.**[4], dig., dios.,
dros., dulc., **EUP-PER.**, euph.,
ferr., ferr-ar.[1], **fl-ac., gels.**[3], glon.,
graph., guaj., halo.[14], hell., **hep.**,
hom.[12], ictod.[4], ign., iod., **IP.**,
kali-bi., kali-c., **kali-i.**[2, 8, 11],
kali-s., kreos., lach., led., **lyc.**,
lyss., m-arct.[4], mag-c., mag-m.,
mang., mang-m.[12], **MERC.**,
merc-c.[8], merc-i-f., **mez., mur-ac.**[4],
nat-c., nat-m., **nat-s.**[2], nat-sil.[1'],
NIT-AC., nux-m.[3, 4], nux-v.[4],
oci-s.[9], ol-an.[3], olnd., op., petr.,
PH-AC., phos., phyt.[1', 3, 8], plb.,
PULS., pyrog.[1', 3], ran-s., raph.[11],
rhod., rhus-t., RUTA, sabad.,
sabin., sacch.[11], samb., sarr.[11, 12],
sars., sec., **sep., sil.**, sol-t-ae.[11],
spig., spong., **staph.**, still.,
stront-c., sul-i.[1'], **sulph., symph.**[8],
syph.[8], teucr., ther., thuj., valer.,
verat., viol-t., vitr.[8], wildb.[12],
zinc.

morning[16]/matin/morgens
sil.

night/nuit/nachts
asaf.[1], **AUR.**, caust., **cham.**,
cinnb., **fl-ac.**, guare.[11], hep.[8],
iod.[8], **KALI-I.**, kalm., **mang.**,
MERC., merc-i-f., mez., NIT-AC.,
ph-ac., phyt., rhod.[8], **sars.**, sil.[1'],
staph.[1'], still.[8], syph.[8], thuj.,
verat.

long, in[8]
longs, dans les os
langen, in den
    cinnb., eup-per., staph., stront-c.,
    syph.

weather, change of[3]
temps, changement de
Wetterwechsel, bei
    am-c.

blood vessels, of[6]
vaisseaux sanguins, des
Blutgefäße, der
    ham., zinc.

cancerous affections, in[8]
cancéreuses, dans les affections
kanzerösen Erkrankungen, bei
    acon.[7], **apis,** anthraci., **ars.,** aster.,
    bry., bufo[7], calc., **calc-a.**[8, 12],
    calc-o-t., calc-ox., carb-an.[1'], carc.,
    cedr., cinnm., **cit-ac.**[2], coloc.[2], **con.,**
    cund., echi.[7, 8], **euph., hydr.,** mag-p.,
    merc.[1'], morph., op., ph-ac.[7, 8], sil.

cartilages, of[8, 12]
cartilages, des
Knorpel, der
    arg-m., lob-s.[12], ruta

chill, during[16]
frissons, pendant les
Fieberfrost, bei
    ars., petr.

eructation am.[7]
renvoi am.
Aufstoßen am.
    jal.

glands, of
glandes, des
Drüsen, der
    acon., all-s.[11], **alum., am-c.,** ambr.,
    ant-c., ant-t., apis[3], **ARN.,** ars.,
    ars-i., arund.[2, 11], asaf.[3], **aur.,**
    aur-ar.[1'], aur-i.[1'], aur-s.[1'], **bar-c.,**
    bar-i.[1'], bar-m., bar-s.[1'] **BELL.,**
    berb.[4], bor.[4], **bry.,** calc., calen.[4],
    cann-s., canth. **carb-an., carb-v.,**
    carbn-s., caust., cham., chin., cic.,

clem., **coloc.,** con., cor-r.[4], dulc.,
graph., ham.[3, 6], hell., hep., ign.,
iod., kali-c., kali-s., lach.[3, 6], **LYC.,**
m-arct.[4], mag-c., mag-m.[4], **MERC.,**
murx.[4], **nat-m., nit-ac.,** nux-v.,
petr., **ph-ac., PHOS., puls.,**
rheum, rhus-t., sel., sep., sil.,
spig., spong., squil., stann., staph.,
stram., **sul-ac.,** sul-i.[1'], **sulph.,**
THUJ., verat.

half sleep, during[16]
demi-sommeil, dans le
Halbschlaf, im
    nit-ac.

joints, of[1]
articulations, des
Gelenke, der
    acon., **acon-c.**[11], aesc., agar.,
    agar-ph.[11], all-c., **alum.,** anh.[9],
    apis., apoc., apoc-a.[11], aran.,
    ARG-M., ARN., ars., ars-i., asaf.,
    asc-t., aster., aur., bar-c., bar-m.[3],
    bell., berb.[3], **bol-la., BRY.,** caj.,
    calc., CALC-P., calc-s., cann-i.,
    caps., carb-ac., carb-an., **carbn-s.,**
    casc.[2], **caust.,** cedr., **cham., chin.,**
    chin-ar., **cimx, cinnb.,** cist., **cit-v.**[2],
    cocc., colch., coloc., con., cop.,
    croc., crot-t., cycl., daph., dig.,
    dios., **dulc., ferr., ferr-ar.,** ferr-i.,
    ferr-p., gels., **guaj.,** harp.[14], hell.,
    hist.[9], hydr., hydrc., ign., **iod.,** ip.,
    iris, jac-c., jatr., **kali-bi., kali-c.,**
    kali-n., kali-p., **kalm., lac-ac., lac-c.,**
    LED., lyc., lyss., mag-f.[14], mand.[9, 14],
    mang., merc., mez., morph., **nat-ar.,**
    nat-f.[14], nat-m., **nat-s.,** nit-ac.,
    NUX-V., ol-an., par., **ph-ac., phos.,**
    phyt., PLB., PULS., ran-s., raph.,
    rheum, rhod., RHUS-T., ruta,
    sabad., **sabin., sang.,** sel., senec.,
    sil., sol-n., sol-t-ae., **staph.,**
    stroph-s.[14], sul-ac., **sulph.,** syph.[1'],
    ter., thala.[14], thuj., tub-r.[14], verat-v.

muscles, of[8, 12]
muscles, des
Muskeln, der
    achy.[14], **acon.,** agav-t.[14], alet.[12],
    am-caust.[11], **ant-t., arn.**[6, 8], ars.[8],

aster.[14], bell.[8], bell-p.[8, 9, 12],
brach.[11], **bry.**[6, 8, 12], carbn-s.[8],
caust.[6, 8, 12], **cimic., colch.**[6, 8, 12],
dulc.[6, 8, 12], eryt-j.[11], ferr-p.[6],
form.[11], **gels.**[6, 8, 12], harp.[14], hist.[9],
ign.[6], lat-m.[9], led.[8], lyc.[11], **macro.,**
mag-s.[9, 14], mand.[9, 14], merc.[8],
merc-c.[11], morph.[8], nat-f.[9, 14],
nat-m.[6, 11], op.[11], **phyt.**[6], plb.[11],
puls.[6], **ran-b.**[8], rham-cath.[8],
rauw.[9], **rhus-t.**[6, 8], **ruta**[8], sal-ac.[8],
sil.[6], staph.[6], stram.[8], stroph-s.[14],
stry.[8, 11], sulfa.[14], tab.[11], tarax.[14],
thal.[6, 14], thuj.[11], valer.[8],
verat.[6, 8, 11], **verat-v.,** zinc.[11]

hot bathing am.[9]
bains très chauds am.
Heißbaden am.
   lat-m.

motion agg.[9]
mouvement agg.
Bewegung agg.
   bell-p.

stretching, on[9]
étirant, en s'
Strecken, beim
   mag-s.

paralyzed parts, of
paralysées, des parties
gelähmter Teile
   agar., arn., **ars.,** bell., cadm-f.[1'],
   calc., **caust.,** cina[1], **cocc.,** crot-t.,
   kali-n. lat-m., nux-v., phos., **plb.,**
   rhus-t., sil., sulph.

paralysis–painful/paralysie–
   douloureuse/Paralysis–schmerz-
   hafte

parts, of affected[16]
parties souffrantes, des
Teile, der leidenden
   con.' dig.

injured long ago[7]
blessées il y a longtemps, dans les
verletzten T., in den vor langem
   glon.

lain on, in[16]
couché, où il est
liegt, auf denen er
   caust., hep., kali-c., phos., sep., sil.

lying–pain/couché–douleur/
   Liegen–Schmerz

recently lain on
sur lesquelles on vient de
   s'appuyer
auf denen man gerade gelegen
   hat
   PULS.

uncovered, of[16]
découvertes, des
unbedeckten, der
   bell.

periosteum
périoste, du
Periost, des
   AM-C.[7], ant-c., **ARN.**[7], **ASAF.,**
   aur., **AUR-M.**[7], bell., bry., **camph.,**
   cann-s.[7], **cham., chin., colch.,**[1, 7]
   coloc., cycl., graph., guare.[7], hell.,
   ign., kali-c.[7], **KALI-I.**[7], **kalm.,** led.,
   mang., merc., merc-c.[7], **mez.,**
   mur-ac.[7, 16], **nit-ac.**[7], **PH-AC.,** phyt.,
   puls.[1, 7], **rhod.,** rhus-t., **RUTA**[1, 7],
   sabad., sabin., **sil.,** spig., **staph.**[1, 7],
   symph.[12], syph.[1', 7]

small spots, in
localisées
kleinen Stellen, an
   agar.[3], **alum.**[3], am-c.[3], am-m.[3],
   ambr.[3], apis[3], arg-m.[3], arg-n.[3], arn.[3],
   ars.[3], asaf.[3], bell.[3], **berb.**[3], bry.[3],
   bufo[3], calc.[3], **calc-p.**[3, 7], cann-s.[3],
   canth.[3], carb-v.[3], caust.[3], cham.[3],
   chel.[3], **cist.**[3], coff.[8], **colch.**[3, 6], **con.**[3],
   croc.[3], cupr.[3], dios.[3, 6], ferr.[3], fl-ac.,
   gels.[3], glon.[3], graph.[3], hep.[3], hist.[9],
   ign., iod.[3], **KALI-BI., LACH.**[3], led.[3],
   lil-t., lith-c., lyc.[3], mag-c.[3], mag-m.[3],
   mag-p., meny.[3], merc.[3], mosch.[3],
   nat-m.[3], nit-ac.[3], nux-m., ol-an.[3, 6],
   ol-j.[3], **onos.,** ox-ac., petr.[3], ph-ac.[3],
   phos.[3], psor., puls.[3], ran-b., ran-s.[3],
   rhod.[3, 6, 11], rhus-t.[3], rhus-v.[11],

sabin.[3], samb.[3], sars.[3], sel.[3], **sep.**[3], sil.[3], spig.[16], squil.[3], sul-ac.[3], **SULPH.**[3], **thuj.**, verat.[3], zinc.[3]

tendons, in[3]
tendons, des
Sehnen, in den
am-m., arn., benz-ac., berb., **bry.**[2], caust., colch., coloc., harp.[14], iod., kali-bi., kalm., mag-f.[14], prun., **RHUS-T.**[2, 3], **ruta**[1'-3], sabin., thuj., zinc.

benumbing
engourdissantes
betäubende
acon., agar., agn., am-c., anac., ant-c., ant-t., arg-m., arn., asaf., asar., aur., bell., bov., bry., **calc.**, cann-s., carb-an., carb-v.[3], **CHAM.**, chin., cic., **cina**, cocc., con., croc., cupr., cycl., dros., dulc., euph., euphr., **gnaph.**[7], **graph.**, hell., hep., hyos., ign., **iris**, kali-n., laur., led., mag-c., mag-m., mang., meny., **mez.**, mosch., mur-ac., nat-c., nat-m., nux-m., nux-v.[3], **OLND.**, op., par., ph-ac., phos., **PLAT.**, **puls.**, **rheum**, rhus-t., ruta, **SABAD.**, sabin., **samb.**, seneg., sep., stann., staph., sul-ac., sulph., tarax., valer., **verat.**, **VERB.**, zinc.

right side, in[16]
droite, dans la
rechten Seite, in der
ars.

biting
mordicantes
beißende
acon., agar., agn., aloe[11], alum., am-c., **ambr.**, ang.[3], ant-c., ant-t., arg-m., arn., ars., asar., aur., bar-m.[4], bell., **berb.**[4], **bov.**[4], bry., calad., calc., camph., cann-s., **canth.**, **caps.**, carb-an., **CARB-V.**, caust., cham., chel.[4], **chin.**, **clem.**, cocc., colch., coloc., con., croc., **dros.**, dulc., euon.[11], **euph.**, **euphr.**, graph., grat.[4], **hell.**, hep., hyos., **ign.**, iod., **ip.**, **kali-c.**, kali-m.[1'],

kali-n., **kreos.**, lach., lact.[4], lam.[4], laur., led., lyc., m-arct.[4], m-aust.[4], mag-c., mang.[4], **merc.**, **mez.**, mosch., mur-ac., nat-c., nat-m., nicc.[4], **nit-ac.**, nux-m., **NUX-V.**, ol-an.[4], olnd., op., paeon., par., petr., **PETROS.**, ph-ac., phos., plat.[4], **prun.**, **puls.**, **ran-b.**, **RAN-S.**, rheum, rhod., **rhus-t.**, **ruta**, sabad., sabin., sars., sel., seneg., **sep.**, sil., spig., **spong.**[4], squil., stann., **staph.**, stram., stront-c., sul-ac., **SULPH.**, **teucr.**, thuj., valer., verat., viol-t., voes.[11], **ZINC.**, **ZINC-P.**[1']

boring
forantes
bohrende
acon., **agar.**, aloe, alum., alum-p.[1'], alum-sil.[1'], am-c., am-m., anac., ang.[3], ant-c., ant-t., apis, **arg-m.**, **ARG-N.**, arn., ars., **asaf.**, **AUR.**, aur-ar.[1'], **aur-s.**[1'], bar-c., bar-s.[1'], **BELL.**, **BISM.**, bor., bov., **calc.**, calc-sil.[1'], cann-i., canth., caps., carb-an., carb-v., carbn-s., **caust.**, chin., cimic., **cina**, clem., coc-c., cocc., colch., coloc., con., cupr., cycl., dig., dios., dros., **dulc.**, euph., euphr., **hell.**, **hep.**, ign., ip., **kali-c.**, kali-n., kreos., **lach.**, laur., led., lyc., m-arct.[3], mag-c., mag-m., mang., meny., **merc.**, merc-i-f.[11], **mez.**, mur-ac., **nat-c.**, **nat-m.**, nat-sil.[1'], nit-ac., nux-m., nux-v., olnd., par., petr., **ph-ac.**, phos., plan.[3,], plat., **plb.**, **PULS.**, ran-b., **RAN-S.**, **rhod.**, rhus-t, ruta, sabad., sabin., sel., **seneg.**, **sep.**, **sil.**, **SPIG.**, spong., stann., staph., stram., stront-c., **sulph.**, **tarax.**, **thuj.**, valer., **zinc.**, **zinc-p.**[1']

inward/vers le dedans/nach innen
alum., bell., calc., cocc., **kali-c.**, mang., zinc.

outward/vers le dehors/nach außen
ant-c., asaf., bell., **bism.**, bov.,
calc., dros., **dulc.**, ip., puls.,
sep., **spig.**, spong., **staph.**

bones/os/Knochen
agar., anac.[4], ang.[3, 4], aran., **asaf.,**
AUR., bar-c., bell., brom., **calc.**,
carb-an., clem., dulc., hell., hep.,
kali-c.[4], kali-i.[3], lach., **lyc.**, mang.,
MERC., mez., nat-c., nat-m.,
nit-s-d.[11], ph-ac., phos., **puls.**,
ran-s.[4], rhod., rhus-t., sabad.,
sabin., **sep., sil., spig.**, staph.,
sulph., **thuj.**

glands/glandes/Drüsen
bell., lyc.[3, 4], puls., sabad., sabin.[4]

small spots, in[11]
localisées
kleinen Stellen, an
fl-ac.

broken, as if bones
fracturés, comme si les os étaient
gebrochen seien, als ob die Knochen
agar.[1'], am-c.[1'], **ang.**[2, 3], arg-m.[11],
arn.[1', 3], ars.[1'], **aur., BELL.**[3], bor.[3],
bov.[3], **bry.**, calc.[3], calc-p.[3],,
caust.[3], **cham.**[2, 3], **chel.**[2, 3], cina[3],
coc-c.[2], **COCC.**[2, 3], cupr., **dros.**[2, 3],
EUP-PER[1', 3, 7], graph.[3], guaj.[3],
hep., hyos.[3], **IGN.**[2, 3], kreos.[3],
lyc.[3], lyss.[2], m-arct.[3], mag-m.[2, 3],
merc.[2, 3, 7], mez.[3], mosch.[3],
nat-m., nux-v.[1', 3], par.[3], ph-ac.[3],
PHOS.[2, 3], puls., rhus-t[1', 3], **ruta,**
samb.[2, 3], sep., sil.[11], sulph.[3],
symph.[2], **tarant.**[11], ther., **thuj.**[2],
valer.[3], **verat., vip.**, zinc.[3]

joints, in[3]
articulations, dans les
Gelenken, in
bov., calc., carb-an.[3, 11], caust.,
dros., hep., merc., mez., par.[2, 3, 11],
sep.

part on which he was lying, in[11]
partie sur laquelle on était couché,
sur la

Teil, auf dem man gelegen hatte,
in dem
mosch.

bruised see sore

burning externally
brûlantes, externes
Brennen, äußerliches
acet-ac.[11], achy.[14], **acon.**,
acon-f.[12], **agar.**, all-c.[6], aloe,
alum., **alum-p.**[1'], **alum-sil.**[1'],
am-c., **am-m.**, ambr., anac.,
ang.[3, 11], ant-c., ant-t., **anthraci.**,
APIS, arg-m., **arn., ARS.**,
ars-i., **ARS-S-F.**[1'], **ARUM-T.**,
asaf., asar., atro.[11], aur.[4],
aur-ar.[1'], **aur-m.**[1'], **bapt.**,
bar-c., bar-m., bar-s.[1'], bell.,
berb., bism., **bor.**, bov.,
brom.[11], **BRY.**, bufo, buni-o.[14],
calad., calc., calc-ar.[1'], calc-i.[1'],
calc-p., camph., cann-s.,
canth., caps., carb-ac.[3, 11],
carb-an., **CARB-V.**, carbn-o.[11],
CARBN-S., CAUST., cham.,
chel., chin., chin-s.[4, 11], cic.,
cimic., cina, **clem.**, coc-c.,
cocc., coff., colch., **coloc.**,
com.[6], **con.**, convo-d.[11], cop.[11],
corn., croc., crot-c.[11], crot-h.,
crot-t., culx.[1'], cupr., **cycl.**,
dig., **dros., dulc.**, eucal.[7],
euon.[4], euph., euph-l.[11],
EUPHR., fago.[11], **ferr.**,
fl-ac.[1', 3, 6], **gels.**[2], **graph., grat.**,
guaj., hell., helon., hep.,
hist.[9, 10, 14], **hyos.**[3, 4], **ign.**, iod.,
ip., **IRIS**, juni.[11], kali-ar.,
kali-bi., kali-br.[11], **kali-c.**,
kali-m.[1'], kali-n., kali-s.,
kali-sula.[11], **kreos.**, lac-ac.[6],
lach., lachn.[11], lap-a.[6], lat-m.[9],
laur., led., lil-t.[11], lob., **lyc.**,
m-arct.[3, 4], m-aust.[3, 4], mag-c.,
mag-m., mag-s.[4], **manc.**,
mand.[10], mang., meny., **MERC.**,
merc-c., merc-sul.[2], merl.[11],
mez., mosch., **mur-ac., nat-ar.**,
nat-c., NAT-M., nat-s.[4],
nat-sil.[1'], nicc.[4], **nit-ac.**, nux-m.,
NUX-V., ol-an.[4], **olnd., op.**,

ox-ac.[1'], paeon., par., petr.,
PH-AC., phel.[4], **PHOS.**, phyt.,
pic-ac.[6], plat., plb., **prun., psor.,
puls., ran-b.**[2, 4, 11], ran-s.,
raph.[4], **RAT.**, rauw.[9], **rheum,**
rhod., **RHUS-T.**, rhus-v.[11],
rumx., ruta, **sabad.**, sabin.,
sal-ac., samb., sang.[4, 6], sars.,
SEC., sel., seneg., **SEP., SIL.,**
sol-n.[11], spig., spong., squil.,
STANN., staph., stram.,
stront-c., sul-ac., sul-i.[1'],
SULPH., tab.[4], **tarax.,
tarent.**[1', 2, 11], tarent-c.[6], teucr.,
thuj., til.[11], trib.[11], valer.,
verat., **viol-o.**[4], viol-t.,
vip.[3, 6, 1], wies.[11], **zinc.,**
zinc-p.[1']

left upper part of body
gauche supérieure, de la
    partie
linken Oberkörpers, des
    kreos.

heat am.[3, 7]
chaleur am.
Hitze am.
    alum., **ARS., caps.**, carb-v.,
    lyc.

right side of body[8]
droite, dans la
rechten Seite, der
    phos.

internally
internes
innerliches
    abies-c., acet-ac., achy.[14],
    ACON., acon-f., aesc.[3, 6], **agar.**,
    aloe[6], **alum.**, alumn., **am-br.**,
    am-c., **am-m.**, ambr., amor-r.[14],
    ang.[3], ant-c., ant-t., **apis**, arg-m.,
    arg-n., arn., ARS., ars-i.,
    ARS-S-F.[1'], **ARUM-T.**, asaf.,
    asar., **aur.**, aur-i.[1'], **bapt., bar-c.**,
    bar-m., **BELL., BERB.**, bism.,
    bor., bov., brom.[3, 6], **BRY., bufo,**
    calad., **calc., calc-p.**, calc-sil.[1'],
    camph., **CANN-I.**, cann-s.,
    CANTH., caps., carb-ac.,

carb-an., **carb-v., CARBN-S.,**
caust., cedr., cham., **chel., chin.,**
cic., cina, **clem.**, cocc., coff.,
colch., coloc., **com., con.**, crot-t.,
cund., **cupr.**, dig., **dios.**, dol.,
dros., dulc., equis., eucal.[6],
eup-pur., **euph.**, euphr., **fl-ac.**,
form.[6], **gamb., GRAPH.**, hell.,
hep., hist.[14], hydr., hyos., ign.,
iod., ip., **iris**, kali-ar., **KALI-BI.,**
kali-c., **kali-i.**, kali-n., kali-s.,
kalm.[6], **kreos.**, lac-ac.[6], **lach.**,
laur., led., **lil-t., lith-c., lob., lyc.,**
m-arct.[3], m-aust.[3], mag-c.,
mag-m., mang., **MERC.,**
MERC-C., merc-i-f., MEZ.,
mosch., mur-ac., **nat-ar., nat-c.,**
nat-m., NIT-AC., nux-m.,
NUX-V., oena.[6], ol-j.[6], **op., osm.,**
ox-ac., par., **petr., ph-ac., PHOS.,**
phyt., plat., plb., **PRUN.**, psor.,
PULS., pyrog.[6], **ran-b.**, ran-s.,
rat., **rhod., RHUS-T.**, rob., **rumx.**,
ruta, **SABAD.**, sabin., **SANG.,**
sang-n., **sars., SEC.**, seneg.,
SEP., sil., sin-n., **SPIG., SPONG.,**
stann., staph., stram., stront-c.,
sul-ac., **SULPH.**, tab.[3], tarax.,
tarent.[1'], **tell., ter., thuj.**, uran.,
ust., uva, **verat.**, verat-v.,
viol-o., viol-t., wye., **ZINC.,**
ZINC-P.[1']

with external coldness[3]
avec froid extérieurement
mit äußerer Kälte
    ars., verat.

as from
comme par brûlure
wie durch Brennen
    agar., aloe, alum., ambr., **apis,**
    arum-t., bapt., bar-c., bell.,
    berb., bry., cann-s., caust., chin.,
    coloc., ferr., hyos., **ign.**, IRIS,
    kali-c., **lil-t., mag-m.**, merc.,
    mez., mur-ac., nat-c., **nux-v.**, op.,
    osm., par., phos., **phyt., plat.,**
    puls., ran-s., sabad., sang., **sep.,**
    still., sul-ac., tarent., thuj., verat.

as from glowing coals[16]
comme par des charbons ardents
wie durch glühende Kohlen
 ars., carb-v.

as from hot coals[16]
comme par des charbons brûlants
wie durch heiße Kohlen
 sabad.

blood-vessels, in
vaisseaux sanguins, dans les
Blutgefäßen, in
 agar., **ARS., aur.,** brom.[3], **bry.,**
 calc., carb-v.[3], chin.[3], com.[3],
 hyos., med., nat-m., nit-ac., **op.,**
 phos.[3], plb.[3], **RHUS-T.,** sec.[3],
 sulph., syph.[3], verat., xan.[3]

night[16]/nuit/nachts
 ARS.

bones, in
os, dans les
Knochen, in
 ang.[3], ant-t.[4], arn.[4], ars., **asaf.,**
 aur., bell.[11], bry., **carb-v.,**
 caust., chel.[3], coloc.[3], con.,
 dros.[3], **euph.,** fl-ac.[8], form.,
 hep., ign., kali-i.[3, 8], **lach.,** lyc.,
 mang., merc., **MEZ.,** nat-c.,
 nit-ac., par., **ph-ac.,** phos.,
 puls., **rhus-t., ruta,** sabin., **sep.,**
 sil., staph., **sulph.,** tarent.[2],
 thuj., **ZINC.**

night/nuit/nachts
 mez.[2], ph-ac., phos.[11]

menses, during
menstruation, pendant la
Menses, während der
 carb-v.

cold parts, in[3]
froides, dans les parties
kalten Körperteilen, in
 sec., verat.

glands, in
glandes, dans les
Drüsen, in
 alum., ant-c., arn., **ARS., bell.,**
 brom., bry., calc., **cann-s.,**
 carb-v., caust., cic., clem., cocc.,
 con., graph., **hep., ign.,** kali-c.,
 laur., merc., mez., nat-m., nux-v.,
 phos., phyt., plat., **PULS.,**
 rheum[3, 4], rhus-t., **sep., sil.,**
 staph., sul-ac., sulph., ter.[4],
 teucr., **zinc.**

joints, in[3]
articulations, dans les
Gelenken, in
 abrot.[3, 11], anac.[14], ant-t.[3, 11],
 arg-n., berb., carb-v., caust.,
 cimic., guare.[11], hist.[14], ign.[4],
 kali-n., lyc., nit-ac.[3, 4, 11], plat.,
 rhus-t., sabin.[1'], sulph.,
 thuj.[3, 11], zinc.

spots[2]/par endroits/stellenweise
 mang.

parts grasped with the hand
parties saisies avec la main, aux
Körperteile, die mit der Hand
 umfaßt sind, der
 bry., **CAUST.**

on which he lies at night[11]
sur lesquelles il se couche la nuit
auf denen man nachts liegt
 sulph.

spots, in[11]
endroits, par
stellenweise
 agar.[3, 11], ambr., apis, atha.,
 carb-v., chin., coloc., glon.[3], ign.,
 lim., lyc., mand.[14], nat-s., plat.,
 raph.[.] sang.[3], **SULPH.**[3, 11], viol-o.

constricting, externally
constrictives, externes
zusammenziehende, zusammen-
 schnürende, äußerlich
 acon., acon-c.[11], agar., alum.,
 alum-sil.[1'], **am-c.,** ambr.,
 AML-NS.[3,] anac., ang.[3], **ant-c.**[3],

apis[3], arg-m., **arg-n.**, arn., ars.[3],
asaf.[3], **asar.**[3], **aur.**[3], bar-c., **bell.**,
bism.[3], bor.[3], brom.[3], bry.,
cadm-s.[3], calad., **calc.**, camph.,
cann-s., **canth.**[3, 4], caps.[3],
carb-an.[3], **carb-v.**, caust., cham.,
chel., **chin.**[3], cic., **cina**, coc-c.[3],
cocc., coff.[3], colch., coloc.,
CON.[3, 4], croc., crot-h.[3], **cupr.**[3],
cycl., **dig.**, dros., dulc., euphr.,
ferr.[3], **gamb.**[11], gels.[3], glon.[3],
graph., guaj.[3], hell.[3], hep.[3],
hist.[9, 10], hydr-ac.[3], hyos., **IGN.**[4],
iod., kali-c., **kali-n.**, kreos.,
lach.[3], laur.[3], led., lob.[3], lyc.,
mag-c.[3], mag-m.[3, 4], manc.[3],
mang., meny., merc., mez.,
mosch., mur-ac.[3], nat-c.,
nat-m.[3, 4], **nit-ac.**, **NUX-M.**[3],
nux-v., oena.[3], olnd., **op.**[3], par.[3],
petr., ph-ac., **phos.**, phys.[3],
PLAT., **PLB**[3], pneu.[14], **PULS.**,
ran-b., ran-s.[3], rheum[3], rhod.,
rhus-t., ruta, sabad., sabin.[3], sars.[3],
sec.[3], sel.[3], sep., sil., spig.,
spong.[3], squil., **stann.**[3], staph.[3],
stram.[3], stront-c., **sul-ac.**[3], sulph.,
sumb., tab.[3], teucr., thuj., valer.,
verat., verb., viol-o.[3], viol-t.,
zinc.

constriction/Zusammenschnüren

internally
internes
innerlich
  acon., agar.[3], agn., **alum.**[3],
  am-c.[3], am-m., **AMBR.**, anac.,
  ang.[3], ant-c.[3], ant-t., arg-m., arn.,
  ars., asaf., asar., aur., bar-c.,
  bell., bism., bor., bov.[3], bry.,
  bufo[3], cact.[1', 3], calad.[3], **calc.**,
  camph., cann-s.[3], canth., caps.,
  carb-an., **carb-v.**, caust.[3], cham.,
  chel., chin., cic.[3], cina, clem.[3],
  cocc., coff.[3], **colch., coloc.**, con.,
  croc., cupr.[3], cycl., dig., dros.,
  dulc., euph.[3], ferr., graph.,
  guaj.[3], hell.[3], hep.[3], hyos., **IGN.**,
  iod., ip.[3], **kali-c.**, kali-n.[3], lach.,
  laur.[3], led., lyc., mag-c., mag-m.[3],

mang.[3], meny., merc., **mez.**,
mosch.[3], mur-ac., nat-c.[3], nat-m.,
nit-ac.[3], **nux-m.**[3], **nux-v.**, olnd.,
op.[3], par.[3], petr., **PH-AC.**, phos.,
PLAT., **PLB.**[3], puls., ran-s.,
rheum, rhod., rhus-t., ruta[3],
sabad.[3], sabin., samb.[3], sars.,
sec.[3], sel., seneg., sep., sil.,
spig.[3], spong., squil., stann.,
staph., stram., stront-c., sul-ac.,
sulph., tab.[3], tarax.[3], **teucr.**, thuj.,
valer., verat., verb.[3], viol-t.[3],
zinc.

bones, in
os, dans les
Knochen, in
  alum., am-m.[3], anac., **apis**[8],
  aur.[3], carb-ac.[8], chin.[3], cocc.[3],
  con.[3], gels.[3], **graph.**[3], hep.[8],
  kreos.[3], lyc.[3], merc.[3], nat-m.[3],
  NIT-AC.[3, 8], nux-v.[3], petr.[3],
  phos.[3], **PULS.**[3], rhod.[3], **rhus-t.**[3],
  ruta[3], sabad.[3], sep.[3], sil.[3],
  stront-c.[3], **SULPH.**[3, 8], valer.[3],
  zinc.[3]

glands, in
glandes, dans les
Drüsen, in
  acon.[3, 4], alum.[3, 4], am-c., anac.,
  arn.[3, 4], bell., **bor.**[3, 4], **calc.**,
  carb-v., caust., chin., cocc.[3, 4],
  con.[3, 4], ign., iod., kali-c., lyc.,
  mang.[3, 4], nat-c., **nit-ac.**[3, 4],
  nux-v., ph-ac., phos.[3, 4], **plat.**,
  plb.[3, 4], **puls., rhus-t.**[3, 4], sabad.,
  sep., sil., spong., sul-ac.[3, 4],
  sulph.[3, 4]

joints, in[3]
articulations, dans les
Gelenken, in
  acon., am-m., **ANAC., AUR.**,
  calc., carb-an., chin., coloc.,
  ferr., **GRAPH.**, kreos., lyc.,
  meny., **NAT-M., NIT-AC.**,
  nux-m., nux-v., **petr.**, pyrus[11],
  ruta, sil., spig., squil., stann.,
  stront-c., sulph., zinc.

orifices, of; sphincter spasm[3]
orifices, des; spasmes
  sphinctériens
Körperöffnungen, der;
  Schließmuskelkrämpfe
    alum., ars., **bell.**, calc., carb-v.,
    chel., cocc., colch., con., dig.,
    dulc., ferr., graph., hep., hyos.,
    ign., iod., ip., lyc., mez., nat-m.,
    nux-v., phos., plat., plb., rhod.,
    sabad., sars., sep., staph., stram.,
    sulph., tarax, thuj., verat.

cramping in joints[3]
crampoïdes dans les articulations
krampfhafte, in Gelenken
    acon., am-m., **anac., ANG.,** arn.,
    ars., aur., bar-c., **bell.**, bov., **bry.,**
    CALC., camph., cann-s., canth.,
    carb-an., caust., cham., chel.,
    chin., cic., cocc., colch., coloc.,
    con., cupr., dulc., euph., hep.,
    hist.[14], hyos., ign., kali-c., kali-n.,
    kreos., lach., laur., led., lyc.,
    m-arct., mez., nux-v., olnd., op.,
    par., petr., ph-ac.[2], phos., **PLAT.,**
    plb., rhus-t., sarcol-ac.[14], **sec.,**
    sel., spig., spong., staph., stram.,
    sulph., tab., verat., verb.,

muscles, in[3]
muscles, dans les
Muskeln, in
    acon., agar., alum., am-c., am-m.,
    ambr., **ANAC.**[2, 3]**, ANG.,** arg-m.,
    arn., ars., asaf., asar.[3, 14], aur.,
    bar-c., **BELL.**[1', 3], bism, bov.,
    bry., bufo, **CALC., CAMPH.**[2, 3],
    cann-s., caps., carb-an., carb-v.,
    carbn-s.[11], **caust.**[2, 3], cham., chin.,
    cic., cimic., **CINA,** clem.,
    cocc.[2, 3], colch., **COLOC.**[2, 3]**, con.,**
    conin.[11], croc., **CUPR.**[2, 3], cupr-a.[2],
    cyt-l.[14], dig., dios.[2], dros., **dulc.,**
    euph., euphr., ferr., **gels.**[2],
    graph.[2, 3], hell., hep., hist.[14],
    hyos., **ign.**[2, 3], iod., ip., **kali-br.**[2],
    kali-c., kali-n., kreos., lach.,
    lat-m.[9], **LYC.,** mag-c., **mag-m.,**
    mag-p., mang., meny., **MERC.,**
    mez., morph.[11], mosch., **mur-ac.,**

nat-c., nat-f.[14], nat-m., **nit-ac.,**
nux-m., **nux-v.**[2, 3], olnd., **op.**[2, 3],
petr., ph-ac., phos., phyt.[1', 3],
PLAT., plb.[2, 3, 11], puls., ran-b.,
rhod., **rhus-t.,** ruta, sabad., samb.,
sang., sarcol-ac.[14], sec., **SEP., sil.,**
spig., spong., squil., **stann.,**
staph., stram., stront-c., sul-ac.,
sulph., tab.[2, 3]**, thuj., valer.,**
VERAT., verb., viol-o., viol-t.,
zinc.[2, 3]

crushed, as if
écrasé, comme
zerquetscht, als ob
    anh.[9], apis[11], **canth.**[11], ran-b.[3],
    verb.[3]

cutting, externally
coupantes, externes
schneidende, äußerlich
    acon., **alum.,** alum-p.[1'],
    alum-sil,[1'], **alumn.**[2], ambr.,
    anac., ang.[2, 3, 4], ant-c.,
    arg-m., arn., ars-s-f[1'], asaf.,
    asar., aur., aur-ar.[1'], aur-s.[1'],
    BELL., berb.[3], bism., bor.,
    brom., bry., **calad.**[2]**, CALC.,**
    calc-i.[1']**, CALC-SIL.**[1'], camph.,
    cann-s., canth., carbn-s., caust.,
    chin., chin-s.[4], cimic., cina[3],
    clem., colch., **coloc., CON.,**
    conv., dig., **DROS.,** dulc., euph.,
    graph., hell., hep., hyos., **ign.,**
    kali-c., **kali-m.**[1'], kali-s., led.,
    lyc., mag-c.[1'], mag-m., mang.,
    meny., **merc.,** mez., mosch.,
    mur-ac., NAT-C., nat-m.,
    nat-sil.[1'], nit-ac., **nux-v.,** olnd.,
    osm., ox-ac.[1'], oxyt., par., **PETR.,**
    ph-ac., phos., plat., puls., ran-b.,
    rheum[2], rhod., **rhus-t.,** ruta,
    sabad., **samb.,** sang.[1'], sars.,
    seneg., **sep., sil.,** spig., stann.,
    staph., stram., **stront-c.**[2]**, sul-ac.,**
    sul-il.[1'], **sulph.,** teucr., thuj.,
    verat., **viol-t.,** zinc., **ZINC-P.**[1']

internally
internes
innerlich
   abies-n., acon., aesc., aeth.,
   agar., agn., all-c., alum., am-c.,
   am-m., ambr., anac., **ang.**[3],
   ant-c., ant-t., arg-m., arg-n.,
   arn., ars., asaf., asar., aur., bar-c.,
   bar-m., **BELL.**, **berb.**, bism., bor.,
   bov., bry., **calad.**, **CALC.**, calc-p.,
   camph., cann-i., cann-s.,
   CANTH., caps., carb-an., carb-v.,
   caust., cham., **chel.**, **chin.**, cic.,
   cina, clem., coc-c., cocc., coff.,
   colch., **coll.**, **COLOC.**, **CON.**,
   conv., croc., crot-h., crot-t.,
   cub., cupr., cycl., dig., **DIOS.**,
   dros., **dulc.**, **elat.**, **equis.**, ferr.,
   gamb., gels., graph., guaj., hell.,
   hep., hydr., **HYOS.**, ign., iod.,
   ip., iris, **KALI-C.**, kali-chl.,
   kali-n., **kali-s.**, lach., laur., led.,
   LYC., m-arct.[3], m-aust.[3], mag-c.,
   mag-m., mang., meny., **MERC.**,
   merc-c., mez., mosch., **mur-ac.**,
   nat-c., **NAT-M.**, nit-ac., nux-m.,
   NUX-V., **op.**, **par.**, petr., ph-ac.,
   phos., plat., plb., **PULS.**, ran-b.,
   ran-s., **rheum**, rhod., rhus-t.,
   ruta, sabad., sabin., samb., sars.,
   sel., seneg., **sep.**, **SIL.**, **spig.**,
   spong., squil., **stann.**, **staph.**,
   stront-c., sul-ac., **SULPH.**, teucr.,
   thuj., valer., **VERAT.**, verb., **vib.**,
   viol-t., **ZINC.**, zing.

blood-vessels, in[3]
vaisseaux sanguins, dans les
Blutgefäßen, in
   calc.

bones, in long
os longs, dans les
Knochen, in langen
   anac.[2, 4], aur-m.[3], calc., dig.[2, 4],
   kali-bi.[3], kali-m.[3], osm., sabad.

glands, in
glandes, dans les
Drüsen, in
   arg-m., **bell.**, calc., con., graph.,
   ign., **lyc.**, nat-c., ph-ac., **sep.**,
   sil., staph., sulph.

around glands[16]
autour des ganglions
um die Drüsen herum
   con.

joints, in[2, 11]
articulations, dans les
Gelenken, in
   cadm-s., guare., hyos.[4, 11],
   sabad.[4, 11], vesp.[11]

digging up (burrowing, rooting
   sensation)
creusantes, fouillantes, sensation
   fouissante
grabende, wühlende
   acon., agar., alum., alum-p.[1'],
   alum-sil.[1'], am-c., **am-m.**, ambr.,
   anac., ang.[3], ant-c., ant-t., arg-m.,
   arg-n., **arn.**, ars., **asaf.**, asar.,
   aur., bar-c., bar-m., **bell.**, bism.,
   bor., **bov.**, **bry.**, calc., cann-s.,
   canth., caps., carb-an., carb-v.,
   caust., cham., chel., chin., **cina**,
   clem., cocc., colch., **coloc.**, con.,
   croc., dig., dros., **DULC.**, euph.,
   ferr., graph., guare.[11], hell., hep.,
   ign., **kali-bi.**, **kali-c.**, kali-n.,
   kreos., laur., led., lyc., m-arct.,[3]
   m-aust.[3], mag-c., mag-m., mang.,
   merc., mez., mur-ac., **nat-c.**,
   nat-m., nux-m., nux-v., olnd.,
   petr., ph-ac., **phos., plat.**, puls.,
   rheum, **RHOD., rhus-t., ruta,**
   sabad., sabin., samb., seneg.,
   sep., sil., **SPIG.**, spong., squil.,
   stann., staph., stront-c., sul-ac.,
   sulph., thuj., valer., zinc.

bones, in
os, dans les
Knochen, in
   aran., arg-m.[11], asaf., **aur.**[8], calc.,
   carb-ac.[8], **carb-an., cocc.**, dulc.,

kali-i.[8], **mang.**, merc.[8], rhod.,
ruta, sep., spig., symph.[8], thuj.

night[16]/nuit/nachts
  mang.

glands, in
glandes, dans les
Drüsen, in
  acon., am-m., arn., asaf., bell.,
  bov., bry., calc., **dulc.**, kali-c.,
  nat-c., phos., plat., **rhod.**, rhus-t.,
  ruta, sep., spig., stann.

joints, in
articulations, dans les
Gelenken, in
  bell.[11], colch.[3]

drawing
tiraillantes
ziehende
  acon., adon.[6], agar.[4], aloe,
  alum.[4], am-c., ambr.[4], anac.,
  ang.[4], ant-t.[4], aphis[4], aran-ix.[10],
  arg-m., arn.[3, 4], ars.[3, 4], asar.[4],
  aur-m.[1'], bar-a.[11], bar-c.,
  bell.[1', 3, 4], bor.[4], **bry., calad.**[3],
  calc.[4, 6], calc-p.[1'], calen.[4],
  camph., cann-s.[4], canth.[4],
  caps.[4], carb-ac.[6], carb-an.[4],
  CARB-V., card-m.[1'], **caul.**,
  caust., **cham.**[3, 4, 6], **CHEL.**,
  chin.[1', 3, 4], chin-ar., chin-s.[4],
  cic.[4], cimic.[1', 3], cist.[4], clem.,
  coc-c., cocc.[4], colch., **COLOC.**,
  con.[3], **crot-t.**, cycl.[1', 4], dig.,
  digin.[11], **dros.**[3], **dulc.**[3, 4, 6],
  esp-g.[13], euon., euph.[3], euphr.[3],
  eupi., ferr-ar., **gamb.**, goss.,
  GRAPH., guaj.[1'], guare.,
  hell.[3], hep.[3, 4], hist.[10], hydrc.,
  hyos.[4], ip.[4], kali-bi., kali-c.,
  kreos., lach., lact., lam.[4],
  laur.[3], led.[4], lup.[4], lyc.,
  m-arct.[4], mag-c.[10], mag-m.[1', 4],
  mang., med.[1'], merc., merc-c.[4],
  mez., **mosch.**[3, 4], mur-ac.[3, 4],
  nat-c.[3, 4], **NIT-AC.**, nux-m.[4],
  nux-v., ol-an., olnd.[4], petr.[4],
  ph-ac.[4, 6], phos., phyt.[1'], plat.,
  PLB.[1', 3, 4], **puls.**, ran-s.[4], raph.,

rhod., **RHUS-T.**[1', 3, 4], ruta[3],
sabad.[4], sabin.[4], samb.[4],
sars.[4, 16], sec., sep., **sil.**[3, 6, 16],
stann., staph., stram.[4], sul-ac.[4],
sulph., tab., ter.[4], thuj., tub.[1'],
VALER., verat.[4], verb.[3],
viol-o.[4], **zinc.**[1', 3, 6], zinc-o.[4]

left side night[16]
gauche nuit, le côté
linken Seite, nachts auf der
  lyc.

right side[16]
droit, le côté
rechten Seite, auf der
  sep.

morning, after rising
matin après le lever
morgens nach dem Aufstehen
  graph.

  after waking
  après le réveil
  nach dem Erwachen
    coloc.

evening/soir/abends
  coc-c., raph.

  20 h
    rhus-t.

  22 h
    bry.

night/nuit/nachts
  coc-c.

alternating with heart symptoms
alternant avec des symptôms
  cardiaques
abwechselnd mit
  Herzsymptomen
  acon.

backward as by a cord[3]
en arrière comme par un cordon
rückwärts wie durch eine Schnur
  crot-t., par., plb.

chill, during[16]
frissons, pendant les
Fieberfrost, während
   lyc.

cold, as from a[16]
froid, comme par un
Erkältung, wie von einer
   plat.

cramplike[16]
crampoïdes
krampfartig
   plat.

eating, after[16]
mangé, après avoir
Essen, nach dem
   camph.

increasing and decreasing
   rapidly[16]
d'apparition et de disparition
   rapide
schnell zu- und abnehmend
   nit-ac.

menses, during
menstruation, pendant la
Menses, während der
   phos.

motion, on
mouvement, au
Bewegung, durch
   calc., cycl.

paralytic
paralytiques
lähmend
   coc-c., staph.[16]

rest, during[1']
repos, pendant le
Ruhe, während der
   tub.

rheumatic
rhumatismales
rheumatische
   am-c.[16], carb-v., chel., sul-ac.

rising, after
levé, après s'être
Aufstehen, nach dem
   coloc.

sitting, while
assis, en étant
Sitzen, im
   samb., **VALER.**

upwards
en montant
aufwärts
   ol-an.

walking, agg.
marcher agg.
Gehen agg.
   calc., coca
am.
   rhus-t.[16], tub.[1']

weather agg., bad
temps agg., mauvais
Wetter agg., schlechtes
   rhod.

wrong position, from[16]
mauvaise position, par une
unbequeme Lage, durch
   staph.

extending to fingers
irradiant aux doigts
erstreckt sich zu den **Fingern**
   apis

toes
orteils
Zehen
   apis

bones, in[3]
os, dans les
Knochen, in
   acon.[4], agar.[3, 4], agn., anac.[4],
   ang.[4], ant-t., asaf.[4, 8], atha.[4],
   aur.[3, 4], **bar-c.**[4], bry.[3, 4], calc-f.,
   cann-s., canth., **carb-v.**[4],
   caust.[4], cham.[3, 11], **chin.**[3, 4, 11, 16],
   cocc.[3, 11], colch., crot-h.[4], cupr.[4],
   cycl., gels.[3, 11], graph.[16], hell.,

ign.[4], indg.[4], ip., kali-bi.,
kali-c.[3, 4], kreos.[4], led., **lyc.**[4],
m-arct.[4], mang.[4], meny.[4],
merc.[3, 4, 11], nat-m., nit-ac.[8],
nux-m., olnd., par.[3, 4], petr.[16],
ph-ac.[4], plb.[4], puls., rhod.[3, 4],
sabad., **SABIN.**[3, 4], samb.[3, 4],
seneg.[3, 4], sil., spig., stann.[4],
staph.[3, 4], sulph., ter.[4], teucr.,
thuj.[4], valer., verat., zinc.[16],
zinc-o.[4]

thread, as from a
linéaires
Faden, wie von einem
   bry.

threads/fils/Fäden

glands, in[3]
glandes, dans les
Drüsen, in
  agn., alum.[4], **bell.**, bov., calc.,
  cann-s., cham., **chin.**, cycl.,
  guaj.[11], **ign.**[3, 4], **merc.**[4], mez.,
  nit-ac., phos.[3, 11, 16], **puls.**[3, 4],
  seneg., sil.[3, 4], sulph., thuj.

joints, in[3]
articulations, dans les
Gelenken, in
  acon.[2, 3], agn., am-c.[4], ang.,
  ant-c., ant-s-aur.[11], **ant-t.**[3, 11],
  arg-m.[3, 11], asaf., asar., bar-c.,
  bell., **bry.**[11], calc.[4], cann-s.,
  canth., caps., **carl.**[11], **caul.**,
  cham.[3, 11], chel., chin., cina,
  cist.[4, 11], clem.[11], coc-c., cocc.,
  colch., cupr., cycl., graph.[4], hep.[4],
  hyos.[3, 4, 11], ign., kali-c.[4], led.,
  lyc.[4, 11], **m-aust.**, meny., merc.,
  mez.[3, 4, 11], nat-c., nat-m.[11],
  nat-s.[11], nit-ac.[4, 11], nit-s-d.[11],
  nux-m.[2], nux-v., olnd., par.,
  phos.[11], plat.[3, 4], plb., puls.[3, 4],
  rheum, **rhod.**[3, 4, 11], rhus-t.,
  sabad.[3, 4], sabin.[3, 4], sec.[3, 4, 11],
  seneg., sep.[4], spig., spong.,
  STAPH.[3, 4], tarax., teucr., valer.,
  verat., viol-o.

muscles, in[3]
muscles, dans les
Muskeln, in
  acon., agn., alum., ambr., anac.,
  ang., **ANT-C., ANT-T.**, apis,
  arg-m., arn., asaf., asar., aur.,
  bar-c., **BELL.**, berb., bism., bov.,
  bry., calc., **camph.**, cann-s.,
  canth., **caps.**, carb-ac., **carb-v.**,
  caust., CHAM., chel., chin.[1', 3],
  cic., **cina, clem., COCC.**, coff.,
  colch., croc., cupr., **CYCL.**, dig.,
  dros., dulc., euph., ferr.,
  GRAPH., hell., hep., hydr.[11],
  hyos., **ign.**, ip., kali-bi., kali-c.,
  kali-n., led., **lyc., meny.**, merc.,
  mez., morph.[11], **mosch.**, nat-m.,
  nit-ac., **nux-m.**, nux-v., olnd.,
  par., petr., ph-ac., phos., **PLAT.**,
  plb., PULS., ran-b., ran-s.,
  raph.[11], **RHOD., rhus-t.**, ruta,
  sabad., sabin., samb., sec., sep.,
  sil., spig., spong., **squil.**, staph.,
  stram., sul-ac., **sulph.**, tarax.,
  teucr., thuj., VALER., verat.,
  verb., viol-o., viol-t., **zinc.**

tendons, in[3]
tendons, des
Sehnen, in
  am-m.[1'], kali-bi., nat-m., rhus-t.,
  thuj.

gnawing
rongeantes
nagende
  agn.[6], alum-sil.[1'], **ars.**, bar-s.[1'],
  caust., lach.[6], **MERC.**, mez.[6],
  nat-m.[6], sil., staph., sulph.

externally
externes
äußerlich
  acon., agar., **AGN.**, alum.,
  alumn.[2], am-c., ambr., arg-m.,
  arn., aur., **bar-c.**, bar-m., bell.,
  bry., calad., calc., calc-p.[11],
  canth., caps., **cham., crot-t.**,
  cycl., dig., **dros.**, dulc., euph.,
  ferr., gamb.[11], **glon.**, graph., hell.,
  hyos., ign., **kali-c.**, kreos., laur.,

led., lyc., mag-c., mag-m., mang.,
meny., merc., mez., mur-ac.,
nat-c., nux-v., olnd., op., **par.**,
ph-ac., phos., PLAT., plb., **puls.**,
RAN-S., rheum, rhod., rhus-t.,
ruta, samb., sep., sil., spig.,
SPONG., stann., **STAPH.**,
stront-c., sulph., **tarax.**, thuj.,
verat., zinc.

internally
internes
innerlich
    agar., alum., am-m., arg-m.,
    arg-n.[3], **ars.**, bar-c., **bell.**, calad.,
    calc., cann-s., canth.[1], carb-an.[3],
    carb-v., CAUST., chel., cocc.,
    coloc., con., cupr., dig., dros.,
    dulc., **gamb.**, glon.[3], hep., iod.,
    kali-bi., kali-c., kali-i.[3], **kreos.**,
    lach., **lyc.**, merc., mez., nat-m.[3, 6],
    nux-v., olnd., ph-ac., phos., **plat.**,
    psor.[3], **PULS.**, ran-b.[3, 6], **ran-s,,**
    rhod., **RUTA**, seneg., **SEP.**, sil.,
    stann., staph.[6], stront-c.[6], sulph.,
    teucr., verat.

bones, in
os, dans les
Knochen, in
    am-m., arg-m., **aur.**[8], **BELL.**,
    brom., canth., carb-ac.[8], **con.**[1],
    dros., graph., kali-bi.[3], kali-i.,
    lyc., **mang.**, merc.[8], nat-s.[3, 11],
    ph-ac., phos., plb.[11], puls., rhod.[3],
    ruta, samb., **staph.**, stront-c.,
    sulph.[3, 6], symph.[8]

glands, in
glandes, dans les
Drüsen, in
    bar-c., cham., mez., ph-ac., **plat.**,
    ran-s., **spong.**, staph.

joints, in
articulations, dans les
Gelenken, in
    am-c., aur-m.[1'], canth., colch.,
    dros.[2, 3, 11], dulc., graph., mag-c.,
    mang., phos., **RAN-S.**, stront-c.,
    zinc.

growing pains[3]
croissance, douleurs de
Wachstumsschmerzen
    acon.[11], agar.[1', 3], bell.,
    calc-p.[1', 3, 8], **ferr-a.**[3, 6],
    guaj.[3, 6, 8, 12], mang.[3, 8], ol-an.,
    PH-AC.[2, 3, 6, 8], phos.[3, 6], sil.[7]

    legs, in
    jambes, dans les
    Unterschenkeln, in
        bell., **calc-p.**[7], cimic., **eup-per.**,
        GUAJ., kali-p.[7], m-aust.[7],
        mag-p.[7], mang.[7], **PH-AC.**

intolerable[16]
intolérables
unerträgliche
    ars., **cham.**, nux-v.

    sensitiveness–pain/sensitivité–
    douleur/Empfindlichkeit–
    Schmerzempfindlichkeit
    Vol. I: *sensitive–pain/sensible–*
    douleurs/empfindlich–Schmerzen

jerking externally
saccades externes, par
ruckartige, äußerlich
    acon., agar., agn., **alum.**,
    alum-p.[1'], alum-sil.[1'], **alumn.**[2],
    ambr., anac., ang.[3], ant-c., ant-t.,
    arg-m., **arn.**, ars., **ASAF.**, asar.,
    aur., bar-c., **bar-m.**, bar-s.[1'],
    bell., bism., bor., bov., **bry.**,
    CALC., calc-a.[6], calc-i.[1'],
    calc-sil.[1'], camph., **cann-s.**[2, 6],
    canth., caps., carb-v.,
    carbn-s., CAUST., cham.,
    chin., cic., cimic.[1'], **cina, clem.**,
    cocc., coff., colch., coloc.,
    con.[3], croc.[3, 6], cupr.[6, 16], cycl.[3],
    dig.[3], dros.[3], dulc.[3], **graph.**[2, 3, 6],
    hell.[3], hep.[3], hyos.[3], **IGN.**[2, 3, 6],
    iod., kali-bi.[3], kali-c., kali-m.[1'],
    kali-s., kreos., lach., laur., led.,
    lyc., mag-c., **mag-p.**, mang.,
    MENY., merc., mez., mosch.,
    mur-ac., **nat-c., NAT-M.**,
    nit-ac., nux-m.[2], **NUX-V.**,
    olnd., op., par., **petr., petros.**[2],
    ph-ac., phos., phyt., plat., plb.,

PULS., **ran-b.**, ran-s., rheum,
rhod., **RHUS-T.**, ruta, sabad.,
sabin., sec., **sep., sil.**, spig.,
spong., **squil., stann.**, staph.,
stront-c., sul-ac., sul-i.[1]',
sulph., **TARAX.**, teucr., thuj.,
VALER., verat., verb., viol-t.,
zinc.

affected parts, of
affectées, des parties
leidenden Teile, der
arn.[16], **merc.**

on rising from bed[16]
en se levant du lit
beim Aufstehen aus dem Bett
mag-c.

internally
internes
innerlich
acon., agar., aloe, am-m., ambr.,
anac., ang.[3], arn., ars., **BELL.**,
bor., bry., **calc.**, cann-s., carb-v.,
caust., cham., **CHIN.**, clem.,
cocc., colch., con., croc., graph.,
IGN., KALI-C., lyc., mang.,
meny., **merc.**, mez., nat-m.,
NIT-AC., nux-v., petr., ph-ac.,
plat., plb., **PULS.**, ran-b., ran-s.,
rhus-t., **sep., SIL., spig., stann.**,
stront-c., sul-ac., **SULPH.**, teucr.,
THUJ., valer.

bones, in
os, dans les
Knochen, in
anac.[4], **ASAF.**, aur., bell., **calc.**,
caust., **chin.**, clem., colch., lyc.,
mang.[3], merc., **nat-m.**, nux-v.,
ol-an.[3], petr., phos., **puls.**, rhod.,
rhus-t., sep., sil., sul-ac.[4],
SULPH., symph.[2], **valer.**

glands, in
glandes, dans les
Drüsen, in
arn., asaf., aur., bell., bry.,
calc., caps., caust., chin., **clem.**,
graph., lyc., meny., merc., nat-c.,
nat-m., nit-ac., nux-v., petr.,
puls., rhus-t., sep., sil., sulph.

right side, of[16]
droite, de la
rechten Seite, der
cupr.

paralytic
paralytiques
lähmende
acon., agar., agn., alum.,
alum-sil.[1]', am-c., am-m., ambr.,
ang.[3], ant-c., arg-m., arg-n.[3],
ars., ars-i., asaf., asar., **aur.**,
bar-c., **BELL., bism.**, bov., **bry.**,
calc., cann-s., canth., caps.[4],
carb-v., caust., **cham.**, chel.,
chin., CINA, COCC., coff.,
COLCH., coloc., con., croc.,
crot-h., **CYCL.**, dig., dros.,
dulc., eug.[4], euph., euphr., **ferr.**,
ferr-ar., ferr-m.[4], gels.[3], graph.,
grat.[3], hell., hep., hyos., ign.,
iod., kali-c., kali-n., kali-p.,
kreos., lach.[4], **laur.**, led., lyc.,
m-arct.[4], mag-c., mag-m., mang.,
meny., meph.[4], merc., **mez.**,
mosch., mur-ac., nat-c., **nat-m.**,
NUX-V., olnd., par., petr., ph-ac.,
phos., plat., plb., puls., ran-s.,
raph.[11], rheum[4], rhod., **rhus-t.**,
ruta, sabad., **SABIN.**, sars., sel.,
seneg., sep., **sil.**, spig., stann.,
staph., stram., stront-c., sul-ac.,
sulph., teucr., thuj., valer.,
verat., verb., zinc.

bones, in
os, dans les
Knochen, in
AUR., bell., chin., **cocc., crot-h.**[4],
cycl., dig., **lach.**[4], led., mez.,
nat-m., nux-v., petr., phos.[3],
puls., rhus-t., sabin., **sil.**, staph.,
verat., zinc.

joints, in[3]
articulations, dans les
Gelenken, in
acon., agn., am-c., ambr., anac.,
arg-m., **arn.**[3, 4], ars., **asar., AUR.**,
bell., bism., **bov.**, calc.,
CAPS.[2, 3, 4], **carb-v.**, caust.,

cham., **chin.**, cina, cocc., colch., coloc., con., **croc.**, dig., **dros.**, **EUPH.**[3, 4], ferr., graph., hell., ign., kali-c., kali-n., laur.[4], **led.**[2, 3, 4], lyc., mag-m., meny., merc., **mez.**, nat-c., nat-m., nux-v., **par.**, petr., ph-ac., phos.[3, 4], **plb.**[2, 3], **puls.**[3, 4], rhus-t.[3, 4], ruta, sabad., **sabin.**[3, 4], samb., sars., **seneg.**, sep., stann., **STAPH.**[3, 4], stram., stront-c., sulph., **VALER.**, verat., verb., zinc.

pinching
pinçantes
kneifende

agar., alum., alum-sil.[1'], **am-c.**[2], ambr., anac., **ARN.**, **ars.**, ars-i., asar., bar-c.[11], **BELL.**, bov., bry., **calc.**, calc-i.[1'], cann-s., canth., **caps.**, carb-an., **carb-v.**, caust., **cham.**, chel.[2], chin.[2], cina, clem., cocc., **colch.**, coloc., con., croc., dros., dulc., **euph., gamb.**[11], graph.[2], guaj., hell., hep., hyos.[2], ign., iod., kali-c., kali-i.[11], kali-m[1'], kali-n., kreos., **laur.**, lyc., mag-m., mang., meny., **merc.**, **mez.**, mur-ac., **nat-c.**, nat-m., nit-ac., nux-m.[1], **NUX-V.**, op., par., petr., **phos., plat., puls.**, ran-b., ran-s., **rheum**, rhod., **rhus-t.**, ruta, **sabad.**, sabin., sars., seneg., sep., sil., spig., **spong.**, stann., staph., stront-c., **sulph.**, teucr., thuj., tub.[1'], valer., verat., verb., zinc.

right side, of
droite, de la
rechten Seite, der
    sep.

externally
externes
äußerlich

acon., anac., ang.[3], ant-c., arg-m., arn., bell., bry., **calc.**, cann-s., caps., carb-v., caust., chel., chin., cina, **clem.**, cocc., con., croc., dig., dros., dulc., euph., euphr., **hyos., ip.**, kali-c., kreos., led.,

mang., **MENY., mur-ac.**, nat-c., nit-ac., nux-v., olnd., **osm.**, par., ph-ac., phos., **RHOD., rhus-t.**, ruta, **SABAD.**, sabin., samb., sars., sil., **spig. SPONG., STANN.**, staph., sul-ac., **sulph.**, thuj., verat., **VERB.**, viol-t., zinc.

internally
internes
innerlich

acon., **agar.**, agn., alum., **am-c.**, am-m., anac., ang.[3], ant-c., ant-t., arg-m., arn., ars., ars-i., asaf., asar., aur., bar-c., **bell., bism.**, bor., bov., **bry., CALC.**, camph., **cann-s., canth.**, caps.[1], carb-an., **carb-v.**, caust., cham., **CHEL., chin.**, cic., **cina**, coc-c., **COCC.**, coff., **colch., COLOC.**, com., con.[3], croc., cupr., cycl., dig., dros., **dulc.**, euph., euphr., **gamb., GRAPH.**, guaj., **hell.**, hep., hyos., **IGN.**, iod., **ip.**, kali-c., kreos., **LYC.**, mag-c., mag-m., mang., **meny., merc.**, mez., mosch., **mur-ac., nat-c., nat-m.**, nit-ac., nux-m., nux-v., olnd., **par., petr.**, ph-ac., **phos.**, plat., **plb., puls., ran-b.**, ran-s., rheum, **rhod., rhus-t., ruta, sabad.**, sabin., samb., sars., seneg., **sep.**, sil., **spig., spong.**, squil., **stann., staph.**, stront-c., sul-ac., **sulph.**, tarax., teucr., **thuj.**, valer., verat., **VERB.**, viol-t., **zinc.**

bones, in
os, dans les
Knochen, in
    bell., calc., cina, ign., mez., nux-m.[11], osm., petr., **ph-ac.**, plat., **VERB.**

glands, in
glandes, dans les
Drüsen, in
    bry., **calc.**, m-arct.[4], meny., mur-ac., prun.[4], **rhod.**, rhus-t., sabad., stann., sulph., verat.

muscles, in[4]
muscles, dans les
Muskeln, in
  bruc., cann-s., lyc.,. m-aust.,
  sulph.[4, 11]

spots, in[11]
endroits, par
stellenweise
  caust., daph., lyc.

pressing, externally
pressives, poussantes externes
drückende, äußerlich
  abrot., **acon., aesc., AGAR.,** agn.,
  aloe, alum., **alum-p.**[1'], **alum-sil.**[1'],
  am-m., ambr., **ammc., anac.,**
  ang.[3], ant-c., **ant-t., APOC.,**
  arg-m., arn., ars., ars-i.,
  ARS-S-F.[1'], **asaf.,** asar., **aspar.,**
  aur., aur-i.[1'], aur-m.[1'], **aur-s.**[1'],
  bapt., bar-c., bar-i.[1'], bar-m.,
  bar-s[1]., **bell.,** berb.[4], bism., bor.,
  bov., **bry., calad., calc.,** calc-i.[1'],
  calc-p., calc-sil.[1'], calen.[4],
  camph., CANN-I., cann-s.,
  canth., caps., **carb-ac.,** carb-an.,
  carb-v.[3], carbn-s., **CAUST.,** cedr.,
  cham., chel., chin., **CHIN-S.,** cic.,
  cimic., cina, cinnb., clem., cob.,
  coc-c., **cocc.,** coff., **colch., coloc.,**
  con., crot-t., cupr., **cycl.,** daph.[4],
  dig., dios., **DROS., dulc.,** elaps,
  EUP-PER., euph., euphr., **FERR.,**
  ferr-ar., **gels., glon., graph.,**
  guaj., hell., hep., **hyos., ign.,** iod.,
  ip., KALI-BI., kali-c., kali-m.[1'],
  kali-n., kali-p., **kalm., kreos.,**
  lach., **laur., led., lil-t.,** lyc., mag-c.,
  mag-m., mang., meny., merc.,
  mez., MOSCH., mur-ac., nat-ar.,
  nat-c., **nat-m.,** nat-sil.[1'], **NIT-AC.,**
  nux-m., **NUX-V.,** olnd., **ox-ac.,**
  par., pareir., **petr., ph-ac.,**
  PHOS., phyt., plat., plb., **PODO.,**
  prun., **psor., PULS.,** ran-b., ran-s.,
  rheum, **RHOD., RHUS-T., RUTA,**
  sabad., sabin., **samb., sang., sars.,**
  sec., seneg., SEP., SIL., SPIG.,
  spong., **squil., STANN., STAPH.,**
  stict., stront-c., sul-ac., **sul-i.**[1'],
  SULPH., tab., **tarax.,** teucr., thuj.,

ust., valer., **verat.,** verb., vib.,
viol-o., viol-t., **zinc.,** zinc-p.[1']

internally
internes
innerlich
  acon., aesc., agar., agn., **ail.,**
  aloe, alum., am-c., am-m., **ambr.,**
  anac., ang.[3], ant-c., ant-t., arg-m.,
  ARG-N., ARN., ARS., ars-i.,
  arum-t., ASAF., asar., **aur.,**
  aur-ar.[1'], aur-i.[1'], bar-c., **BELL.,**
  berb., **bism., bor.,** bov., **BROM.,**
  bry., cact., calad., **CALC.,**
  camph., cann-i., cann-s.,
  CANTH., caps., **carb-an.,**
  CARB-V., carbn-s., **caust., cedr.,**
  cham., chel., chen-a., **CHIN.,** cic.,
  CIMIC., cina, clem., **coc-c.,**
  cocc., cod., coff., **colch., COLOC.,**
  con., cor-r., croc., crot-t., **CUPR.,**
  cycl., **dig.,** dios., dros., dulc.,
  elaps, euph., euphr., **ferr., gamb.,**
  gels., glon., goss., **graph.,** guaj.,
  HAM., hell., hep., hydr.,
  hydr-ac., hyos., hyper., **ign.,** iod.,
  ip., iris, kali-bi., **kali-c., kali-i.,**
  kali-n., **kalm.,** kreos., **LACH.,**
  laur., led., **lept., LIL-T., lith-c.,**
  LYC., mag-c., mang., **MENY.,**
  merc., merc-c., merc-i-f., **mez.,**
  mosch., mur-ac., murx., naja,
  nat-ar., nat-c., **NAT-M., nit-ac.,**
  nux-m., **NUX-V.,** olnd., onos.,
  OP., osm., **ox-ac.,** par., **PETR.,**
  ph-ac., PHOS., phys., phyt.,
  pic-ac., plat., plb., **podo., prun.,**
  psor., **PULS., RAN-B.,** ran-s.,
  rheum, rhod., **RHUS-T., rumx.,**
  RUTA, sabad., **sabin.,** samb.,
  SANG., SANG-N., sars., **SEC.,**
  SENEG., SEP., SIL., SPIG.,
  SPONG., squil., STANN., staph.,
  stict., stram., stront-c., sul-ac.,
  SULPH., tab., **tarax.,** tarent.,
  ter., teucr., thuj., ust., **VALER.,**
  VERAT., verat-v., verb., vesp.,
  vib., viol-o., viol-t., vip., xan.,
  ZINC., ZINC-P.[1']

inward
en dedans
nach innen
  acon., agar., alum., **ANAC.,**
  ant-c., ant-t., asaf., asar., aur.,
  bar-c., bell., bism., bor., bry.,
  calc., cann-s., carb-an., caust.,
  chel., chin., **cocc.,** coff., croc.,
  cycl., **dulc., hell.,** hep., ign.,
  kali-c., **kreos.,** laur., mez.,
  mosch., **nit-ac.,** nux-m., nux-v.,
  olnd., ph-ac., **PLAT.,** prun.[7],
  ran-s., rheum, rhod., rhus-t.,
  ruta, sabad., sabin., sars., sep.,
  sil., **spig., STANN., staph.,**
  sul-ac., **sulph.,** tarax., teucr.,
  thuj., valer., verb., viol-t.,
  zinc.

deep inward with instruments
interne profonde comme par un
  instrument
tief nach innen wie durch ein
  Instrument
  bov., verat.

load, as from a
poids, comme par un
Gewicht, wie von einem
  abies-n., ACON., aesc., agar.,
  aloe, alum., am-c., **am-m., ambr.,**
  ant-t., aran., arg-m., **arg-n.,** arn.,
  ars., asaf., asar., aur., **bar-c.,**
  BELL., bism., bor., bov., **BROM.,**
  BRY., cact., calad., calc., camph.,
  cann-s., carb-an., carb-v., caust.,
  cham., **chel.,** chin., cina, cinnb.,
  cocc., colch., coloc., **com., con.,**
  croc., corn., crot-t., **cupr.,** dig.,
  ferr., gels., graph., hell., hep.,
  hyos., ign., iod., **IP.,** kali-c.,
  kali-chl., kali-n., **kreos.,**
  laur., led., **LIL-T.,** lyc.,
  mag-c., mag-m., mang., **meli.,**
  MENY., merc., mosch., **nat-c.,**
  nat-m., nit-ac., nux-m., **NUX-V.,**
  olnd., **op., PAR.,** petr., **ph-ac.,**
  PHOS., plat., plb., **psor., puls.,**
  RAN-B., rheum[1], rhod., **RHUS-T.,**
  sabad., sabin., **samb.,** sars., **sec.,**
  seneg., **SEP., sil., spig.,** spong.,
  squil., stann., staph., **STICT.,**

stront-c., sul-ac., **SULPH.,** thuj.,
valer., **verb.,** viol-o., zinc., zing.

together
compressives
zusammendrückende
  acon., aeth.[3], agar., **alum.,** am-m.,
  ambr., **anac.,** ang.[3], ant-c., ant-t.,
  arg-m., arg-n.[3], **arn., ars.,** asaf.,
  ASAR., aur. bar-c., **bell., bov.,**
  bry., cact.[3], calc., camph.,
  cann-s., canth., caps., carb-an.,
  carb-v., caust., cham., chel.,
  chin., cic., cimic.[3], cina, **COCC.,**
  coff., coloc., con., cupr., dig.,
  dros., dulc., euph., ferr., graph.,
  guaj., **hell.,** helon.[3], hydr-ac.[3],
  hyos., ign., iod., **ip.,** kali-c.,
  kali-i.[3], kali-n., laur., led., lil-t.[3],
  lyc., mag-c., mag-m., meny.,
  merc., mez., **mosch., nat-m.,**
  nit-ac., nux-m., **NUX-V.,** olnd.,
  op., petr., ph-ac., phos., **PLAT.,**
  plb., puls., ran-s., rhod., rhus-t.,
  ruta, sabad., sabin., **sars.,** seneg.,
  sep., sil., spig., **spong.,** squil.,
  stann., staph., stram., stront-c.,
  sul-ac., SULPH., tarax., teucr.,
  thuj., valer., verat., verb.[1],
  viol-t., zinc.

upward[3]
vers le haut
aufwärts
  calc-p.

within outward, from
de dedans en dehors
von innen nach außen
  acon., **aloe,** alum., am-c., am-m.,
  anac., ang.[3], ant-c., ant-t.[3],
  arg-m., arg-n.[3], arn., ars.[3],
  ASAF., asar., **aur.,** bar-c., **bell.,**
  berb., bism., bor., bov.[3], **BRY.,**
  calc., camph., cann-s., canth.,
  caps., carb-an.[3], carb-v., caust.,
  cham.[3], chel., chin., **CIMIC.,**
  cina, clem., cocc., coff.[3], colch.,
  coloc., con., **cor-r.,** croc., cupr.,
  dig., **dros.,** dulc., euph., **ferr.,**
  graph., guaj., ham.[3], hell., hep.,
  hyos.[3], **ign.,** iod.[3], ip., iris[3],

kali-c., **kali-i.,** kali-n., kreos.,
lach., laur., led., **lith-c.,** lyc.,
mag-c.[3], mag-m., mang., meli.,
meny., **merc., merc-c., mez.,**
mosch.[3], **mur-ac.,** nat-c., **nat-m.,**
nit-ac., nux-m., **nux-v.,** olnd., op.,
par., petr., ph-ac., **phos.,** plat.,
plb.[3], **prun., PULS.,** ran-b., ran-s.,
rheum, rhod., **rhus-t.,** ruta,
sabad., **sabin.,** samb., sars.[3],
seneg., **sep., sil., spig., spong.,**
squil., stann., staph., stront-c.,
sul-ac., **SULPH.,** tarax., **teucr.,**
thuj., usn.[3], **VALER.**[1], verat.[3],
verb., viol-t., zinc.

bones, in
os, dans les
Knochen, in
    alum., am-m.[4], anac., ang.[3, 4],
    anis.[4], **arg-m.,** arn.[4], ars., asaf.,
    aur., **bell., bism.,** bry., cann-i.,
    cann-s.[4], canth., carb-v.[4],
    carbn-s., cham., chel.[4], cocc.,
    colch., **coloc.,** con., **cupr.,**
    cycl., daph.[4], dros., graph.,
    guaj., hell., hep., ign., kali-bi.[3],
    kali-c., kali-n., **led.**[4], m-arct.[4],
    m-aust.[4], mang-o.[11], merc.,
    mez., nux-m., nux-v.[4], **olnd.,**
    petr.[16], phos., plat., puls., rhod.,
    rhus-t., ruta, sabin., sil.,
    spong., stann., **staph.,** teucr.[4],
    thuj., valer., verat., viol-t.,
    zinc.

    on going to sleep[16]
    en s'endormant
    beim Einschlafen
       graph.

sticking
piquantes, avec douleurs
Stechen mit
    anac.[3], mez., ruta[3], staph.

tearing
déchirantes, avec douleurs
Reißen, mit
    arg-m., bell., cham., coloc.,
    thuj.

glands, in
glandes, dans les
Drüsen, in
    alum.[4], arg-m., ars., asar., aur.,
    bell., calc., carb-v., caust.,
    chin., cina, cocc., con.[4], cycl.,
    hyos., ign., kali-c., **lyc.,**
    m-arct.[4], mag-m.[4], mang.,
    meny., **MERC.,** mur-ac.,
    nat-m.[4], nit-ac.[4], osm., par.,
    ph-ac., puls., rheum, rhust-t.,
    sabin., **spong.,** stann., **staph.,**
    stram., **sulph.,** teucr.[3], verat.,
    zinc.

  inward
  vers l'intérieur
  nach innen
      aur., **calc.,** cocc., cycl., rheum,
      staph., zinc.

  outward
  vers l'extérieur
  nach außen
      arg-m., cina, ign., lyc., mang.,
      meny., **merc.,** par., puls.,
      rhus-t., **spong.,** sulph., teucr.[3]

joints, in[3]
articulations, dans les
Gelenken, in
    agn., alum.[1', 3, 4, 11], anac.,
    arg-m., asaf., asar., bar-c.,
    bell., calc.[3, 4], camph., carb-an.,
    caust., cham., chel., chin.,
    clem., colch., coloc.[11], dulc.,
    graph., hep., hyos., ign., iod.,
    kali-c.[2, 3, 4], **led.**[3, 11], lyc.[4],
    meny., merc., mez., mosch.,
    nat-s.[11],, nit-ac.[3, 4], nit-s-d.[11],
    nux-v., petr., rhust-t., sabad.,
    sabin., sep., sil., spong., stann.,
    staph., stront-c., sulph., tarax.,
    thuj., viol-o., viol-t., zinc.

  sticking[3]
  piquantes, avec douleurs
  Stechen, mit
    ph-ac., sars., staph., zinc.

tearing
déchirantes, avec douleurs
Reißen mit
    agn.³, anac., ang.³, arg-m.³,
    arn., asaf., bell., bism., carb-v.,
    caust., cham., chin.³, coloc.³,
    graph.³, guaj.³, hyos., kali-c.³,
    led., lyc., mez.³, ph-ac.³, ruta,
    sabad.³, sars.³, sep.³, spong.,
    stann., staph.³, zinc.³

muscles, in
muscles, dans les
Muskeln, in
    agar., agn., am-m., **anac.**, ang.³,
    arg-m., arn., **asaf., asar.,** aur.,
    bell., bism., bry., calc., camph.,
    cann-s., **caps., carb-an.,** caust.,
    chel., chin., cina, clem., cocc.,
    con., **cupr., CYCL.,** dig., dros.,
    euph., euphr., graph., hell., hep.,
    ign., kali-n., **led.,** lyc., mag-c.,
    mag-m., mang., meny., merc.,
    mez., **mosch.,** mur-ac., nat-c.,
    nat-m., nitro-o.¹¹, **NUX-M.,**
    nux-v., **olnd.,** petr., **ph-ac.,**
    phos., plat., plb., puls., ran-b.,
    ran-s., rheum, rhod.³, rhus-t.,
    RUTA, sabad., sabin., samb.,
    sil., spig., spong., **stann.,**
    staph., stront-c., **sul-ac.,** sulph.,
    tarax., teucr., thuj., **valer.,**
    verat., VERB., viol-t., zinc.

sticking
piquantes, avec douleurs
Stechen, mit
    am-m.³, anac., arg-m.³, arn.³,
    , asaf., bar-c.³, bell., calc.,
    chin.³, colch.³, coloc., cycl.,
    dios.³, dros., euph., **ign.,**
    kali-c.³, mez.³, **mur-ac.,** olnd.,
    phos.³, plat., rhus-t.³, ruta³,
    sabad³., sars., sep., spong.³,
    stann.³, staph.³, sul-ac., tarax.³,
    thuj., verb.³, viol-t.³, **zinc.³**

tearing
déchirantes, avec douleurs
Reißen, mit
    agar., anac., **ang.³,** arg-m.,
    arn., asaf., asar., aur.,

bell., bism., calc., **camph.,**
cann-s., carb-v., chin., colch.,
cupr., cycl., hyos., led., meny.,
petr., ph-ac., ruta, sars., sep.,
spig., spong., stann., sulph.,
zinc.

twitching¹⁶
soubresautantes, avec douleurs
Zucken, mit
    petr.

parts lain on, in¹⁶
parties où il est couché, dans les
Teilen, auf denen er liegt, in
    kali-c.

spots, in¹¹
endroits, par
stellenweise
    bar-a., sul-ac.

upward³
vers le haut
aufwärts
    calc-p.

radiating
irradiantes
ausstrahlende
    agar.⁶, apis⁶, **arg-n.,** ars.⁶, berb.,
    cupr.⁶, dios., kali-c.⁶, lil-t.⁶,
    mag-m.³, **mag-p.,** plb.³, spig.⁶, **tell.**

scraped, as if
griffure, comme une
kratzend, schabend, wie
    acon., aesc., alumn., **arg-n.,** arn.,
    asaf., **asar.²,** bell., **BROM.,** bry.,
    carbn-s., cham., **chin., coc-c.,**
    coloc., **con.,** crot-t., dig., **DROS.,**
    kali-bi., kali-chl., lach., led.,
    lepi.¹¹, **lyc., mez.,** NUX-V., osm.,
    par., ph-ac., **phos.,** phyt., **PULS.,**
    rhus-t., rumx., sabad., sel.,
    seneg., spig., **stann., SULPH.,**
    tell., **VERAT.**

bones, in², ³
os, dans les
Knochen, in
    asaf., berb.², bry.³, **CHIN.,**

coloc.[3], nat-m.[3], **PH-AC.**, puls.,
RHUS-T., sabad.[2, 3, 11], spig.,
thuj.[3]

long, in
longs, dans les
langen, in den
bry., **sabad.**

periost, of
périoste, du
Periost, des
asaf., CHIN., coloc., **PH-AC.,**
puls., **RHUS-T., sabad.,** spig.

sore, bruised
meurtrissantes, contuses
Wundschmerz, wie gequetscht, wie
zerschlagen
acon.[6], adon.[6], aesc., agar.[1], agn.,
aloe, **alum.**, alum-p.[1]', alum-sil.[1]',
alumn., **am-c.,** am-m.[3], ammc.,
anac.[3], **ang.**[2, 3], ant-c., ant-t.,
apis, **ARG-M.,** arg-n.[6], **ARN.,**
ars.[6], ars-i.[1]', arum-t., **asar.,**
aur.[2, 3], aur-ar.[1]', **bad., bapt.,**
bar-a.[11], bar-c., bar-i.[1]', bar-m.,
bell.[3], bell-p.[6, 9, 14], berb., bor.,
bov., **brom.**[2], **bry.,** calc.,
calc-sil.[1]', calen., **camph.**[2, 11],
cann-s.[3], **canth.,** caps.[3, 6],
(non[1]: carb-ac.), carb-an.,
carb-v., carbn-o.[11], **carbn-s.,**
caust., cedr., cent.[11], cerv.[11],
cham., chel., **CHIN.**[2, 3, 6], chlor.,
CIC., CIMIC., CINA, cinnb.[1]',
clem., cob., cob-n.[9], **COCC.**[2],
colch.[6], coloc., con., cot.[11],
croc.[2], crot-h., crot-t., culx.[1]',
cund.[11], cupr., cycl., dig., **DROS.,**
dulc., echi.[3, 6], elaps, eucal.[3, 6],
EUP-PER.[2, 3, 11], euph., eupi.,
fago., **FERR.**[2], ferr-ar., ferr-p.,
form.[11], gamb., **GELS.**[2, 3, 6], glon.[3],
goss., graph.[1', 3], grat., guare.[11],
HAM., hedeo.[11], **hell.**[2], helon.[3, 6],
hep., hip-ac.[9], hipp., hist.[9], hyos.,
hyper.[2, 3], **hydrc.**[2], iber.[11], ign.,
ind.[11], iod., ip., juni.[11], kali-c.,
kali-i.[3, 6], kali-m.[1', 3], kali-n.,
kalm., kreos.[3, 4, 6], lach., lap-a.[3],

lec., **led.,** lil-t., **lith-c.,** lyc.,
lyss.[2, 11], **mag-c.**[2, 11], mag-m.,
mag-p.[1]', mag-s., **mang., med.,**
merc., **merc-i-f.**[2], merc-i-r., mez.[3],
mit.[11], morph.[11], mosch., **myric.**[2],
narcin.[11], **nat-ar.,** nat-c., nat-m.,
nat-n.[3], nat-p.[1], nat-s.[1]', nat-sil.[1]',
nicc.[2], nit-ac., **nux-m.,** nux-v.,
oci-s.[9], ol-an.[3], **olnd.,** onos.[3],
ox-ac.[1]', pall.[3, 6], par., paull.[11],
petr., **ph-ac.**[2, 3, 6], **phos.,** phys.[11],
phyt., pic-ac.[1]', plan.[3], **PLAT.,**
plb., plect.[11], prun.[3], ptel.[3, 6],
puls., puls-n.[11], **PYROG., ran-b.,**
raph., rat.[4], rhod., **RHUS-T.,**
rhus-v.[11], **RUTA,** sabad., sabin.,
sars.[3], sec.[11], sel.[3], seneg., sep.,
SIL., sin-n.[11], sol-n., sol-t-ae.[11],
spig., spong., **stann.**[2], staph.[2, 3, 6],
stict.[3], still.[11], stry.[11], **sul-ac.,**
sul-i.[1]', sulph., tarax.[3], tarent.,
tart-ac.[11], tell., ter.[3], teucr., thuj.,
til.[3], **tub.,** uva[2], **valer.**[2], verat.,
verb., viol-o., wies., x-ray[9], zinc.,
zinc-p.[1]'

externally
externes
äußerlich
acon., aesc., agar., aloe, **alum.,**
am-c., am-m., anac., **ang.**[3], ant-t.,
apis, **ARG-M., ARN.,** ars., asaf.,
asar., aur., bad., **BAPT.,** bar-c.,
BELL., berb., bism.[3], bor.[3, 4], bov.,
bry., calad., **calc.,** calc-p.[3],
camph., cann-s., canth., caps.,
carb-an., carb-v., carbn-s., **caust.,**
cedr., **cham.,** chel., **CHIN.,** cic.,
cimic.[1', 3], **cina, clem.,** COCC.,
coff., **colch.,** coloc., con., **croc.,**
cupr., cycl., **daph.**[4], dig., dros.,
dulc., EUP-PER., euph., euphr.[3],
ferr., fl-ac., form., **gran.,** graph.,
guaj., **HAM.,** hell., **HEP.,** hyos.,
ign., iod.[3], ip., kali-bi.[3], kali-c.,
kalm., kreos., lach., laur., **led.,**
lith-c., lyc., m-aust.[3, 4], **mag-c.,**
mag-m., **mang.,** med., meny.,
merc.[1], mez., mosch.[3, 4], mur-ac.,
nat-c., NAT-M., nit-ac.[1], **nux-m.,**
NUX-V., olnd.[3, 4], **ox-ac.,** par.,
petr., **ph-ac., phos., phyt.,** plat.,

plb., podo.[3], **puls., PYROG.,
RAN-B.,** ran-s., rheum, **rhod.,
RHUS-T.,** rhus-v.[4], **RUTA,
sabad., SABIN.,** samb., sars.,
sec.[3], sel.[4], seneg., **sep., SIL.,
spig., SPONG.,** squil., **stann.,**
staph., stict.[3], stram., stront-c.,
sul-ac., **SULPH.,** tab.[3, 4], tarax.,
teucr.[3, 4], thuj., **valer., VERAT.,**
viol-t., **zinc.**

internally
internes
innerlich
    acon., **aesc.,** agar., alum.,
    am-c.[1', 3], am-m., ambr., anac.,
    ang.[3], ant-c.[3], ant-t.[3], **apis,
    arg-m.**[3], arg-n.[3], arn., **ars.,** ars-i.,
    asaf., asar.[3], **aur.,** aur-i.[1'], **BAPT.,**
    bar-c., bar-m., bell.[3], bell-p.[3],
    bism.[3], bor.[3], bov., bry., **calc.**[3],
    calc-sil.[1'], **CAMPH.,** cann-i.,
    cann-s., canth.[3], caps.[3], carb-ac.,
    carb-an., carb-v., carbn-s., caust.,
    cham., **CHIN.,** cic.[3], cina, clem.,
    cocc., coff., colch.[3], **coloc.,** con.,
    croc.[3], **cupr.,** dig.[3], **dros., eup-per.**[3],
    euph., euphr., ferr., **GELS.,** glon.,
    graph., **hell.,** hep., ign., iod., **ip.,**
    kali-c., kreos., lach., **laur.,** led.,
    lyc., m-arct.[3], m-aust.[3], mag-c.,
    mag-m., **mang.,** meny., merc.,
    MERC-C., mez.[3, 4], mosch.,
    mur-ac., nat-c., **nat-m.**[3], nit-ac.,
    nux-m.[3], **nux-v.,** olnd.[3], **op.,**
    petr.[3], ph-ac., phos., phyt., plat.[3],
    plb.[3], **PULS., PYROG., RAN-B.,**
    ran-s., rhod., rhus-t., rumx., ruta,
    sabad.[3], sabin., samb., **sang.**[3],
    sars., seneg.[3], sep., **sil.,** spig.,
    spong., **STANN.,** staph., stram.,
    stront-c., sul-ac., **sulph.,** teucr.[3],
    thuj., valer., **verat.,** viol-o.[3],
    viol-t., **zinc.**

morning/matin/morgens
    aesc., bry., carb-an., chin.[16],
    cob.[11], euphr., form., lyc., lyss.[2],
    mag-m.[16], nat-c.[16], ox-ac.,
    phyt.[11], polyp-p.[11], sarr.[11], tab.,
    thuj.

bed, in
lit, au
Bett, im
    anac.[11], grat., rhod., nat-m.,
    petr.[16], viol-o.[11]

insufficient sleep, after
sommeil insuffisant, après un
ungenügendem Schlaf, nach
    mag-m.

rising, on
se levant, en
Aufstehen, beim
    nat-ar., sulph.[16]

    am.[11]
       anac., crot-h., viol-o.

    after
    après s'être levé
    nach dem
       am-m., mag-c.[16], phos., sulph.

waking, on
réveil, au
Erwachen, beim
    aesc., bar-c., calc.[16], crot-h.[11],
    thuj., til., zinc.[16]

    after/après le/nach dem
    bry.[11], carb.-ac.[1], crot-h.,
    sep.[1], sulph.[11]

forenoon[11]/matinée/morgens
    mag-m.[16], mag-s., sars.[16]

afternoon[11]/après-midi/nachmittags
    sang.

evening/soir/abends
    agar.[16], am-c., caust.[16], lyc.,
    par.[6]

23 h
    fago.

lying down, after
couché, après, s'être
Hinlegen, nach dem
    mag-m., mag-s.

sitting, on
assis, étant
Sitzen, im
  brom.

night/nuit/nachts
  carb-an.[16], caust.[16], ferr-i., **sil.**

midnight, after
minuit, après
Mitternacht, nach
  caust.

air am., in open
air, am. en plein
Freien am., im
  caust.

chill, during
frissons, pendant les
Fieberfrost, während
  tarent.

coition, after
coït, après le
Koitus, nach
  SIL.

cramp, after[16]
crampe, après une
Krampf, nach einem
  plat.

exertion, as after great
effort, comme après un gros
Anstrengung, wie nach großer
  clem.

headache, during
maux de tête, pendant les
Kopfschmerzen, bei
  seneg.

heat, during[16]
chaleur fébrile, pendant la
Fieberhitze, bei
  agar., mang.

heated walk and rapid cooling,
  after
échauffé en marchant et rapidement refroidi, après s'être
Erhitzung beim Gehen und
  schneller Abkühlung, nach
  bry., RHUS-T.

march, as after a long
marche, comme après une longue
Marsch, wie nach einem langen
  chel.

menses, during
menstruation, pendant la
Menses, während der
  nat-c., petr.[16], sep.[16]

motion, on
mouvement, par
Bewegung, bei
  aesc.[2, 11], **arn.**[2], bapt., bov.[11],
  bry., chel., **hep.**[2], lach.,
  merc-c.[11], phyt., plb., staph.[16]

  am.
    ars-h.[2], caust., **pyrog., rhus-t.,**
    tub.

  bed, in
  lit, au
  Bett, im
    sol-t-ae.

parts affected with cramp-like pain
parties affectées, douleurs
  crampoïdes des
Teilen mit krampfartigen Schmerzen, in den betroffenen
  PLAT.

parts lain on
partie sur laquelle on est couché,
  sur la
Teilen, auf denen man liegt, in
  ARN., bapt., caust.[16], graph.[16],
  hep., mosch., nux-m., (non[1]:
  pyrog.) **PYRUS**[1]**, RUTA, sep.,**
  sil.[16], thuj.

pressure, on
pression, par la
Druck, bei
    alum-sil.[1]', **PLAT.**, plb.

red hard nodules
nodules rouges et durs
roten harten Knötchen, in
    petr.

rising, on[11]
se levant, en
Aufstehen, beim
    bar-a.[16], pic-ac., ptel.

    am.
        grat., mag-c.

siesta, during[11, 16]
sieste, pendant la
Mittagsruhe, bei der
    graph.

    after/après la/nach der
    bar-c.[16], eug.

sitting, on[11]
assis, étant
Sitzen, beim
    agar., am-m., caust.[11, 16]

    from[7]
    position assise, par
    durch
        spig.

somnambulism, after[16]
somnambulisme, après
Schlafwandeln, nach
    sulph.

spots, in
endroits, par
stellenweise
    aloe, **ARN.**, calc-p., carb-ac.[1],
    colch.[1], **KALI-BI.**, nux-v., ox-ac.,
    petr., plat., **SABAD.**

stool, after
selle, après la
Stuhlgang, nach
    calc.[16], grat.

stooping, after
penché en avant, après s'être
Bücken, nach
    berb.

stormy weather, in
temps orageux, pendant
stürmischem Wetter, bei
    cham.

touch, on[11]
touche, quand on le
Berührung, bei
    acon., alum-sil.[1]', ars-s-f.[1]', bov.,
    brach., **bry.**, calc-p., calc-sil.[1]',
    caust.[11, 16], clem., **colch.**,
    mang.[11, 16], nat-m., nicc., nux-v.,
    rhus-t., ruta, sil., spig., stram.,
    stry., thuj.

waking, on
réveil, au
Erwachen, beim
    aesc.[2], (non: carb-ac.), hydrc.,
    ptel.[2], spong., sulph., thuj.

    after/après le/nach dem
        mag-s., (non: sep.), sulph.[11]

walking, while
marchant, en
Gehen, beim
    staph.

    am.
        coloc.

working am.
travailler am.
Arbeiten am.
    caust.

bones, in
os, dans les
Knochen, in
    acon., **agar.**, am-m., ang.[3, 4],
    apis.[3], **ARG-M., asaf.**, aur., bar-c.,
    bov., **bry.**[2, 3, 4, 6], bufo[3], **calc.**,
    calc-sil.[1]', cann-s., canth.[3, 4],
    carb-v.[3], chin., **COCC.**,

con., conch.[8], **cor-r.**, **crot-h.**[2],
cupr., dros.[2, 4], **EUP-PER.**[2, 3, 6, 8, 11],
graph., **HEP.**, **ign.**, **IP.**, jab.[2],
kali-bi., kreos.[2], lac-d.[7], lach.[3],
led., **lith-c.**, lyss.[2, 8], m-aust.[4],
mag-c., **mang.**, meph.[4], merc.[2, 3, 4],
mez., nat-m., nit-ac.[2, 3], nux-m.[11],
nux-v., **par.**, petr., ph-ac.[1], **phos.**,
phyt.[8], **puls.**, **rhus-t.**[2-4, 8], **RUTA**,
sabad., sabin.[4], sarr.[2], sep., **sil.**,
spig., staph.[4], sulph.[2], syph.[1'],
teucr.[3], ther.[2], thuj.[2], tub.[1'],
valer., **verat.**, zinc.

menses, during[16]
menstruation, pendant la
Menses, während der
  carb-v.

cartilages, in
cartilages, dans les
Knorpel, im
  ARG-M., rhod., rhus-t.

glands, in
glandes, dans les
Drüsen, in
  alum., ant-c., arg-m., **arn.**, ars.,
  bry., calc., **carb-an.**, caust., **cic.**,
  clem.[3, 4], **CON.**, cupr., graph.[1],
  hep., **ign.**[3, 4], iod., kali-c., merc.,
  mez., nat-m., nicc.[11], nux-v.[3],
  petr.[3], phos., plat., **psor.**, puls.,
  rhod., rhus-t., **ruta, sep.,** staph.,
  sul-ac., sulph., teucr., zinc.

joints, in[11]
articulations, dans les
Gelenken, in
  abrot., agar.[3, 11], alumn.[2],
  apoc.[3, 11], **ARG-M.**[2, 3],
  ARN.[1', 3, 11], aur.[3], berb.[1'],
  calad.[2], carb-an.[3, 11], **cham.**[2, 3, 11],
  chlf., clem., coff.[1'], coloc.[3, 11],
  con.[2, 3], **crot-h.**[2], guaj.[1'], hipp-ac.[9],
  hyos.[3, 11], **hyper.**[2, 11], kali-i.,
  lith-c.[2], mang.[4], **mez.**[2, 3, 11],
  mur-ac.[2, 3, 11], **nat-p.**[2, 11],
  nit-ac.[3, 11], petr.[1'], phys., phyt.[1'],
  PULS.[3, 11], ran-a.[4, 11], **RHUS-T.**[2, 3],
  sulph.[3], tub.[1'], viol-o.[3]

muscles, in[16]
muscles, dans les
Muskeln, in
  kali-c., verat.

veins, in[3]
veines, dans les
Venen, in
  ham., puls.

splinters, sensation of
échardes, sensation d'
Splitterschmerzen
  aesc., **AGAR.**, **alum.**, ANAG.[7],
  ARG-N., asaf.[3], **bar-c.**, **carb-v.**, cic.,
  colch., coll., **dol.**, **fl-ac.**, **HEP.**,
  kali-c.[3], **NIT-AC.**, petr., plat.,
  ran-b., **sil.**, stann.[3], sulph.

stinging–wounds see wounds–
  stinging

stitching[11]
piquantes
stechende
  ACON.[2, 3, 6, 7], aconin., ail.,
  alum-p.[1'], **alum-sil.**[1'], **alumn.**[2],
  am-m.[2], amgd-p., anac.,
  apis[1', 3, 6, 11], arg-n.[6], arist-cl.[9],
  arn.[2, 3], ars., **ars-s-f.**[1'], **ASAF.**[2, 11],
  astac., aur-ar.[1'], aur-i.[1'], aur-m.[1'],
  aur-s.[1'], bar-c., bar-i.[1'], bar-s.[1'],
  bart., **BELL.**[2, 3], benz-ac.[6], berb.[6],
  bor.[3], **bov.**[2], **BRY.**[2, 3, 6, 11], bufo[6],
  buni-o.[14], **CALC.**[2, 11], calc-f.[6],
  calc-i.[1'], **calc-sil.**[1'], camph.[3],
  cann-i.[6, 11], **CANTH.**[2, 4, 6],
  caust.[2, 3, 11], cham.[3, 11], **chel.**[2, 11],
  CHIN.[3, 3], cina[6], **cocc.**[2, 3], coff.[1'],
  colch.[2, 3], **coloc.**[3, 6], **CON.**[2, 6, 11],
  culx.[1'], cupr., dig., **dros.**[2],
  esp-g.[13], eucal., ferr-ar.[1'], ferul.,
  gamb., gast., **graph.**[2, 11], **hell.**[2],
  hist.[9, 10], hydr.[6], hydroph.[14],
  hyos., hyper.[1', 3], **IGN.**[2], jac-c.,
  kali-ar.[1'], **KALI-C.**[2, 3, 6, 11, 14],
  kali-i.[6], kali-m.[1', 3], kali-n.,
  kali-sil.[1'], **kreos.**[2], lac-c., lach.,
  lat-m.[3], **laur.**[2], led.[6, 11], lyc.,
  mag-c.[2, 11], **mag-m.**[2], manc.,
  meny.[2], **MERC.**[2, 3], merc-c.[1', 6],
  merc-i-f., mez., mosch.,

mur-ac.[2, 11], naja, **nat-c.**[2],
nat-m.[2, 11], **nat-sil.**[1]',
NIT-AC.[2, 3, 6, 11], nux-v.[3, 6, 7],
op.[5], **par.**[2], **ph-ac.**[2, 11], **PHOS.**[2, 11],
plat., **plb.**[2], plb-i.[6], pneu.[14],
PULS.[2, 3, 6], pulx.[3], ran-b.[3, 6],
ran-s.[2], rauw.[9], **RHUS-T.**[2, 3, 6, 11],
sabad.[2], **sabin.**[2, 3], sang.[6],
sars.[2, 11], scut., **SEP.**[2], sil.[2, 11],
SPIG.[2, 3, 6], **spong.**[2, 3, 11], squil.[3, 6],
stann.[2], **STAPH.**[2, 3, 6], stict.[6],
stroph-h.[3], stroph-s.[9], sul-ac.[6],
sul-i.[1]', **SULPH.**[2, 3, 6], symph.[3],
tarax.[2], tarent., **THUJ.**[2, 6, 11],
tub.[1]', urt-c., verat., **VERB.**[2],
verin., vip.[6, 11], zinc.[2, 3, 6],
ZINC-P.[1]'

left side[11]
gauche, sur le côté
linken Seite, auf der
  aesc., all-c., ant-s-aur., coc-c.,
  crot-h., **IGN.**, lach., lepi., merc.,
  nicc., **sil.**, sphing., **SQUIL.**,
  stann., **sulph.**, sumb., tax., zinc.

right side[11]
droit, sur le côté
rechten Seite, auf der
  bad., carb-an., chel., con., hura,
  hyos., kali-bi., mosch., phos.,
  plect., sil., sin-n., sol-t-ae.

morning in bed[6]
matin au lit
morgens im Bett
  stann.

night[16]/nuit/nachts
  euphr.

ascending[16]
montantes
aufsteigende
  spig.

crawling[16]
reptation, avec
kribbelndes
  lyc.

one-sided[16]
d'un côté
einseitig
  stann.

parts lain on, in[16]
parties où il est couché, dans les
Teilen, auf denen er liegt, in
  carb-v.

externally
externes
äußerlich
  abrot., **acon.**, **agar.**, agn., **aloe**,
  alum., am-c., **am-m.**, ambr.,
  anac., ang.[3], ant-c., ant-t., apis,
  arg-m., arg-n.[6], **arn.**, ars., ars-i.,
  ASAF., asar., aur., **bar-c.**,
  bar-m., **BELL.**, benz-ac.[6], **berb.**,
  bism., bor., bov., **BRY.**, bufo[6]
  calad., **CALC.**, calc-f.[6], **calc-p.**,
  camph., **cann-i.**, cann-s., canth.,
  caps., carb-ac., carb-an.,
  carb-v., **CARBN-S.**, **caust.**,
  cedr., cham., **chel.**, **chin.**, chin-ar.,
  chin-s.[4], **CIC.**, **cimic.**, cina,
  cinnb., **clem.**, **cocc.**, coff.[3, 4],
  colch., **coloc.**, **CON.**, croc.,
  crot-h., crot-t., cupr., cycl.,
  daph.[4], dig., **dios.**, **dros.**, dulc.,
  euonin.[4], euph., euphr., **ferr.**,
  ferr-ar., ferr-ma.[4], ferr-p.,
  fl-ac.[3], form., **gels.**, **graph.**,
  guaj., **hell.**, hep., hydr., hyos.,
  ign., **indg.**, iod., ip., kali-ar.,
  kali-bi., **KALI-C.**, kali-i.[6],
  kali-n., **KALI-P.**, **KALI-S.**,
  kreos., lach., lact.[4], laur., **LED.**,
  lith-c., **lob.**, **LYC.**, m-arct.[4],
  m-aust.[4], mag-c., mag-m.,
  manc., mang., **med.**, **meny.**,
  MERC., merc-c.[4, 6], **mez.**,
  mosch., **mur-ac.**, naja, nat-ar.,
  nat-c., **nat-h.**, **nat-m.**, **nat-p.**,
  nat-s., nicc.[4], **NIT-AC.**, nux-m.,
  nux-v., **ol-an.**, olnd., op.[4],
  ox-ac., **par.**, petr., **ph-ac.**,
  phel.[4], **phos.**, **phyt.**, plat., **plb.**,
  plb-i.[6], prun.[4], psor., **PULS.**,
  RAN-B., **ran-s.**, **rat.**, rheum,
  rhod., **RHUS-T.**, ruta, **sabad.**,
  sabin., samb., sang., sars., sel.,
  seneg., **sep.**, **sil.**, **SPIG.**, **spong.**,
  squil., **stann.**, **STAPH.**, stict.[6],
  still., stram., stront-c., sul-ac.,
  SULPH., tab.[4], **TARAX.**, teucr.,
  THUJ., **valer.**, verat., verb.,

viol-o., **viol-t.,** vip.[4, 6], vip-r.[4],
ZINC.

here and there[3, 6]
ici et là
hier und da
   BAR-C.[7], sul-ac., zinc.

perspiration, during[7]
transpiration, pendant la
Schwitzen, beim
   cann-s.

rest, during[1']
repos, pendant le
Ruhe, während der
   tub., valer.

vexation, after
contrariétés, après
Ärger, durch
   rhus-t.

internally
internes
innerlich
   abrot., **acon., aesc., agar.,** agn.,
   all-c., aloe, **alum.,** am-c.,
   am-m., ambr., ammc., anac.,
   ang.[3], ant-c., ant-t., apis,
   arg-m., arg-n., arn., **ars.,** ars-i.,
   ASAF., asar., aspar., aur.,
   bar-c., bar-m., **bell., BERB.,**
   bism., **BOR., bov., BRY., cact.,**
   calad., **calc.,** calc-p., camph.,
   CANN-I., CANTH., caps.,
   carb-an., carb-v., **CARBN-S.,**
   card-m., **caust.,** cham., **CHEL.,**
   CHIN., chin-ar., cic., cimic.,
   cina, clem., **coc-c.,** cocc., coff.,
   colch., coll., **coloc., con., croc.,**
   crot-t., cupr., cycl., dig., dios.,
   dol.[1], dros., **dulc.,** euph.,
   euphr., **ferr., gamb.,** gels.,
   glon., graph., **guaj.,** hell., hep.,
   hydr., hyos., **IGN.,** iod., ip.,
   kali-ar., **kali-bi., KALI-C.,**
   kali-i., kali-n., **KALI-S.,** kalm.,
   kreos., LACH., laur., **LED.,**
   lyc., mag-c., mag-m., mang.,
   meny., **MERC., MERC-C.,**

merc-i-r., merc-ns., mez.,
mosch., mur-ac., **naja,** nat-ar.,
nat-c., nat-m., nat-s., NIT-AC.,
nux-m., **nux-v., ol-an.,** olnd.,
op., ox-ac., **par.,** petr., **ph-ac.,**
phel., **PHOS.,** phyt., plan.,
plat., **PLB.,** prun., psor., **PULS.,**
RAN-B., ran-s., rheum, rhod.,
rhus-t., rumx., ruta, **sabad.,**
sabin., samb., sang., **sars.,** sec.,
sel., **seneg., SEP., SIL., SPIG.,**
spong., **SQUIL.,** stann., **staph.,**
stram., stront-c., sul-ac., **sulph.,**
tab., **tarax.,** teucr., **thal., ther.,**
thuj., valer., verat., verb.,
viol-t., zinc., ziz.

night[16]/nuit/nachts
   euphr.

cold needles like
aiguilles froides, comme des
kalte Nadeln, wie durch
   AGAR.

burning[3]
brûlantes, et
Brennen, mit
   am-m.[4], ant-c., **apis, ars.,**
   bell.[3, 4], berb.[3, 11], **con.,** dig.[4],
   dulc., gamb.[11], **glon.,** ign.[3, 4],
   iris, lyc., m-aust.[4], mez.,
   nat-s.[4], ph-ac., **phos.,** rat.[4],
   rhod.[4], rhus-t., sil., **urt-u.**

externally[4]
externes
äußerlich
   acon., alum., **anac.,** arg-m.,
   arn., ars., **asaf.,** aur., **bar-c.,**
   bell., berb., **bry.,** cann-s., caps.,
   caust., cina, **cocc., con., dig.,**
   hep., hyos., ign., **lach., lyc.,**
   m-arct., m-aust., mag-c., meny.,
   merc., mez., mur-ac., nat-s.,
   nicc., **nux-v., ph-ac.,** phel.,
   phos., plat., **puls., ran-b.,**
   ran-s., rhus-t., sabad., sel., **sep.,**
   sil., spig., **spong.,** squil., **stann.,**
   staph., sul-ac., sulph., thuj.,
   viol-t.

internally
internes
innerlich
  ARS., aur., **mez., ol-an.**, spig.

bones, in[3]
os, dans les
Knochen, in
  arg-m., euph., zinc.

joints, in[3]
articulations, dans les
Gelenken, in
  ign.[11], mez., plat., plb., sul-ac.,
  thuj.

muscles, in
muscles, dans les
Muskeln, in
  acon., alum., am-m., anac.,
  apis, **arg-m.**, arn., **ASAF.**,
  aur., bar-c., bry., bufo[3], calc.,
  caust., cic., cina, **COCC.**,
  colch.[3], **dig.**, euph., glon.[3],
  ign., laur., lyc., mag-c.,
  mang., merc., **MEZ.**, mur-ac.,
  NUX-V., olnd., par., phyt.,
  plat., plb., rhod., **RHUS-T.**,
  sabad., sabin., samb., sep.,
  spig., stann., **STAPH.**,
  SUL-AC., tarax., **THUJ.**,
  viol-t., zinc.

like hot needles
comme des aiguilles chaudes
wie durch heiße Nadeln
  alum.[3], apis[3], **ARS.**, bar-c.[3],
  kali-c.[7], mag-c.[3], naja[3],
  nit-ac.[3], ol-an., rhus-t.[3],
  spig.[3], vesp.[3]

drawing[16]
tiraillantes
ziehende
  mang.

dull[16]
sourdes
dumpf
  mang.

downward
vers le bas
abwärts
  ant-c., arn., **asc-t.**, bell., bor.,
  canth., caps., **CARB-V., caust.**,
  chel., cimic., cina, coloc., dios.,
  dros., **FERR.**, gels., kreos., lyc.,
  mang., mez., nit-ac., nux-v., pall.,
  petr., ph-ac., **phyt., puls., ran-s.**,
  RHUS-T., sabin., sars., sep.,
  squil., still., **sulph.**, tarax., ust.,
  valer., zinc.

inward
ver l'intérieur
nach innen
  acon., alum., am-m., arg-m.,
  ARN., asaf., bar-c., bell., bov.,
  bry., calc., cann-s., **CANTH.**,
  caps., carb-v., caust., cina, clem.,
  cocc., coloc., croc., dros., guaj.,
  hyos., **ign.**, ip., **laur.**, mang.,
  meny., mez., nux-v., olnd., par.,
  petr., ph-ac., phos., **phyt., plb.**,
  RAN-B., rhus-t., **sabin.**, samb.,
  sel., squil., staph., sul-ac., tarax.,
  thuj., verb.

itching[16]
pruriantes
juckende
  carb-v., euphr., stann.

jerking
saccades, par
ruckartig
  ang.[3], arn., **bry., calc.**, carbn-s.,
  caust., **CINA**, cocc., coff., **coloc.**,
  euph., guaj., **lyc.**, mang., **meny.**,
  mez., mur-ac., **NUX-V.**, ph-ac.,
  plb., sep., sil., spong., **SQUIL.**,
  stann., zinc.

outward
vers l'extérieur
nach außen
  alum., am-m., ant-c., **ARG-M.**,
  arn., **ASAF.**, asar., **bell., bry.**,
  calc., cann-s., canth., carb-v.,
  caust., cham., **CHEL., CHIN.**,
  clem., cocc., coff., colch.,
  CON., dros., **dulc.**, hell., hyos.,

kali-c., kali-m.[1]', **lach., laur.,**
lith-c., lob., lyc., mang., meny.,
MERC., mez., mur-ac., **nat-c.,**
nat-m., nit-ac., **ol-an.,** olnd.,
ph-ac., **PHEL.,** phos., phyt.,
PRUN., puls., rhod., **rhus-t.,**
sabad., sabin., sil., **SPIG.,**
SPONG., STANN., staph.,
stront-c., **SULPH., tarax.,** ther.,
thuj., **VALER.,** verat., verb.,
viol-o., viol-t.

to tips of fingers
jusqu'au bout des doigts
bis zu den Fingerspitzen
lob.

paralytic[16]
paralysantes
lähmende
sep.

tearing in bones[3]
déchirantes dans les os, et
Reißen in Knochen, mit
acon., **ars.,** bell., calc.[11],
camph.[11], chel., merc., mur-ac.,
phos., sabin.[3, 11], thuj.

joints, in[3]
articulations, dans les
Gelenken, in
ang., ars., asaf., **asar.,** calc.[11],
camph.[11], carb-v., caust., clem.,
dulc., ferr., merc., mur-ac.,
puls., sabin.[3, 11], stann.,
STAPH., sul-ac., sulph., tarax.,
thuj., verb., zinc.

muscles, in
muscles, dans les
Muskeln, in
acon., agn., alum., am-c.,
am-m., ambr., **ANAC.,** ang.[3],
arg-m., **ars.,** asaf., asar., aur.,
bell., bism., bor., **CALC.,**
camph., cann-s., canth., caps.,
caust., chel., **chin.,** cina, clem.,
coloc., con., cycl., dig., dros.,
GUAJ., hell., kali-c., kreos.,
led., **MANG.,** merc., mez.,
mur-ac., nat-m., nux-v., olnd.,

ph-ac., phos., **PULS.,** rheum,
rhus-t., ruta, sabin., samb.,
sars., sep., sil., spig., spong.,
squil., staph., sul-ac., tarax.,
THUJ., verb., zinc.

wandering[16]
erratiques
wandernde
euphr.

transversely
transversalement
querverlaufend
acon., ambr., anac., arg-m.,
asc-t., atro., BELL., bov., bry.,
calc., canth., caust., cham., **chin.,**
cimic., cocc., cupr., dig., **kali-bi.,**
kali-c., kali-m.[1]', laur., lyc.,
merc., mur-ac., phos., **plb., ran-b.,**
rhod., rhus-t., seneg., **sep., spig.,**
stict., stront-c., sul-ac., **sulph.,**
tarax.

upward
vers le haut
aufwärts
acon., alum., arn., ars., bar-c.,
BELL., bry., calc., canth., carb-v.,
caust. cham., chin., cimic., cina,
coloc., dios., **dros.,** euphr., gels.,
glon., guaj., kali-c., **lach., lith-c.,**
mang., **meny.,** merc., nat-s., petr.,
PHYT., plb., puls., rhus-t., rumx.,
ruta, **SEP., spong., stann., sulph.,**
tarax., thuj.

bones, in
os, dans les
Knochen, in
abrot.[3], acon., aeth.[4], agar., agn.,
am-c., anac., ant-c., arg-m., ars.,
asaf., aur., **BELL.,** berb.[4], **BRY.,**
CALC., canth., carb-v., **CAUST.,**
cedr., chel., **chin.,** cocc., colch.,
CON., daph.[4], **dros.,** dulc., euph.,
euphr.[4], graph., **HELL.,** iod.,
kali-bi.[2], kali-c., kali-n.[4], **kalm.,**
lach., laur.[4], lyc., mag-c.,
mag-m.[4], mang., **MERC.,** mez.,
mur-ac.[4], nat-c.[4], nat-s.[4], nit-ac.,
nit-s-d.[11], nux-v., ol-an.[4], par.,

petr., ph-ac., phel.[4], phos., **phyt.**[6],
prun.[4], **PULS., ran-s.,** raph.[4], **ruta,**
sabin., samb., **SARS., SEP.,** sil.,
spig., staph., stront-c., **SULPH.,**
tarax.[4], tax.[4], **thuj.,** valer., verb.,
viol-t., zinc.

glands, in
glandes, dans les
Drüsen, in
    acon., agn., alum., **am-m.,** ang.[3, 4],
    apis[3], arg-m., arn., **asaf.,** bar-c.,
    bar-m., **BELL.,** berb.[4], bor., **bry.,**
    calc., carb-an., caust., chin.,
    cocc., con., cupr., cycl., euph.,
    euphr.[4], graph., grat.[4], hell., hep.,
    ign., iod., kali-c., kali-m.[1'], kreos.,
    lach., lyc., m-arct.[4], **MERC., mez.,**
    mur-ac., murx.[4], **nat-c., nat-m.,**
    NIT-AC., nux-v.[1], ol-an.[4], ph-ac.,
    phos., plb., **PULS., ran-s.,** raph.[4],
    rheum, **rhus-t.,** sabad., sang.[4],
    sep., sil., spig., **spong.,** stann.,
    staph., sul-ac., **sulph.,** thuj.,
    verat., zinc.

around glands[16]
autour des ganglions
um die Drüsen herum
    con.

joints, in[3]
articulations, dans les
Gelenken, in
    acon.[2, 3, 4], agar.[2, 3], **agn.,** aloe[11],
    alum., am-c., am-m., anac., ang.,
    ant-c., ant-t., apis, arg-m., arg-n.,
    arist-cl.[9], **arn.**[3, 4, 11], ars., **asaf.,**
    asar., **bar-c.**[3, 11], **bell.,** benz-ac.,
    berb., **bov., BRY.**[2, 3, 4], bufo,
    CALC.[3, 11], calc-f., camph.,
    cann-s., canth., caps., carb-an.,
    carb-v., carl.[11], **caust.**[3, 4], cham.[11],
    chel., chin., cina, clem.[3, 11], **cocc.,**
    colch.[2], coloc., **con.,** crot-t.,
    dros.[2, 3, 4, 11], dulc., euph., euphr.,
    ferr., gast.[11], **graph.,** guaj.[3, 4],
    HELL.[3, 4], **hep.**[2, 3, 4], hydr., hyos.,
    ign.[3, 4], indg.[11], iod.,
    KALI-C.[2, 3, 4, 11], kali-i., **kali-n.,**
    kreos.[2, 3, 4, 11], lac-ac.[11], laur.,
    led.[3, 4], lyc., mag-c., **mag-m.,**

MANG.[3, 4], **meny.**[3, 4], **MERC.,**
merc-c., mez., mosch., mur-ac.,
nat-c.[3, 4], **nat-m.**[3, 11], nit-ac.,
nit-s-d.[11], nux-m., nux-v.[3, 4], olnd.,
par.[3, 11], petr., ph-ac., **phos.**[3, 11],
plat., plb., plect.[11], **puls.,** ran-b.,
rheum, **rhod., RHUS-T.**[3, 4], ruta,
sabad., **sabin.**[3, 4], samb., sang.,
sars., sep., SIL.[3, 4, 11], **SPIG.**[3, 4],
spong., squil., **stann., staph.,**
stict., **stront-c.,** stroph-s.[9], **sul-ac.,**
sulph.[3, 4], **TARAX., THUJ.**[2, 3, 4, 11],
valer., verat., verb., viol-t., vip.,
zinc.[2, 3, 4, 11]

muscles, in
muscles, dans les
Muskeln, in
    acon., agar., agn., **alum.,** am-c.,
    am-m., ambr., anac., ang.[3],
    ant-c., ant-t., arg-m., **arn.,** ars.,
    ars-i., ASAF., asar., aur.,
    bar-c., bar-m., **BELL.,** bism.,
    bor., bov., **BRY.,** calad., **CALC.,**
    camph., cann-s., canth., caps.,
    carb-an., carb-v., **caust.,** cham.,
    chel., **chin.,** cic., cina, clem.,
    cocc., colch., coloc., **con.,** croc.,
    cupr., cycl., dig., dros., dulc.,
    euph., euphr., ferr., **graph.,**
    guaj., hell., hep., hyos., **ign.,**
    iod., **KALI-C., kali-m.**[1'], kali-n.,
    kreos., lach., **laur.,** led., lyc.,
    mag-c.[1], mag-m., mang., **meny.,**
    MERC., merc-c.[3], merc-i-r.[11],
    mez., mosch., **mur-ac., nat-c.,**
    nat-m., nit-ac., nux-m., nux-v.,
    olnd., **par.,** petr., ph-ac., **phos.,**
    plan.[11], plat., plb., prun.[11],
    PULS., ran-b., **ran-s.,** rheum,
    rhod., **RHUS-T.,** ruta, **sabad.,**
    sabin., samb., sang.[3], **sars.,**
    sep., sil., SPIG., spong., squil.,
    stann., STAPH., stront-c.,
    stry.[11], sul-ac., **SULPH.,**
    TARAX., teucr.[3], **THUJ.,**
    valer., verat., verb., **viol-t.,**
    zinc.

jerking[3]/secousses, avec/
    ruckartige
    ang.

warm in bed, while
chaleur du lit, à la
Bettwärme, in der
carb-v.

tearing externally
déchirantes externes
reißende, äußerlich
ACON., adon.[6], aesc., **agar.,** agn.,
alum., alum-p.[1'], **ALUM-SIL.**[1'],
alumn.[2], **am-c., am-m., ambr.,**
anac., ang.[3], ant-c., ant-t., aphis[4],
apis[3], arg-m., **ARN., ars.,** ars-s-f.[1'],
asaf., asar., aur., aur-ar.[1'], aur-i.[1'],
aur-m.[1'], aur-s.[1'], bar-a.[6], bar-c.,
bar-i.[1'], bar-m., bar-s.[1'], **BELL.,**
BERB., bism., bor., bov., brom.,
bruc.[4], **BRY.,** cact., calad., **calc.,**
calc-caust.[6], calc-i.[1'], calc-p.,
calc-sil.[1'], camph., cann-s., canth.,
caps., carb-an., **carb-v.,**
CARBN-S., caust., cedr., **cham.,**
chel., CHIN., chin-ar., chin-s.[4],
cic., **cimic.**[6], cina, cist.[4], clem.,
coc-c.[3, 4], cocc., coff., **COLCH.,**
coloc., con., croc., **crot-t.**[1], cupr.,
cycl., cyt-l.[10], dig., dros., **dulc.,**
euph., euphr., **ferr., ferr-ar.,**
ferr-m.[4], ferr-p., **gamb., gels.,**
graph., **guaj.,** hell., hep., hera.[4],
hist.[10], hyos., **HYPER.,** ign., **indg.,**
iod., ip., kali-ar., **kali-bi.,**
KALI-C., kali-i., **kali-n., KALI-P.,**
KALI-S., kali-sil.[1'], **kalm.**[6], **kreos.,**
lach., lact.[4], lam.[4], laur., **LED.,**
LYC., lyss., **mag-c.,** mag-m.,
mang., med.[1'], meny., **merc.,**
merc-c.[1'], **mez.,** mosch., mur-ac.,
nat-ar., nat-c., NAT-M., nat-p.,
NAT-S., nat-sil.[1'], **nicc., NIT-AC.,**
nux-m., **nux-v.,** olnd., op.,
ox-ac.[1'], par., petr., ph-ac.,
phos.[1'-3, 4], phyt., plan.[2], plat.,
plb., **PULS., ran-b.,** ran-s., **rat.,**
rheum, **rhod., rhus-t.,** ruta,
sabad., sabin., samb., sang.[1'],
sars., sec., **sel.,** seneg., **SEP., SIL.,**
spig., spong., squil., stann.,
staph.[1], stram., **stront-c.,** sul-ac.,
sul-i.[1'], **SULPH.,** tarax., teucr.,
thuj., ton.[4], **tub.**[1', 7], **valer.,** verat.,

verb., vinc.[4], viol-o., viol-t.,
ZINC., zinc-o.[4]

internally
internes
innerlich
acon., aesc., **agar.,** agn., aloe,
alum., am-c., am-m., **ambr.,** anac.,
ang.[3], ant-c., **ant-t.,** apis, **arg-m.,**
arn., ars., ars-i., asaf., asar., **aur.,**
bar-c., **BELL., BERB.,** bism., bor.,
bov., **BRY.,** calad., calc., calc-p.[3],
camph., cann-s., canth., **caps.,**
carb-an., **CARB-V., carbn-s.,**
caust., **cham., chel.,** chin.,
chin-ar., cic., cina, clem., cocc.,
coff., colch., **coloc., CON.,** croc.,
crot-h., cupr., cycl., dig., dios.,
dros., dulc., euph., euphr., ferr.,
gran., graph., guaj., hell., hep.,
hyos., **ign.,** iod., ip., kali-ar.,
kali-bi.[3], kali-c., **kali-n., KALI-S.,**
kalm., kreos., **lach.,** laur., **LED.,**
LYC., mag-c., mag-m., mang.,
meny., MERC., mez., mosch.,
mur-ac., nat-ar., nat-c., **nat-m.,**
nit-ac., nux-m., **NUX-V.,** olnd.,
op., par., petr., ph-ac., **phos.,**
plat., plb., **PULS.,** ran-b., ran-s.,
rhod., rhus-t., ruta, sabad., sabin.,
samb., sang., sars., sec., sel.,
seneg., **SEP., SIL., SPIG.,** spong.,
squil., **stann.,** staph., stram.,
stront-c., sul-ac., **SULPH., tarax.,**
teucr[3], thuj., uva, valer., verat.,
verat-v., verb., viol-o., viol-t.,
zinc.

asunder
en deux
auseinanderreißende
agar., alum., am-m., anac., arn.,
ars., asar., calc., carb-an., carb-v.,
caust., **COFF.,** colch., con., dig.,
ferr., graph., ign., **mez.,** mur-ac.,
nat-m., **NIT-AC., NUX-V.,** op.,
puls., rhus-t., sabin., sep., spig.,
staph., sul-ac., sulph., **teucr.,**
thuj., zinc.

away
arrachantes
abreißende
  act-sp., coloc., dig., hep.,
  KALI-BI., kreos.[3], led., mosch.,
  nux-v., paeon., petr., phos., **plb.,**
  RHUS-T., sep., sulph., thlas.[3],
  thuj., urt-u.[3], uran-n.[3]

downward
en descendant
von oben nach unten
  acon., agar., agn., alum., anac.,
  ant-c., ant-t., arg-n.[1]', ars.,
  ars-s-f.[1]', asaf., aur., aur-s.[1]',
  bar-c., bar-i.[1]', bar-m., bar-s.[1]',
  BELL., bism., **bry.,** calc., canth.,
  CAPS., carb-v., carbn-s., caust.,
  chel., **chin.,** cina, colch., **coloc.,**
  con., croc., dulc., euphr., **ferr.,**
  ferr-p., **graph.,** ign., **kali-c.,**
  kali-m.[1]', kali-n., kali-p., **kali-s.,**
  kalm.[3], laur., **LYC.,** mag-c.,
  meny., merc., mez., mur-ac.,
  nat-ar., **nat-c.,** nat-m., nit-ac.,
  nux-v., ph-ac., phos., **puls.,** rhod.,
  RHUS-T., sabin., sars., seneg.,
  sep., sil., **spĭg.,** squil., stann.,
  staph., **SULPH.,** thuj., valer.,
  verat., verb., zinc.

outward
en dehors
nach außen
  all-c., am-c., bell., bov., **bry.,**
  calc., cann-s., caust., **cocc.,** cycl.,
  elaps, euph., ip., mang., mez.,
  mur-ac., nat-c., par., ph-ac.,
  PRUN., puls., **rhus-t., sil., spig.,**
  spong., stram.

rest, during[1]'
repos, pendant le
Ruhe, in der
  tub.

upward
en montant
von unten nach oben
  acon., alum., **anac.,** ant-c., arn.,
  ars., asaf., aur., **BELL.,** bism.,
  bor., calc., carb-v., caust., chin.,

clem., colch., **con., dulc.,** euphr.,
mag-c., meny., merc., **nat-ar.,**
nat-c., nat-m., **nit-ac., nux-v.,**
ph-ac., phos., puls., rhod.,
rhust-t., samb., sars., **SEP., SIL.,**
SPIG., spong., **stront-c.,** sulph.,
thuj., valer.

bones, in
os, dans les
Knochen, in
  acon., **agar.,** alum., **am-m.,**
  anac., ang.[11], **arg-m.,** arn., ars.,
  asaf., **AUR., aur-m.,** aur-s.[1]',
  bar-c., bell., berb., bism., bor.,
  bov., bry., calc-p., cann-s.,
  canth., **caps., carb-v., caust.,**
  cham., chel., **CHIN., cina,**
  cocc., colch.[8], coloc., con.,
  crot-t., **cupr., cycl.,** dig., **dros.,**
  dulc., **ferr.,** fl-ac.[8], gamb.[11],
  graph., hell., hep., ign., iod.,
  kali-bi.[11], **KALI-C., kali-n.,**
  kalm.[2], **LACH.,** lact.[4], laur.,
  lyc., lyss.[2], **mag-c.,** mag-m.,
  mang., meph.[4], **MERC., merc-c.,**
  mez., mur-ac.[4], nat-c., nat-m.,
  nicc.[4], **nit-ac.,** nit-s-d.[11], nux-v.,
  ph-ac., phos., plb., puls.,
  RHOD., rhus-t., **ruta,** sabad.[4],
  sabin., samb., sars., sep., **SPIG.,**
  spong., stann., **staph., stront-c,**
  sul-ac., sulph., **tab., teucr.**[4],
  thuj., valer., verat., verb., **zinc.**

burning
brûlantes, et
Brennen, mit
  sabin.

cramp-like
crampe, comme une
krampfartig
  aur., olnd., **verat.**

jerking
secousses, avec
ruckartig
  ang., **bry., CHIN.,** cupr., mang.

paralytic
paralytiques
lähmende
    bell., **bism.**, chel., chin., **cocc.**,
    dig.

pressive
pressives
Drücken, mit
    ARG-M., arn., asaf., bism.,
    bry., coloc., **CYCL.**, staph.,
    teucr.

sticking
piquantes
Stechen, mit
    bell., cina, mur-ac., sabin.

epiphyses, in[16]
épiphyses, des
Epiphysen, in
    arg-m.

periost, in
périoste, dans le
Periost, im
    bry., **mez.**, ph-ac., **rhod.**

glands, in
glandes, dans les
Drüsen, in
    agn., am-c., **ambr., arn.,** bar-c.,
    bar-s.[1'], **bell.,** bov., **bry., calc.,**
    cann-s., **caps., carb-an., carb-v.,**
    caust., **cham., CHIN.,** cocc., con.,
    cycl., **dulc.,** ferr., graph., grat.[4],
    ign., **kali-c.,** kali-s., kreos., **lyc.,**
    MERC., mez., nat-c., nit-ac.,
    nux-v., ol-an.[4], phel.[4], phos.,
    PULS., rhod., rhus-t., sel., seneg.,
    sep., **sil.,** staph.[1'], **sulph.,** thuj.,
    zinc.

joints, in[3]
articulations, dans les
Gelenken, in
    acon., agar., **agn.,** alum., am-c.,
    am-m., **ambr.**[3, 4], anac., ang.,
    ant-s-aur.[11], ant-t.[2, 3, 11],
    ARG-M., arist-cl.[9], arn.[3, 4], ars.,
    ars-i.[1'], asaf., asar., **aur.,** bar-c.,
    bell.[2, 3], bism., **bov., bry.,**

cact.[11], **calc.**[2, 3, 4], camph.[2, 3],
canth., carb-an., carb-v., **carl.**[11],
CAUST.[3, 4, 11] cham., chel.,
chin., cic., cina, cist.[2, 4, 11],
clem., cocc., **colch.**[2, 3], con.,
cupr., cycl., dig., dros., dulc.,
euphr., ferr., graph.[3, 4], grat.[11],
guaj.[3, 4], hell., hep., hera.[4],
hyos.[3, 4], ign., iod.[3, 4], **KALI-C.,**
kali-n., kreos., lach.[4], laur.,
mag-m., mang., meny., **MERC.,**
mez., mosch., mur-ac., nat-c.[3, 4],
nat-m., nat-s.[11], nit-ac.[3, 4, 11],
nit-s-d.[11], nux-m., **nux-v.**[3, 4],
olnd., par., petr., **ph-ac.,**
phos.[3, 4], plb., puls., ran-b.,
rheum, rhod.[3, 4], **RHUS-T.,**
ruta, sabad., sabin.[3, 4], samb.,
sars.[3, 4, 11], sec.[3, 4, 11], **sep.**[3, 4],
sil.[3, 4], spig.[2, 3, 4], spong., stann.,
staph., **STRONT-C.**[3, 4], **SULPH.,**
tarax., **teucr.,** thuj.[3, 11], valer.,
verat., verb., viol-o., **ZINC.**

burning, and[3]
brûlantes, et
Brennen, mit
    carb-v., caust., nat-c., nit-ac.

cramp-like[3]
crampe, comme une
krampfartig
    anac., ars., aur., bov., kali-c.,
    OLND., phos., **plat.**

jerking, and[3]
secousses, avec
ruckartig
    acon., caust., **CHIN.,** cupr.,
    laur., mang., olnd., **puls.,**
    rhus-t., sulph.

paralytic[3]
paralytiques
lähmende
    bell., carb-v., chel., chin., cocc.,
    con., dig., **kali-c.,** meny.,
    nat-m., nit-ac., phos., sars.,
    stann., **STAPH.**

pressive[3]
pressives
Drücken, mit
   agn., anac., ang., arg-m., arn.,
   asaf., bell., bism., **CARB-V.,**
   caust., cham., chin., coloc.,
   graph., guaj., hyos., kali-c.,
   led., lyc., mez., ph-ac., ruta,
   sabad., sars., sep., spong.,
   stann., staph., zinc.

sticking[3]
piquantes
Stechen, mit
   agn., anac.[3], bar-c., calc., chin.,
   colch., dulc., graph., guaj.[3],
   hyos., **LED.**[3, 11], mag-c., mang.[3],
   merc., mur-ac., nat-c., nat-m.,
   puls., sabin., sep., staph.,
   thuj.[3], **zinc.**

muscles, in
muscles, dans les
Muskeln, in
   acon., adon.[3], aesc.[3], agar.,
   agn., alum., am-c., **am-m.,**
   ambr., anac., ang.[3], ant-c.,
   ant-t., **arg-m.,** arn., **ars., ars-i.,**
   ars-s-f.[1'], **asaf.,** asar., **aur.,**
   aur-s.[1'], bar-c., bar-i.[1'], bar-m.,
   bell., bism., bor., bov., **bry.,**
   CALC., camph., **canth.,** caps.,
   carb-an., CARB-V., CARBN-S.,
   CAUST., cham., **chel., chin.,**
   cic., cimic.[3], **cina,** clem., cocc.,
   colch., coloc., con., croc.,
   cupr., cycl., dig., dros., **dulc.**[3],
   euph., ferr., **graph.,** guaj., hell.,
   hep., hyos., ign., iod., ip.,
   KALI-C., kali-m.[1'], **kali-n.**[1],
   kali-s., kreos., lach., laur., led.,
   LYC., mag-c., mag-m., mang.,
   meny., **MERC.,** mez., mosch.,
   mur-ac., nat-c., nat-m.,
   NIT-AC., nux-v., olnd., par.,
   petr., ph-ac., **phos.,** plat., plb.,
   puls., ran-b., rheum, **RHOD.,**
   rhus-t., **ruta,** sabad., **sabin.,**
   samb., sars., sec., sel., seneg.,
   SEP., SIL., spig., spong.,
   squil., **stann., STAPH.,**
   STRONT-C., sul-ac., **SULPH.,**

   tarax., **teucr.,** thuj., valer.,
   verat., verb., viol-o., viol-t.,
   ZINC., ZINC-P.[1']

burning
brûlantes, et
Brennen, mit
   bell., **carb-v.,** caust., kali-c.,
   led., lyc., **nit-ac.,** ruta, sabin.,
   tarax., zinc.

cramp-like
crampe, comme une
krampfartig
   ANAC., ang.[3], ant-c., arg-m.,
   asaf., aur., bism., **calc.,** caust.,
   chel., **chin.,** dulc., euph.,
   graph., iod., kali-c., mang.,
   meny., mosch., **mur-ac.,**
   NAT-C., nat-m., nux-v., **petr.,**
   ph-ac., phos., **PLAT.,** ran-b.,
   ruta, samb., sil., stann.,
   stront-c., thuj., valer.

jerking
secousses, avec
ruckartig
   acon., agar., agn., alum., bell.,
   calc., camph., **CHIN.,** cina,
   cupr., dig., dulc., guaj., lyc.,
   mang., merc., nat-c., ph-ac.,
   phos., plat., **PULS.,** rhus-t.,
   spig., **staph.,** stront-c., sul-ac.,
   sulph.

paralytic
paralytiques
lähmende
   agn., ant-c., asaf., carb-v.,
   cham.[1]**, chin.,** cic., **cina,** cocc.,
   con., dig., graph., **hell.,**
   KALI-C., mez., mosch., nat-m.,
   nit-ac., phos., **sabin., sars.,**
   seneg., sil., stann., verb.

pressing
pressives
Drücken, mit
   acon., ambr., anac., ang.[3],
   ant-c., arg-m., arn., asar.,
   bism., camph., cann-s.,
   CARB-V., caust., chin., colch.,

cupr., cycl., dig., euph., guaj.,
kali-c., kali-n., laur., led., lyc.,
ph-ac., ran-b., ruta, sabin.,
sars., sep., spig., **STANN.,**
staph., stront-c., sulph., teucr.,
viol-t., zinc.

sticking
piquantes
Stechen, mit
    acon., agn., ambr., ang.[3], ant-t.,
    arg-m., arn., bar-c., bell., bry.,
    camph., cann-s., canth., caps.,
    chin., cic., **colch.,** coloc., con.,
    dros., dulc., **euph.,** guaj., hyos.,
    ign., iod., kali-c., **lyc.,** mag-c.,
    mang., merc., mur-ac., nat-m.,
    ph-ac., phos., rheum, sars.,
    spong., staph., sulph., teucr.,
    thuj., **ZINC.**

thread, like a long, evening agg.[7]
fil, comme un long, le soir agg.
Faden, wie ein langer, abends agg.
    all-c.

twinging
lancinantes
schießende
    acon.[6], **agar.[6],** aloe, alum., **AM-M.,**
    ant-c., apis, arg-n.[6], **ars.[6],** aur., bell.,
    berb., **bov.,** canth., carb-an., caust.,
    cham.[6], chel., cimic.[6], cocc., coff.[6],
    coloc., **crot-t., dios.,** dros., **ferr.,**
    iod., iris[6], **kali-bi.[6],** kali-c., **kali-i.[6],**
    kali-m.[1]′, **kalm.[6],** lact.[11], **LAUR.,**
    lyc., **mag-c.,** mag-m., **mag-p.[6],**
    merc., **mez.[6], MOSCH.,** mur-ac.,
    nat-p., nux-v.[6], ph-ac., phos.,
    phys.[11], plan., **PLB.,** plb-i.[6], **prun.,**
    puls.[6], **rhus-t.,** sabin., sang.[6], sars.,
    seneg., **sep.[6],** sieg.[10], sil., **spig.[6],**
    staph., stel.[6], stront-c., sul-ac.,
    tab.[6], valer.

twisting
tordantes, d. en vrille
drehende
    agar., alum., am-m., anac., ant-c.,
    ant-t., **arg-n.,** arn.[3], ars., asaf.,
    bar-c., **bell.,** berb., bor., **bry.,**
    calad., calc., **caps.,** canth., cham.,

cina, clem.[3], **coloc.[3],** con., dig.,
dios., dros., dulc., **ign.,** ip., kali-c.,
kali-n., led., **merc.,** mez., nat-c.,
nat-m., nux-m., **nux-v.,** olnd.,
ox-ac., ph-ac., phos., **plat.,** plb.,
podo., ran-b., ran-s., **rhus-t.,** ruta,
sabad., sabin., sars., seneg., sep.,
SIL., staph., sul-ac., sulph., thlas.[3],
thuj., valer., **VERAT.**

ulcerative[2]
ulcérantes
geschwürige
    alum-sil.[1]′, **AM-M.,** bry., **cann-s.,**
    caust., cic., cycl., graph., hep.,
    ign., iodof., **kali-c.,** kali-m.[1]′,
    KALI-S.[1]′, LACH., mang., merc.,
    mur-ac., nat-m., nux-v., PHOS.,
    PULS., RAN-B., RHUS-T., zinc.

externally
externes
äußerlich
    acon., agar., alum., am-c.,
    AM-M., ambr., anac., ang.[3],
    ant-c., arg-m., arn., ars., aur.,
    bar-c., bell., bov., **BRY.,** calc.[4],
    camph., cann-s., **canth.,** caps.,
    carb-an., carb-v., **caust.,** cedr.,
    cham., chin., **cic.,** cocc., colch.,
    cycl., dros., dulc., ferr., **graph.,**
    hep., **ign., kali-c.,** kali-n.,
    KALI-S., kreos., lach., laur.,
    mag-c., mag-m., **mang.,** merc.,
    mur-ac., nat-c., **nat-m.,** nit-ac.,
    nux-v., petr., ph-ac., phos., plat.,
    PULS., RHUS-T., ruta, sars., **sep.,**
    SIL., spig., spong., staph., sul-ac.,
    sulph., teucr., thuj. verat., **zinc.**

internally
internes
innerlich
    acon., **am-c., arg-n.,** ars., bell.,
    bor., bov., **bry., cann-s.,** canth.,
    caps., carb-an., carb-v., carbn-s.,
    caust., cham., chel., cocc., **coloc.,**
    cupr., dig., **gamb.,** hell., hep.,
    kali-c., kreos., **LACH.,** laur.,
    mag-c., mag-m., mang., **merc.,**
    mur-ac., nit-ac., **nux-v.,** ph-ac.,
    phos., **psor., PULS., RAN-B.,**

rhus-t., ruta, sabad., sep., **SIL.,**
spig., stann., staph., stront-c.,
sulph., valer., verat.

bones, in
os, dans les
Knochen, in
am-c., am-m., **bry.,** bufo[3], caust.,
cic., graph., ign., mang., nat-m.,
puls., rhus-t.

glands, in
glandes, dans les
Drüsen, in
am-c., **am-m.,** aur., bell., bry.,
calc., canth., caust., cham., chin.,
cic., cocc., graph., hep., ign.,
kali-c., merc., mur-ac., nat-c.,
nat-m., nit-ac., petr., **PHOS.,**
puls., rhus-t., ruta, **SIL.,** staph.,
sul-ac., teucr., **zinc.**

undulating
ondulantes
wellenartige
acon., anac., ant-t., arn., asaf.,
chin., cocc., dulc., mez., olnd.,
plat., rhod., sep., spig., sul-ac.[16],
teucr., viol-t.

wandering
erratiques
wandernde
acon., adon.[6], aesc., agar.[3, 6],
agav-t.[14], alum-sil.[1'], **am-be.[6],**
am-c., **am-m.,** ambr.[6], aml-ns.[11],
ant-t.[3], **apis.[2, 3, 6, 8],** apoc.,
apoc-a.[11, 12], arg-m., **arn.,** ars.,
ars-s-f.[2], arund.[11], asaf., **aur.,**
aur-ar.[1'], bapt.[11], bar-c., **bell.,**
benz-ac., **berb.[1'-3, 6],** berb-a.[6], bry.,
buni-o.[14], calc.[3], calc-caust.[6],
calc-p., camph., caps., **carb-v.,**
carbn-s., caul., **caust.,** cedr.,
chel., **chin., cimic.[3, 6],** cina[3], clem.,
COCC.[3], colch., coloc.[11], com.[6],
con.[4, 6], croc., **cupr.[3, 6],** daph.[2, 4, 7],
dios., elat.[11], ery-a.[2], eup-per.[6],
eup-pur., ferr.[3], ferr-p.[1', 6], fl-ac.[11],
form.[6], gels., goss., graph.[3, 11, 16],
hydr.[3, 6], hyper.[6], ictod.[2], ign.,
iod., **iris, KALI-BI.,** kali-c.,

kali-fcy., kali-n.[3], **KALI-S., kalm.,**
LAC-C., lach., lact.[4], **LED.,** lil-t.,
lyc.[3, 6], lycps., mag-c.[3, 16],
mag-m.[3], **mag-p.,** magn-gr.[8],
manc., mang., meny.[3], meph.[11],
merc.[3, 11], merc-i-r.[3, 6], mez.[11],
myric.[11], naja[11], nat-m., nat-s.,
nit-s-d.[2, 11], **nux-m.,** nux-v.[6], op.[3],
ox-ac.[6], pall.[3], ph-ac.[3], phos.[3],
phyt., plan.[3, 11], plat., **plb.,**
polyg-h., prun.[3, 6], **PULS.,**
puls-n.[12], pyrog.[6], pyrus[11], rad.[3],
rad-br.[3], **ran-b.,** rat.[3], rhod.,
rhus-t.[3, 6, 11], rhus-v.[11], rumx.[3],
sabad.[6], **sabin.,** sacch.[11], **sal-ac.,**
sang., sars., sec.[3, 4, 6, 11], senec.[6],
sep., sil.[3], **spig.,** spong.[6], stann.[3],
staph.[3], **stel.[1]** (non: still.), sulph.,
syph.[1', 7, 8], tab.[3], tarent., tax.[4],
tell.[11], **thuj.[3, 6, 11], tub.,** valer.,
verat.[2, 6], verat-v.[3, 6], zinc.

suddenly[3]
soudain
plötzlich
ambr., colch., rad-br.

touch agg.[16]
attouchement agg.
Berührung agg.
graph.

joints, in[2]
articulations, dans les
Gelenken, in
ang., **ant-t., hyper.,** kali-bi.[1'],
tub.[1']

PAINLESSNESS of complaints usually
painful
ABSENCE de DOULEURS de manifesta-
tions en général douloureuses
SCHMERZLOSIGKEIT gewöhnlich
schmerzhafter Beschwerden
ant-c.[3, 7], ant-t.[3], **hell., OP., STRAM.**

analgesie/analgésie/Analgesie

PARALYSIS agitans
PARALYSIE agitante
LÄHMUNG, Paralysis agitans
　　agar.[3, 6, 8], ant-t.[12], aran.[10, 14],
　　aran-ix.[10, 14], arg-m.[6, 14], **arg-n.**[3],
　　ars.[6, 8], aur.[6], **aur-s.**[1', 8, 12], aven.[7, 8],
　　bar-c., bufo, **camph-br.**[6, 8], cann-i.[8],
　　chlorpr.[14], cimic.[14], cocain.[8],
　　cocc.[3, 6, 8], **con.**[3, 6, 8, 10], dub.[6],
　　dub-m.[8], gels., halo.[14], helo., **hyos.**,
　　hyosin.[8, 12], **kali-br.**, kres.[10],
　　lath.[6, 8, 12], levo.[14], **lol.**[3, 6, 8, 12], lyc.[12],
　　mag-p., mang.[6, 8], **MERC.**, nicot.[8],
　　nux-v.[3], perh.[14], **phos.**,
　　phys.[2, 3, 6-8, 12], **plb.**, prun.[3], psil.[14],
　　rauw.[9, 14], reser.[14], **RHUS-T.**, scut.[8],
　　tab., **tarent.**, thiop.[14], **ZINC.**,
　　zinc-cy.[8, 12], **zinc-pic.**[6, 8, 12]

alcohol, after abuse of[2]
alcool, par abus d'
Alkoholmißbrauch, durch
　　ant-t., **ars.**, calc., **lach.**, nat-s.,
　　nux-v., OP., ran-b., sep., **sulph.**

anger, after
colère, après
Zorn, nach
　　nat-m., **nux-v.**, staph.

　　one-sided[2]
　　côté, d'un
　　einseitige
　　　　staph.

atrophy, with[2]
atrophie, avec
Atrophie, mit
　　cupr., **GRAPH.**, kali-p., plb., sec.,
　　sep.

change of weather from warm to
　　cold-wet[7]
changement de temps du chaud au
　　froid humide, par
Wetterwechsel von warm zu naßkalt,
　　durch
　　caust., dulc., rhus-t.

coition, after
coït, par
Koitus, durch
　　phos.

cold, after taking
refroidissement, après avoir pris un
Erkältung, nach einer
　　dulc., rhod.

　　bathing am.[3]
　　bains froids am.
　　kaltes Baden am.
　　　　con.

　　wind or draft, after[15]
　　vent froid ou courant d'air, après
　　kaltem Wind oder Zugluft, nach
　　　　caust.

exertion, after
exercice physique, après un
Anstrengung, nach
　　ars., **caust., gels.**, nux-v., **rhus-t.**

extends from above **downwards**
bas, vers le
absteigende
　　bar-c., merc., zinc.[3]

　　upwards
　　haut, vers le
　　aufsteigende
　　　　agar., **ars.**, bar-c.[15], **con.**,
　　　　hydr-ac., **kali-c.**, karw-h.[14],
　　　　lyss.[10, 12], mang., phos.[7], plb.[3],
　　　　sulfon.[12]

fright, as if from[16]
frayeur, comme par
Schreck, wie durch
　　nat-m.

gradually appearing
graduellement, apparaît
allmählich auftretende
　　CAUST.

intermittend fever, after
intermittente, après une fièvre
Wechselfieber, nach
　　arn.[2], **ars.**[2], **lach.**[2], **NAT-M.**, nux-v.[2]

internally
interne
innerliche
    acon., ant-c., arg-n.[3], **ars.**, bar-c.,
    BELL., calc., cann-s., canth., caps.,
    caust., chin., cic., **cocc.**, coloc.,
    con., cycl., dig., **DULC.**, euphr.,
    gels., graph., helo.[3], **HYOS.**, ip.,
    kali-c., lach., **laur.**, lyc., meny.,
    merc., mur-ac., nat-m., **nux-m.**,
    nux-v., **op.**, petr., phos., plb., **puls.**,
    ran-b.[3], rheum, **rhus-t.**, sec., sel.[3],
    seneg., sep., sil., spig., **STRAM.**,
    sulph.[3], tab[3], tarent., zinc.[3]

Landry's ascending p.[12]
p. ascendante aiguë
Landry' Syndrom
    aconin., con., lyss.

lower half of body, of[1']
inférieure du corps, de la partie
unteren Körperhälfte, der
    alum-p., alum-sil., ars.[11], graph.

lying on a moist ground[15]
couché sur un sol humide
Liegen auf feuchtem Boden, nach
    rhus-t.

masturbation, from/par/durch
chin.[2], stann.

mental shock, from
choc mental, par
seelischen Schock, durch
    apis, caust.[15]

mental emotion, after
excitation émotionelle, par
Gefühlserregung, durch
    apis, **IGN.**, nat-m., nux-v., stann.

muscles, extensor
muscles extenseurs, des
Streckermuskeln, der
    alum., ars., calc., **cocc., crot-h.**,
    cur.[7], **PLB.**

flexor m.
m. fléchisseurs
Beugermuskeln
    caust., **nat-m.**

neuralgias, with
névralgies, avec
Neuralgien, mit
    abrot.

nicotinism, from[10]
nicotinisme, par
Nikotinvergiftung, durch
    nux-v.

old people, of
vieillards, chez les
alten Menschen, bei
    bar-c., con., kali-c., **OP.**[2, 7]

one-sided
unilatérale
einseitige
    acon., acon-c.[11], adren.[7], agar.,
    alum., alum-p.[1'], alumn.[2, 8],
    am-m., ambr.[8], **anac., apis,** arg-m.,
    arg-n., arn., **ars.,** ars-s-f.[1'], asar.,
    aur.[8], bapt., bar-c., bar-m.,
    bar-s.[1'], **bell., both.,** bov.,
    cadm-s., caj.[2, 7], calc., carb-v.,
    carbn-o.[11], carbn-s., **CAUST.**,
    chel., chen-a.[8, 12], chin., chin-s.[4],
    cob-n.[14], **coc-c., cocc.,** colch.,
    conin.[12], cop., cur.[8], cycl., dig.,
    dulc., **elaps, graph.,** guaj., hell.,
    hep., **hydr-ac.**[2, 8, 12], hyos., ign.,
    irid.[8], **kali-c., kali-i.,** kali-m.[1'],
    kali-p., **lach.,** laur., led., lyc.,
    merc., mez., **mur-ac.,** nat-c.,
    nat-m., nit-ac., nux-v., olnd., **op.**,
    ox-ac., perh.[14], petr., **ph-ac.**,
    phos., phys.[8], pic-ac.[8, 12], plb.,
    podo., rhod., **rhus-t.,** sabin., **sars.**,
    sec.[8], sep., spig., stann., staph.,
    stram., stront-c., stry.[8, 12], **sul-ac.**,
    syph., tab., tarax., thuj.,
    verat-v.[8], vip.[4, 8], xan.[8, 12], zinc.,
    zinc-p.[1']

left
gauche, du côté
linken Seite, der
    acon., **all-c.**[2], ambr.[8], **anac., apis,**

arg-n., **arn.**, ars., art-v.², bapt.,
bar-m., bell., brom., caust., cocc.,
cupr-ar.⁸, ¹², elaps, gels., hydr-ac.,
karw-h.¹⁴, lacer.¹¹, **LACH.**, lyc.,
nit-ac., **NUX-V.**, op.³, ox-ac.,
petr., phys.⁸, ¹¹, ¹², **plb.**², ¹¹, podo.,
RHUS-T., santin.¹², stann., **stram.**,
stront-c.³, sulph., verat-v.⁸, vip.³,
xan.⁸

right
droite, du côté
rechten Seite, der
    acon.¹¹, apis, **arn.**, **bell.**, both.¹¹,
    calc., **canth.**, carbn-s.¹¹,
    CAUST., **chel.**³, chen-a.⁸, colch.,
    CROT-C., crot-h., cur.⁸, **elaps,**
    graph., irid.⁸, ¹², iris-fl.¹²,
    iris-foe.¹¹, kali-i., merc-i-r.³,
    nat-c., nat-m.³, **op.**, phos.,
    plb., **rhus-t.**, sang., sil.,
    stront-c., sulph., thuj.³, vip.⁴

anger, after¹⁵
colère, après
Zorn, nach
    staph.

aphasia, with⁷
aphasie, avec
Aphasie, mit
    cench.

apoplexy, after
apoplexie, après
Apoplexie, nach
    acon.³, ⁶, **alum.**, anac., apis,
    arn., ars.³, ⁶, **bar-c.**, bell., both.¹⁰,
    cadm-s., caj.⁷, calc-f.³, ⁶, calen.⁷,
    caust., **cocc.**, con., **crot-c.**,
    crot-h., crot-t.³, ⁶, **cupr.**, form³, ⁶,
    gels., glon.³, ⁶, **hyos.**², ⁴,
    kali-br.³, ⁶, lach., laur., merc.³, ⁶,
    nux-v., **OP.**, **PHOS.**, **plb.**, sec.,
    sep.³, ⁴, ⁶, stann., stram.,
    stront-c.³, ⁶, sulph.³, ⁶, verat-v.³, ⁶,
    vip.³, ⁶, zinc.

coldness of the paralyzed part, with
froid des parties paralysées,
    avec sensation de
Kälte im gelähmten Teil, mit
    ars., **caust.**, **cocc.**, **dulc.**, **graph.**,
    nux-v., plb., **RHUS-T.**, zinc.

convulsions of the well side
convulsions du côté sain
Konvulsionen der gesunden Seite
    apis, **art-v.**, bell., hell., **stram.**

paralyzed side, of
paralysé, du côté
gelähmten Seite, der
    phos., sec.

convulsions, after
convulsions, après
Konvulsionen, nach
    ars.², **bell.**², **CAUST.**, **CIC.**²,
    cocc.², ³, con.⁷, **CUPR.**², ³, ⁷,
    elaps³, **hyos.**, **ip.**², ⁷, laur.²,
    nux-v.², **plb.**², ⁴, ⁸, **sec.**², ³, ⁸, **sil.**²,
    stann.², **stram.**², **sulph.**², **vib.**²

headache, after¹⁶
maux de tête, après
Kopfschmerzen, nach
    ars.

heat in the paralyzed part, with
chaleur dans la partie paralysée,
    avec
Hitze im gelähmten Teil, mit
    alum.¹, ⁷, phos.

hyperesthesia of the well side
hyperesthésie du côté sain, avec
Überempfindlichkeit der gesunden
    Seite, mit
    plb.

involuntary motion of the para-
    lyzed limb¹⁶
involontaire du membre paralysé,
    mouvement
unwillkürliche Bewegung des
    gelähmten Gliedes
    arg-n., merc., phos.

mental excitement, after
excitation mentale, après
seelischer Erregung, nach
    stann.

    shock, after
    choc mental, après
    seelischem Schock, nach
      apis

now here, now there[16]
tantôt ici, et tantôt là
bald hier, bald dort
    bell.

numbness of the paralyzed side,
    with[2]
engourdissement du côté
    paralysé, avec
Taubheit der gelähmten Seite, mit
    apis, cann-i.[7], **caust., coc-c.,**
    rhus-t., staph.[7]

    well side, of
    sain, du côté
    gesunden Seite, der
      cocc.

pain, from
douleurs, par
Schmerzen, durch
    nat-m.

spasms, after
spasmes après
Krämpfen, nach
    stann.

    of the other side[15]
    de l'autre côté
    Krämpfe auf der anderen Seite
    bell., lach., phos., stram.

suppression of eruption, from
suppression d'une éruption, par
Unterdrückung eines Haut-
    ausschlages, durch
    caust., dulc., hep., **psor., sulph.**

twitching of the well side
soubresauts de la partie saine, avec
Zucken der gesunden Seite, mit
    apis, art-v., **bell., stram.**

of the paralysed side
du côté paralysé
der gelähmten Seite
    apis, **arg-n.,** merc., nux-v.,
    phos., **sec.,** stram., stry.

nettle rash, after disappearance of
urticaire, après disparition d'
Urtikaria, nach Verschwinden der
    cop.

organs, of
organes, des
Organen, von
    absin., **acon.,** agar., agn., alum.,
    alum-p.[1]', am-c., am-m., ambr.,
    anac., ang.[3], ant-c., ant-t., arn., ars.,
    asaf., asar., aur., aur-s.[1]', **bar-c.,**
    bar-s.[1]', **BELL.,** bism., bor., bov.,
    bry., calc., camph., cann-s., canth.,
    caps., carb-ac., carb-an., carb-v.,
    carbn-s., **caust.,** cham., chel., chin.,
    cic., **cocc.,** colch., coloc., con.,
    croc., cupr., cycl., dig., dros.,
    DULC., euphr., gels., graph., hell.,
    hep., hydr-ac., **HYOS.,** ign., iod.,
    ip., kali-br., kali-c., kali-m.[1]', kreos.,
    lach., laur., led., **lyc.,** mag-c.,
    mag-m., mang., meny., merc., mez.,
    mur-ac., nat-c., nat-m., **nit-ac.,**
    nux-m., nux-v., **olnd., op.,** par.,
    petr.[1], ph-ac., **phos., plb., PULS.,**
    rheum, rhod., **rhus-t., ruta,** sabad.,
    sabin., sars., **SEC.,** seneg., **sep.,**
    SIL., spig., spong., squil., stann.,
    staph., **stram.,** stront-c., **sul-ac.,**
    sulph., thuj., **verat.,** verb., zinc.,
    zinc-p.[1]'

painful
douloureuse
schmerzhafte
    agar., alum-sil.[1]', arn., **ars.,** bell.,
    cadm-s.[1]', calc., **caust.,** cina, **cocc.,**
    crot-t., **kali-n., lat-m.,** phos., **plb.,**
    sil., sulph.

pain – paralyzed/douleurs – paraly-
sées/Schmerzen – gelähmter

painless
indolore
schmerzlose
  abies-c., absin., acon., aeth., alum.,
  alum-p.[1'], ambr., **anac.**, ang.[3],
  arg-n., arn., **ars.**, ars-s-f.[1'], **aur.**,
  aur-ar.[1'], aur-s.[1'], **bapt., bar-c.**,
  bar-s.[1'], bell., bov., **bufo**, bry.,
  cadm-s., calc., camph., **CANN-I.**,
  cann-s.[3], carb-v., **carbn-s.**,
  caust., cham., chel., chin., chin-s.,
  chlor., cic., **COCC.**, colch., coloc.,
  CON., crot-h., **cupr.**, cur., ferr.,
  GELS., graph., hell., hydr-ac., **hyos.**,
  ign., ip., kali-c., kalm., karw-h.[14],
  laur., led., **LYC.**, m-arct.[4], **merc.**,
  nat-m., nux-m., nux-v., **OLND., op.**,
  ph-ac., phos., **PLB., puls.**, rhod.,
  RHUS-T., sec., sil., staph., stram.,
  stront-c., sulph., **verat.**, zinc.,
  zinc-p.[1']

paraplegia[12]
paraplégie
Paraplegie
  anh., arg-n.[3], ars.[3], caul.[2, 12], gels.,
  kali-t., kalm., lath., mang., nux-v.[3],
  phys., pic-ac., pip-m., rhus-v., stry.,
  thal., thyr., wildb.

parturiton, after[2]
accouchement, après l'
Entbindung, nach der
  PHOS., RHUS-T.

perspiration, from suppressed
transpiration supprimée, par
Schweiß, durch unterdrückten
  colch., **gels.**[7], **lach.**[7], rhus-t.

poliomyelitis[7]
poliomyélite
Poliomyelitis
  acon.[2, 7, 8], aeth.[8], alum., arg-n.,
  arn.[2, 7], ars., bell.[2, 7, 8], **bung.**[8],
  calc.[8], carb-ac., **caust.**[2, 7, 8],
  chin-ar., chr-s.[8], cur., dulc.,
  ferr-i., ferr-p., **GELS.**[2, 7, 8],
  hydr-ac., hydroph.[14], hyos.[2, 7],

kali-i., kali-p.[7, 8], karw-h.[14],
kres.[10], lach., lath.[7, 8, 10],
merc.[2, 7, 10], nux-v.[2, 7, 8], phos.[7, 8],
phys., **plb.**[7, 8], plb-i., rhus-t.[1', 2, 7, 8],
sec.[7, 8], stry-p., sulph.[2, 7, 8], verat.,
verat-v.

paralysis of diaphragm, with
paralysie du diaphragme, avec
Zwerchfellähmung, mit
  cupr., op., sil.

post-diphtheric
post-diphtérique
Diphtherie, nach
  ant-t., apis, arg-m., **arg-n.**[2, 3, 6, 8],
  arn., **ars.,** aur-m.[8], aven.[8], **bar-c.**[2],
  botul.[8], camph., carb-ac., **caust.**,
  COCC., con., crot-h., diph.[3, 6, 8, 12],
  gels., helon.[2], **hyos.,** kali-br.,
  kali-i.[8], kali-p., **lac-c., lach., nat-m.,**
  nux-v., **phos., phys.**[2, 3, 6], phyt.,
  plb., plb-a.[8], rhod.[8, 12], **rhus-t.**[2, 3, 6, 8],
  sec., sil., sulph.[2], thuj.[2], zinc.[2]

river bath in summer, from
bain de rivière en été, par un
Baden im Fluß im Sommer, durch
  caust.

sensation of[16]
sensation de
Gefühl von
  phos.

senses, of[16]
sens, des
Sinne, der
  kali-n.

sexual excesses, from
sexuels, par excès
sexuelle Ausschweifungen, durch
  nat-m., nux-v., PHOS.[2], **rhus-t.,** sil.[3]

single parts
isolées, de parties
einzelner Teile
  anac., **ars., CAUST.,** dulc., plb.[1', 3]

spastic spinal p.[8, 12]
spasmodique spinale, par p.
spastische Spinalparalyse
ben-d., gels., hyper., kres.[10], lachn.,
lath.[10], **nux-v.,** phos.[1'], plect., sec.

suppressed eruptions
supprimées, par éruptions
unterdrückte Hautausschläge, durch
caust., **dulc.,** hep., **psor., sulph.**

toxic
toxique
Vergiftung, durch
apis, ars., bapt., crot-h.[2], gels.,
lac-c., **lach.,** mur-ac., rhus-t.

arsenic[2]/Arsen
chin., ferr., graph., **hep., nux-v.**

lead[8]/plomb/Blei
alumn., ars.[2], cupr.[2, 8], kali-i.,
nux-v., **op.**[2, 8], pipe.[12], **plat.**[2], plb.,
sul-ac.[8, 12]

mercurial[7]/mercure/Quecksilber
HEP., nit-ac., staph., stram.,
sulph.

typhoid, in
typhoïde, au cours de la
typhusähnlicher Erkrankung, bei
agar., caust.[15], **lach., rhus-t.**

wet, after getting
mouillé, après s'être
Durchnässung, nach
CAUST., rhus-t.

paresis–convulsions see convulsions–
paresis

parturiton see Vol. I index, Vol II
index, Vol. III

PERIODICITY
PÉRIODICITÉ
PERIODIZITÄT
acon., **agar.**[1], aloe[7], **ALUM.,**
alum-sil.[1'], **ALUMN.**[2], am-br.,
ambr.[2, 7], **anac., ant-c.,** ant-t.,
ARG-M., aran., **arn., ARS.,**
ars-met.[8], ars-s-f.[1'], **asar., bar-c.,**
bell., benz-ac.[6], bov., bry., bufo,
cact., calc., calc-sil.[1'], cann-s.,
canth., caps., carb-v., CARBN-S.[2, 7],
carl.[8], **CEDR.,** cent.[7, 11], chel.[6],
CHIN., CHIN-AR., CHIN-S.,
chr-ac.[8], cina, clem., cocc., colch.,
croc., crot-h., cupr., dros., **eucal.**[7],
eup-per.[3, 8], ferr., ferr-ar., **gels.,**
graph., hep.[3], **ign., IP., kali-ar.,**
kali-bi., kali-c.[3], kali-n., lac-d.[1', 7],
lach., lact.[4], lil-t.[6], **lyc., mag-c.,**
mag-s.[10], meny., merc., nat-ar.,
NAT-M., nat-n.[6], **nat-s.,** nicc.[8],
nicc-s.[7], **NIT-AC., nux-v.,** petr.,
phos., plb., prim-o.[8], **puls.,**
ran-s.[4, 6, 8], **rhod., rhus-t.,**
rhus-v.[7, 11], **sabad.,** samb., **sang.,**
sec., senec.[6], **SEP., SIL., spig.,**
stann., staph., sul-ac.[7], **sulph.,**
tarent.[3, 6-8, 11], **tela**[8], thal.[14], **tub.,**
urt-u.[8], valer., **verat.,** vip.[4, 6], zinc.

Vol. I: *absent-minded/distrait/*
zerstreut
anxiety/anxiété/Angst
confusion/Verwirrung
delirium/délire/Delirium
despair/désespoir/Verzweiflung
dullness/esprit gourd/Stumpfheit
ecstasy/extase/Ekstase
fancies/fantaisies/Phantasien
forgetful/oublieux/vergeßlich
indifference/indifférence/Gleich-
gültigkeit
insanity/folie/Geisteskrankheit
memory, weakness of/mémoire,
faiblesse de/Gedächtnisschwäche
restlessness/agitation/Ruhelosig-
keit
sadness/tristesse/Traurigkeit
unconsciousness/inconscience/
Bewußtlosigkeit
weeping/pleurer/Weinen

Vol. II: *chorea/chorée/Chorea*
convulsions/Konvulsionen
faintness/évanouissement/Ohn-
macht
menses/menstruation/Menses
moon/lune/Mond
seasons/saisons/Jahreszeiten
weakness/faiblesse/Schwäche

Vol. III: *sleepiness/somnolence/*
Schläfrigkeit
sleeplesness/insomnie/Schlaflosig-
keit
yawning/bâille/Gähnen
abortion/avortement/Fehlgeburt

annually
annuelle
jährliche
am-c.[3, 7], **ant-t.**[3], **ARS.**[1, 7],
buth-a.[9, 14], carb-v.[3, 8], carc.[9],
cench., crot-h.[3-4, 6, 8], echi.[3], elaps[3],
gels.[3], kali-bi.[3], **lach.**[3-4, 7, 8], lyc.[3],
naja[3], nat-m.[3], nicc.[3, 7, 8], psor.[3, 7],
rhus-r.[8], **rhus-t.**[3], rhus-v.[7, 11],
sulph.[3, 8], tarent., thuj., urt-u.[3, 6-8],
vip.[3, 6]

same hour, complaints return at
même heure, les troubles se
produisent toujours à la
selben Stunde, Beschwerden kommen
zur
ant-c., **aran.**, ars.[3], bov.[3], **cact.**,
CEDR.[1, 7], cench.[7], chin.[1'],
chin-s.[3, 4], cina[3], cocc.[4], ign.,
ip.[6], kali-bi.[1'], kali-br.[7], lyc.[3],
nat-m.[3], sabad., sel.[1] (non: sil.),
tarent.[7], tub.[7]

neuralgia every day at
névralgie tous les jours à la
Neuralgien jeden Tag zur
KALI-BI., sulph.[1']

regular intervals, complaints return
at[7]
réguliers, les troubles se produisent
à des intervalles
regelmäßigen Abständen,
Beschwerden kommen in
CARBN-S.

daily[3]
quotidienne
täglicher
aran., ars., caps., ip., nux-v., puls.

every other day[4, 6]
tous les 2 jours
jeden 2. Tag
alum.[4, 6-8, 15, 16], anac.[6], ars.[1', 3],
calc.[4, 6, 16], cham.[6],
chin.[3, 6, 8, 15, 16], chin-s.[4],
crot-h., fl-ac.[8], **ip.**[6, 7], lyc.[15],
lycps.[7], nat-c.[16], nat-m.[3, 6, 16],
nit-ac.[8], nux-v.[16], oxyt.[8],
psor.[7], puls.[16]

morning[2]/matin/morgens
alumn.

evening[4, 7]/soir/Abend
puls.

third day[6]
3 jours
3. Tag
anac., aur., chin-s.[4], kali-ar.[1'],
kali-br.[7]

pregnancy, in
grossesse, pendant la
Schwangerschaft, in der
lyc.[7], **mag-c.**[2]

fourth day[3]
4 jours
4. Tag
ars.[1', 3, 4, 6], aur.[6], eup-per.[6],
kali-br.[7], lyc., puls., sabad.

seventh day
7 jours
7. Tag
am-m., ars.[1', 3, 6], ars-h.[2, 7],
aur-m.[6], canth., cedr.[6], **chin.**,
croc.[6], eup-per.[6], gels.[3], **iris**[3, 6],
lac-d.[3, 6], lyc., nux-m.[6], phos.[3, 6],
plan., rhus-t., sabad.[6], sang.[3, 6],
sil.[3, 6], **SULPH.**[1, 7], tell.[7, 11], tub.

tenth day[6]
10 jours
10. Tag
   kali-p., lach.[3, 6], phos.[3]

fourteenth day
14 jours
14. Tag
   am-m., ARS., ars-met.[2, 7, 8], calc.,
   canth.[7], chel.[6], chin., chin-s.,
   con., ign.[6], kali-br.[7], LACH.,
   nicc.[3, 6, 8], phyt.[6], plan., psor.,
   puls., sang.[3], sulph.[3, 6]

twenty-first day
21 jours
21. Tag
   ant-c., ars.[8], ars-met.[8], aur.,
   chin-s., mag-c.[1'], psor., sulph.,
   tarent., tub.

twenty-eighth day
28 jours
28. Tag
   mag-c.[4], nux-m.[1], NUX-V., puls.,
   SEP., tub.

forty-two day[3]
42 jours
42. Tag
   mag-m.

PERSPIRATION, agg. during
TRANSPIRATION, agg. pendant la
SCHWEISS, agg. beim Schwitzen
   acon., ant-t., arn., ARS., calc.,
   CAUST., CHAM., chin., chin-ar.,
   cimx., croc., eup-per., ferr., ferr-ar.,
   FORM., ign., ip., lyc., MERC.,
   nat-ar., nat-c., nux-v., OP., phos.,
   puls., psor., RHUS-T., SEP., spong.,
   STRAM., SULPH., VERAT.

am.
   acon., aesc., aeth., ars., apis, bapt.,
   bell., bov., BRY., calad., calc.,
   camph., canth., cham., chin-s.,
   cimx., CUPR., elat., eup-per.,
   fl-ac.[7], GELS., graph., hep., lach.,
   lyc., nat-c., NAT-M., psor.,
   RHUS-T., samb., sec., stront-c.,
   tere-ch.[14], thuj., verat.

gives no relief
ne soulage pas
erleichtert nicht
   acon., anac., ant-c., ant-t., apis[1'],
   arn., ARS., ars-s-f.[1'], bar-c., bell.,
   benz-ac., calc., camph., cann-s.,
   carb-v., CAUST., CHAM., chel.,
   chin., chin-ar.[6], cimx., cina, cinnb.,
   cocc., coff., colch.[1], coloc., con.,
   croc., dig., dros., dulc., eup-per.,
   ferr., ferr-ar., FORM., graph., hep.,
   hyos., ign., ip., kali-c., kali-n.,
   kreos., lach.[3, 6], led., lyc., mang.,
   MERC., mez., mosch., mur-ac.,
   nat-ar., nat-c., nat-m., nit-ac.,
   NUX-V., OP., par., ph-ac., phos.,
   plb., psor., puls., pyrog.[3], ran-b.,
   rhod., RHUS-T., sabad., sabin.,
   sal-ac.[3, 6], samb., sel., SEP., spong.,
   stann., staph., STRAM., stront-c.,
   sul-ac.[3], SULPH., tarax., tarent-c.[3],
   thuj., til., tub.[3], valer., VERAT.,
   verat-v.

after p. agg.
après la t. agg.
nach dem Schw. agg.
   acon., ant-t., arn.[2], ars., ars-i.[6],
   ars-s-f.[1'], bell., bry., calc., canth.[6],
   carb-an.[16], carb-v., cast.[6], cham.,
   CHIN., chin-s.[8], cinnb.[1'], con.,
   ferr.[2], hep.[6, 8], ign., iod., ip.,
   kali-c., kali-i.[6], lyc., merc.,
   merc-c.[8], mur-ac.[1', 2], nat-c.,
   nat-m., nit-ac.[3, 8], nux-v., op.[8],
   petr., PH-AC., phos., psor.[6],
   puls., samb.[6], sel., SEP., sil.,
   spig., spong.[2], squil., stann.[6],
   staph., stram.[8], sulph., tub.[6],
   verat.[8]

am.
   acon., aesc., am-m., ambr., ant-t.,
   apis[2], ars., aur.[3, 6], bapt.[3], bar-c.,
   bell., bov., bry., calad., calc.[3, 6],
   camph.[2, 3, 6], canth., CHAM.,
   chel., cimx.[2], clem., cocc., coloc.,
   cupr.[3, 6, 8], elat.[2], ferr-p.[3, 6], fl-ac.[2],
   franc.[8], GELS., glon.[3], graph.,
   hell., hep., hyos., iod.[3, 6], ip.,
   kali-i.[3, 6], kali-n., lach.[2], led., lyc.,
   lyss.[2, 10], mag-m., NAT-M.,

nit-ac., nux-v., **olnd.**, op., **PSOR.,**
puls., ran-b.[3, 6], rhod., **RHUS-T.,**
sabad., sabin., samb., sel., spong.,
stram., **stront-c.**, sul-ac., **sulph.,**
tab.[3], tarax., **thuj.**, urt-u.[3, 6],
valer., **verat.**, vip.[3, 6], vip-a.[14],
visc.[3, 6]

acrid
âcre
scharfer
all-s., **caps., CHAM.**, coff.[3], **con.,**
fl-ac., graph., **hell.**[3], iod., ip.,
lac-ac., lyc., merc., nat-m.[3],
nit-ac.[3, 6], par., ran-b.[3], rhus-t., sil.[3],
tarax., tarent.[3], zinc.[3]

burning/brûlante/brennender

bloody
sanguinolente
blutiger
anag.[2], arn., ars.[3, 6], calc.,
cann-i.[6], cann-s.[3], cham., chin.,
clem., cocc.[2], **CROT-H.**, cur.,
hell.[3, 6], **LACH., lyc., nux-m.,**
nux-v., petr., phos.[3, 6]

night/nuit/nachts
cur.

burning
brûlante
brennender
merc., **mez., NAT-C.**, verat.

acrid/âcre/scharfer

clammy, sticky, viscid
collante, visqueuse
klebriger, zäher
absin.[11], acet-ac., acon., act-sp.[2],
agar., aloe[3, 6], aml-ns., anac.,
ant-c., **ant-t.**, anthraci., anthraco.,
apis, arn., **ARS.**, ars-s-f.[1'],
ben-n.[11], both., brom., **bry.**[2, 3],
calc., CAMPH., cann-i., canth.,
carb-ac.[3, 6], carb-an., carb-v.,
carbn-h.[11], caust., **cench.**[7, 11],
CHAM., chin., chlor., cimic.,
cocc., coff., coff-t.[11], colch.,
coloc.[3], **corn., crot-c.**, crot-h.,

crot-t., cub.[11], cupr., **cupr-ar.**[2, 11],
daph., dig., elat., fago., **FERR.,**
FERR-AR., ferr-i., FERR-P., fl-ac.,
gast.[11], glon., guat.[9], **hell., hep.,**
hydr.[11], hydr-ac.[2, 11], hyos., iod.,
jatr., kali-bi., kali-br., kali-cy.[11],
kali-n.[11], kali-ox.[11], lach., lachn.,
lil-t.[3, 6], lob.[11], **LYC., MERC.,**
merc-c., merc-pr-r.[11], merc-sul.[11],
mez., morph., **mosch.**, mur-ac.[11],
naja[3, 11], napht.[11], nat-m.[3],
nat-sil.[1'], **nux-v.**, op., ox-ac.,
PH-AC., phal.[12], **PHOS.**, phys.[11],
plb., psor., rauw.[14], **sec.**, sol-t.[11],
spig., spong., stann., stry.[11],
sul-ac., sul-i.[1'], sulph.[11], sumb.,
tab., tanac.[11], tax., ter., trach.[11],
tub., VERAT., verat-v.[3], vip.,
wies.[11], zinc., zinc-m.[11], zinc-s.[11]

morning/matin/morgens
mosch.

evening/soir/abends
anthraco., clem., fl-ac., sumb.

night/nuit/nachts
cupr., fago., hep., **lyc.**[2], **merc.**[2]

bed, in[2]
lit, au
Bett, im
plb.

climacteric period, at[7]
ménopause, pendant la
Klimakterium, während des
crot-h., lach., lyc., sul-ac., ter.

falling asleep[2]
s'endormant, en
Einschlafen, beim
daph.

starting from sleep, with
tressaillant au cours du sommeil,
en
Aufschrecken aus dem Schlaf, beim
daph.

cold
froide
kalter

acet-ac., **acon.**, act-sp., aeth.,
agar., agar-ph.[11], ail., alco.[11],
aloe[3, 6], **AM-C.**, ambr.[3], **anac.**,
anh.[9], **ant-c., ANT-T., anthraci.**,
apis, aran.[14], **arn., ARS.**, ars-i.,
ars-s-f.[1], asaf.[3], aur.[3], **aur-m.**,
bar-c., bar-m., bar-s.[1], bell.,
benz-ac., bol-lu.[11], both., **bry.**,
bufo[1], buth-a.[9], cact.[1], cadm-s.[1],
calad., **calc.**, calc-p.[3], calc-s.,
calc-sil.[1], **CAMPH., cann-i.**[2],
cann-s., canth., caps., **carb-ac.**,
CARB-V., carbn-s., cast.[3], **cench.**[7],
cent.[11], cham., **CHIN., CHIN-AR.**,
chlol.[2], **chlor.**, cimic., **cina**[1], **cist.**,
COCC., coff., coff-t.[11], colch.[1],
coloc., con.[3], convo-s.[14], corn.,
croc., **crot-c.**, crot-h., cupr.,
cupr-a.[2, 11], **cupr-ar.**[2], **cur.**,
cyt-l.[9, 14], dig., digin.[11], **dros.**,
dulc., **elaps**, esp-g.[13], **euph.**[3],
euphr., **FERR., ferr-ar., ferr-i.**,
ferr-p.[3], frag.[11], gels., **graph.**[3],
hell., HEP., hydr.[2], **hydr-ac.**[3, 6],
hyos., hura, **ign.**, iod., **IP.**, jatr.,
kali-ar., kali-bi.[1, 3], **kali-c.**[1, 14],
kali-cy.[11], kali-n., kali-p.[3, 6],
kalm., lac-c.[1] (non: lac-ac.),
lachn., laur., lil-t.[3, 6], **lob.**,
lol.[11], **LYC.**, manc., mang.[3],
med.[1], **merc., MERC-C.**,
merc-pr-r.[11], **mez.**, morph.,
mur-ac., **naja**[3], narcot.[11], **nat-ar.**,
nat-c., nat-m., nat-p., nit-ac.,
nux-v., op., ox-ac., paeon.[2],
penic.[13], **petr., ph-ac.**[2, 3, 11], **phos.**,
plan., plb., podo., **psor., puls.**,
pyrog., ran-s.[3], **rheum**[2, 3], rhus-t.,
ruta, sabad.[3], sang., **SEC.**, seneg.,
SEP., sil., **spig., spong.**, stann.,
staph., stram., sul-ac., sul-i.[1],
sulo-ac.[14], **sulph.**, sumb., **tab.**,
ter., tere-ch.[14], thea[11], **ther., thuj.**,
tub., VERAT., VERAT-V., vip.,
vip-a.[14], wye.[11], zinc.

Vol. I: *anxiety-perspiration/*
   anxiété-transpiration/Angst-
   Schweiß

---

faintness – perspiration/
   évanouissement – transpira-
   tion/Ohnmacht – Schweiß

morning/matin/morgens
   ant-c., canth., chin., esp-g.[13],
   euph., ruta

afternoon/après-midi/nachmittags
   GELS., phos., verat-v.

evening/soir/abends
   anac., hura, phos.[11]

   18 h
      psor.

night/nuit/nachts
   am-c., buth-a.[14], chin., coloc.,
   croc., cupr., cur., **dig.**, fago., iod.,
   lob., mang.[16], op., rhus-t., **SEP.**,
   thuj.

am.
   nux-v.

cigar, after[11]
cigare, après avoir fumé un
Zigarre, nach einer
   op.

clammy sweats with haemorrhage
collante avec hémorrhagie, et
klebriger, kalter Schweiß bei
   Blutungen
      CHIN.

   chill
   frissons, pendant les
   Fieberfrost, während
      corn., cupr.[2], lyss.[2], **VERAT.**[2]

coffee, after[11]
café, après avoir bu un
Kaffee, nach
   digin.

convulsions, during
convulsions, pendant les
Konvulsionen, bei
   camph.[1], **cupr.**[2]; **ferr.**, stram.,
   verat.[2]

diarrhoea, in[2]
diarrhée, pendant la
Diarrhoe, bei
    aeth., ant-t., **ars.**, calc., **camph.,**
    cupr., hell., jatr., pic-ac., **sec.,**
    sil., sulph., **tab.**, ter., **verat.**

dysmenorrhoea, in[2]
dysménorrhée, pendant la
Dysmenorrhoe, bei
    sars., verat.

eating, while
mangeant, en
Essen, beim
    MERC.

    after/après avoir mangé/ nach
      dem
      digin.[11], sul-ac.

exertion of body, or mind, after the
    slightest
exercice physique ou
    mental, après le moindre
Anstrengung, nach der geringsten
    körperlichen oder geistigen
    act-sp., **calc., HEP., SEP.**

headache, with
maux de tête, avec
Kopfschmerzen, mit
    GELS.[2], graph., **verat.**[2]

heat, with sensation of internal[14]
chaleur interne, avec sensation
Hitzegefühl, mit innerlichem
    anac.

lying, while[11]
couché, en étant
Liegen, beim
    thea

menses, during
menstruation, pendant la
menses, während der
    ars., coff., phos., **sars., sec.,**
    VERAT.

motion, on
mouvement, par
Bewegung, bei
    ant-c., sep.

nausea, with[2]
nausée, avec
Übelkeit, bei
    calc., ip., lach., **PETR., tab.,**
    verat., verat-v.

    and vertigo
    et pendant les vertiges
    und Schwindel
      ail.

over the body, warm sweat on the
    palms
sur tout le corps avec paumes des
    mains chaudes et transpirantes
am ganzen Körper, warmer
    Schweiß in den Handtellern
    dig.

perspiration increases the coldness
    of the body
transpiration augmente le froid
    du corps
Schweiß verstärkt die Kälte des
    Körpers
    cinnb., cist.

rising from bed, on[11]
sortant du lit, en
Aufstehen vom Bett, beim
    bry.

stool, during
selle, pendant la
Stuhlgang, bei
    merc., sulph., thuj., verat.

sudden attacks of
accès subits de
plötzliche Anfälle von kaltem Schw.
    crot-h.

urination, after
uriner, après
Urinieren, nach
    bell.

walking, on[14]
marchant, en
Gehen, beim
   rhus-t.

in cold open air[16]
au grand air froid
in kalter Luft
   rhus-t.

vertigo, with[2]
vertiges, pendant les
Schwindel, bei
   ail., **merc-c.,** ther.

vomiting, with[2]
vomissement, avec
Erbrechen, mit
   CAMPH., ip., thea[11], **VERAT.,**
   verat-v.

colliquative
colliquative, extrèmement abondante
   et épuisante
erschöpfender, reichlicher
   acet-ac., **ANT-T.,** ars., ars-h.[2],
   camph., **carb-v., CHIN., EUPI.,**
   iod.[2], jab.[2], **lach., lyc.,** mill., **nit-ac.,**
   psor., sec.

critical
critique
kritischer
   acon.[6], bapt., bell.[6], bry., **canth.**[6],
   chlor., pneu.[6], **pyrog.,** rhus-t.[6]

hot
très chaude
heißer
   ACON., aesc., aml-ns.[3, 6], anac.[3],
   ant-c.[3], asar.[3], asc-t., aur.[3, 6], **bell.,**
   bism.[3, 6], bry., calc., calc-sil.[1'],
   camph.[3], canth.[3], **caps.**[2], **carb-v.,**
   CHAM., chel., chin., cocc.,
   coff.[3, 6], **CON.,** corn., dig., dros.[3],
   hell.[2, 3], **IGN., IP.,** kreos.[3], lach.[3],
   led.[3], lyc.[3], **merc.**[2], merc-i-r.,
   nat-c., **NUX-V., OP.,** par.[3],
   penic.[13], **ph-ac.**[2], phos., pip-n.[3],
   PSOR., puls., **pyrog.,** rauw.[9],
   rhus-t.[2], sabad., sang.[3], **SEP.,** sil.,

stann., staph., **stram., sulph.,**
thuj., verat., viol-t.

gives no relief[7]
ne soulage pas
erleichtert nicht
   til.

odor, aromatic
odeur aromatique
odeur, aromatique
Geruch, aromatischer
   all-c.[3], benz-ac., guare., petr.[3],
   rhod., sep.[3]

bitter[3]
amère
bitterer
   dig., **verat.**

morning/matin/morgens
   verat.

blood, like
sang, de
Blut, wie
   lyc.

bread, like white[2]
pain blanc, de
Weißbrot, wie
   ign.

burnt
brûlée, comme
verbrannt, wie
   BELL.[2, 3], **bry.**[3], mag-c.[3], sulph.,
   thuj.[3]

cadaverous, carrion
cadavérique, charogne
aashafter
   ars., art-v., lach.[15], **psor.**[2], thuj.

camphora, like[2, 3, 7]
camphre, comme le
Kampfer, wie
   camph.

cheesy
fromage, de
käsiger
con.[3], **hep.,** plb., sulph.

drugs, like corresponding
drogue employée, correspondant
à la
Arzneien, ähnlich den entsprechen-
den
asaf., ben., camph., carbn-h.,
chen-a.[11], iod., ol-an.[11], phos.,
sulph., tab., ter.[11], valer.

eggs, like spoiled
œufs, comme pourris
Eier, wie verdorbene
plb.[3], staph., sulph.

elder-blossoms, like
sureau, comme fleurs de
Holunderblüten, wie
sep.

fetid
fétide
stinkender, fötider
aesc., all-s.[2], aloe[2], am-c.,
am-m.[3], ambr.[2], anac., arn.,
ars.[2, 3], aur-m.[2], **bapt.**[2, 3, 6],
BAR-C.[2, 3, 6], bell.[3], bov.[3, 6],
canth.[2, 3], **carb-ac.,** carb-an.,
carb-v.[3, 6], cimic.[2], coloc.[3], con.,
crot-h.[3, 6], **cycl.**[2, 3], dios.[3], **dulc.,**
eucal.[2], **euphr.**[2, 3], ferr.,
fl-ac.[3, 6], **GRAPH.**[2, 3, 6],
guaj.[2, 3, 6], **HEP., kali-c.**[2, 3, 6],
kali-p.[2, 3, 6], lac-c.[3, 6], lach.[3],
led., lyc., **mag-c.**[2, 3], mag-m.[3, 6],
merc., merc-c.[2],
NIT-AC.[2, 3, 6, 12], **NUX-V.**[2, 3],
petr.[3, 6], **PHOS.**[2, 3], plb.[3], **psor.,**
PULS.[2, 3], pyrog., **rhod.**[2, 3],
rhus-t.[2, 3], rob., **SEL.**[3], **sep.**[1'-3, 6],
SIL.[2, 3, 6, 7], spig.[2, 3],
STAPH.[2, 3, 6], stram.[3, 6],
sulph.[2, 3, 6], tell., thuj., **tub.,**
vario.[2], **verat.**[2, 3], zinc.

coughing, after
toux, après la
Husten, nach
hep.

eruptions, with
éruptions, avec
Hautausschlägen, mit
dulc.

garlic, like
ail, d'
Knoblauch, wie
art-v.[2-3', 7, 11], lach.[2], sulph.[7],
thuj.[1']

honey, like
miel, de
Honig, wie
thuj.

leek, like[7]
poireaux, comme
Lauch, wie
thuj.

lilac, like[8]
lilas, de
Flieder, wie spanischer
sep.

mice, like[7]
souris, de
Mäuse, wie
tub.

musk, like
musc, de
Moschus, wie
apis, bism.[3], mosch., puls., **sulph.,**
sumb.

musty
moisie
schimmeliger
arn., **cimx.,** merc.[3], merc-c.[3],
nux-v., psor., **puls., rhus-t.,**
stann., syph.[15], thuj.[3], thyr.[3]

offensive
repoussante, malodorante
widerlicher

> acon.[3], aloe, all-s., am-c.,
> ambr.[3], apis, **ARN., ars.,**
> ars-s-f.[1'], art-v., asar.[3], aur-m.,
> **bapt.,** bar-c.[3], **BAR-M.,** bar-s.[1'],
> bell., bov.[3], bry.[3], calc-sil.[1'],
> camph.[3], **canth.[3], CARB-AN.,**
> **carb-v., CARBN-S.,** caust.[3],
> cham.[3], cimic., cimx., cocc.,
> coloc.[3], con., cycl., daph., **dulc.,**
> euphr., **ferr.,** ferr-ar., **fl-ac.,**
> **GRAPH.,** guaj., **HEP.,** hyos.[3],
> ign.[3], iod.[3], ip.[3], kali-a.[11],
> kali-ar., kali-c., kali-p., **lach.,**
> led., **LYC.,** mag-c.[1, 7], mand.[9],
> med., **MERC., merl.,** mosch.[3],
> murx.[1'], nat-m.[3], **NIT-AC.,**
> **NUX-V.,** oci-s.[9], oena.[11], **PETR.,**
> **phos.,** plb.[3], podo.[1'], **psor.,**
> **PULS., pyrog.,** rheum[3], rhod.,
> **rhus-t.,** rob., sacch-l.[12], **sel.,**
> **SEP., SIL.,** sol-t-ae.[12], spig.,
> stann., **staph.,** stram.[3], **SULPH.,**
> syph.[1'], tarax., tax.[11], **tell.,**
> **THUJ.,** vario.[3, 7], **verat.,**
> wies.[12], zinc.[3]

morning/matin/morgens
> carb-v., dulc., merc-c., nux-v.

afternoon/après-midi/nach-
mittags
> **fl-ac.**

night/nuit/nachts
> ars., **CARB-AN.,** carb-v.,
> con., cycl., dulc., euphr.,
> **ferr.[2],** graph., **guaj.[2], lyc.[2],**
> mag-c., **MERC.,** nit-ac.,
> nux-v., puls.[16], rhus-t., **sep.[2],**
> spig., staph., **tell.,** thuj.

during sleep
pendant le sommeil
im Schlaf
> cycl.

midnight/minuit/Mitternacht
> mag-c., merl.

cough, after
toux, après la
Husten, nach
> hep., merl.

exertion, on
exercice physique, par
Anstrengung, bei
> nit-ac.

menses, during
menstruation, pendant la
Menses, während der
> stram.

motion, on
mouvement, au
Bewegung, bei
> eupi., mag-c.

on one side
unilatérale
auf einer Seite
> **BAR-C.**

onions, like[3]
oignons, d'
Zwiebeln, wie
> art-v.[3, 6], bov.[2, 3, 6, 7], **calc.[16],**
> lach., kali-p., **lyc.[2, 3, 6, 7, 16],** osm.,
> phos., sin-n., tell.

pickled herring, like[7]
hareng salé, de
Salzhering, wie
> vario.

pungent[2]
piquante
stechender
> **cop.,** gast.[11], **ip.,** rhus-t.[3], **sep.[2, 11],**
> sulph.[1'], thuj.[1']

putrid
pourri, de
fauliger
> **bapt., CARB-V.,** con., led.,
> **mag-c.[1, 7],** nux-v.[3], **PSOR.,** rhus-t.,
> sil.[3], **spig., STAPH.,** stram., verat.

rancid, at night
rance pendant la nuit
ranziger, nachts
  thuj.

rank
forte
starker
  art-v., **bov.**, cop., ferr., goss.,
  lac-c.², **lach.**, **lyc.**, **sep.**, **tell.**

during menses
pendant la menstruation
während der Menses
  stram., **tell.**

rhubarb, like[3, 7]
rhubarbe, de
Rhabarber, wie
  rheum

sickly
maladive
kränklicher
  chin., cinch.[11], thuj.

smoky
fume, de
rauchiger
  bell.

sour
acide
saurer
  acon., alco.[11], all-s.[11], **arn.**,
  ARS., ars-s-f.[1'], **asar.**, **bell.²**, ³,
  BRY., bufo³, calc., calc-s.,
  calc-sil.[1'], **carb-v.**, **carbn-s.**,
  caust., **cham.**, chel., chin.³,
  cimx., clem.⁷, **COLCH.**, **cupr.²**,
  ferr., ferr-ar., ferr-m., **fl-ac.¹**,
  gast.[11], **graph.**, **HEP.**, hyos.,
  ign., **IOD.**, **ip.**, iris¹, kali-c.,
  kalm.², lac-ac., **lach.²**, led.,
  LYC., **MAG-C.**, **MERC.**, nat-m.,
  nat-p., **NIT-AC.**, **nux-v.**, pilo.[11],
  PSOR., puls., **rheum**, **rhus-t.**,
  ruta², samb.², **SEP.**, **SIL.**, spig.³,
  staph.³, sul-ac., sul-i.[1'], **SULPH.**,
  sumb., tarent., tep.[11], **thuj.**,
  VERAT., zinc.

morning/matin/morgens
  bry., **carb-v.**, **iod.**, lyc., nat-m.,
  rhus-t., sep.[16], **sul-ac.**, **SULPH.**

forenoon/matinée/vormittags
  sulph.

afternoon/après-midi/nach-
  mittags
  fl-ac.

night/nuit/nachts
  arn., ars., asar.², bry.,
  carbn-s., **caust.**, cop.[11],
  graph., **HEP.**, iod., **kali-c.²**, [16],
  lyc., mag-c., **MERC.²**, nat-m.,
  nit-ac., **phyt.²**, plect.[11], **sep.**,
  sil.[16], **sulph.**, **thuj.**, **zinc.**[16]

during sleep
pendant le sommeil
im Schlaf
  bry.

sour-sweet
aigre-douce
süß-saurer
  bry.[3, 7], **PULS.**[2, 3, 7]

spicy
épice, d'
gewürziger
  rhod.

sulphur, like/de/wie
  phos., **sulph.**[11]

sulfuricum acidum, like³/comme/
  wie
  plb., **staph.**, sulph.

sweetish
douceâtre
süßlicher
  apis, **ars.²**, **calad.**, merc., puls.,
  sep.², thuj., **uran-n.²**

urine, like
urine, d'
Urin, wie
  berb., bov.⁷, **CANTH.**,
  card-m.³, caust., coloc., ery-a.,

graph.[3, 7], lyc.[3, 7], nat-m.[3],
NIT-AC., plb.[3], rhus-t.[3], sec.[3],
thyr.[3], urt-u.[3]

horse's
cheval, de
Pferde-Urin
NIT-AC., nux-v.[2]

vinous[3]
vin, de
Wein, wie
sec.

oily
huileuse
öliger
agar., arg-m., arn.[3], **ars.**[2],
aur.[2, 3, 6], **BRY.,** bufo, calc.,
CHIN., fl-ac.[3], lyc.[7], **MAG-C.,**
med.[3], **MERC., nat-m.**[2, 3], nux-v.,
ol-j.[11], petr.[3], plb.[2, 3], **psor.**[2],
rhus-t.[3], **rob., sel., STRAM.,**
sumb., **THUJ.,** thyr.[3]

daytime/pendant la journée/tags-
über
bry.

morning/matin/morgens
bry., chin.

night/nuit/nachts
agar.[2], bry., croc., mag-c.[16],
MERC.

periodical at the same hour[16]
périodique à la même heure
periodisch zur selben Stunde
ant-c.

single parts, of:
certaines parties, de:
einzelner Teile:
affected parts, on
affectées, de parties
erkrankter Teile
AMBR., ANT-T., anthraco.[4],
ars., asar.[6], bry., calc.[3, 6],
caust., chin.[6], **cocc., coff.,** fl-ac.,
guaj.[6], hell.[6], kali-c.[3], lyc.[3],
MERC., nat-c., nit-ac., nux-v.,
petr.[6], puls.[6], **RHUS-T., sep.,**

sil., **stann.,** stram., stront-c.,
thuj.[6]

morning/matin/morgens
ambr.

all parts except the head
partout excepté la tête
allgemein außer am Kopf
bell.[1, 7], merc., mur-ac.[16], nux-v.,
RHUS-T., SAMB., sec.[2, 7], sep.,
THUJ.[1, 7]

feet[16]
les pieds
an den Füßen
chin., phos.

legs[16]
les jambes
an den Unterschenkeln
lyc.

lower limbs[16]
les jambes
an den Beinen
lyc.

thights[16]
les cuisses
an den Oberschenkeln
lyc.

back part of body, on[3]
postérieure du corps, de
Körperrückseite, der
ars., calc., caust., **CHIN.**[2, 3], **dulc.,**
ferr., guaj., lach., led., mang.,
mosch., **mur-ac.,** nat-c., **nux-v.,**
par., petr., **ph-ac., puls.**[2, 3], sabin.,
SEP.[2, 3, 8], sil.[2], **stann.,** stram.,
SULPH.[2, 3]

covered parts, on
couvertes, des parties
bedeckter Teile
ACON., BELL., cham., CHIN.,
ferr., led., lyc.[3], **nit-ac.,** nux-v.,
puls., sec., spig., **thuj.**

night/nuit/nachts
bell., **CHAM., CHIN., ferr.,
nit-ac.,** nux-v., sec., **thuj.**

front of body, on
antérieures, des parties
Körpervorderseite, der
agar., ambr.[3], anac.[3], **ARG-M.,**
arn., **asar.**[3], **bell.**[2, 3], **bov.**[2, 3], **calc.,**
canth., cina[3], **COCC.,** dros.[3],
euphr.[2, 3], **graph.,** ip.[3], kali-n.,
laur.[3], merc., merc-c.[3], nat-m.[3],
nux-v., **PHOS.,** plb.[3], rheum[3],
rhus-t.[2], ruta[3], sabad.[3], sec.[3], **SEL.,**
sep.[2], staph.[3]

head, only on the
tête seulement, de la
Kopf, nur am
acon., am-m.[3], **bell.**[3], **calc.,** cham.,
kali-m.[3], phos., **puls.,** rheum[3],
sabad., sanic.[3], sep., **sil.,** spig.,
stann.

left side, on
partie gauche, de la
linken Seite, der
ambr.[3, 6], anac.[3, 7], **BAR-C.,** chin.,
fl-ac., jab.[2], kali-c.[3], phos., **PULS.,**
rhus-t., spig.[3], stann.[3], sulph.

lain on
couché, de la partie sur laquelle
on est
unten liegenden Seite, der
acon., bry., **bell., CHIN.,
NIT-AC.,** nux-v., puls., **sanic.**

one-sided
côté, d'un
einseitige
acon., alum.[3, 7], **ambr.,** anac.[3, 7],
ant-t.[7], arn.[7], aur-m-n., **bar-c.,**
bell., **bry.,** carb-v.[3], **caust.**[3, 7],
cham., **chin., cocc.**[2, 3], fl-ac., ign.[3],
jab.[8], lyc., merc., merl., nux-m.,
NUX-V., PETR., phos., **PULS.,**
ran-b., rheum[3], rhus-t., **sabad.**[2],
sabin., **spig.**[2, 3], stann.[3], stram.,
sulph., THUJ.

lower part of body, on
moitié inférieure du corps, de la
Unterkörpers, des
am-c., am-m., apis, ars., asaf.[3],
aur.[3], bry.[3], calc.[3], cinnb., **cocc.**[2],
coloc., con.[3], **CROC.,** cycl., dros.[3],
euph., ferr.[2], **hyos., iod.**[2], kali-n.[3],
mang., merc., nit-ac., nux-v.[3],
phos.[3, 6, 7, 15], ran-a.[8], sanic.[8],
sep., sil.[3], thuj., **zinc.**[2, 3]

not lain on
n'est pas couché, sur laquelle on
oben liegenden Seite, der
ben., thuj.

right side, on
partie droite, de la
rechten Seite, der
aur-m-n., bell., bry., fl-ac.[3], jab.[2],
merl., nux-v., **phos., puls.,** ran-b.,
sabin.

uncovered parts, on
découvertes, des parties
unbedeckter Teile
bell.[7], puls., **thuj.**

night, except the head
nuit excepté la tête
nachts außer am Kopf
thuj.

upper part of body, on
moitié supérieure du corps, de la
Oberkörpers, des
acon.[3], agar.[3], **anac.**[2, 3], **ant-t.**[2, 3],
arg-m., arn.[3], **ASAR.,** aza.[8],
bar-c.[3], bell.[3], berb., **bov.**[2, 3],
calc.[7, 8], camph., canth.[3], **caps.**[2],
carb-v., caust.[3], **cham.,** chin.,
cina, coc-c.[3], dulc., dig.,
eup-per., euphr.[3], fl-ac.,
graph.[3], **guaj.**[2, 3], **ign.**[2], ip.,
KALI-C., laur., mag-c.[3],
mag-m.[3], mag-s.[4], merc-c.[3],
mosch.[3], mur-ac.[3], nat-c.[3],
nit-ac., nux-v., **OP., PAR.,**
petr.[3], ph-ac.[3], phos.[3], plb.[3],
puls.[3], **ran-s.**[2], **rheum,** rhus-t.[3],
ruta[2, 3], sabad.[3], **samb.**[2], **sars.**[2],
sec., sel.[3], sep., sil., spig.,

stann.[2], sul-ac., thuj., tub.[3], valer., verat.

before sleep
avant le sommeil
vor dem Schlaf
  berb.

spots, in[3]
localisée, par places
stellenweise
  merc., ptel., tell.

salty[3, 7, 14]
salée
salziger
  nat-m.[3], **sel.**

staining the linen
tache, colore le linge
färbt die Wäsche
  arn.[2, 3, 7], ars., bar-c., bar-m.,
  BELL., benz-ac.[7], **calc.**[2, 3, 7],
  carb-an., carl.[7], cham.[3, 7], chin.,
  clem.[3, 7], dulc.[3, 7], **graph.**, lac-c.[7],
  LACH., lyc.[2, 3, 7], mag-c., med.[15],
  merc.[1, 7], nux-m.[3], **nux-v.**[2, 3, 7],
  rheum, **sel.**[1, 7]

bloody
sang, coleur
blutig
  anag.[7], **arn.**[7], ars.[7], calc.,
  cann-i.[7], **cham.**[7], chin.[7],
  clem.[1, 7], cocc.[7], crot-h., **cur.**,
  dulc.[7], hell.[7], **LACH.,** lyc.[1, 7],
  merc.[7], **NUX-M.,** nux-v.[7],
  phos.[7], **sel.**[7]

  night/nuit/nachts agg.[7]
  cur.

blue[7]
bleu, en
blau
  indg., iod., kali-i.

brown[15]
brun, en
braun
  iod., nit-ac., sep., wies.[7, 11]

brownish-yellow
jaune-brun, en
braun-gelb
  ars., **bell.**[1, 7], carb-an., graph.[3],
  lac-c.[7], **lach.**[2, 3, 7], mag-c.[3],
  sel.[2, 3, 7], thuj.[2, 3, 7]

dark[7]
foncé
dunkel
  bell.

difficult to wash off
difficile à laver
schwer auszuwaschen
  lac-d.[2, 7], **mag-c.**[1, 7], **merc.**

green
vert, en
grün
  agar.[3], cupr.

red
rouge, en
rot
  arn.[1, 7], **calc.**[2, 7], **carb-v.**, cham.[2, 7],
  chin.[2, 7], clem.[2, 7], **crot-h.**[3, 7],
  dulc.[1, 7], ferr.[7], gast.[2, 7, 11], **LACH.,**
  lyc.[2, 7], **NUX-M., nux-v.**[1, 7], thuj.

yellow
jaune, en
gelb
  ars., **bell.**, ben-n.[11], bry., cadm-s.,
  CARB-AN., carl.[11], **chin.**, chin-ar.,
  crot-c., ferr., ferr-ar., **GRAPH.,**
  guat.[9], hep.[3], **ip.**[1, 7], lac-c.[7], lac-d.,
  LACH., mag-c., MERC.,
  rheum[2, 3, 6, 7, 11], **SEL., thuj.,** tub.,
  verat.[2, 3, 7]

white[2, 3]
blanc, en
weiß
  sel.

stiffening the linen
empèse le linge
steif, macht die Wäsche
  MERC.[1, 7], nat-m.[3], sel.

suppression of, complaints from*
supprimée, troubles à la suite de
unterdrücktem Schw., Beschwerden
infolge von
acon., am-c., anthraci., apis,
arn., **ars., aspar.**[2], atro.[11],
aur-m-n.[2], **BELL.,** bell-p.[8], **BRY.**[1],
cadm-s., **caj.**[2, 12], **CALC.,**
CALC-S., calc-sil.[1'], cann-s.,
carb-v., carbn-s., cary.[11], caust.[3],
CHAM., CHIN., clem., coff.,
COLCH., coloc., cupr., **DULC.,**
eup-per., ferr., ferr-p.[12], **graph.,**
hep., hyos., iod., ip., kali-ar.,
KALI-C.[1], kali-sil.[1'], lach.[3], led.,
lyc., mag-c., **merc.,** mill.[6], nat-c.,
nat-m., nat-s., nit-ac., **NUX-M.**[1],
nux-v., olnd., op., ph-ac., **phos.,**
plat., **plb., PSOR.,** puls., **RHUS-T.,**
sabad., sec., sel., senec.[6], seneg.,
SEP., SIL., spong., squil., staph.,
STRAM., SULPH., teucr., thuj.[3],
verat.[3], verb., viol-o.

paralysis–perspiration/
  paralysie–transpiration/
  Lähmung–Schweiß

foot, of*
pieds, des
Fußschweiß
am-c., apis, ars., bad., **BAR-C.,**
bar-m., bar-s.[1'], cham., coch.,
colch., **cupr., form.,** graph., haem.,
kali-c., lyc., merc., nat-c., **nat-m.,**
nit-ac., ol-an.[3, 12], ph-ac., phos.,
plb., psor.[8], **puls.,** rhus-t.,
sal-ac.[12], sanic.[8], sel., **SEP., SIL.,**
sulph. **thuj., ZINC.,** zinc-p.[1']

warm
chaude
warme
acon., ant-c., asar., ben., camph.,
carb-v., cham., cocc., dig.[4], dros.,
ign., kali-c., kreos.[4], lach., led.,
nat-m., nux-v., op., phos., puls.[4],
sep., sil.[4], staph., stram., thuj.[4, 16],
verat.[4]

morning[4]/matin/morgens
carb-v.

every other morning[4]
tous les 2 jours le matin
jeden 2. Morgen
ant-c.

evening[4]/soir/abends
anac., puls.

night[4]/nuit/nachts
staph., thuj.

causing uneasiness
provoquant de l'inconfort
verursacht Unbehagen
CALC., cham., nux-v., **puls.,**
SEP., sulph.

convulsions with[4]
convulsions avec
Konvulsionen mit
sil.

epilepsy, after[15]
épilepsie, après les crises d'
epileptischen Anfällen, nach
sil.

sitting, in[4]
assis, étant
Sitzen, beim
asar.

somnolence with[4]
somnolence avec
Schlafsucht mit
op.

waking, am. on[4]
réveil, am. au
Erwachen, am beim
thuj.

wash off, difficult to
lavage, difficile à enlever par
abzuwaschen, schwer
lac-d.[2], **mag-c., merc.,** sep.[15]

PINCHING am.[3]
PINCEMENT am.
KNEIFEN am.
apis, ars., pip-n.

pressure – hard/pression – dure/
  Druck – harter

PLAYING piano*
JOUER du piano, troubles par
KLAVIERSPIEL, Beschwerden durch
anac., calc., cham.[7], kali-c., **nat-c.,**
phos.[1, 7], **sep.,** zinc.

weariness – playing/fatigué – jouer/
Müdigkeit – Klavierspiel

PLETHORA
PLÉTHORE
BLUTÜBERFÜLLE
acon., aesc.[1'], aloe[1', 3, 6], alum.,
am-c., am-m.[3], ambr., ant-t.[3], apis[3],
arn., ars., AUR., aur-ar.[1'], aur-i.[1'],
aur-s.[1'], **bar-c.,** bar-i.[1'], **BELL.,**
bov., brom.[1'], **BRY., CALC.,** canth.,
caps.[3], **carb-an., carb-v., carbn-s.,**
caust., cham., chel., **chin.,** clem.,
cocc., coloc., con., **croc.,** cupr., dig.,
digin.[11], dulc., **ferr.,** ferr-ar.,
ferr-i.[2, 11, 12], ferr-p., glon.[1', 12],
graph., guaj., hep., **HYOS.,** ign.,
iod., ip., **KALI-BI., kali-c.,** kali-n.,
lach., led., **LYC.,** mag-m., **merc.,**
mosch., nat-c., **NAT-M.,** nit-ac.,
nux-v., op., perh.[14], petr., **ph-ac.,**
PHOS., puls., rauw.[14], rhod., **rhus-t.,**
sabin., sacch.[11], sars., sec., sel.,
seneg., **SEP., SIL.,** spig., spong.,
stann., staph., **stram., stront-c.,**
sul-i.[1'], **SULPH., thuj.,** tus-fr.[12],
valer., verat., zinc.

plethoric constitution[2]
constitutions pléthoriques
plethorische Konstitution
ACON., aur., BELL., bry.[1'], cact.[2, 7],
calc., glon., nux-v., op., ruta,
seneg., **verat-v.**

portal stasis, pylestasis[2]
stase portale
Pfortaderstauung
aesc., aesc-g.[8], asaf., apoc., card-m.,
cimx., ham.[1'], **kali-m., NUX-V.,**
SULPH.[2, 12]

PLUG externally, sensation of
CHEVILLE extérieure, d'un bouchon
sensation d'une
PFLOCKES, äußerlich Gefühl eines
agar., ang.[3], arn., bufo[3], coloc.[3],
crot-t., hell., hyper.[3], **kali-bi.,** lach.,
plat., ruta

internally
intérieure
innerlich
acon., **agar., ALOE,** am-br., am-c.,
ambr., **anac., ant-c.,** apoc.[3, 6],
arg-m., arg-n.[3], **arn., asaf.,** aur.,
bar-c., bell., bov., bufo[3], calc.,
caust., cham., chel., cimic.[3],
coc-c., cocc., coff., con., croc.,
dros., ferr., graph., hell., **hep., IGN.,**
iod., **kali-bi.[3, 6],** kali-c., kreos.,
lach., led., lith-c.[3], lyc., merc., mez.,
mosch.[3], mur-ac., nat-m., **nux-v.,**
olnd., par., plat., plb., ran-s., rat.[3],
rhod., **ruta,** sabad., sabin., sang.,
sep., spig., **spong.,** staph., **sul-ac.[3, 4],**
sulph., THUJ.

POLYPUS
POLYPES
POLYPEN
all-c.[7, 8], alum.[3, 6], alumn.[12], ambr.,
ant-c., **aur.,** bell., berb.[12], cadm-s.[3, 6],
CALC., calc-i.[3, 6], **CALC-P.,** calc-s.,
carb-an., caust., coc-c.[3], **CON.,**
form.[3, 6, 8], graph., **hep., kali-bi.[3, 6, 8, 12],**
kali-i.[3, 6, 8], kali-m.[6], kali-n.[6, 12],
kali-s.[6, 12], lem-m.[8, 12], **lyc.,** med.[3, 12],
merc., merc-i-r.[6], **mez.,** nat-m., nit-ac.,
petr., ph-ac., **PHOS., psor.[3, 6, 8, 12],**
puls., sang., **sang-n.[8, 12],** sep., **sil.,**
STAPH., sul-ac., sulph., **TEUCR.,**
thuj.

POUNDING, foreign hammering side
  lain on[16]
PILONNAGE, martèlement extérieur
  du côté sur lequel on est couché
SCHLAGEN, fremdartiges Hämmern
  der aufliegenden Seite
  clem.

PRESSURE agg.
PRESSION agg.
DRUCK agg.
  acon., **AGAR.,** alum., alum-sil.[1]',
  am-br.[1], am-c., am-m., ambr.,
  anac., **ang.**[2, 3], ant-c., **APIS,**
  aq-mar.[14], **arg-m.,** arg-n.[3], arn., **ars.,**
  ars-i., asaf., bapt., **BAR-C.,** bar-i.[1]',
  bar-m., bar-s.[1]', bell., bism., bor.,
  bov., **bry.,** cact., **calad.,** calc.,
  calc-p., camph., **cann-s., canth.,**
  caps., carb-an., **carb-v.,** carbn-s.,
  card-m., caust., cench.[8], **chel.,** chin.,
  cimic.[14], **CINA,** coc-c., cocc., coloc.,
  cortiso.[14], crot-t., culx.[1]', cupr., dig.,
  dros., dulc., equis.[8], ferr.[3], fl-ac.[3],
  guaj., hecla[14], hell., **HEP.,** hyos.,
  ign., **IOD.,** ip., **kali-bi., kali-c.,**
  kali-i., kali-n., kali-p., kali-sil.[1]',
  LACH., laur., led., **LIL-T., LYC.,**
  mag-c., mag-m., mang., meny.,
  merc., MERC-C., mez., **mosch.,**
  mur-ac., nat-ar., nat-c., **nat-m.,**
  nat-s., nit-ac., nux-m., **nux-v., olnd.,**
  onos.[8], **op.,** ovi-p.[8], ox-ac., ph-ac.,
  phos., phyt.[3, 8], **plat.,** psor.[3], puls.,
  ran-b., ran-s., rhus-t., **ruta,** sabad.,
  sabin., samb., sars., **sel.,** seneg.,
  sep., **SIL.,** spig., **spong., stann.,**
  staph., stram., stront-c., sul-ac.,
  sul-i.[1]', sulph., **teucr.,** thal.[14], **ther.**[8],
  thuj., **valer., verb.,** vib.[3], vip-a.[14],
  zinc.

  am.
    abies-c., acon., agar., **agn.,**
    alum., alum-p.[1]', alum-sil.[1]',
    alumn.[2], **am-c., am-m.,** ambr., anac.,
    ant-c., **apis,** arg-m., **arg-n.,** arn.,
    ars., **asaf.,** atra-r.[14], **aur.,** bar-m.[1]',
    bell., bell-p.[7, 14], bism., **bor.,** bov.,
    BRY., cact., cadm-met.[14], calc.,
    calc-f., camph., **canth., caps.**[8],

carb-ac., **carbn-s.,** cast.[3], caust.,
chel., CHIN., cina, cinnb., **clem.,**
cocc.[2, 3], **COLOC., CON., croc.,**
crot-t., cupr-a.[8], cupr-ar.[3], dig.,
dios., **DROS., dulc.,** esp-g.[13], euon.[8],
form., **glon., graph.,** guaj., hell.,
hip-ac.[14], hist.[10, 14], ign., indg.[4, 8],
ip., **kali-bi.,** kali-c., **kali-i.,** kali-p.,
kreos., **lac-d.**[1', 7], **lach.,** laur., led.,
LIL-T., mag-c., **MAG-M., MAG-P.,**
mang., med.[7], **MENY.,** merc., mez.,
mosch., **mur-ac., NAT-C.,** nat-f.[10, 14],
nat-m., nat-p., **nat-s.,** nat-sil.[1]',
nit-ac., nux-m., nux-v., olnd., **par.,**
ph-ac., phos., pic-ac.[8], **PLB., PULS.,**
rad-br.[8], **rhus-t.,** ruta, sabad., sabin.,
sang., **sep., SIL., spig.,** stann.,
sul-ac., sulfonam.[14], sulph., thuj.,
tril., verat., verb., vip-a.[14], zinc.

hard edge am., over a[3]
rebord dur am., sur un
scharfe Kante am., über eine
  bell., **chin., COLOC.,** con., ign.,
  lach., samb., sang., stann., zinc.

hard p. agg.[3]
forte agg.
harter D. agg.
  pip-n., spig., tell.

  am.[3]
    achy.[14], arg-n., arn., coloc.,
    culx.[1]', ign.[1]', mag-m.[14], plb.,
    rauw.[14], sep.[1]', stann.[14]

painless side agg., on
indolore agg., sur le côté
schmerzlose Seite agg., auf die
  ambr., arn., bell., **BRY.,** calc.,
  cann-s., carb-an., carb-v., **caust.,**
  cham., coloc., fl-ac.[3], **IGN., kali-c.,**
  lyc., nux-v., **PULS., rhus-t., sep.,**
  stann., viol-o., **viol-t.**

slight p. agg., hard p. am.[3]
légère agg., forte am.
leichter D. agg., harter D. am.
  aloe, bell., **cast.**[3], caust., **CHIN.,**
  culx.[1]', ign., kali-c., lac-c.[1]',

lach.[1',3,10], **mag-p., nux-v.,** plb., sulph.

rubbing – am., gentle/frottement – am., toucher légèrement/ Reiben – am., leises Streicheln

PRICKLING externally
PICOTEMENTS externes
PRICKELN, äußerliches
abrot.[3], acon., agar., **ail.,** alum., ant-c., ant-t., **apis**[2,3,11], arn.[2], ars.[3,11], arum-t.[1'], bar-c.[3], bell., bor.[3], brom.[11], bry.[3], calc., cann-i., cann-s., caps., carbn-s., carl.[11], caust., chin.[11], cimic., coloc., con., croc., **crot-c.,** crot-h.[3], delphin.[11], **dros.,** elaps[11], ferr-m.[11], ferr-ma.[4], glon., grat.[4], ham.[3], hep., hydr-ac.[11], hyos.[11], ign.[3], ip.[2], kali-bi.[3], kali-br., kali-p.[3], laur., linu-c.[11], **lob.,** lyc., med., **mez.,** mosch., nat-m.[3], **nit-ac.[3]**, **nux-m.,** nux-v.[3], onos., **phos.[2]**, **PLAT., RAN-S.,** rhod.[3], rhus-t.[3], ruta, sabad., **sec.,** sep., sil.[3], spira.[11], staph., stram.[11], sul-ac., sulph., symph.[3], tarent.[2,3], tep.[11], thuj.[4], urt-u.[3], verat.[3,11], verat-v.[3], xan.[2], zinc.

internally
internes
innerliches
abrot., acon., **ail.,** arum-t.[1'], aur., cann-s., dios., lach., **NIT-AC., osm.,** ph-ac., **phos.,** plat., **ran-b., sabad., sang.,** sec., seneg., verb.[1], viol-o.

PSORA[7]
acon., adlu.[14], aesc., **agar.[3,6,7,16]**, alco.[11], aln.[12], alum.[3,6,7,16], alumn.[1'], ambr.[3,7], am-c.[3,6,7,16], am-m.[3,6,7,16], amyg.[3,7], anac.[3,7,16], ang., anh.[14], **ant-c.[3,6,7,16]**, ant-t.[3,7], apis[3,7,16], aran.[14], arg-m.[7,16], arg-n.[3,6,7], arn.[3,7], ars.[3,6,7], **ars-i.[2,7]**, ars-s-f.[1'], asaf.[3,6,7], asar.[3,7], astra-e.[14], aur.[3,6,7,16], aur-m.[3,7], bac.[12], **bar-c.[3,6,7,16]**, bell.[3,7,16], berb., berb-a.[14], beryl.[14], bism., bor.[3,6,7,16], bor-ac.[16], bov.[3,6,7], bry.[3,7], bufo, buni-o.[14], **calc.[2,3,6,7,16]**,

calc-ac.[3,7], calc-f.[14], **calc-p.[6,7,16]**, calc-s.[3,7], camph.[3,7], cann-s.[3,7], canth.[3,7], caps.[3,7], **carb-an.[3,6,7,16]**, **carb-v.[3,6,7,12]**, caust.[3,6,7,12,16], cham.[3,7], chel.[3,7], chin.[3,7], cic.[3,7,14], cina[3,7], cinnb.[7], clem.[3,6,7,16], coc-c.[7], coca, cocc.[3,7], coff., colch.[3,7,14], coloc.[3,6,7,16], con.[3,6,7,16], cortiso.[14], croc.[3,7], **cupr.[3,6,7,16]**, cycl.[3,7], cyna.[14], daph., des-ac.[14], dig.[3,6,7], dros., dulc.[3,6,7,16], euph.[3,6,7,16], euph-cy., euph-l., euphr., ferr.[3,7], ferr-ar.[1'], ferr-ma., ferr-p., fl-ac., flav.[14], galph.[14], graph.[2,3,6,7,16], guaj.[3,6,7,16], guat.[14], halo.[14], ham., harp.[14], hell., helon., **hep.[2,3,6,7,16]**, hip-ac.[14], hir.[14], hist.[14], hydr., hydr-ac., hyos., hypoth.[14], iber.[14], ign., iod.[3,6,7,16], ip., kali-ar.[1'], kali-bi.[6,7,11], **kali-c.[3,6,7,16]**, kali-i., kali-n.[3,6,7,16], kali-p., kreos.[2], kres.[14], lac-c., lac-d., lach., laur., led., levo.[14], lil-t., lob., **lyc.[3,6,7,16]**, m-arct., m-aust., **mag-c.[3,6,7,16]**, **mag-m.[3,6,7,16]**, mag-s.[14], mand.[14], mang.[3,6,7,16], **merc.,** merc-c., mez.[3,6,7,16], mill., mim-p.[14], morph., mosch., mur-ac.[3,6,7,16], murx., **nat-c.[3,6,7,16]**, **nat-m.[3,6,7,16]**, nicc.[3,7], **nit-ac.[3,6,7,16]**, nux-v., oci-s.[14], okou.[14], **ol-j.[6,7,11]**, olnd.[6,7], onop.[14], op., orig., palo.[14], par., paraph.[14], ped.[12], perh.[14], pers.[14], **petr.[3,6,7,16]**, ph-ac.[3,6,7,16], phenob.[14], phos.[3,6,7,16], plat.[3,6,7,16], plb.[3,7], plb-a., plb-m., pneu.[14], podo., prot.[14], **PSOR.[2,3,6,7,12]**, puls., ran-b., rauw.[14], reser.[14], rheum, rhod.[3,7,16], rhus-t.[3,7], rib-ac.[14], rumx., ruta, sabad.[3,7], sabin., samb., saroth.[14], sarr., sars., sec., sel.[3,7], seneg.[3,7,16], **sil.[3,6,7,16]**, spig.[3,7], spong.[3,7], squil., stann.[3,6,7], staph., stram., stront-c.[3,7], sul-ac.[3,6,7,16], **SULPH.[2,3,6,7,12,16]**, tarax., tell.[14], teucr., thala.[14], thiop.[14], thuj., thyr.[14], trif-p., trios.[14], tub., tub-r.[14], ven-m.[14], verat., visc.[14], zinc.

PTOMAINE POISONING, ailments from[12]
PTOMAÏNES, troubles à la suite d'empoisonnement par
PTOMAINE, Beschwerden infolge von Vergiftung durch
    ars.[3], pyrog.

PUBERTY ailments in[3, 6] ✱
PUBERTÉ, troubles de la
PUBERTÄT, Beschwerden in der
    acon.[2, 12], agar.[3], **ant-c.**[3], apoc.[12],
    aur.[6, 12], bell.[3, 12], **calc.**[2, 6],
    calc-p.[3, 6, 12], caust., cimic.[3], croc.,
    cupr.[6], ferr., **ferr-p., GELS.**[2, 12],
    graph., guaj.[3], hell.[3], helon., ign.[12],
    iod., **jug-r.**[3, 6], kali-br.[3], **kali-c.,**
    lach.[3], mag-p.[12], mill.[12], **nat-m.,**
    ph-ac., **PHOS.,** plat., **PULS.**[3, 4, 6, 12],
    senec.[3], sep.[12], sil., stram.[12], ther.[4],
    verat.[12], viol-o.[3]

    girls, in[2]
    jeunes filles, chez les
    Mädchen, bei
        aur.[2, 12], **bar-c., bell., calc-p.**[1', 2, 12],
        ferr., fil., hyoth.[14], **LACH., phos.,**
        puls.

PULSATION, externally
PULSATIONS externes
PULSIEREN, äußerliches
    acet-ac.[1'], **acon.,** acon-s.[11], **aesc.,**
    agar., alum., alumn., am-c.,
    am-m., **ambr.,** ammc., anac.,
    ang.[3], **ant-t., arg-m., arg-n.,** arn.,
    ars., ars-i., ars-s-f.[1'], **asaf.,** asar.,
    aster.[3], **bar-c.,** bar-i.[1'], bar-m.,
    bar-s.[1'], **bell.,** benz-ac., berb.,
    bov., brom., bry., bufo[3], **cact.,**
    calad., **CALC.,** calc-i.[1'], **calc-p.,**
    calc-s., calc-sil.[1'], **cann-s.,** canth.,
    caps., carb-an., **carb-v., carbn-s.,**
    caust., cham., chel., chin., chin-ar.,
    chlol., chlor.[11], cina, clem., coc-c.,
    cocc., coff., **coloc., con.,** cop.,
    croc., cupr., dig., dros., dulc.,
    euph.[3], euphr., **FERR.,** ferr-ar.,
    FERR-I., ferr-p., **fl-ac.,** gamb.,
    gast.[11], gels., **GLON., GRAPH.,**
    guaj., hell., helo., hep., hyos.,

ign., iod., jab.[3], kali-ar., **kali-bi.,**
KALI-C., kali-m.[1'], kali-n.,
kali-p., **KALI-S.,** kali-sil.[1'], kiss.,
KREOS., LACH., laur., led.[1'],
lil-t., lyc., lyss., macro.[11], mag-c.,
mag-m., manc., mang., med.,
MELI., merc., mez., mosch.,
mur-ac., nat-ar., **nat-c., NAT-M.,**
nat-p., nat-s., nat-sil.[1'], **nit-ac.,**
nitro-o.[11], nux-m., **nux-v., OLND.,**
op., par., petr., ph-ac., **phos.,**
phys., phyt., **plat.,** plb., polyg-s.[3],
PULS., ran-b., rheum, **rhod.,**
rhus-t., **rumx., ruta, SABAD.,**
sabin., samb., sang., sars., sec.,
sel., seneg., **sep., sil.,** spig.,
spong., squil., stann., staph.,
still., stram., stront-c., stroph-h.[3],
sul-ac., sul-i.[1'], **SULPH., tarax.,**
teucr., **thuj.,** til., **urt-u.,** verat.,
zinc., zinc-p.[1']

morning, on waking
matin au réveil
morgens beim Erwachen
    bell.

14.30 h
    pall.

evening/soir/abends
    arn., **carb-an.,** caust., nat-m.,
    sep.

during rest
au repos
in Ruhe
    nat-m.

sleep, before going to[16]
s'endormir, avant de
Einschlafen, vor dem
    sil.

night/nuit/nachts
    am-m., **bry.,** cact., nat-m., **sil.,**
    sulph.

coughing, from
toux, par la
Husten, durch
    calc.

half awake, while
moitié éveillé, à
halbwachem Zustand, in
    sulph.

midnight/minuit/Mitternacht
    phys.

        after/après/nach 4 h
            iris, trios.[11]

air am., in open
air am., en plein
Freien am., im
    aur.

bed, in
lit, au
Bett, im
    arn., carb-an., caust., nat-m.,
    sep., upa.

coition, after[4]
coït, après le
Koitus, nach
    nat-c.

cough, during
toux, pendant la
Husten, bei
    calc.

dreams, after[4]
rêves, après des
Träumen, nach
    nit-ac.

eating, after
mangé, après avoir
Essen, nach dem
    arn., camph., **clem.,** lyc., **SEL.**

excitement agg.
excitation agg.
Erregung agg.
    ferr, kreos.

exertion, on
exercice, par
Anstrengung, bei
    ferr., iod.

after[16]/après/nach
    anac.

fever, during[11, 16]
fièvre, pendant la
Fieber, beim
    urt-u.[3], zinc.

haemorrhage from anus, after[16]
hémorrhagie anale, après
Analbluten, nach
    kali-c.

headache, during
maux de tête, pendant les
Kopfschmerzen, bei
    lach.

lying, while
couché, étant
Liegen, im
    calad., coloc.[16], **glon.,** sel.[3]

    on right side[1']
    sur le côté droit
    auf der rechten Seite
        arg-n.

menses, before
menstruation, avant la
Menses, vor den
    cupr., thuj.

motion agg.
mouvement agg.
Bewegung agg.
    ant-t., **graph., iod.**

    am.
        kreos., nat-m.

music agg.
musique agg.
Musik agg.
    kreos.

    Vol. I: *music/musique/Musik*

    plaintive/triste/traurige
        kreos.

pregnancy, during
grossesse, dans la
Schwangerschaft, in der
  kali-c.

rest, in[11]
repos, pendant le
Ruhe, in der
  kreos.

sitting, while
assis, étant
Sitzen, im
  anac.[16], eupi., phys., **sil.**

sleep, during
sommeil, pendant le
Schlaf, im
  aesc.[1'], nat-m., sulph.

speaking in company, while
parlant en société, en
Sprechen in Gesellschaft, beim
  , carb-v.

standing, while
debout, étant
Stehen, beim
  alum.

starting, on[11]
tressaillant, en
Auffahren, beim
  camph.

touches anything, when body
touche n'importe quoi, lorsque le
  corps
berührt, wenn der Körper irgend
  etwas
  glon.

tremulous
tremblotantes
zittriges.
  nat-c.

waking, on
réveil, au
Erwachen, beim
  bell.[2], ferr-i., **nat-m.**[2, 4], nit-ac.[4],
  sulph.[4]

walking, on
marchant, en
Gehen, beim
  dig., ferr.

in open air, after
en plein air, après une marche
im Freien, nach dem
  ambr.

wandering[3]
erratiques
wanderndes
  puls.

internally
internes
innerliches
  ACON., aesc.[6], aeth., agar., aloe,
  ALUM., alum-p.[1'], alum-sil.[1'], am-c.,
  am-m., ambr., **aml-ns.,** anac.,
  ang.[3, 11], ant-c., **ANT-T.,** apis[3],
  arg-m., **arg-n.,** arn., **ars., ars-i.,**
  asaf., asar., **atro.**[6], **aur.,** aur-ar.[1'],
  aur-i.[1'], aur-s.[1'], bar-c., bar-i.[1'],
  bar-m.[1'], bar-s.[1'], **bell.,** berb.[4], **bor.,**
  bov., **BRY., cact.,** calad., **CALC.,**
  calc-p., calc-sil.[1'], **camph., CANN-I.,**
  cann-s., canth., **caps.,** carb-an.,
  carb-v., carbn-s., caust., cedr.,
  cench.[1'], **cham.,** chel., chin.,
  chin-ar., chin-s.[4], **cic.,** clem.[4, 6, 16],
  COCC., coff., colch., **coloc., con.,**
  croc., crot-h., crot-t., cycl., **dig.,**
  dros., dulc., **FERR.,** ferr-ar.[1'],
  FERR-I., ferr-s.[6], gels., **GLON.,**
  graph., ham.[6], hell., hep., hyos.,
  ign., iod., ip., kali-ar.[1'], kali-bi.[3],
  kali-c., kali-i.[3], kali-m.[1'], kali-n.,
  kreos., lach., **laur.,** led., lil-t.[6], lyc.,
  mag-c., mag-m., mang., **MELI.,**
  merc., merc-c., mez., mosch., murx.,
  nat-c., **nat-m.,** nat-p., **nat-s.,**
  nat-sil.[1'], nit-ac., nux-m., **nux-v.,**
  ol-an.[4, 6], **olnd.,** op., par., petr.,
  ph-ac., PHOS., phys., phyt.[3],
  pic-ac., **plan., plat., plb., psor.,**
  PULS., pyrog.[6], ran-b., rheum,
  rhod., **rhus-t.,** ruta, **sabad.,** sabin.,
  sang., sars., sec., **SEL.,** seneg., **SEP.,**
  SIL., spig., spong., stann., **stram.,**
  stront-c.[6], sul-ac., sul-i.[1'], **sulph.,**

tab.[6], **thuj.**, verat., verat-v., verb.,
zinc., zinc-p.[1']

bones, in
os, dans les
Knochen, in
   asaf., calc., carb-v., lyc., **merc.,**
   nit-ac., phos., rhod., ruta, sabad.,
   sep., sil., **sulph.,** thuj.

glands, in
glandes, dans les
Drüsen, in
   am-m., arn., asaf., bell., bov., bry.,
   calc., caust., cham., clem., con.[3],
   kali-c., lach.[4], lyc., **MERC.,** nat-c.,
   nit-ac., **phos.,** rhod., **sabad.,** sep.,
   sil., sulph., thuj.

joints, in[3]
articulations, dans les
Gelenken, in
   am-m., arg-m., dros., led.[11],
   merc.[3, 11], mez., olnd., ph-ac., rhod.,
   rhus-t., **ruta,** sabad., spig., thuj.

upper part of body[16]
moitié supérieure du corps
Oberkörper, des
   nit-ac.

venous see venous pulsations

PULSE abnormal
POULS anormal
PULS, abnormer
   ACON., agar., agn., am-c., am-m.,
   ambr., ang.[3], ant-c., **ant-t.,** arg-m.,
   arg-n., arn., ARS., ARS-I., asaf.,
   asar., aur., bar-c., **BELL.,** bism.,
   bor., bov., **bry., CACT.**[3], calad.,
   calc., **camph.,** cann-s., canth., caps.,
   carb-an., **carb-v., carbn-s.,** caust.,
   cham., chel., **chin.,** chin-s.[3], cic.,
   cina, cocc., colch., coloc., **con.,**
   croc., **CUPR., DIG.,** dulc., ferr.,
   gels., glon., graph., guaj., hell.,
   hep., **HYOS.,** ign., **IOD.,** ip., **kali-c.,**
   kali-n., kalm.[3], **KREOS., LACH.,**
   laur., led., lyc., mang., **meli.**[3],
   meny., **merc.,** mez., mosch., mur-ac.,

nat-m., nit-ac., nux-m., nux-v.,
olnd., **OP.,** par., petr., **PH-AC.,**
PHOS., plat., plb., puls., ran-b.,
ran-s., rheum, rhod., **RHUS-T.,**
sabad., sabin., samb., sang.[3], **sec.,**
seneg., **sep., SIL.,** spig., spong.,
squil., stann., staph., **STRAM.,**
stront-c., sul-ac., **sulph.,** thuj.,
valer., **VERAT.,** viol-o., viol-t.,
zinc.

audible
hörbarer
   ant-t., **camph.**[3], con.[3], **dig.**[3], hell.[3],
   iod.[3], kali-c.[3], kreos.[3], merc.[3], op.[3],
   phos.[3], plb.[3], sep.[3], **SPIG.**[3], sulph.[3],
   thuj.[3]

bounding
bondissant
schnellender
   acon.[2], aether[11], alco.[11], ars., atro.[11],
   bell.[2, 7], benz-ac., camph., cann-i.,
   canth., chin-s., chlor.[11], colch.[2],
   corn-f.[11], dulc.[2], eup-per., **eup-pur.**[2],
   fago.[11], glon., iod., jatr.[11], kali-chl.,
   lil-t., naja, paro-i.[14], plan., raph.,
   trif-p.[11], visc.[11]

ascending stairs, on[16]
montant un escalier, en
Treppensteigen, beim
   petr.

walking, on[16]
marchant, en
Gehen, beim
   petr.

contracted
contracté
zusammengezogener
   acet-ac., acon., agar., ant-t., arn.,
   ars., **asaf.,** aster., bell., bism.,
   bor.[3, 16], calc., calth.[11], cann-i.,
   canth., chin.[3], cina, colch., crot-t.,
   cupr.[3], cupr-a.[11], hyos., iod., **kali-bi.,**
   kali-br.[2], kali-s.[11], kiss.[11], lach.[3],
   laur., merc-cy., morph.[11], nit-ac.,
   op., ox-ac., paeon.[11], petr., phos.,
   plb., russ.[11], **sec.,** spira.[11], squil.[11],

stann., stram.[11], stry.[11], sul-ac.,
tarent.[2], vip.[11], zinc., zinc-m.[11]

hard/dur/harter
spasmodic/spasmodique/
    spastischer
thready/filiforme/fadenförmiger
wiry/en fil de fer tendu/Drahtpuls

discordant with temperature
discordant avec la température
widersprechend dem Fieber
    lil-t.[8], **PYROG.**[3, 7, 8]

double, dicrotism
bigéminé, dicrotisme
Pulsus bigeminus, Dikrotie
    acon.[3, 11], agar., aml-ns.[3], amyg.[3],
    anan.[2], apis[3], apoc.[3, 11], bell., cycl.,
    ferr.[3], gels.[3], glon., iber.[3, 11],
    kali-c.[3, 7], **phos.,** pilo.[11], plb., rhod.[3],
    stram., zinc.[3], zinc-s.[11]

empty
vide
leerer
    alco.[11], camph., chin., ferr.[3], **lach.**[2],
    petr., **sec.**[2], **verat.**[2]

excited
excité
erregter
    ant-t., anth.[11], cyt-l.[11], dig.[3], iod.,
    nux-v., petr., plumbg.[11], sol-t-ae.[11]

febrile
fébrile
Fieberpuls
    acon., alum., alumn.[11], anthraco.[2, 11],
    ars., bell., bov., croc.[2], gins.[11],
    lac-ac., merc-c., mez., morph.[11],
    plb., sars., sec., **stram., sulph.**[2],
    thuj., vip.[11]

fluttering
battement d'ailes, comme un
flatternder
    apis, **arn., ars.,** cann-i.[1'], carb-ac.[11],
    cimic.[1'], coff.[1'], colch., **crot-h.,**
    dig.[1'], gels., gins.[11], juni.[11], **kali-bi.,**
    kali-n., morph.[11], **NUX-V.,** op.,
    ph-ac., **phos.,** ptel.[11], pyrog., sec.[1],

stann., stram., sul-h.[11], thea[11],
verat.[2], zinc., zinc-m.[11]

frequent, accelerated, elevated,
    exalted, fast, innumerable, rapid
fréquent, rapide, incomptable
frequenter, jagender, unzählbarer,
    schneller
    abies-n.[8], abrot.[11], acal.[7], **ACON.,**
    adon.[8], adren.[7, 8], aesc., **aeth.,**
    aether[11], **agar.,** agar-pa.[11],
    agar-se.[11], **agn.**[8], **ail.,** alco.[11],
    aloe, all-c., alum., alum-p.[1'],
    alum-sil.[1'], alumn.[2], am-be.[2],
    am-br.[11], am-c., am-m., am-val.[8],
    ambr., **aml-ns.**[2, 11], ammc.[2],
    amyg.[2, 11], anac., anan.[2], **ang.**[2, 3],
    ant-ar.[2, 8, 11], ant-c., ant-m.[2], **ant-t.,**
    anthraco.[2, 11], antip.[8], aphis[2, 11],
    APIS, apoc.[8], apom.[11], aq-pet.[11],
    arg-m., **arg-n., ARN., ARS.,**
    aran-ix.[14], **ars-h.**[2], **ARS-I.,**
    ars-s-f.[1', 2], arum-d.[2, 11], arum-i.[11],
    arum-t.[2], **arund.**[2], **asaf.,** asar.,
    asc-c.[2], asc-t.[11], asim.[2, 11], aster.,
    atro.[2, 11], **AUR.,** aur-ar.[1'], aur-i.[1'],
    aur-m., AUR-S.[1'], aza.[14], **bapt.,**
    bar-a.[11], bar-c., bar-i.[1'], bar-m.,
    BELL., benz-ac., ben-n.[11], **BERB.,**
    beryl.[9], bism., bor., both.[11], bov.,
    brom., **BRY.,** bux.[11], **cact.**[8], cain.[11],
    caj.[11], calad., calc., calc-ar.[1', 7],
    camph., cann-i., cann-s.[3], **canth.,**
    carb-ac.[2, 11], **CARB-AN.**[1', 3],
    carb-v., carbn-h.[11], carbn-o.[11],
    carbn-s.[1'], cary.[11], catal.[11], caust.,
    cedr., celt.[11], **cham.,** chel., **chim.**[2],
    chin., chin-ar., chin-b.[2], **chin-s.,**
    chlol.[2], chlor.[2], chloram.[14],
    chlorpr.[14], chr-ac.[2], cic.[11, 14],
    cimic.[1', 11], **cina,** cinch.[11], cinnb.[11],
    clem., coc-c., coca[2, 11], cocc.,
    coch.[2], cod.[11], coff., coff-t.[11],
    colch., COLL., coloc., **CON.,**
    conv.[8], convo-s.[9], cop.[2], corn.[2, 11],
    crat.[8], **CROC.**[2, 3], **CROT-C.,**
    crot-h.[1], crot-t., cub.[2, 11], cund.[11],
    CUPR., cupr-a.[11], cupr-ar.[2],
    cupr-n.[11], cupr-s.[2], cur.[7], cycl.,
    cyna.[14], cyt-l.[9, 14], daph.[2], dat-m.[11],
    DIG., digin.[11], diph.[8], dor.[2, 11],

dubo-m.[11], dulc.[11], **echi.**, equis.[11], erech.[11], erio.[11], ery-a.[11], eucal.[2, 11], euph., fago.[11], fagu.[11], **ferr.**, ferr-i., ferr-m.[11], **FERR-P.**, fl-ac., foll.[14], **form.**[2], gad.[11], gamb.[11], gast.[11], **GELS.**, gins.[11], **GLON.**, gran.[11], grat., guaj., guat.[9], gymno.[11], hall.[11], halo.[14], ham., hed.[14], **hell.**, hep., hipp., hippoz.[2], hist.[9], hoit.[14], hydr-ac.[11], hydrc.[11], **hyos.**, **hyper.**, **iber.**[2, 8, 11, 14], ign., **IOD.**, ip., iris[11], jab.[11], jatr.[11], jug-r.[11], kali-ar.[11], kali-bi., kali-br.[2], kali-c., kali-chl.[8, 11], kali-i., **kali-m.**[2], kali-n., kali-ox.[11], **kali-p.**[2], kalm.[8], keroso.[11], kreos., **lac-c.**[2], **lach.**, lapa.[11], lat-m.[8, 9, 14], **laur.**, **LED.**[2, 3, 8, 11], levo.[14], lil-s.[11], **lil-t.**[8], linu-c.[11], lipp.[11], lob., lyc., **lycps.**, lyss.[2], **mag-c.**[3], **mag-m.**[3], **manc.**, mang., med.[2], **meny.**[3], **MERC.**, merc-c., merc-cy., merc-d.[11], merc-i-f.[11], merc-pr-a.[11], merc-sul.[2], merl.[2], meth-ae-ae.[11], methys.[14], **mez.**, mill., mom-b.[11], **morph.**[8, 11], **mosch.**, **mur-ac.**, mygal.[2, 11], myric.[11], **naja**, narcot.[11], nat-ar., **nat-c.**, nat-f.[9, 14], **NAT-M.**, **nat-s.**, nicc., **nit-ac.**, nit-s-d.[11], nitro-o.[11], **nux-m.**, **NUX-V.**, oena.[11], **ol-j.**[2, 11], olnd., onos., **OP.**, osm., ox-ac., par., penic.[13, 14], petr., **PH-AC.**, phase.[8], phel., **PHOS.**, **phys.**, **phyt.**, pic-ac., pilo.[8, 11], **plat.**, plat-m.[11], **plb.**, plect.[11], podo., prun.[7], **psor.**[2], **ptel.**[2, 11], **puls.**, pyre-p.[11], **PYROG.**, ran-b., **ran-s.**, raph.[11], rham-f.[11], rheum, rhod., rhodi.[11], **RHUS-T.**, **rhus-v.**, ric.[11], **rumx.**[2], rumx-a.[11], **ruta**[3], sabad., sabin.[3], samb., **sang.**, santin.[11], sapin.[11], saroth.[9, 14], sarr.[2, 11], sars., scroph-n.[11], scut.[7], **SEC.**, **sel.**[3], seneg., **sep.**, ser-ang.[8], **SIL.**, sin-n.[11], sol-n.[11], sol-t-ae.[11], solin.[11], **SPIG.**, spig-m.[11], **spong.**, **STANN.**, staph., still.[2], **STRAM.**, **stront-c.**[3], stroph-h.[8], stry.[11], stry-p.[8], sul-ac., sul-h.[11], sulfa.[9], sulo-ac.[14], **SULPH.**, sumb.[11], **tab.**,

tanac.[11], tarax.[11], **TARENT.**[2, 7, 11], tax.[11], **tell.**, tep.[11], ter., **teucr.**[3], thal.[14], thea[8, 11], ther.[11], thiop.[14], thlas.[2], thuj., thymol.[9, 14], **thyr.**[3, 7, 8], til.[11], tox-th.[11], throm.[11], urt-u.[11], vac.[2, 11], **valer.**, vario.[2], **verat.**, **VERAT-V.**, vesp., viol-o.[2], **VIOL-T.**[2, 3, 11], vip.[11], vip-a.[14], visc.[9, 11, 14], wies.[11], xan.[11], **ZINC.**, zinc-m.[11], **ZINC-P.**[1'], zinc-s.[11]

daytime/pendant la journée/tags-über
nat-ar., nat-m.

morning/matin/morgens
agar., ail., **ars.**, **ars-met.**[2], asaf., atro.[11], **canth.**, cedr., chin., chin-s.[1] (non: chin-ar.), fago.[11], **graph.**, ign., **kali-c.**, merc-c., **mez.**[2], mit.[11], myric.[11], oena.[11], onop.[14], ox-ac., phos., phys., podo., sang., sulph., sumb.[11], ther.[11], thuj., upa.[11]

slow during the day and in the evening, but[3]
lent pendant la journée et le soir, mais
langsam tagsüber und abends, aber
AGAR., alum., **ARS.**, calc., canth., chin., graph., **ign.**[2, 3], **KALI-C.**, lyc., mez., nux-v., phos.

waking, on[11]
réveil, au
Erwachen, beim
alumn.

forenoon/matinée/vormittags
aphis[11], calc., chin., com.[11], lyc.[11], merc-sul.[11], mez., nat-p.[11], oena.[11], op., plan., ptel.[11], trom.[2]

noon[11]/midi/mittags
mit., oena., ox-ac.

afternoon/après-midi/nachmittags
agar.[2], bapt.[2], chel.[11], chin-s.[11],
chr-ac.[2], ferr-i.[11], gels.[11], gins.[11],
kali-chl.[11], kali-n.[16], lyc.,
merc-sul.[11], nat-m.[11], oena.[11],
phos.[11], phys.[11], phyt.[11], podo.[3],
ptel.[11], sumb.[11]

slow in the morning, but[3]
lent le matin, mais
langsam morgens, aber
KALI-N., thuj., zinc.

evening/soir/abends
acon., alum-sil.[1'], am-caust.[11],
anth.[11], anthraco.[2], aphis[2],
arg-m., arg-n., ars.[11], arum-i.[11],
aster.[11], atha.[11], bry.,
carb-an., CAUST., chin-s.[11],
cinnb., crot-h., dulc., euph.,
euphr.[11], ferr., gent-l.[11], ham.[11],
hell., hyper.[11], jug-r.[11], lach.,
lyc., mez., mill.[11], mur-ac.,
murx., nat-c., nat-sil.[1'], nux-v.,
oena.[11], olnd., ox-ac.[11], ph-ac.,
phos., plan., puls., ran-b.,
rheum[2], sars., sep., sil., sulph.,
sumb.[11], teucr.[11], thuj., tub.,
upa.[11], zinc.

in bed[16]
au lit
im Bett
sul-ac.

slow in the morning, but[3]
lent le matin, mais
langsam morgens, aber
arg-m., arn., asar., carb-an.,
caust., chin., kali-c., KALI-N.,
lyc., mez., OLND., petr., phos.,
puls., RAN-B., sars., sep.,
SPIG., teucr., THUJ., ZINC.

night[11]/nuit/nachts
alum-sil.[1'], anthraco., arum-i.,
aster., cinnb.[1'], con., nat-sil.[1'],
nux-v., plect., ptel.

slow by day, but[3]
lent pendant la journée, mais
langsam tagsüber, aber
am-c., bor., bry.[2, 3], calc.,
carb-an., dulc., hep., kali-n.,
mag-c., merc.[2, 3], mur-ac.,
nat-c., nat-m., phos., ran-s.,
sabin., SEP., sil., sulph.

midnight, after/minuit, après/
Mitternacht, nach
benz-ac., hyper.[11]

chill, during[11]
frissons, pendant les
Fieberfrost, während
chin-s., coloc., crot-t., gels., zinc.

convulsions, during[11]
convulsions, pendant les
Konvulsionen, bei
oena., op., stry.

drinking, after[16]
bu, après avoir
Trinken, nach dem
nat-m.

eating, after
mangé, après avoir
Essen, nach dem
arg-n., iod., LYC., mez.[11, 16],
nat-m.[16], nux-v., phos., puls.,
rhus-t., sulph.

excitement, from[2]
excitation, par
Erregung, durch
anthraco., bar-m., cain., con.[11],
digox.[11], merc.[11]

faster than the heart-beat
plus rapide que les pulsations
cardiaques
schneller als der Herzschlag
acon., arn., rhus-t., spig.

motion agg.
mouvement agg.
Bewegung agg.
  alum-sil.[1]', ant-t., **arn., bry., dig.,**
  digin.[11], fl-ac., **gels.,** glon.[11],
  graph., iod., lycps., NAT-M.,
  nux-v., petr., **phos.,** sep., staph.,
  stram.

noticing it, when
prête attention, lorsqu'on y
achtet, wenn man darauf
  arg-n.

rest, during
repos, pendant le
Ruhe, in der
  mag-m.

rising up, on
levant, en se
Aufstehen, beim
  bry., dig.

sitting, while
assis, étant
Sitzen, im
  aspar.[11], gins.[11], indg.[11], **mag-m.,**
  nat-m.[11], oena.[11]

standing, on[16]
debout, étant
Stehen, beim
  nat-m.

stool, after
selle, après la
Stuhlgang, nach
  agar., CON., glon.[11]

supper, after[16]
souper, après le
Abendessen, nach dem
  cupr.

thinking of past troubles
penser à ses troubles passés
Denken an vergangene Schwierig-
  keiten, beim
  sep.

urin, with copius[16]
polyurie, avec
Urinflut, mit
  dig.

vexation, after
contrariété, par
Ärger, nach
  acon., arg-n., **CHAM.,** coloc.,
  ign., **nat-m., nux-v., petr., SEP.,**
  staph.

warm applications, from
chaudes, par des applications
warme Umschläge, durch
  sulph.

and intermittent
et intermittent
und intermittierender
  acon., agar., aloe, alum., am-m.,
  ars., **aur.,** bell., benz-ac., bism.,
  cann-i., canth., chin., chin-s.,
  colch., cupr., **dig.,** gels., glon.,
  grat., hyos., ign., kali-chl., lob.,
  merc-c., merc-cy., mez., mur-ac.,
  nat-ar., nit-ac., nux-m., **nux-v.,**
  olnd., op., ox-ac., phos., phys.,
  plb., sep., stram., **sulph.,** tab.,
  verat-v., zinc.

and small
et petit
und kleiner
  ACON., aeth., alum., apis,
  arn., **ARS.,** ars-i.[1], asaf., **aur.,**
  aur-m., bell., benz-ac., bism.,
  bry., cain.[2], **camph.,** canth.,
  chin., cocc., colch., coloc.,
  con., crot-t., **dig.,** ferr-m.[2],
  fl-ac., gels., glon., grat., **hell.,**
  hyos., ign., **iod.,** kali-bi.,
  kali-chl., kali-n.[16], **lach.[1],**
  LAUR., led., lob., lyc., **lycps.,**
  merc-c., merc-cy., **mur-ac.,**
  nat-m., nit-ac., **nux-m.,**
  NUX-V., olnd., op., ox-ac.,
  petr., phos., phyt., pic-ac.,
  puls., ran-s., raph., rhod.,
  rhus-t., samb., **SIL.,** sol-t-ae.[11],
  staph., **STRAM.,** sul-ac., tab.,
  VERAT., zinc.

and irregular[7]
et irrégulier
und unregelmäßiger
visc.

strong and small
fort, petit et
kräftiger, kleiner und
acon., apis, arn., ars., bell., chin.,
crot-t., gels., hyos., merc-c.,
merc-cy., op., raph., stram.

full
plein
voller
acet-ac., **ACON.**, aesc., aether[11],
agar.[2], agar-pa.[11], alco.[11], **all-c.**,
aloe, **ALUM.**[3], alumn.[2], am-m.[8],
aml-ns.[2, 8], **amyg.**[2, 11], anan.[2],
ANT-T., anth.[11], antip.[8], apis,
apoc., aq-pet.[11], **arn.**, ars.,
ars-h.[2, 11], ars-i., ars-met.[2, 11],
arum-d.[2, 11], arum-t.[2], asaf., asar.,
asc-c.[2], asim.[11], atro.[2, 11], **aur.**[1', 3, 8],
bapt., bar-c., bar-i.[1'], bar-m.,
BELL., benz-ac., **BERB.**, bism.,
brom., **BRY.**, **cact.**[8], cain.[2, 11],
caj.[11], **CALC.**[3, 8], camph., **canth.**,
carb-ac.[11], carbn-o.[11], cedr.,
celt.[11], cent.[11], cham., **CHEL.**,
chin., chin-ar.[2], chin-s., chlf.[11],
chr-ac.[2, 11], cimic., coff., colch.,
coloc., con., cor-r., cori-r.[11],
crot-c.[11], crot-h., crot-t., cub.[2, 11],
cupr., cupr-a.[11], cupr-s.[2, 11], cycl.,
cyt-l.[11], daph., dat-f.[11], **DIG.**,
digin.[11], dirc.[11], dor.[11], **dulc.**,
eup-per., **eup-pur.**[2], fago[8, 11], ferr.,
ferr-p., gast.[11], **GELS.**, gins.[11],
glon., **GRAPH.**[3], ham., hell., **hep.**,
hydr-ac.[11], **HYOS.**, iber.[2, 11],
ictod.[8], **ign.**[1], iod., jab.[11], jug-r.[11],
juni.[11], kali-bi., **kali-c.**, kali-chl.,
kali-i., kali-m.[1', 2], **KALI-N.**,
kali-ox.[11], kreos.[3, 11], lac-ac.[11],
lach., laur., **led.**, **lil-t.**[8], linu-c.[11],
lipp.[11], lyc., menth.[11], **merc.**,
merc-c., merc-cy., merc-pr-a.[11],
merl.[2], **mez.**, mill., morph.[11],
mosch., mur-ac., myric.[11], **naja**,
nat-m., **nat-n.**[6], nit-ac., nitro-o.[11],
nux-v., ol-an.[11], olnd., onos.[8], **op.**,

ox-ac., par., **petr.**, **ph-ac.**, phel.,
phos., **phys.**[8, 11], phyt., pilo.[8, 11],
plan , plb., plect.[11], puls.[3, 8],
ran-b., ran-s., raph.[11], rat.[11],
rhus-t., sabad., **sabin.**, samb.,
sang., sarr., sars., scroph-n.[11],
sec.[3], seneg., **sep.**, **sel.**, sin-n.[2, 11],
sium[11], sol-n.[11], **spig.**, spira.[11],
spong., **STRAM.**, stront-c.,
sul-ac., **sulph.**, sumb.[11], **tab.**,
tanac.[11], tarax.[11], tarent., tell.,
tep.[11], thea[11], thuj., til.[11], toxi.[11],
trif-p.[11], trom.[11], valer., **verat.**,
verat-v., vinc.[11], viol-o., vip.[11],
visc.[11], yuc.[11], zinc., zing.[11]

morning/matin/morgens
canth.[2], jac-c.[11], phos., phyt.,
sep., zinc.

forenoon[11]/matinée/vormittags
nat-ar., trom.[2], zing.

afternoon/après-midi/nachmittags
iod., nat-ar.[11], phyt.[11], zinc.,
zing.[11]

evening/soir/abends
acon., anth.[11], anthraco.[2], hell.,
myric.[11], olnd., ran-b., scut.[11],
seneg., sulph., thuj., zinc., zing.[2]

night/nuit/nachts
com.[11], **merc.**, sep.[2]

hard
dur
harter
ACON., aesc., aether[11],
agar-cps.[11], agar-pa.[11], agro.[11],
alco.[11], **all-c.**, all-s.[2], am-c.,
am-caust.[11], am-m., **aml-ns.**[2],
ammc.[2], **amyg.**[2, 11], anan.[2], ant-c.,
ant-m.[2], **ant-t.**, apis[3], **arn.**, ars.,
ars-h.[2, 11], ars-i., ars-s-f.[2, 11],
arum-d.[2, 11], asaf., asar., aster.,
atro.[11], **bar-c.**, bar-i.[1'], bar-m.,
BELL., benz-ac., **BERB.**, bism.,
brom., **BRY.**, **cact.**, calad.,
calth.[11], camph., **canth.**,
carb-ac.[11], carbn-s.[11], cent.[11],

cham., **CHEL., chin.,** chlor.[11],
cimic., **cina,** clem.[3], cocc., coff.,
colch., coloc., con., cor-r.,
corn.[2, 11], crot-h.[11], **cupr., cupr-a.**[11],
cupr-s.[2, 11], cycl., cyna.[14], daph.,
dig., digin.[11], **dulc., ferr.,** gast.[11],
gels., glon., gran.[11], **GRAPH.**[3],
ham., hell., **hep., HYOS.,**
hyper.[2, 11], iber.[11], **ign.,** indg.[11],
iod., jatr.[11], kali-bi., **kali-c.,**
kali-i., kali-m.[1'], **kali-n., kreos.,**
lach., laur.[3], **led.,** lyc., **lycps.**[2],
merc., merc-c., merc-cy.,
merc-d.[11], **merc-pr-r.**[11], mez.,
morph.[11], **mosch.,** mur-ac.,
nat-c.[11], nat-m., **nit-ac.,** nit-s-d.[11],
nitro-o.[11], **nux-v.,** olnd., op.,
ox-ac., par., petr., ph-ac., phel.,
phos., phyt., plb., plect.[11],
plumbg.[11], puls.[3], ran-b., ran-s.,
rauw.[9], sabin., samb., sang.[2],
sec., seneg., **sep.,** serp.[11], **sil.,**
sin-a.[11], sol-m.[11], sol-t-ae.[11], spig.,
spira.[11], spong., squil., **STRAM.,**
STRONT-C.[2, 3], stroph-s.[9], **stry.**[11],
sul-h.[11], **sulph.,** tab., tanac.[11],
tarent. tep.[11], **ter.,** thuj.[11], til.[11],
uva[11], valer., verat., verat-v.,
vinc.[11], viol-o., vip.[11], wies.[11],
zinc., zinc-m.[11]

morning/matin/morgens
petr., phyt., zinc.

11 h[11]
zing.

noon/midi/mittags
ox-ac.

evening/soir/abends
all-c., **bapt.,** dulc., plb., plumbg.[11],
ran-b.[2], zing.[2]

climbing, after[9]
ascension, après
Steigen, nach
rauw.

excitement, with[9]
excitation, avec
Erregung, mit
stroph-s.

exertion, after sudden[9]
exercice soudain, après un
Anstrengung, nach plötzlicher
rauw.

old people, in[2]
âgées, chez les personnes
alten Menschen, bei
ANT-T.

slow, and[9]
lent, et
langsamer, und
stroph-s.

heavy
lourd
schwerer
crot-c.[11], phos., stram., **verat-v.**[2],
yuc.[11]

night[11]/nuit/nachts
com.

imperceptible
unfühlbarer
ACON., aeth.[15], agar.[11], agn.,
amyg.[2, 11], anil.[11], ant-t., **apis**[3],
arg-n.[2], arn.[3], **ars.,** ars-h.[2],
ars-s-f.[2], bell., benz-ac., **cact.,**
cadm-br.[11], **CAMPH.**[3, 11], cann-i.,
cann-s., **canth., carb-ac., CARB-V.,**
carbn-h.[11], chel., chin., chlor.[11],
cic. cic-m.[11], cit-l.[2, 11], **cocc.,**
COLCH., coloc., con.[2, 3, 16], crot-h.,
CUPR., cupr-ar.[11], cyt-l.[9, 11], digin.[11],
dulc., ferr., gins.[11], gels.[7], guaj.,
hell., **HYDR-AC.**[2, 3, 6, 11], hyos.,
ip., kali-cy.[11], kalm., kreos., lach.,
laur., **led.**[3], mand.[9], **merc.,** merc-c.,
morph.[11], **mosch.**[2, 3], **naja,** nux-v.,
oena.[11], **op.,** ox-ac., petr.[11], ph-ac.,
phos., **phyt.**[2], plb., plat., **podo.**[2],
puls., rhus-t., **sec., SIL.,** stann.,
stram., stry.[11], sul-ac., sulph., tab.,
tax.[11], **VERAT.,** zinc.

imperceptible, almost
impercetible, presque
kaum fühlbarer
    ACON., aeth.[15], agar.[16],
    agn.[11], am-c., aml-ns.[11],
    CAMPH., carbn-o.[11], chin.,
    chlor.[11], cic-m.[11], coff-t.[11], crot-h.,
    cyt-l.[9], dig., digin.[11], ferr., GELS.,
    glon., ham., hell., hydr-ac.[6, 11],
    hydrc.[11], ip., kali-bi., lach., laur.,
    mand.[9], mang., merc., merc-c.[11],
    morph.[11], naja, olnd., op., ox-ac.,
    ph-ac., phos., plb., podo., puls.,
    rhus-t., ric.[11], seneg., sol-n.[11],
    sol-t.[11], spong., stram., tab.,
    tere-ch.[14], thea[11], ther., verat.,
    vip.[11], zinc.

convulsions, during
convulsions, pendant les
Konvulsionen, bei
    nux-v., olnd.

stupor, during
stupeur, pendant la
Stupor, bei
    hep.

intermittent
intermittent
intermittierender
    acet-ac., acon., aeth., agar.,
    agar-pa.[11], aloe, alum.,
    am-c., am-m., amyg.[2], ang.,
    ant-t.[3, 11], apis, apoc.[3, 6, 8, 11],
    arg-n., arn.[2, 3, 6], ars., ars-h.[2],
    ars-i.[1'], ars-s-f.[1'], asaf., atro.[2],
    aur., bapt.[3, 6], bell., ben-n.[11],
    benz-ac., bism., brom., bry.,
    cact.[3, 6, 8], calth.[11], camph.,
    cann-i.[11], canth., caps., carb-ac.,
    carb-an.[11], carb-v., cedr., CHIN.,
    chin-s., chlol.[2], chlor.[11], cic-m.[11],
    cimx., cinnb.[11], coff., colch., con.,
    conv., crat.[6, 8], crot-h., cupr.,
    cupr-ac.[11], daph., DIG., digin.[11],
    digox.[11], fago.[11], ferr., ferr-m.[8],
    frag.[11], gast.[11], gels., glon., grat.,
    hep., hura[11], hydr-ac.[11], hyos.,
    iber.[6, 8, 14], ign., iod., jatr.[11],
    juni.[11], kali-bi., kali-c., kali-chl.,
    kali-i., kali-m.[1'], kali-p., kalm.,

keroso.[11], kreos.[2], lach., lapa.[11],
laur., lil-t., lipp.[11], lob., lycps.,
lyss.[2], mag-p.[3], meny.[3], MERC.,
merc-c.[1], merc-cy.[1], merc-sul.[11],
meth-ae-ae.[11], mez., morph.[11],
mur-ac., murx.[3], naja, nat-ar.,
NAT-M., nit-ac., nit-s-d.[2],
nitro-o.[11], nux-m., nux-v., olnd.,
op., ox-ac., PH-AC., phos.,
phys.[11], phyt., pip-n.[8], plan.[11],
plb., prun-v.[7], ptel.[2, 11], ran-s.[2],
rhus-t., sabin., samb., scut.[11],
SEC., sep., spig., staph.[3], stram.,
stroph-h.[6, 8], stry.[11], sul-ac.,
sulph., tab., tarent.[2], ter.[3, 6, 8],
thea, thuj., trif-p.[11], trom.[2, 11],
verat., VERAT-V.[1, 7], vip.[11], zinc.,
zinc-p.[1']

every other beat[3]
tous les 2 battements
jeden 2. Schlag
    nat-m., ph-ac., spig.[2]

third beat[2]
3 battements
3. Schlag
    apis[2, 3], arum-t.[3], ars-h.,
    cimic.[3, 7, 14], dig. [3,8], iber.,
    kali-c.[6], mur-ac.[1'-3, 6-8],
    nat-m.[2, 3, 6, 7, 15], nit-ac.[3, 6],
    phas.[15], sulph., vib.

third or fourth beat[3, 6]
3 ou 4 battements
3. oder 4. Schlag
    apis[15], cimic.

fourth beat[2, 3]
4 battements
4. Schlag
    apis[2], calc-ar.[1', 2, 7, 15],
    cimic.[3, 7, 14], dig.[3, 8], iber.,
    NIT-AC., nux-v., sulph.[2], tab.[3]

third or fifth beat[2, 6]
3 ou 5 battements
3. oder 5. Schlag
    crot-h.[6], nit-ac.

fourth or fifth beat[3, 6, 15]
4 ou 5 battements
4. oder 5. Schlag
  nux-v.

fifth beat[2]
5 battements
5. Schlag
  ars-h., **chel., coca**[2, 15], crot-h.[6],
  dig.[8], nit-ac.[6], **nux-v.**[2, 3]

sixth beat
6 battements
6. Schlag
  acon.[3], ars-h.[2], **chel.**[2], dig.[8],
  mur-ac.[8]

seventh beat[8]
7 battements
7. Schlag
  dig., **mur-ac.**

tenth beat after exertion or
  vexation[6]
10 battements après exercice ou
  contrariété
10. Schlag nach Anstrengungen
  oder Ärger
  gels.

tenth to thirtieth beat[2]
10–30 battements
10.–30. Schlag
  agar.[2, 3], **cina,** kali-m., lach.[3]

fortieth to sixtieth beat[2]
40–60 battements
40.–60. Schlag
  agar., ars-h.

dinner, after[16]
déjeuner, après le
Mittagessen, nach dem
  nat-m.

menses, before[7]
menstruation, avant la
Menses, vor den
  kali-c.

old people, in[7]
âgées, chez les personnes
alten Menschen, bei
  tab.

irregular
irrégulier
unregelmäßiger
  acetan.[8], **acon.**[1], acon-c.[11],
  adon.[3, 6, 8], **adren.**[7, 8], aeth.[15],
  agar., agar-pa.[11], agarin.[8], aloe,
  alum., alum-p.[1'], am-caust.[11],
  aml-ns., anac.[14], ang., anh.[14],
  anil.[11], **ANT-C.,** ant-t., antip.[8],
  apis[1], apoc., arg-m., **arg-n.,** arn.,
  ARS., ars-h.[2], **ars-i.,** ars-s-f.[1'],
  arum-d.[2, 11], **asaf.,** arar.[14], **aspar.,**
  atro.[2, 11], **aur.,** aur-ar.[1'], **aur-s.**[1'],
  bapt., bar-a.[11], bar-c.[2], bar-m.[11],
  bell., bell-p.[9, 14], ben-n.[11],
  benz-ac., bism., bol-lu.[11], **bry.,**
  bufo[3], **cact.,** cael.[14], calc., calen.[2],
  camph., cann-i., cann-s.[3], canth.,
  caps., carb-ac., carb-an., carb-v.,
  carbn-o.[11], caust.[3], cham., chel.,
  CHIN., chin-s., **chlol.**[2], chlor.[11],
  chlorpr.[14], chr-ac.[11], **cimic.**[14],
  cimx., cinch.[11], clem.[11], coff.,
  coffin.[8], **colch., con., conv.**[6, 8],
  convo-s.[9, 14], cor-r., cortico.[14],
  crat.[6, 8], **crot-h.,** cub.[2, 11], cupr.,
  cupr-a.[11], cyt-l.[11, 14], **DIG., digin.**[11],
  digox.[11], dulc.[11], euph.[11], fago.[11],
  ferr.[1', 3, 8], ferr-p.[3], form.[11], **gels.,**
  gins.[11], glon., guare.[11], ham.,
  hed.[14], hell., **hep.,** hir.[14], hist.[14],
  home.[11], **hydr-ac.**[8, 11], **hyos.,**
  iber.[2, 8, 11, 14], ign., iod., jab.[11],
  jatr.[11], juni.[11], **kali-bi., kali-c.,**
  kali-chl., kali-cy.[11], **kali-i.,**
  kali-m.[1'], kali-n.[11], kali-p.,
  kali-s.[11], **kalm., LACH.,** lachn.[2],
  laur., **lil-t.**[6, 8], lob., lol.[11], **lycps.,**
  mag-p.[3], mag-s.[9, 14], manc.[2, 3, 6, 11],
  mang., meny., meph.[14], **merc.,**
  merc-c., merc-cy., merc-i-f.[2, 11],
  merc-sul.[2, 11], mez., morph.[11],
  mur-ac.[3, 6, 8], myric.[2], **naja,**
  nat-ar., nat-f.[9, 14], **NAT-M.,**
  nat-n.[6], nat-s.[11], nicc.[11], nit-ac.,
  nit-s-d.[11], nux-m.[3, 6, 8], nux-v.,
  oena.[11], **olnd.,** onop.[14], **op.,** ox-ac.,

penic.[14], **PH-AC., phase.**[8], **phos.**,
phys., **phyt.**, pic-ac.[11], pilo.[8],
pip-n.[3], **plan., plb.**, prun-v.[7],
ptel.[11], puls.[3, 8], pyrog., rauw.[9],
rhus-t., sabad., sabin., sacch.[11],
samb., sang., santin.[11], **saroth.**[8, 9],
SEC., seneg., **sep.**, ser-ang.[8], **sil.**,
sol-n.[11], sol-t-ae.[11], **spig., squil.**[3, 6],
stann.[3], **still., STRAM.**,
stroph-h.[3, 8], stroph-s.[9], stry.[11],
stry-ar.[8], stry-p.[8], sul-ac., sul-h.[11],
sulfa.[14], sulo-ac.[11], **sulph.**,
sumb.[2, 3, 6, 8, 11], **tab.**, tanac.[11],
tarent.[11], tax.[11], thea, thiop.[14],
thuj., trach.[11], trif-p.[11], **tub.**[7],
uva[11], valer., **verat., VERAT-V.**,
vib.[2], vip.[3, 6, 11], vip-a.[14], visc.[9],
wies.[11], xan.[11], yuc.[11], zinc.,
zinc-p.[1']

morning[16]/matin/morgens
caust.

exertion, on slight
mouvement, au moindre
Anstrengung, bei der geringsten
arg-n., meny., **nat-m.**

lying down, on[11]
s'étendant, en
Hinlegen, beim
lycps., still.

lying on back, while
couché sur le dos, en position
Rückenlage, bei
arg-n.

on left side[2]
sur le côté gauche
linken Seite, bei Lage auf der
nat-m.

stool, after
selle, après la
Stuhlgang, nach
agar.

and slow
et lent
und langsamer
acon., arn., ars., asaf., bell.,

camph., cann-i., chel., chin.,
cimic., colch., **DIG.**, dulc., ham.,
hell., hyos., iod., **KALM.**, laur.,
lob., merc-c., merc-cy., mez.,
naja, nit-ac., nux-v., olnd., op.,
ox-ac., ph-ac., phys., phyt., plb.,
rhus-t., seneg., sul-ac., tab.,
verat., **VERAT-V.**, zinc.

irritable
reizbarer
arg-m., ars., colch., dig., iod.,
kali-bi., meny., ox-ac., stram., tab.

jerking
saccadé
ruckartiger
acon., agar.[3], aml-ns.[2, 3, 11], **arn.**[3],
ars.[3, 11], arum-d.[2, 3, 11], aur., bar-c.,
calad.[2, 3, 11], canth.[3], con.[3], dig.[3],
digin.[11], dulc., fago.[3, 11], gins.[3, 11],
glon.[3, 11], **IBER.**[2, 11], jatr.[3, 11], nat-m.[3],
nat-p.[3], nux-v.[3], plb., thuj.[3]

labored
fatigué
mühsamer
crot-h.[2], cupr., cupr-a.[11], hydr.[11],
iris, kreos., merc., merc-c.[11],
merc-i-f.[2, 11], mit.[11], morph.[11], op.,
stram.

large[3]
Pulsus magnus
ACON., ant-t., **APIS**[2], **arn.**, asaf.,
asar., atro.[11], bar-c., **BELL.**[2, 3, 11],
bism., **bry.**[3, 11], camph.[3, 11], canth.,
cench.[11], **chel.**[3, 11], chin., chin-s.[11],
colch.[2, 3], coloc., **CON.**[2, 3, 11], **cupr.**,
cupr-a.[11], dig., dulc., ferr.[3, 11],
ferr-p., gels., glon., hell., hep.,
HYOS., ign., **IOD.**[2, 3], ip.[2], jatr.[11],
kali-cy.[11], **KALI-N.**, lach., led.,
lycps.[3], manc.[3], merc., mez.,
mosch., mur-ac., nat-m., nat-p.,
nux-v., olnd., op.[3, 11], par., petr.,
ph-ac., phos., plb.[3, 11], ran-b., ran-s.,
sabin., samb., **sep.**, sil., **spig.**,
spira.[11], spong., **STRAM.**, stry.[11],
sul-ac.[11], sulph., syph.[3], **tab.**[2],
verat., **verat-v.**, viol-o.

slow
lent
langsamer

abies-n.[8], acet-ac., achy.[14], **acon.,**
acon-c.[11], acon-f., acon-l.[11],
adon.[8], adren.[8], aesc.[3, 6, 8], aeth.,
aether[11], **agar.,** agar-cps.[11],
agar-pa.[11], agn., **all-c.**[2],
am-caust.[11], aml-ns.[2, 11], **amyg.,**
anan.[2], anh.[9, 14], anil.[11], ant-c.,
ant-t., apis[3], apoc., arn., ars.,
ars-met.[2], ars-s-f.[2], asaf., asc-t.[2],
aspar., atro.[11], bapt., bar-a.[11],
bar-i.[1'], **bell.,** ben-n.[11], benz-ac.,
BERB., both.[11], brom., cact.[8],
cain.[11], **camph., CANN-I.,**
cann-s., canth., caps.,
carb-ac.[2, 11], carbn-o.[11], carbn-s.[1'],
catal.[11], caust., cench.[11], **chel.,**
chin., **chin-s.,** chlor.[2, 11], chr-ac.[11],
cic., cimic., coca[11], coff-t.[11],
colch., coloc., **con.,** croc.[11],
crot-h., cryp.[11], cub.[2, 11], cund.[11],
cupr., cupr-am-s.[11], cur.[7], cyt-l.[11],
daph.[2], dat-f.[11], delphin.[11], **DIG.,**
digin.[11], digox.[11], dubo-m.[11], dulc.,
ery-j.[11], esin.[8], euph-c.[11], eupi.[7, 11],
fago.[11], ferr., ferr-ma.[11], gast.[11],
GELS., gins.[11], glon., grat.[11], ham.,
hell., helo.[8], hep., hippoz.[2],
home.[11], hydr.[3, 11], hydr-ac.,
hyos., ign., iod., iris, jab.[11],
jac-c.[11], jatr.[11], juni.[11], kali-bi.,
kali-br.[2], kali-c., kali-chl.,
kali-cy.[11], kali-m.[1'], kali-n,
kali-s.[11], **KALM.,** kreos., kres.[14],
lach., lachn., lact.[11], lat-k.[11],
lat-m.[8, 9, 11], **laur., lob.,** lon-x.[11],
lup.[8, 11], lycpr.[8], **lycps.,** mag-c.[3],
mag-s.[4, 14], **manc., mang.**[3, 11],
mec.[11], meny., meph.[14], merc.,
merc-c., merc-cy., merc-sul.[2],
meth-ae-ae.[11], mez., **morph.**[8, 11],
mosch., mur-ac., myric.,
myrt-c.[3], **naja,** narcot.[11], nat-ar.[2],
nat-c.[3], **nat-m.**[3], nat-n.[6], nit-ac.,
nit-s-d.[11], nitro.[11], **nux-m.,**
nux-v., oena.[11], ol-an.[11], olnd.,
OP., ox-ac., par., pen.[11], petr.,
ph-ac., phel.[11], phos., phys., phyt.,
pic-ac., pip-n.[3, 8], pitu.[9], plb.,

podo., prop.[11], prun.[11], prun-p.[7],
puls., ran-b.[3], raph.[11], rauw.[9],
rhod., rhus-t., ruta, samb., **sang.,**
sars., **sec., SEP.,** sil., sol-n.[11],
solin.[11], spig., spong., squil.,
STRAM., stroph-s.[9], stry.[11],
sulo-ac.[11], sumb.[11], **tab.,** tanac.[11],
tarent.[2], tax.[11], thea[11], thiop.[14],
thuj., thymol.[9, 14], trif-p.[11], trios.[14],
uva[11], upa.[11], valer., **VERAT.**[1, 7],
VERAT-V.[1, 7], verb.[11], vip.[11],
visc.[9, 11, 14], wies.[11], wye.[11], zinc.,
zing.[2]

daytime/journée, pendant la/tags-
über
dulc.[2], mur-ac., sep.

morning/matin/morgens
arg-m., chin-s., grat., jac-c.[11],
lycps.[11], myric.[11], olnd., petr.

forenoon/matinée/vormittags
cinnb., myric.[11]

afternoon/après-midi/nachmittags
chin-s., gins.[11], myric.[11], ox-ac.

evening/soir/abends
ars., cund.[11], **graph.,** myric.[11],
nat-ar., phyt.

night[11]/nuit/nachts
phys.

alternating with frequent[8]
alternant avec p. fréquent
abwechselnd mit schnellem
bell.[3], chin., cic.[14], cimic.[14], dig.,
gels., iod., **morph.**[7, 8], rhus-t.[3, 5],
stroph-h.[3]

bounding, full and[7]
bendissant, plein et
schnellender, voller und
visc.

chill, during[16]
frissons, pendant les
Fieberfrost, während
  mur-ac.

fever with[14]
fièvre avec
Fieber mit
  karw-h.

lying, in[16]
couché, étant
Liegen, beim
  dig.

slower than the beat of heart
plus lent que les pulsations
  cardiaques
langsamer als der Herzschlag
  agar., cann-s., **dig.**, dulc., hell.,
  KALI-I.[3], **kali-n.**, kres.[13], laur.,
  lyc.[3], **nat-m.**[3], sec., verat.

vomiting, on[16]
vomissement, pendant le
Erbrechen, beim
  squil.

small
petit
kleiner
  ACON., acon-s.[11], **aeth.**[2, 11],
  aether[11], **agar.**, agar-pa.[11], agro.[11],
  ail.[11], ald.[11], alco.[11], alum., am-c.[3],
  am-caust.[11], ammc.[2], amyg.[11], ant-c.,
  ant-m.[2, 11], **ant-t.**, apis, apoc.[1'], arn.,
  ARS., ars-h.[2, 11], **ars-i.**, ars-s-f.[1', 2, 11],
  arum-d.[2, 11], asaf., asc-t.[2, 11], aspar.[11],
  aster.[2], atro.[11], **aur.**, aur-ar.[1'],
  aur-m., **aur-s.**[1'], bar-c., bar-i.[1'],
  bar-m., **bell.**, ben-n.[11], benz-ac.,
  bism., bol-lu.[11], bry., caj.[11], calad.,
  calc., calth.[11], **CAMPH.**, cann-i.,
  cann-s., canth., carb-ac., carb-an.[3],
  CARB-V., carbn-h.[11], catal.[11],
  cham., **CHEL.**[2, 3], **chin.**, **chin-ar.**[2],
  chin-s.[2], **chlor.**[2, 11], cic., **cina**[2, 3, 11],
  clem.[3], coca[2], **cocc.**, cod.[11], coff.[2],
  colch., **coloc.**[2, 3, 11], **con.**, conin.[11],
  cop.[11], croc.[3], **crot-h.**[2], crot-t.[11],
  cub.[2, 11], cund., **CUPR.**, cupr-ar.[2],
  cuprs.[2], cyt-l.[11], delphin.[11], **DIG.**,

digin.[11], **dulc.**, euph-l.[11], ferr.,
ferr-m.[11], fl-ac.[11], frag.[11], gels.,
glon.[2, 11], graph.[3], grat., **GUAJ.**,
gymno.[11], haem.[11], **hell.**, helo.[11],
hippoz.[2], hydr-ac.[11], **hyos.**, iber.[11],
ign., **iod.**, ip., juni.[11], kali-ar.[11],
kali-bi., **kali-br.**[2], **kali-c.**, kali-chl.,
kali-cy.[11], kali-fcy.[11], kali-i.,
kali-m.[1', 2], kali-n., **kali-p.**[2], kali-s.[11],
keroso.[11], **kreos.**, lac-ac., **lach.**, led.,
LAUR., lil-t.[11], **lob.**, lyc., **lycps.**[2],
mang., meny., **merc.**, merc-br.[11],
merc-c., merc-cy., merc-d.[11],
merc-pr-r.[11], merc-n.[11], merc-sul.[2],
meth-ae-ae.[11], **mez.**[2], morph.[11],
mosch.[3], **mur-ac.**, naja[3], narcot.[11],
nat-br.[11], nat-m., nat-n.[11], nat-s.[11],
nit-ac., nit-s-d.[11], **nux-m.**, nux-v.,
oena.[11], **ol-j.**[2], olnd.[11], **op.**, ox-ac.,
past.[11], peti.[11], petr., **ph-ac.**, **phos.**,
phys., phyt., pic-ac., **plat.**, plb.,
plumbg.[11], podo., prun.[11], prun-p.[7],
ptel.[11], puls., ran-a.[11], ran-b., ran-s.,
raph., rhod., rhus-t., ric.[11],
rumx-a.[11], russ.[11], ruta[11], sabad.,
sal-ac.[2], **samb.**, **sang.**[2], sarr.[2, 11],
SEC., seneg., serp.[11], **SIL.**, sol-n.[11],
sol-t.[11], sol-t-ae.[11], solin.[11], spig.,
spirae.[11], spong.[2, 3], squil., **stann.**,
staph., **STRAM.**, stroph-h.[3], stry.[11],
sul-ac., **sulph.**, tab.[3, 11], tanac.[11],
tarent.[2], tax.[11], **ter.**, thea[11], thuj.,
til.[11], upa.[11], uva[11], valer., **VERAT.**,
vesp.[2, 11], viol-o., vip.[11], visc.[7, 11],
wies.[11], zinc., **zinc-m.**[11], **zinc-p.**[1'],
zinc-s.[11]

soft
mou
weicher
  acal.[8], acet-ac., **acon.**, aesc., aeth.,
  aether[11], agar., agn., ant-c.,
  ant-s-aur.[11], **ANT-T.**, anth.[11], apis,
  apoc., arn., **ars.**, ars-h.[2], arum-d.[11],
  aspar.[11], aster., atro.[11], **aur.**, bapt.,
  bar-c., bar-m., bell., bism., bry.,
  calc-ar.[7], calc-i.[11], camph., cann-i.,
  cann-s., canth., **carb-ac.**, **CARB-V.**,
  carbn-o.[11], carbn-s.[11], cham., chin.,
  chlor.[2, 11], cic., cit-l.[11], cocc.,
  coffin.[8], **colch.**, con., conv., crot-h.,
  cub.[2], **CUPR.**, cuprs.[2], cyt-l.[11],

DIG., digin.[11], digox.[11], dulc., ery-a.[11], euph., ferr., ferr-m., **ferr-p.**[3, 6-8], **gels.**, glon.[11], **guaj.**, ham., hell., hep., hydr-ac., hyos., iber.[2], iod., ip., jab.[11], jal., jatr.[11], juni.[11], kali-bi., kali-br., kali-c., kali-chl., kali-cy.[11], **kali-m.**[1', 2], kali-n., **kalm.**, kreos., lac-ac., **LACH.**, lat-m.[14], laur., **lob.**, lyc., **lycps.**[2], **manc.**[2], mang., **merc.**, merc-cy., mez., morph.[11], **MUR-AC.**, **naja**, narcot.[11], nat-ar., nat-m., nat-n.[11], nitro-o.[11], nux-v., oena.[11], **ol-j.**[2], olnd., **OP.**, **ox-ac.**, ph-ac., **phos.**, phys., phyt., **plat.**, plb., polyp-p.[11], puls., ran-s., rhod.[3], rhus-t., **sang.**, santin.[11], sec., seneg., sil., sin-n.[11], sol-n.[11], **spig.**, spirae.[11], **STRAM.**, stry.[11], sul-ac., **sulph.**[2], **sumb.**[2, 11], syph.[3], **tab.**, tarax.[11], **TER.**, thuj., toxi.[11], trios.[14], uva[11], valer., **VERAT.**, **verat-v.**, vip.[11], zinc., zinc-m.[11]

spasmodic
spasmodique
spastischer

ang.[2, 3], arn.[3], ars., bism., carbn-s.[1', 2], chin.[3], **COCC.**[2, 3], cupr., cupr-a.[11], **dig.**[2, 3], indg.[11], iod.[3], kali-bi.[3], merc., **merc-c.**[2, 3, 11], nux-m., nux-v.[11], plb.[3], sabad., **sec.**[3], sep., **stram.**[2], zinc., zinc-s.[11]

contracted/oppressé/zusammen-gezogener

strong
fort
kräftiger

achy.[14], acon., aether[11], agar.[2], agar-pa.[11], alco.[11], aloe, am-c., aml-ns.[2, 11], amyg.[2, 11], ant-t., apis, arn., ars.[11], ars-h.[2], ars-i.[2, 11], asar., aster.[14], aza.[14], **bell.**, bism.[3], **bry.**[3], caj.[11], cann-i., canth.[3], catal.[11], chel.[3], chin., chin-ar.[2], cinnb.[11], coca[11], con., crot-t., **cupr.**[2, 3], dig.[3], fago.[11], ferr-p.[1'], gast.[11], gels., gins.[11], hell.[3], hoit.[14], hydrc.[11], hyos., iber.[11], iod.[3], jatr.[11], **kali-m.**[2], kreos.[3], lach.[3], lappa[11], laur.[3],

lycps.[11], **merc.**[3], merc-c., merc-cy., merc-i-r.[11], mill., morph.[11], nat-s.[11], op., par.[11], paro-i.[14], petr.[3], **PH-AC.**[3], phys., **puls.**[2], ran-b.[3], raph., sabad., **SABIN.**[2, 3], sang., sarr.[2, 11], seneg., serp.[11], sium[11], sol-t-ae.[11], **SPIG.**[3], stram., stront-c.[3], stry.[11], tanac.[11], ter.[2], uva[11], valer.[3], **verat.**[3], **VIOL-O.**[3]

tense
tendu
gespannter

acon.[3], adren.[7], agro.[11], all-c., all-s.[11], am-c., **am-m.**, ammc.[2], **ant-t.**, aphis[11], ars., atro.[11], bell., ben-n.[11], bism., **BRY.**[2, 3], cann-i., camph., canth., cham., chel.[3], chin., clem., coca[11], coff-t.[11], colch., con., corn-f.[11], **cupr.**[2, 3], dig.[3], **DULC.**[3], ferr., hyos., kali-i., merc-c.[3], **mez.**, morph.[11], nat-c., nit-ac., ox-ac., petr., plb., sabad., **SABIN.**[3], sang., sec., sol-t-ae.[11], spira.[11], squil.[3, 11], stram.[3], til.[11], **valer.**[2, 3, 11], verat.[11], verat-v., zinc.[2, 3, 11]

thready
filiforme
fadenförmiger

acon., agar-pa.[11], **ail.**[3, 6], alum., aml-ns.[3, 6], amyg.[2, 11], **apis**[3, 6], arn., **ars.**, ars-s-f.[2], ars-s-r.[2], bell., camph., canth., carb-v., carbn-h.[11], chlf.[11], colch., cop.[11], crat.[6, 11], **crot-h.**[2], cupr., dig., digin.[11], hell., **hydr-ac.**[3, 6], hyos., iod., jatr.[11], kali-bi., kali-n.[11], lach.[3, 6], **LAT-M.**[7, 9, 14], merc-c.[3], merc-ns.[11], morph.[11], naja, nat-f.[9, 14], olnd., op., ox-ac., petr., phos., phys.[11], phyt., **plat.**[2], plb., ptel.[11], **pyrog.**[3, 6], raja-s.[14], rhus-t., sal-ac.[6], santin.[11], sec.[1'], sol-t-ae.[11], solin.[11], **spig.**[3, 6], stram.[2, 3], sul-ac.[11], sulph., tab.[3, 6], tax.[11], **ter.**[2, 11], **VERAT.**[2, 3, 6], verat-v.[3, 6], **verb.**[2], vip.[11], **zinc.**[2], zinc-m.[11]

tremulous
tremblant
zittriger
  acon., ambr., **ANT-T.,** apis², **ars.,**
  bell., CALC., camph., cann-i.,
  canth., carb-ac., **cic.,** cina,
  cinnb.¹¹, cocc., colch.², crot-h.,
  dig., fago.¹¹, gels., gins.¹¹, **hell.,**
  iber.² ¹¹, iod., kali-c., **kreos.,**
  lach., merc., merc-c.,
  merc-sul.² ¹¹, nat-m., nux-m., op.,
  ox-ac., phos., plat.², plb., **rhus-t.,**
  ruta, **sabin., sep., SPIG., staph.,**
  stram., sul-ac., valer.

  night/nuit/nachts
  calc., narc-po.¹¹

  eating, after
  mangé, après avoir
  Essen, nach dem
    calc.

undulating
ondulant
wellenförmiger
  agar. ¹¹, ¹⁶, amyg.¹¹, **ars.,** camph.,
  carb-ac.¹¹, carbn-o.¹¹, chlf.¹¹, crot-h.,
  dig., digin.¹¹, gins.¹¹, iber.¹¹, op.,
  plb.

weak
faible
schwacher
  acet-ac., acon., acon-f.¹¹, aesc.,
  aeth., aether¹¹, agar.² ³ ¹⁶,
  agar-cps.¹¹, agar-em.¹¹, **AGN.³,**
  ald.¹¹, aloe, alum-p.¹',
  am-caust.¹¹, am-m., amyg.² ¹¹,
  ampe-qu.¹¹, **ant-ar.⁶,** ant-c.³ ⁶,
  ant-m.², **ANT-T.,** anth.¹¹, apis,
  apoc.¹', apom.¹¹, **arn., ARS.,**
  ars-h.² ¹¹, ars-s-f.¹', arum-d.¹¹, asaf.,
  asc-c.², **aspar.,** aster.², **atro.**² ¹¹,
  AUR., aur-ar.¹', aur-m.¹', **aur-s.¹',**
  aza.¹⁴, bapt., **BAR-C.¹' ³ ⁶,** bar-s.¹',
  bell., benz-ac.², **BERB.,** bism.³, bry.,
  buth-a.⁹, cact.², caj.¹¹, calad.¹¹,
  CAMPH., cann-i., **CANN-S.**² ³ ⁶,
  canth., carb-ac.², carb-an.,
  CARB-V., carbn-chl.¹¹, carbn-o.¹¹,
  cass.¹¹, catal.¹¹, cedr., cench.¹¹,

cham.³, chen-a.¹¹, **chin., chin-ar.,**
chlol.², chlor.¹¹, **CIC.³,** cimic.,
cimx., cinch.¹¹, coca² ¹¹, **cocc.²,**
cod.¹¹, coff.² ³, coff-t.¹¹, colch.,
coloc.² ³, con.³, conin.¹¹, **crat.⁶,**
CROT-H., crot-t., cub.², **cupr.,**
cupr-a.² ¹¹, cupr-ar.² ¹¹, cycl.,
cyt-l.¹¹, **dig.,** digin.¹¹, digox.¹¹,
dios.², dirc.¹¹, dor.¹¹, erio.¹¹, ery-a.¹¹,
eryt-j.¹¹, fago.¹¹, fagu.¹¹, ferr-m.,
gast.¹¹, **GELS., glon.,** guaj.³, ham.,
hell., hydr-ac.⁶ ⁷ ¹¹, hydrc.¹¹, hyos.,
iber.² ¹¹, **ign., iod., ip.,** iris, jasm.¹¹,
jatr.¹¹, juni.¹¹, kali-ar.¹¹, **kali-bi.,**
kali-br., kali-c.² ³ ⁶ ¹¹, kali-n.¹¹,
kali-ox.¹¹, kali-t.¹¹, **kalm.,** keroso.¹¹,
kreos., lac-ac., **lac-c.², LACH.,**
lact.¹¹, lat-k.¹¹, **LAT-M.⁷ ¹⁴, LAUR.,**
lil-t., lob., lyc.³, **lycps., lyss.²,**
manc., mang., **merc., merc-c.,**
merc-cy., merc-i-f.², merc-ns.¹¹,
merc-pr-r.¹¹, merc-sul.¹¹,
meth-ae-ae.¹¹, mez.¹¹, mom-b.¹¹,
morph.¹¹, **mosch.³ ¹¹, mur-ac.,**
NAJA, narcot.¹¹, nat-f.⁹ ¹⁴, nat-m.,
nit-ac.¹¹, nit-s-d.¹¹, **nux-m.**² ³ ⁶,
nux-v., oena.² ¹¹, olnd., op., ox-ac.,
past.¹¹, peti.¹¹, **PH-AC., phos.,**
phys., phyt., **PLAT.**² ³, plb.,
plumbg.¹¹, podo., polyp-p.¹¹, prop.¹¹,
psor.², **puls.,** pyre-p.¹¹, raja-s.¹⁴,
rhod., **rhus-t.,** rhus-v., ric.¹¹,
rumx-a.¹¹, sabin.¹¹, sacch.¹¹,
sal-ac.², sal-p.¹¹, **sang.,** santin.¹¹,
sapin.¹¹, **sec.,** seneg., sep., sil.³ ⁶,
sol-t-ae.¹¹, solin.¹¹, **spig.,** spira.¹¹,
spong.², **staph., still.**² ¹¹, **stram.,**
stront-c.³, stry.¹, sul-ac., sul-h.¹¹,
sulo-ac.¹¹, **sulph.²,** sumb.¹¹, **tab.,**
tanac.¹¹, **tarent.²,** tart-ac.¹¹, tax.¹¹,
ter.² ¹¹, tere-ch.¹⁴, thea¹¹, **thuj.³ ¹¹,**
thymol.⁹, trif-p.¹¹, upa.¹¹, **ust.²,**
uva¹¹, **valer.**² ³ ¹¹, **vario.²,** verat.,
verat-v., verb.¹¹, vesp.² ¹¹,
vip.³ ⁶ ¹¹, vip-a.¹⁴, xan.¹¹, zinc.,
zinc-m.¹¹, zinc-p.¹', zinc-s.¹¹,
zing.¹¹

morning¹⁶/matin/morgens
  sep.

motion, on[1']
mouvement, en
Bewegung, bei
    bar-s.

wiry
en fil de fer tendu
Drahtpuls
    amyg.[2, 11], ars., ben-n.[11], bol-la.[11],
    cupr., cupr-a.[11], dig., gels., **glon.**[1', 2],
    ham., iber.[11], kreos., **lac-c.**[2], **lycps.**[2],
    oena.[11], ox-ac., phos., phys., sec.,
    tax.[11], ter.[2], zinc.

tense/tendu/gespannter

PUNISHMENT agg.[3]*
CHÂTIMENTS agg.
BESTRAFUNG agg.
    ambr., con., dig., lach., stann., staph.

PURGATIVES, abuse of[3]
PURGATIVES, abus des
ABFUHRMITTELN, Mißbrauch von
    hydr., **nux-v.**[3, 6], op.[3, 6], sulph.

pus see abscesses–pus

QUININE, abuse of*
QUININE, abus de
CHININ-MISSBRAUCH, Folgen von
    am-c., **ant-t., apis, ARN., ars.,**
    ars-s-f.[1'], asaf., aza.[12], **bell.,** bry.
    CALC., calc-ar.[7], caps., carb-an.[12],
    CARB-V., cham., chelo.[12], **cina,**
    coloc.[8], cupr., cycl., dig., eucal.[8, 12],
    FERR. , ferr-ar., gels., hell., **hep.**[2], **IP.,**
    kali-ar.[1'], **lach.,** mang.[3], meny.[3, 8, 12],
    merc., **NAT-M.,** nat-p.[7], nat-s.[1'],
    nux-v., parth.[8], **ph-ac.,** phos.[1], plb.,
    PULS., ran-s.[3], samb., sel.[3, 8], **sep.,**
    stann., sul-ac., **sulph., verat.**

china/quinquina/Chinarinde

QUIVERING
FRÉMISSEMENT
BEBEN
    agar.[3, 11], agn.[3], alum.[3], **am-c.,**
    am-m.[3], ambr.[3], **ang.**[3], ant-c.[3], ars.[3],

ASAF.[3], bapt.[1'], bar-c.[3], **BELL.,**
berb., bism., bov.[3], bry.[3], **calc.,**
calc-p.[11], camph.[3], **cann-s.**[3], canth.[3],
caps., carb-v.[3], caust., chel.[3], chin.[3],
cic.[3], **clem.,** cocc.[1'], colch.[3], coloc.[3],
com., **CON.,** croc.[3], cupr.[3], dig.,
dros.[3], gels.[12], graph.[3], guaj.[3], hell.[3],
hep., hyos., ign., iod., ip.[3], kali-c.,
kali-n., kali-s.[1'], kreos.[3], lyc., mag-c.,
mag-m.[3], med.[1'], meny.[3], merc.[1', 3],
MEZ.[3], mosch., mur-ac.[3], **NAT-C.**[3],
nat-m.[3], **nit-ac.,** nux-v., par.[3], petr.,
phos.[3], plat.[1', 3], plb.[3], puls.[3], rhod.[3],
rhus-t.[3], ruta[3], sabin.[3], sars., sel.[3],
seneg.[3], **sep.,** sil., **spig.**[3], stann.,
stram.[3], stront-c., sul-ac.[1'], **SULPH.,**
tarax.[3], thuj.[3], valer.[3], verb.,
viol-t.[3], **zinc.**[1', 3]

all over, followed by vertigo
général, suivi de vertiges
am ganzen Körper, gefolgt von
    Schwindel
    calc.

lying, while
couché, étant
Liegen, im
    clem.

glands
glandes, dans les
Drüsen, in
    bell., calc., kali-c., mez., nat-c., sil.

REABSORBENT action[3]
ABSORBANTE, action
RESORBIERENDE Wirkung
    arn., kali-i., sul-i., **sulph.**

REACTION, lack of
RÉACTION, manque de
REAKTIONSMANGEL
    aeth.[3], agar., **alum., AM-C., AMBR.,**
    anac., ant-c., ant-t., apis[7], arn., **ars.,**
    ARS-I.[1], ars-s-f.[1'], **asaf., bar-c.,**
    bar-m.[3], bar-s.[1'], bell.[7], bism., **brom.,**
    bry.[1, 7], **CALC.,** calc-f.[3, 6], **calc-i.,**
    calc-s., camph., CAPS., carb-an.,
    CARB-V., carbn-s.[8], **cast.,** caust.,
    cham., **chin.,** cic., **cocc.,** coff.,

coloc.[3], **CON.**, **cupr.**, cypr.[7], dig.[3],
dulc., euph., **ferr.**, ferr-i., **fl-ac.**,
gaert.[7], **GELS.**, **graph.**, **guaj.**, **HELL.**,
hep.[3, 6], **HYDR-AC.**, hyos., **iod.**, **ip.**,
kali-bi.[3, 6], **kali-br.**, **kali-c.**, kali-i.[3],
luf-o.[14], **lyc.**, mag-c., mag-f.[10],
mag-m., **MED.**, **merc.**, mez., **mosch.**,
mur-ac., nat-ar.[7, 8], nat-c., nat-m.,
nat-p., nat-s.[8], nit-ac.[3, 6], **nux-m.**,
OLND., **OP.**[1,7], ped.[7], petr., **PH-AC.**,
phos., plb., prot.[7], **PSOR.**, puls.[3, 6],
rhod., scut.[7], **sec.**, seneg., **sep.**,
spong., **stann.**, **stram.**, stront-c.,
sul-i.[1'], **SULPH.**, **syph.**, **TARENT.**,
thal.[14], **thuj.**, **TUB.**[1', 3, 6-8], **valer.**,
vario.[6], **verat.**, verb.[1], x-ray[7, 8],
ZINC.[1, 7], **zinc-p.**[1']

*irritability – lack/hypersensibilité –
    insensibilité/Reizbarkeit –
    Unempfindlichkeit
weakness – reaction/faiblesse –
    réaction/Schwäche – Reaktions-
    mangel*

acute danger[3]
danger imminent, lors d'un
akuter Gefahr, in
    ambr., ars., camph., lyc.

chill, after[3]
frissons, après les
Fieberfrost, nach
    camph., dulc.

climacteric period, at[3]
ménopause, pendant la
Klimakterium, während des
    con.

convalescence, in[3]
convalescence, pendant la
Rekonvaleszenz, in der
    cast., ph-ac.

*convalescence–ailments/
    convalescence–troubles/
    Rekonvaleszenz–Beschwerden*

exanthemas, in[3]
exanthèmes, au cours d'
Exanthemen, bei
    ant-t., **bry.**, cupr., dulc., psor.,
    stram., **sulph.**, zinc.

loss of fluids, after[3]
perte de fluides vitaux, par
Säfteverlust, durch
    chin.

remedies, to[3]
remèdes, aux
Arzneimitteln, gegenüber
    carb-v., laur., op.[12], teucr.[2, 12]

nervous patients, in[3]
nerveux, chez les malades
nervösen Patienten, bei
    ambr., laur., op., **VALER.**[2, 3], zinc.

old age, in[3]
personnes âgées, chez les
Alter, im
    con.

suppression, after[3]
suppression, par
Unterdrückungen, durch
    lach.

eruptions, of[1']
éruptions, d'
Hautausschlägen, von
    ars-s-f.

*suppressed – eruptions/suppri-
    mées – éruptions/unterdrückte
    Hautausschläge*

suppuration, in[3]
suppuration, au cours de
Eiterung, bei
    calc-f., hep.

*abscesses–chronic/abcès–
    chroniques/Abszesse–chronische*

REACTION, violent[3]
RÉACTION, violente
REAKTION, heftige
   bell., **cupr.**, **nux-v.**, zinc.

REBELS against poultice[15]
SE RÉVOLTE contre un cataplasme
REBELLIERT gegen Umschläge
   bor., bry., **calc.**, carb-v., **cham.**, **lyc.**,
   merc., mur-ac., nit-ac., nux-v., phos.,
   puls., rhus-t., sep., spig., staph.,
   sulph.

REFLEXES, diminished[3, 6]
RÉFLEXES diminués
REFLEXE, abgeschwächte
   alum., arg-n., cur.[3, 6, 8],
   kali-br.[3, 6, 11], oena, op.[11], oxyt.[8],
   phys., plb.[8], sec.[8]

   increased[3, 6]
   exagérés
   gesteigerte
      anh.[8], bar-c.[11], cann-i.[8], cic., cocc.,
      lath.[3, 6, 8], mang.[8], morph.[11], nux-v.,
      stry.[6]

   lost[11]
   absents
   aufgehobene
      morph., nat-br., sulfon.[8, 12]

RELAXATION of **connective tissue**[12]
RELÂCHEMENT de **tissu connectif**
ERSCHLAFFUNG des **Bindegewebes**
   calc.[1'], calc-br., caps., ferr-i., hep.,
   kali-c., mag-c., merc-i-r., nit-ac.,
   sec., spong.

   complexion-fair-lax/teinte-claire-
   lâche/Aussehen-hell-schlaffen

   muscles, of
   muscles, des
   Muskeln, der
      acet-ac.[7], aeth.[3], **agar.**, alum.[3],
      ambr., amyg.[2], ang.[3], anh.[10], ant-t.,
      arg-m.[1'], arn., **ars.**, asaf., atro.[11],
      bar-m.[11], bar-s.[1'], bell.[2], bor., bry.,
      CALC., calc-sil.[1'], camph., canth.,
      CAPS., carb-ac.[3], carb-an.[11],
      camph., canth., **CAPS.**, carb-an.[11],

carbn-o.[11], carbn-s.[11], caust[1', 3],
cham., chin., chin-ar., chlor.[11], cic.,
clem., coca[3], **COCC.**, colch.[1'], **con.**,
croc., **crot-c.**, cupr., cur.[3], cycl.[1'],
dig., **dios.**, dros.[3], euph., **ferr.**,
ferr-ar., ferr-i.[12], fl-ac.[3], **GELS.**,
graph., guare.[11], **hell.**, helo.[3], hep.[12],
hydr., hydr-ac.[11], **hyos.**, **iod.**, **ip.**,
jug-r.[11], kali-ar.[1'], **KALI-C.**,
kali-m.[1'], kali-n.[3], kali-p.[3], kali-s.[1'],
lach., laur., **lyc.**, **mag-c.**, mang.[1'],
merc., morph.[11], mur-ac., murx.[1'],
nat-c., nat-p.[1', 7], nit-ac.[12], nux-m.,
nux-v.[11], olnd.[3], op., oxyt., ph-ac.[3],
PHOS., phys.[11], plat., plb., puls.,
rheum, sabad., **sec.**, **seneg.**, **sep.**,
sil., sol-n., spig., **spong.**, stram.[3],
sul-ac., sul-h.[11], **sulph.**, tab.[3, 11],
ter.[11], thuj., **verat.**[3, 11, 12], verat-v.,
viol-o., zinc.[3]

physical[3]
physique
körperliche
   acon., agar., agn., alum.,
   ant-t.[3, 11], arn., ars., asar., aur.,
   bell., bism., bry., camph., caust.,
   cham., chel.[3, 11], chin.[3, 11], cic.,
   cina, cocc., coff., colch., cupr.,
   cycl., dig., dulc., euph., ferr.,
   hydr-ac.[11], hyos., ign.[3, 11], ip.,
   kali-c., kali-n., lach.[3, 11], linu-c.[11],
   lyc., meny., merc., morph.[11],
   nat-c., nat-m., nit-ac., nux-m.,
   nux-v., olnd., op., par., petr.,
   ph-ac., phos., plat., plb., ran-s.,
   rhod., rhus-t., ruta, sabad.,
   sabin., sel., sep., sil., spig.,
   spong., stann., staph., stram.,
   sulph., tarax., verat., viol-o.,
   viol-t., zinc.

   flabby/mollesse/Erschlaffung
   weakness/faiblesse/Schwäche

   coition, after
   coït, après le
   Koitus, nach
      agar.[2], sep.[11]

REST agg.[2, 3]
REPOS agg.
RUHE agg.
acon.[2, 3, 8], **aesc.**[3, 6], **agar.**[2, 3, 6],
alum.[3], **alumn.**[2], am-c., **am-m.,**
ambr., anac., ang., ant-c., **ant-t.,**
aran-ix.[14], **arg-m.**[1'-3, 6], **arn.**[2, 3, 8],
ars.[2, 3, 6, 8], **asaf.**[1'-3, 6, 8], asar.,
AUR.[2, 3, 6, 8], aur-m.[1'], bar-c., bell.,
bell-p.[14], benz-ac.[3, 6], **bism., bor.,**
bov., bry., calc., calc-f.[8],
CAPS.[2, 3, 8], carb-v., caust.,
cham., chin., cic., cimic.[14], **cina,**
cocc., **coloc.**[1'-3], com.[8], **CON.**[2, 3, 6, 8],
cortiso.[14], cupr., **CYCL.**[2, 3, 8],
dros., DULC.[1'-3, 8], **EUPH.**[2, 3, 8],
euphr., FERR.[1'-3, 6, 8], ferr-ar.[1'],
ferr-p.[1'], fl-ac.[3, 7], foll.[14], gels.[3],
glon.[3], guaj., hecla[14], hep., hyos.,
ign., indg.[8], **iod.**[3, 6], iris[8],
kali-c.[2, 3, 8, 14], kali-i.[3, 6], **kali-n.,**
kali-s.[1'], **kreos.**[2, 3, 6, 8], **lach.**[2, 3, 6],
laur., lith-lac.[8], **LYC.**[2, 3, 6, 8],
mag-c.[2, 3, 6, 8], **MAG-M.**[2, 3, 6],
mang., **meny.**[2, 3, 8], **merc.**[2, 3, 8],
merc-c.[3], merc-i-f.[1'], mez.,
mosch., mur-ac.[2, 3, 6], **nat-c.**[2, 3, 6],
nat-f.[10, 14], **nat-m.,** nat-s.[1', 3, 6],
nit-ac., **nux-m.**[2, 3, 6], olnd.[2, 3, 8],
op., par., petr., **ph-ac.,**
phenol.[13, 14], phos., **plat.,** plb.,
pneu.[14], **PULS.**[1'-3, 6, 8], pyrog.[3],
rhod.[1'-3, 6, 8], **RHUS-T.**[1'-3, 6, 8],
ruta[2, 3, 6], **SABAD.**[2, 3, 8], sabin.,
SAMB.[2, 3, 8], sars., sel.,
seneg.[1'-3, 8], **SEP.**[2, 3, 8], sil., spig.,
spong., stann., staph.,
stront-c.[2, 3, 8], sul-ac.,
sulph.[2, 3, 6, 8], **TARAX.**[2, 3, 8, 14],
tarent.[8], tell.[14], teucr., **thuj.**[1'-3, 6],
tub.[1', 7], tub-r.[14], **VALER.**[1'-3, 6, 8],
verat.[2, 3, 6], **verb., viol-t.**[3],
zinc.[2, 3, 6], zinc-val.[6]

as well as motion agg., during[3]
et mouvement agg.
und Bewegung agg.
am-c., bov., calc., carb-an.,
carb-v., caust., mez., ph-ac.,
phos., sulph.

am.[2, 3]
achy.[14], acon.[2, 3, 7], adlu[14], aesc.[8],
agar., **agn.**[1', 3], alum.[3], alum-sil.[1'],
alumn.[2], **am-c.,** am-m., ambr.,
anac., ang., anh.[14], ant-c.[2, 3, 8],
ant-t., aq-mar.[14], arg-m., **Arn.,**
ars., asaf., **asar.,** aur., bar-c.,
bar-m.[3], **BELL.**[1'-3, 8], bism., **bor.,**
bov., **BRY.**[1'-3, 6, 8], buth-a.[10, 14],
cadm-s.[8], **calad., calc.**[2, 3, 6], calc-f.[1'],
calc-p.[1', 3], **camph.,** cann-i.[1', 8],
cann-s., canth., caps., **carb-an.,**
carb-v., caust., cham., **chel.,** chin.,
cic., cina, coc-c.[3, 6], **cocc., coff.,**
COLCH.[2, 3, 6, 8, 14], **coloc.**[2, 3, 6], con.,
crat.[8], **croc.,** cupr., cycl., des-ac.[14],
dicha.[14], **dig.,** dros., dulc., **echi.**[3, 6],
euph., ferr., fl-ac.[3], **GELS.**[2], get.[8],
gink-b.[14], **graph., guaj.**[1'-3], guat.[14],
gymno.[8], **hell., hep.,** hydr.[1'], hyos.,
ign., **iod., ip.,** kali-bi.[1'], kali-c.,
kali-i.[1'], **kali-n.,** kali-p.[8], kalm.[1'],
kreos.[3], lac-d.[1'], lach., laur., **LED.,**
lyc., mag-c., mag-m., mag-p.[1'],
mand.[14], **mang.,** meny., **merc.**[2, 3, 8],
merc-c.[3, 8], **mez.,** mosch., mur-ac.,
nat-c., **nat-m., nit-ac., nux-m.,**
NUX-V.[2, 3, 6, 8], olnd., onop.[14], op.,
par., penic.[13], **petr.,** ph-ac.[1', 2],
penob.[13, 14], **phos.,** phyt.[8], plat.,
plb., prot.[14], pulx.[8], **ran-b., rheum,**
rhod., rhus-t., ruta, sabad., sabin.,
samb., sang.[3], **sars., sec., sel.,**
seneg., sep.[2, 3, 6], sieg.[10], sil.,
spig.[1'-3], **spong., squil.**[2, 3, 8], stann.,
staph.[2, 3, 8], **stram.,** stront-c.,
stroph-s.[14], stry-p.[8], **sul-ac.,** sulph.,
teucr., ther.[1'], thuj., trios.[14], verat.,
vib.[8], viol-t.[3], zinc.

must rest[3, 6]
doit se reposer
muß ruhen
aesc., alum., alum-sil.[1'], **anac.**[3, 6, 14],
arn., brom., **bry.,** lach., lyc., nux-v.,
op., **ph-ac.,** sabad., **stann.**

REVELING, from night
RÉJOUISSANCES NOCTURNES,
suites de
NACHTSCHWÄRMEN, Folgen von
agar.[3], ambr., ant-c., **ars.,** bry., **carb-v.,**
coff., colch., ip., **laur.,** led., nat-c.[3],
NUX-V., puls., rhus-t., sabin.[3],
staph.[3], sulph.

RICKETS[2, 3]
RACHITISME
RACHITIS
am-c.[3, 12], arg-m.[14], **ars.**[12], **ASAF.,**
bar-c.[3], **bell.,** bufo[3], **CALC.**[2, 3, 8, 10, 12],
calc-p.[2, 3, 6, 10-12], caust.[3], cic.[3], con.[2],
ferr., ferr-i.[2], ferr-m.[2, 12], ferr-p.[2],
guaj.[2], hecla[2, 12], hed.[12], **hep.,** iod.,
ip., iris[8], **kali-i.**[3, 12], lac-c.[2], **lyc.**[2, 3, 6],
MERC.[2, 3, 11, 12], mez., **nit-ac.**[2, 3, 12],
nux-m.[2], **ol-j.**[2], op.[11], petr.[3],
ph-ac.[3, 6, 10], **PHOS.**[2, 3, 8, 10, 12], plb.[3],
psor.[2], **puls.,** rhod.[3], **rhus-t.**[2], ruta,
sacch.[12], sanic.[12], **sep., SIL.**[2, 3, 8, 10, 12],
staph., sulph., tarent.[11], ther.[2, 3, 12],
thuj.[2, 3, 12]

RIDING horseback agg.
MONTER À CHEVAL agg.
REITEN agg.
arist-cl.[9], arg-n.[7], ars., **bell.,**
bor.[3, 6], bry., **graph., lil-t.,**
mag-m., meph., **nat-c.,** nat-m.[4, 16],
psor.[3], **ruta**[2, 3, 7], **SEP.,** sil., spig.,
sul-ac., ther.[12], valer.

ailments from[12]
troubles à la suite de
Beschwerden infolge von
ther.

am.
brom., calc., kali-c.[3, 6], lyc.,
tarent.[3]

cars agg., in a wagon or on the
aller en voiture ou par le train agg.
Fahren im Wagen oder mit der Bahn
agg.
acon.[6], alum-sil.[1'], **arg-m.,**
arg-n., arn., ars., asaf.[1', 3],

aur., bell.[3], berb.[3, 8], **bor.,**
bry., calc., calc-p.[3], carb-v.,
caust.[6, 8], coc-c.[3], **COCC.,**
colch.., **con.,** croc., cycl.[2, 7],
dig.[3], ferr., fl-ac.[3, 6], graph.[2, 3, 7],
grat.[3], **HELON.**[2, 7], **hep.,** hyos.,
ign., iod., iodof.[2], kali-c.,
lac-d.[7], **lach.,** lyc., **lyss.,**
mag-c., mag-s.[9, 10, 14], meph.,
nat-m., **nux-m.,** op., **PETR.,**
phos., plat., **psor.,** puls., rhus-t.,
rumx., sanic.[7, 8], **sel., SEP.,** sil.,
spig.[1'], staph., sul-ac.[3], **sulph.,**
TAB.[3, 7], **ther.,** thuj., tril.[3],
valer.

after r. agg.
après avoir été
nach dem Fahren agg.
graph., kali-n., nat-c., nat-m.,
nit-ac., plat., **SIL.**

aversion to[7]
aversion pour
Abneigung gegen
psor.

down hill agg.
descendre d'une montagne
Abwärtsfahren agg.
BOR., psor.

ailments from[12]
troubles à la suite d'
Beschwerden infolge von
lyc., petr.

am.
arg-n.[6, 7], **ars.,** bar-m.[3], brom.,
bry.[3], des-ac.[14], **gels.**[3, 6], glon.[3],
graph.[2, 3], kali-n., lyc.[3], merc.[3],
merc-c.[3], **naja**[7], nat-m.[3, 4, 16],
NIT-AC., nux-m.[6], phos., puls.[6],
thiop.[14]

ship, ailments form r. in a[12]
voyage par mer, troubles à la suite de
Seefahrt, Beschwerden infolge von
ars., petr.[1', 12] ther.

RISING UP agg.
SE LEVANT agg., en
AUFSTEHEN agg.
   ACON., aesc.[3], agar.[3], alum.,
   alum-sil.[1'], **am-m.**, ambr.[3], anac.,
   ang.[3], ant-c.[3], **ant-t.**, apis[3], arg-m.,
   arg-n.[6, 7], **arn.**, **ars.**, asar., aur.[3],
   bar-c., bar-m., bar-s.[1'], **BELL.**,
   berb.[3, 4], bov., **BRY.**, cact.,
   calad., **calc.**[3], **cann-i.**, **cann-s.**,
   canth.[3], caps., carb-an.,
   CARB-V.[3, 8], caust., **cham.**, **chel.**,
   chin., **cic.**, **cina**[3], clem.[3], **COCC.**,
   colch., coloc., **con.**, croc., **DIG.**,
   dros., dulc.[3], **euph.**[3], ferr., **fl-ac.**[3],
   graph.[3], guaj.[3], hell., hep., hyos.[3],
   ign., kali-bi.[3], kali-c., kali-m.[1'],
   kali-n.[3], kreos.[3], lach., laur., **led.**[3],
   lept.[3], **LYC.**, mag-c.[3], mag-m.,
   mang., meny., merc., merc-i-f.[3],
   mosch.[3], **mur-ac.**, **nat-c.**, **nat-m.**,
   nat-s.[3], **nit-ac.**, **NUX-V.**, olnd.[3],
   OP., osm., par.[3], **petr.**[3], ph-ac.,
   phos., phyt.[6, 8], plat., plb., psor.[1'],
   puls., rad-br.[8], ran-b., **rhod.**[3],
   RHUS-T., rumx., **ruta**[3], sabad.,
   sabin.[3], samb.[3], **sang.**, sars., **sel.**[3],
   seneg., sep., **SIL.**, **SPIG.**[3], spong.,
   squil., stann., staph., stram.,
   stront-c.[3], sul-ac., **SULPH.**, tarax.,
   thuj.[3], valer.[3], verat., verat-v.,
   viol-t., zinc.

am.
   acon., **agar.**[3], agn.[3], alum., **AM-C.**,
   am-m., **ambr.**[3, 8], anac.[3], **ang.**[3],
   ant-c.[3], **ant-t.**, arg-m.[3], ant-c.[3], **ARS.**,
   asaf., asar.[3], aur., bar-c., bell.,
   bism.[3], **bor.**, bov., bry., **CALC.**,
   cann-s., canth., **CAPS.**[3, 6], carb-an.[3],
   carb-v., caust., **cham.**, chel., chin.,
   cic., **cina**[3], cocc.[3], colch.[6], coloc.,
   con., **cupr.**, **CYCL.**[3], **dig.**, **dros.**[3],
   DULC.[3], **euph.**[3], euphr.[3], ferr.,
   graph.[3], guaj.[3], hell., hep., **hyos.**,
   ign., iod.[3], **kali-c.**, kali-n.[3, 6], kreos.[3],
   lach.[3], laur., led.[3, 6], lith-c.[8], **lyc.**,
   mag-c., **mag-m.**[3], mang., **meny.**[3],
   merc., mez.[3], mosch., **mur-ac.**[3], naja,
   nat-c., nat-m., nit-ac.[3], nux-m.,
   nux-v., olnd., op.[3], par.[3], parth.[8],
   petr., **ph-ac.**[3, 4, 6], phos., **PLAT.**[3, 16],

plb.[3], puls., **rhod.**[3], rhus-t., **ruta**[3],
sabad.[3], sabin., **SAMB.**, sars.[3], sel.[3],
seneg.[3], **SEP.**, **sil.**, spig., spong.[3],
squil., stann., staph.[3], sul-ac.,
sulph., **tarax.**[3], teucr., thuj.[3],
valer.[3], **verat.**[3], **VERB.**[3], viol-o.[3],
VIOL-T.[3], zinc.[3]

ROOM full of people agg.
CHAMBRE remplie de monde, agg.
dans une
ZIMMER agg., **volles**
   ambr., ant-c., apis[1', 3], **arg-n.**, ars.,
   bar-c., carb-an., con., **hell.**,
   iod.[1', 3, 6], kali-i.[1', 3, 6], lil-t.[1', 3],
   lyc., **mag-c.**, nat-c., nat-m., petr.,
   phos., plb., puls., sabin., **sep.**,
   stann., stram., **sulph.**

   Vol. I: *fear – narrow place – trains/*
   Furcht – Menschenmenge

close r. agg.[5]
fermée agg.
geschlossenes Z. agg.
   alum.[1'], arist-cl.[14], ars-i.[1'] bar-s.[1'],
   nux-v., puls., rauw.[14], staph.,
   sulph., tub.[7]

   Vol. I: *fear – narrow place – trains/*
   peur – claustrophobie – trains/
   Furcht – engem Raum – Zügen

RUBBING agg.
FROTTEMENT agg.
REIBEN agg.
   am-m., **ANAC.**, arn., ars., **bism.**,
   bor., **calad.**, calc., cann-s., canth.,
   caps., carb-an., **caust.**, cham., chel.,
   coff., **CON.**, cupr., dros., guaj.,
   kreos., **led.**, mag-c., mang., merc.,
   mez., mur-ac., nat-c., par., ph-ac.,
   phos.[2, 3], **PULS.**, seneg., **SEP.**, **sil.**,
   spig., spong., squil., stann., staph.,
   stram. **STRONT-C.**, **SULPH.**,
   thuj.[3]

am.

    acon., agar., agn., **alum., alumn.**[2],
    am-c., **am-m.**, ambr., anac.,
    ang.[2, 3], ant-c., ant-t., **arn., ars.,**
    asaf., bell., bell-p.[10], benz-ac.[2],
    bor., bov., bry., **CALC.**, calc-f.[7],
    camph., cann-s., **CANTH.**, caps.,
    CARB-AC., carb-an., cast.[3, 6],
    caust., cedr., chel., chin., cic.,
    cina, colch., croc.[3], **cupr.**[3], **cycl.,**
    dios., **dros.**, form.[8], **guaj.**, ham.,
    hed.[10, 14], hep., **ign.**, indg.[4, 8],
    iod.[10], kali-c., kali-m.[1'], kali-n.,
    kreos., laur., lil-t., mag-c.,
    mag-m., **mag-p.**[3, 8], mang., meny.,
    merc., mim-p.[14], mosch., **mur-ac.,**
    NAT-C., nit-ac., **nux-v.,**
    OL-AN.[1, 7], olnd., osm., pall.,
    ph-ac., **PHOS.**, plat., **PLB.,**
    podo.[3, 8], puls.[3, 10], ran-b.,
    rhus-t., **ruta**, sabad., sabin.,
    samb., sars., sec., sel., seneg.,
    sep.[3], sil.[3], spig., spong., stann.,
    staph., sul-ac., **sulph.**, tarax.,
    tarent.[1', 3, 6-8], **thuj.**, valer.,
    verat-v.[3, 6], viol-t., **zinc.**, zinc-p.[1'],

clothes am., of[3]
habits am., par f. des
Kleidung am., der
    bufo

gently agg., stroking
légèrement agg., caresser
leise streicheln agg.
    teucr.

but hard r. am.[3]
mais pression forte am.
aber hartes R. am.
    rhus-t.

with hand am.[2]
avec la main am.
mit der Hand am.
    arn., **asaf.**, CALC., caps., cina,
    croc., **CYCL.**, dros., guaj., ign.,
    mang., meny., **merc., mur-ac.,**
    NAT-C., phos., plb., puls., ruta,
    sulph., **thuj.**, zinc.

RUNNING agg.
COURIR agg.
LAUFEN, Rennen agg.
    alum., alumn.[2], **ang.**[2, 3], arg-m., **arn.,**
    ARS., ars-i., ars-s-f.[1'], aur., aur-ar.[1'],
    aur-i.[1'], aur-s.[1'], **bell.**, bor., **BRY.,**
    calc., **cann-s., caust.**, chel., chin.,
    cina, **cocc.**, coff., **con.**, croc.,
    cupr., dros., **ferr.**, ferr-ar.[1'], hep.,
    hyos., **ign.**, iod., ip., **kali-c.**, laur.,
    led., lyc., merc., mez., nat-c.,
    nat-m., nit-ac., nux-m. **nux-v.,**
    olnd., phos., plb., **PULS.**, rheum,
    rhod., rhus-t., ruta, sabin., **seneg.,**
    sep., **sil., spig.**, spong., squil.,
    staph., sul-ac., **SULPH.**, verat.,
    zinc.

walking – fast/marcher – vite/
    Gehen – schnelles

am.
    ars.[3], brom.[3], caust., fl-ac.[3], graph.[3],
    ign., nat-m., nit-ac.[3], **SEP.**, sil.,
    stann., sul-ac.[3], tarent.[3], thlas.[3]

SALT abusus[12]
SEL, abus de
SALZ, Mißbrauch von
    nit-s-d., phos.

SARCOMA
SARCOME
SARKOM
    bar-c., calc-f., carb-ac.[2], **crot-h.**[2],
    cupr-s.[7], graph.[2], hecla[2, 7, 12], **kali-m.**[2],
    lap-a.[2, 7]

SCARLET fever, after
SCARLATINE, troubles à la suite de
SCHARLACH, Folgekrankheiten von
    AM.C.[3], **AM-M.**, aur., bar-c., **BELL.,**
    bry., calc., carb-ac., carb-v.,
    CHAM., con.[3], dulc., euph., **hep.,**
    hyos., **lach.**, lyc., **merc.**, nit-ac.,
    petros.[12], phos., rhus-t., **sulph.**

exanthema repelled[4]
exanthème supprimé, avec
Exanthem, bei unterdrücktem
    phos.

glands swollen[15]
glandes, tuméfaction des
Drüsenschwellungen
   am-c.

SCLEROSIS, multiple[7]
SCLÉROSE en plaques disséminées
SKLEROSE, multiple
   alum.[8], arg-m.[14], arg-n., **aur.**, aur-m.[12],
   bar-c., bell.[8], calc., cann-i.[8], carbn-s.[12],
   caust., **con.**[8], des-ac.[14], gels., halo.[14],
   hyosin.[12], irid.[8], **lath.**[7, 8, 12], lyc.,
   mand.[14], nux-v., **phos.**[7, 8], **phys.**[7, 8, 12],
   pic-ac.[8, 12], **plb.**[2, 7, 8], psil.[14], sil., sulph.,
   tarent.[7, 12], thala.[14], thuj., wildb.[12],
   xan.[8]

SCURVY, scorbutus
SCORBUT
SKORBUT
   acet-a.[8], agav-a.[8, 12], agn.[1] (non: ang.),
   all-s.[12], alum., alumn.[12], **am-c.,**
   am-m.[12], ambr., ant-c., arg-m.,
   aran.[2, 12], **ars.**[1], ars-i., arum-m.[12], aur.,
   bell., bor., bov., brass.[12], bry., **calc.,**
   canth., caps., **carb-an., CARB-V.,**
   cary.[12], caust., cetr.[12], chin., cic.,
   cist., cit-ac.[11], cit-l.[12], cit-v.,
   coca[12], coch.[12], con., **dulc.,** elat.[12],
   graph., **ham.**[12], **hep., iod.,** jug-r.[12],
   kali-c., kali-chl.[12], **kali-m.**[2, 3, 12], kali-n.,
   kali-p.[2], kreos., lach.[12], lyc., mag-m.,
   MERC., MUR-AC., nat-hchls.[12],
   nat-m., nit-ac., nux-m., **NUX-V.,**
   petr., ph-ac., phos., plb.[11], psor.[12],
   rat.[12], rhus-t., ruta, sabin., sacch.[11, 12],
   sanic.[12], sep., **sil.,** sin-n.[12], sol-t-ae.[12],
   stann., **STAPH.,** sul-ac., **sulph.,** tep.[12],
   zinc.

seashore see air–seashore

SEASONS/SAISONS/JAHRESZEITEN

autumn, agg. in
automne, agg. en
Herbst, agg. im
   all-c.[12], **ant-t.,** aur., bapt.,
   bar-m., bry., **calc.,** calc-p.[3, 6, 7],
   chin., cic., **colch.**[1, 7], coloc.[3],

dulc.[1', 3, 7], **graph.**[1, 7], hed.[10], hep.,
   ign.[3, 6, 7], iris[3, 7], **KALI-BI.**[1, 7],
   LACH., merc.[1, 7], merc-c.[3, 7],
   nat-m.[3, 6, 7], nux-v., rhod.[7, 12],
   RHUS-T., stram., verat.

ailments since[12]
troubles depuis l'
Beschwerden seit
   kali-bi.

am.[14]
   flav.

springs, agg. in*
printemps, agg. en
Frühling, agg. im
   acon., all-c.[3, 7, 8, 12], **AMBR.**[1, 7],
   ant-t., apis, ars-br.[8], **aur.**[1', 7],
   bar-m., **BELL.**[1, 7], brom.[1', 7],
   bry.[1, 7], **CALC.**[1, 7], calc-p.[3, 6-8],
   carb-v.[1, 7], **cench., chel.,** cina[16],
   colch., con.[12], **crot-h.**[1', 3, 4, 6-8],
   dulc., **GELS.**[2, 3, 7, 8], ham.[3], hed.[10],
   hep., **iris, kali-bi., LACH.,**
   LYC.[1, 7], merc-i-f.[12], nat-c.[3, 7],
   nat-m.[1, 7], **nat-s.,** nit-s-d.[7, 8],
   nux-v., **puls.,** rhod.[7, 12], **rhus-t.,**
   sars.[1, 7], sec., sel.[3], **sep.**[1, 7], **sil.**[1, 7],
   sulph.[1, 7], urt-u.[3], **verat.**

ailments since[12]
troubles depuis le
Beschwerden seit
   con., kali-bi., merc-i-f.

am.[14]
   flav.

summer, agg. in
été, agg. en
Sommer, agg. im
   acon.[1', 8], **aeth.,** aloe[3, 6-8], **alum.,**
   alum-sil.[1'], **ANT-C.**[1, 7], apis[3, 6, 7],
   arg-n., ars-i., bapt.[2, 7], bar-c.,
   BELL.[1, 7], bor., bov.[2, 3, 7],
   brom.[1', 7], **BRY.**[1, 7], calc.[3],
   CAMPH.[2, 7], **CARB-V.**[1, 7],
   carbn-s., cham., **chion.,** cina[3, 6, 7],
   cinnb., coff.[1'], croc.[8], crot-h.[3, 6, 8],
   crot-t.[7, 8], cupr.[3, 6, 7], dulc.[3],
   FL-AC., gamb.[2, 7], **GELS.**[2-3, 7, 8],

GLON.[1'-3, 6-8], graph., **guaj., iod.,**
iris[3, 7], **KALI-BI.,** kali-br.[7],
kali-c.[6, 7], kali-i.[3], **LACH.**[1, 7],
lyc.[1, 7], mur-ac.[3, 7], **NAT-C.**[1, 7],
nat-m., nit-ac.[8], nux-m.[3, 7],
nux-v., ph-ac.[3, 7], **phos.**[3, 7, 8],
pic-ac.[8], **PODO.**[3, 6-8, 12], **psor.,**
PULS.[1, 7], rheum[7], rhod.[3, 6, 7],
sabin.[8], **sel.,** sep.[3, 6, 7], sin-n.[12],
sul-i.[1'], syph.[1', 7, 8], thuj.,
verat.[2, 7], verat-v.[3, 7]

ailments since[12]
troubles depuis l'
Beschwerden seit
  podo., sin-n.

am.[3]
  aesc.[3, 7], alum.[8], ars-i., aur.[8],
  aur-ar.[1'], calc-p.[8], calc-sil.[1'],
  caust.[7], ferr.[8], kali-sil.[13], **petr.,**
  psor., sil.[7, 8], stront-c.[3, 6]

children, in[7]
enfants, chez les
Kindern, bei
  ip.

cool days in, after[2, 7]
fraîches, troubles en été après des
  journées
kühlen Tagen im, Beschwerden
  nach
  BRY.

summer solstice agg.[7]
solstice d'été agg.
Sommersonnenwende agg.
  apis., **BELL.,** brom., **bry., carb-v.,**
  gels, iris, **kali-bi., LACH.,** lyc.,
  nat-c., **nat-m.,** nux-v., **puls.,** rhod.,
  sep., **verat.**

winter, agg. in ✳
hiver, agg. en
Winter, agg. im
  ACON.[1, 7], **aesc., agar., alum.,**
  AM-C.[1, 7], ammc., **arg-m.,**
  ARS.[1, 7], **AUR.,** aur-ar.[1'], aur-s.[1'],
  bar-c.[1, 7], **bell.,** bor.[7], bov.,
  BRY.[1, 7], **calc., calc-p.,** calc-sil.[1'],
  CAMPH.[1, 7], **caps.**[1, 7], carb-an.,

carb-v.[1, 7], carbn-s.[1'], **caust.,**
cham.[1', 7], cic., cina, cist.[3, 7],
coc-c., cocc.[1, 7], colch., **con.**[1, 7],
DULC.[1, 7], **ferr.,** ferr-ar., **FL-AC.,**
graph.[1', 3, 7], **HELL.**[1, 7], **HEP.**[1, 7],
hyos.[1, 7], **ign.**[1, 7], **ip.**[1, 7], **kali-bi.,**
KALI-C.[1, 7], **kali-p.,** kali-sil.[1'],
kalm.[3, 7], **LYC.**[1, 7], mag-c.,
MANG.[1, 7], **merc., mez.,**
MOSCH.[1, 7], nat-ar., nat-c.,
nat-m., **NUX-M.**[1, 7], **NUX-V.,**
PETR.[1, 7], ph-ac., **phos.,** prot.[14],
PSOR.[1, 7], **PULS.**[1, 7], rhod.[1, 7],
RHUS-T., ruta, **sabad.,**
sang-n.[7, 12], sars., sec.[3], **sep., sil.,**
spig., spong., stann.[3, 7],
STRONT-C.[1, 7], **sulph.**[1, 7],
syph.[1', 7], **VERAT.**[1, 7], viol-t.

ailments since[12]
troubles depuis l'
Beschwerden seit
  sang-n.

am.[1']
  glon., ilx-a.[8], ilx-c.[2, 7], sul-i.

winter solstice agg.[7]
solstice d'hiver agg.
Wintersonnenwende agg.
  aur., bry., **calc.,** calc-p., cic.,
  colch., **dulc.,** graph., hep., ign.,
  kali-bi., merc., nat-m., nux-v.,
  rhod., RHUS-T., verat.,

SEDENTARY habits[8, 12]
SÉDENTAIRES, par habitudes
SITZENDE Lebensweise, durch
  acon., aloe, alum.[5, 12], am-c.[7, 8, 12],
  anac.[7, 8, 12], arg-n.[8], ars.[16], asar.[12],
  bry.[5, 8], **calc.**[5, 12], cocc.[12], con., **lyc.**[5],
  nat-m.[12], **NUX-V.**[3, 5, 7, 8, 12], petr.[12],
  rhus-t.[5], sep., sil.[12], staph.[5],
  sulph.[1', 3, 12], ter.[12]

SENSITIVENESS externally
SENSIBILITÉ externe
EMPFINDLICHKEIT, äußerliche
  acon., aesc., agar., ail.[12], aloe,
  alum., alum-p.[1'], alum-sil.[1'], am-c.,
  am-m., ambr., ang.[3], ant-c., ant-t.,

APIS, arg-m., ARN., ars., asaf., aur., aur-ar.[1'], bapt., bar-c., bar-s.[1'], BELL., bor., bov., bry., calc., calc-p., calc-sil.[1'], camph., cann-s., canth., caps., carb-an., carb-v., caust., chel.[1'], CHIN., CHIN-S., cimic., cina, clem., coc-c., coff., colch., coloc., con., crot-c., cupr., dig., euph-pi.[12], ferr., ferr-p., gels., glon.[12], graph.[1'], ham.[1'], hell., hep., hist.[10], hyos., ign., ip., kali-bi., kali-c., kali-i.[12], kali-n., kali-p., kali-s., kreos., LACH., led., lyc., mag-c., mag-m., menth., meny.[3], merc., merc-c.[3], mez., mosch., mur-ac.[3], nat-ar., nat-c., nat-m., NAT-P., nat-s.[1'], nat-sil.[1'] nit-ac., nux-m., NUX-V., olnd., op., par., petr., ph-ac., PHOS., plb., psor., PULS., RAN-B., ran-s., rhus-t., sabad., sabin., sal-ac., sars., sec., sel., seneg., sep., SIL., SPIG., spong., squil., stann., STAPH., stront-c., sul-ac., sulph., teucr., thuj., valer.[1'], verat., zinc.

internally
interne
innerliche
acon., agar., **alum.**, alum-p.[1'], alum-sil.[1'], **am-c.**, ant-c., ant-t., apis, arn., **ars.**, ars-i., asaf., **asar.**, aur., aur-ar.[1'], **bapt.**, bar-c., **bell.**, bism., **bor.**, bov., **bry.**, calad., **calc.**, cann-s., CANTH., **carb-an.**, carb-v., carbn-s., caust., **cham.**, chin., cic., cimic.[1'], **clem.**, coc-c., **cocc.**, coff., colch., **coloc.**, con., croc., crot-h., cub., cupr., cycl., dulc., **equis.**, ferr., **graph.**, hell., helon., HEP., hyos.[1], **iod.**, ip., **kali-bi.**, **kali-i.**, kali-p., LACH., laur., led., **lil-t.**, mag-c., **mag-m.**, mang., meny., merc., **merc-c.**, **mez.**, mosch., nat-ar., **nat-c.**, NAT-M., **nit-ac.**, **nux-v.**, olnd., **osm.**, par., PHOS., puls., ran-b., rhus-t., **ruta**, sars., **sec.**, sel., seneg., sep., SIL., spong., **squil.**, stann., **stram.**, stront-c., sul-ac., sulph., tarax., tarent., teucr., thuj., valer., verat., zinc.

pain, to
douleur, à la
Schmerzempfindlichkeit
acon., agar., alum., am-c., ambr., anac., ang.[3], ant-c., ant-t., arg-n.[3], arn., ars., ars-i., ars-s-f.[1'], asaf.[1'], asar., AUR., aur-ar.[1'], aur-m.[8], aur-s.[1'], bar-c., bar-i.[1'], bar-s.[1'], bell., bry., cact., calad., calc., calc-p., calc-sil.[1'], camph., cann-s., canth., caps., carb-an., carb-v., carbn-s.[1', 7], CHAM., chin., chin-ar., cimic.[3], cina, cocc., COFF., colch., con., cupr., dig., ferr., ferr-ar.[1'], ferr-p., graph., hell., HEP., hyos., hyper.[8], IGN., iod., ip., kali-ar., kali-c., kali-m.[1'], kali-p., lac-c.[3], LACH., lact.[10], laur., led., LYC., mag-c., mag-m., mag-p.[3, 6, 8], MED., meli.[8], merc., mez.[8], morph.[2, 8, 10], mosch.[8], mur-ac., nat-c., nat-p., nat-s.[1', 7], NIT-AC., nux-m., NUX-V., olnd., petr., ph-ac., PHOS., phyt., plat.[3], plb., PSOR., PULS., ran-s.[8], rhus-t., sabad., sabin., sars., sel., seneg., SEP., SIL., spig., squil., STAPH., stram.[3, 6], sulph., thuj., tub., valer., verat., vesp., viol-o., zinc., zinc-p.[1'], zinc-val.[8]

Vol. I: *sensitive – pain/sensible – douleurs/empfindlich – Schmerzen*

bones, of
os, des
Knochen, der
asaf., aur., bell., bry., bufo[2], calc., carb-an., chel., chin., chin-s., cupr., EUP-PER., guaj., hyper., kali-bi.[3], lach., lyc., merc., merc-c., mez., nat-c., nat-sil.[1'], PHOS., puls., rhus-t., sil., stram., sulph., symph.[3], TELL., zinc.

pain – bones/douleurs – os/ Schmerzen – Knochen

cartilages, of
cartilages, des
Knorpel, der
   ARG-M.

*pain – cartilages/douleurs –
   cartilages/Schmerzen – Knorpel*

glands, of
glandes, des
Drüsen, der
   arn., **aur.,** aur-s.[1]', **BAR-C.,** bar-i.[1]',
   bell., **cham.,** chin., cimic.[1]', clem.,
   cocc., **CON.,** crot-h., cupr., graph.,
   hep., ign., kali-c., laur., **lyc.,**
   mag-c., nat-c.; nat-sil.[1]', nit-ac.,
   nux-v., petr., ph-ac., **PHOS.,** puls.,
   sep., sil., spig., squil., sul-ac., zinc.

*pain – glands/douleurs – glandes/
   Schmerzen – Drüsen*

periosteum
périoste, du
Periost, des
   acon.[3], ant-c., aur., bell., **bry., chin.,**
   chin-s.[3], ign., **LED.,** mang.[3], merc.,
   merc-c.[3], **mez.,** nit-ac.[3], **ph-ac.,**
   puls., rhus-t., ruta, sil., spig.,
   staph., symph.[12], tell.[3]

*pain – periosteum/douleurs –
   périoste/Schmerzen – Periost*

SEPTICAEMIA, blood-poisoning
SEPTICÉMIE, empoisonnement du sang
SEPSIS, Blutvergiftung
   achy.[14], acon.[8], agar.[12], ail.[1', 6],
   am-c.[1', 6, 10], anthraci., ap-v.[8], **apis,**
   arg-m.[14], arg-n., **arn., ARS.,**
   ars-i.[6, 8], arum-t.[6], atro.[8], **bapt.,**
   bell.[6, 8], bor-ac.[12], both.[8], **bry** bufo[6],
   calc.[1', 2, 7], calc-ar.[6, 7], calen.[8],
   carb-ac.[6, 8], **CARB-V., cench.,**
   chin.[10], **chin-ar.**[6, 8, 10], **chin-s.**[8, 10, 12],
   chlorpr.[14], colch.[6], conch.[12],
   CROT-H., dor.[6], **echi.**[3, 6-8, 10, 12],
   elaps[6], **ferr.,** ferr-p.[6], gels.[6], gunp.[8],
   hell.[6], **hippoz.,** hydroph.[14], hyos.[6, 8],
   ip.[6, 10], irid.[8], kali-bi.[2, 6], kali-c.[6],
   kali-p., kreos.[6], **LACH.,** lat-h.[8],

lob-p.[12], **lyc.,** mag-c.[10], **merc.**[8, 12],
merc-cy.[3, 6, 8], methyl.[8], mur-ac.[6, 8],
naja[6], nat-s-c.[8], **nit-ac.**[6], op.[6],
paro-i.[14], ph-ac.[6], **phos.,** phyt.[6],
puls., PYROG., rad-br.[7], raja-s.[14],
rhus-t., sal-ac.[2], **sec.**[6, 8], sieg.[10], sil.[8],
stram.[1', 6], streptoc.[8], sul-ac.[6],
sulfonam.[14], **sulph.,** tarax.[6], tarent.,
tarent-c.[6, 8], **ter.**[3, 6], trach.[12],
verat.[2, 3, 6, 8, 12], **verat-v.**[3, 6, 10],
vip.[6], zinc.[6]

ailments from[12]
troubles à la suite de
Beschwerden infolge von
   agar., gunp., lob-p., pyrog., tarent.

SEXUAL excesses, after*
SEXUELS, par **excès**
SEXUELLEN Ausschweifungen, Folgen
von
   acon., **AGAR.,** agn., alum.,
   alum-p.[1'], anac., ant-c., arg-n.[7, 12],
   arn., **ars.,** asaf., aur., aur-ar.[1'],
   aven.[8, 12], bar-c., bell., bor.,
   bov., bry., **calad.**[1, 7], **CALC.,**
   calc-p.[12], **calc-s.,** cann-s., canth.,
   caps., carb-an., **CARB-V.**[1], caust.,
   cham., **chin., chin-ar.,** cina,
   cocc., coff., **CON., dig.,** digin.[8],
   dulc., ferr., ferr-pic.[12], **gels.,**
   graph., ign., **iod.,** ip.[1], **kali-br.,**
   kali-c., kali-n., **KALI-P.,** led., **lil-t.,**
   LYC., lyss.[8], mag-m., **merc.,** mez.,
   mosch., nat-c., NAT-M., NAT-P.,
   nit-ac., NUX-V., ol-an.[6], onos.[12],
   op., petr., **PH-AC., PHOS.,** plat.,
   plb., **puls.,** ran-b., rhod., rhus-t.,
   ruta, sabad., samb., sec., **SEL., SEP.,**
   SIL., spig., squil., stann., **STAPH.,**
   SULPH., symph.[12], thuj.,trib.[8],
   upa.[12], valer., zinc., zinc-p.[1']

excitement agg.
excitation sexuelle agg.
Erregung agg., sexuelle
   agar.[1'], arg-n.[12], arn.[12], **bufo.,**
   calc.[2], cinch.[12], gins.[12], kali-p.[12],
   LIL-T., sars., sep.[1'], staph.[12]

drunkenness, s. e. during[5]
ivresse, e. s. pendant l'
Trunkenheit, s. E. bei
   canth., **caust.**, chin., nux-v., phos.

suppression of s. desire agg.
suppression de désir sexuel agg.
Unterdrückung des s. Verlangens
agg.
   agn.[3, 6], **APIS**, bell.[3], berb.,
   calc., **CAMPH.**, **carb-v.**[2, 3],
   carbn-o., **CON.**, graph.[3, 6], **hell.**,
   hyos.[3], **kali-br.**[2], kali-p.[12], **lil-t.**,
   lyc.[3, 7], mosch.[2], orig.[7], **ph-ac.**,
   phos.[3, 6], pic-ac., plat., **PULS.**,
   staph.[3, 6], stram.[3]

ailments from[12]
troubles à la suite de
Beschwerden infolge von
   con., kali-p.

am.
   calad.

climacteric period, during[7]
ménopause, pendant la
Klimakterium, im
   con.

SEWER-GAS poisoning[12]
GAZ MÉPHITIQUES des égouts,
empoisonnement par les
FAULSCHLAMMGASVERGIFTUNG
   bapt., phyt., pyrog., **tub.**[7]

SHAVING agg.[3]
SE RASER agg.
SICH-RASIEREN agg.
   ant-c., aur., caps.[3, 6, 8], **carb-an.**[3, 6, 8],
   hep., kalm., mang., ox-ac.[3, 8],
   ph-ac., phos., plb.[8], **PULS.**, rad-br.[3],
   stroph-s.[15]

   am.[3, 6, 8]
   brom.

SHINING objects, ailments from[6]
BRILLANTS, troubles par des
objets
GLÄNZENDEN Gegenständen, Beschwerden infolge von
   bell., canth., glon., hyos., stram.

Vol. I: *shining/brillants/glänzende*

SHOCK agg.[3]
CHOC agg.
SCHOCK agg.
   acet-ac., **acon.**[3, 12], am-c., arn.,
   camph., cham., cic., coff., gels.,
   hep., hyos., hyper.[3, 12], mag-c.[12],
   merc., nat-m., op., ph-ac.[12], puls.,
   sec., stram.[12], stront-c., sulph.,
   verat.

injury see shock–injury

electric-like
électrique, comme un
elektrischer Schlag, wie ein
   acon., **agar.**, ail., alum., alum-p.[1'],
   ambr., anac., ang., apis,
   aran-ix.[10], **ARG-M.**, **arg-n.**, arn.,
   ARS., ars-s-f.[1'], **art-v.**, bar-c.,
   bar-m., bar-s.[1'], bell., bufo,
   calad., calc., **calc-p.**, **camph.**,
   cann-s., carb-ac., carb-v., caust.,
   cic., cimic., **cina**, **clem.**, **cocc.**,
   colch., con., croc., cupr., **dig.**,
   dulc., **fl-ac.**, graph., hell., hep.,
   hydr-ac.[6], kali-c., kreos., **laur.**,
   lyc., mag-m., manc., mang.,
   meph.[11], mez., mur-ac., nat-ar.,
   nat-c., **nat-m.**, nat-p., **nit-ac.**,
   nux-m., **nux-v.**, ol-an., olnd.,
   op.[3], ox-ac.[6], **phos.**, plat., plb.[6, 11],
   puls., **ran-b.**, **ruta**, sang.[6], sep.,
   spig., squil., stram., **stry.**, sul-ac.,
   sulph., sumb., **tab.**, **thal.**, thuj.[3],
   valer.[1', 6], **VERAT.**, verat-v.[6],
   xan., zinc., zinc-p.[1']

right side of body
côté droit du corps
rechte Körperseite
   agar.

morning[16]/matin/morgens
 mang.

evening in bed[16]
soir au lit
abends im Bett
 sulph.

concussion of brain, from
commotion du cerveau, par
Commotio cerebri, durch
 CIC.

 ailments–commotion of brain

convulsions, before
convulsions, avant
Konvulsionen, vor
 bar-m., laur.

 interrupted by painful shocks
 interrompues par chocs
  douloureux
 unterbrochen durch schmerzhafte
  Schläge
  stry.

epilepsy, before
épileptique, avant une attaque
epileptischen Anfall, vor einem
 ars.

lying, while
couché, étant
Liegen, im
 clem.

motion, on beginning of
mouvement, au commencement du
Bewegung, im Anfang der
 arg-n.

 during/pendant le/bei
  colch.[7], graph.

rest, during,
repos, pendant le
Ruhe, in der
 graph.

return of senses, on
en reprenant conscience
Wiedererlangen des Bewußtseins,
 bei
 cic.

sleep, during
sommeil, pendant le
Schlaf, im
 arg-m., ars., iod.[11], kreos., lyc.,
 mez.[16], **nat-m., nux-m.**

 *jerking – sleep/tressaille-
  ments – sommeil/
  Zuckungen – Schlaf*

 on going to
 en s'endormant
 beim Einschlafen
  agar., alum., **ARG-M., ARS.,**
  bell., calc.[16], **ip.,** kali-c.[16],
  nat-ar., **nat-m., nit-ac., phos.,**
  stry., thuj.[16]

slow pulse, with
lent, avec pouls
langsamem Puls, mit
 dig.

touched, when[7]
touche, quand on le
Berührung, bei
 colch.

touching anything
touchant qc., en
berührt, wenn man etwas
 alum.

waking, while
réveil, au
Erwachen, beim
 alum-p.[1'], lyc., **mag-m.,** manc.

wide awake, while
réveillé, étant tout à fait
Wachsein, während des
 mag-m., nat-p.

injury, from
traumatismes, par
Verletzungen, durch
acet-ac.[2], **ACON.,** am-c., **ARN.,**
ars.[2], bell., **calc.**[2], calen.[7],
CAMPH., caps., carb-v., cham.,
chin.[2], chlf.[2], cic., cocc., **coff.,**
cupr., cupr-ar.[6], **DIG.**[2], **gels.,**
hell.[2], hep.[2], **hydr-ac.**[2], hyos.[6],
HYPER., ip., LACH., laur.[2], lyc.[2],
merc., **nat-m.**[2], nit-ac.[2], **nux-m.**[2],
nux-v.[2], **OP., phos.**[2], psor., **ran-b.,**
sec., sep.[2], **staph.,** stront-c.,
stry-p.[6], sulph., **tab.**[2], **VERAT.**

faintness–injury/
évanouissement–choc/
Ohnmacht–Verletzungsschock
injuries/traumatismes/
Verletzungen

fractures, from[7]
fractures, par
Frakturen, durch
acon., arn.

SHORTENED muscles and tendons
RACCOURCIS, muscles et tendons
VERKÜRZTE Muskeln und Sehnen
abrot.[6], ambr., am-c., **am-caust.**[6],
AM-M., anac., ars., aur., **bar-c.,** calc.,
carb-an., carb-v., **CAUST.,** cic., **cimic.,**
coff.[6], **COLOC.,** con., cupr., dig., dros.,
ferr.[6], form.[6], **GRAPH., guaj.,** hell.,
hep., hyos., iod.[6], kali-c., kali-i.[6],
kreos., lach., led., **lyc.,** mag-c., **merc.,**
mez., mosch., **nat-c., NAT-M.,** nit-ac.,
nux-v., olnd.[6], ox-ac., petr., ph-ac.,
phos., plb., puls., ran-b., rheum,
rhus-t., ruta, samb., sec.[6], **sep.,** sil.,
stann., sul-ac., sulph., tell.[6]

SHOT rolling through the arteries,
sensation
GRENAILLES roulant dans les artères,
sensation de
SCHROTKUGELN durch die Arterien
rollen, als ob
nat-p.

SHRIVELLLING
RIDÉ
RUNZLIGWERDEN, Runzeln
abrot.[6], alum.[6], am-c.[4], am-m., ambr.[4],
ant-c.[4, 6], **arg-n.,** arn., **bar-c.**[6], bism.,
bor.[3, 6], bry.[4], **calc.**[1', 4, 6], camph.[4],
cham.[4], chin., cupr., fl-ac.[6], hell.[4],
graph.[4, 6], kali-br.[6], **lyc.**[4-6], merc.,
mur-ac.[4], nux-v.[6], op.[6], ph-ac.[4], plb.[4],
psor.[1'], rheum[4, 6], rhod., rhus-t.[4],
sabad.[4], **sars.**[1', 4], **sec.**[1', 4, 6], **sep.**[1', 4, 6],
sil.[5], spig.[4], stram.[4, 6], **sulph.**[1', 4-6],
verat., viol-o.[4, 6], vip.[4], zinc.

SHUDDERING, nervous
FRISSONNEMENT, grelottement nerveux
SCHAUDERN, nervöses
absin.[11], acon., acon-l.[11], aether[11],
agar.[11], aloe[11], anac., **am-m., ARN.,**
ars.[3], asar.[11, 16], aur., **bell.,** benz-ac.,
blatta-a.[11], bond.[11], bor.[11], **brom.**[11],
bry.[11], caj.[11], calc., camph., cann-s.,
caps.[11], caust., cham.[3, 11], **cimic.**[2, 3, 15],
cina, clem.[11], **cocc.,** cupr.,
cupr-s.[11], cycl.[11], dig.[11], digin.[11],
dios.[3, 11], dros.[11], dulc.[11], elae.[11],
elaps.[11], eup-per.[11], euph.[11],
gast.[11], **gels.,** gins.[11], glon.[3], graph.[11],
haem.[11], hell.[3, 11], hura[11], hydr-ac.[11],
hyos., **hyper.**[3], ign.[3, 11], ip.[11],
iris-fl.[11], junc-e.[11], kali-c.[11],
kali-chl.[11], kali-n.[11], kalm.[11], kiss.[11],
kreos., **lach.**[11], laur., **led.,** linu-c.[11],
lyc., mag-m., mag-s.[11], mang.,
merc.[11], merc-i-r.[11], merc-sul.[11],
mez., morph.[11], mosch.[3, 11], **nat-m.,**
nit-ac.[11], nux-m., **NUX-V.,** op.[11],
osm.[11], ped.[11], ph-ac., phos., phys.[3],
phyt.[11], plat.[11], plb.[11], podo.[11],
polyp-p.[11], **puls.,** ran-b.[3], raph.[11],
rheum[3, 11], **rhus-t.,** ruta[11], samb.[11],
scroph-n.[11], seneg., sep., **sil.,**
sin-n.[11], **spig.,** stann.[11], staph.,
stram.[11], tab.[11], tarent.[11], thuj.[3, 11],
til.[11], upa.[11], valer., verat., viol-t.,
vip.[11], zinc.[3, 11], zinc-s.[11]

morning from rising from bed[16]
matin en se levant
morgens beim Aufstehen
coloc., rhus-t.

alternating with heat[11]
alternant avec chaleur
abwechselnd mit Hitze
  bol-la., mang., merc., puls., raph.,
  stry., tab.

asleep, when falling[11]
s'endormant, en
Einschlafen, beim
  am-c., **BELL.,** calc., ign., merc-c.,
  mez., rhus-t.

bruised, if[3]
meurtri, quand
gequetscht, wenn
  spig.

cold air, in[16]
froid air, en
kalter Luft, in
  cham.

dinner, before[11]
déjeuner, avant le
Mittagessen, vor dem
  ars., cann-i., grat., sulph.

drawing pain in abdomen, with[16]
tiraillantes dans le ventre, avec
  douleurs
ziehenden Schmerzen im Abdomen,
  mit
  nit-ac.

drinking, when[11]
buvant, en
Trinken, beim
  ars., calen.

  after[11]/après avoir bu/nach
  caps., carb-ac.[3]', chin., elaps,
  lyc., nux-v., verat.

  agg.[3]: carb-ac.

eating, when[11]
mangeant, en
Essen, beim
  cham., lyc.[11, 16], staph.

  after[11]/après avoir mangé/nach
  dem
  digin., ign., lyc.[16], rhus-t.[16],
  sulph.[16], tab.

emotions agg.[3]
émotions agg.
Gefühlserregungen agg.
  asar.

emptiness in stomach, after[16]
vide dans l'estomac, après
  sensation de
Leeregefühl im Magen, nach
  phos.

epileptic convulsions, before[15]
épileptique, avant une attaque
epileptischen Anfällen, vor
  cupr.

eructations, with[16]
renvois, avec
Aufstoßen, mit
  ip.

headache, from[16]
maux de tête, par
Kopfschmerzen, durch
  bor., sars.

lying down, on[11]
s'étendant, en
Hinlegen, beim
  cit-v.

menses, before
menstruation, avant la
Menses, vor den
  sep.

  during[11]/pendant la/während der
  nux-v., sapin.

motion, during[11]
mouvement, au
Bewegung, bei
  caps., caust., con., merc., nux-v.

  am.[11]
  dros.

nausea, with[16]
nausée, avec
Übelkeit, mit
  mag-c., stann.

pain, during the[11, 16]
douleur, pendant la
Schmerz, bei
  sep., sil.[16]

  umbilicus[16]
  ombilicale, dans la région
  Nabelegend, in der
    chin., ip.

part touched
parties touchées, des
Teiles, des **berührten**
  spig.

rest, during[11]
repos, pendant le
Ruhe, in der
  dros.

rising, after[11]
levé, après s'être
Aufstehen, nach dem
  lyc.

  am.[11]
    nat-c.

sitting, while[11]
assis, étant
Sitzen, im
  hyper., nat-m.

starting, with[16]
tressaillement sursant, avec
Auffahren, mit
  sulph.

stool, before[11]
selle, avant la
Stuhlgang, vor
  merc.

  during/pendant la/beim
    aesc.[11], alum., bell.[1], calad.,
    calc-s.[11], cast., con.. ind., kali-c.,

mag-m., mez.[11], nat-c., nit-ac.[16],
plat., rheum[11], stann., spig.,
verat.

after[11]/après la/nach
acon-l., grat., mag-m., mez.[16],
plat., ptel.

supper, during[11]
souper, pendant le
Abendessen, beim
  bov.

thinking of disagreeable things
pensant à choses désagréables, en
Denken an Unangenehmes, beim
  benz-ac., phos.

twitching of legs[16]
soubresaut des jambes, avec
Zucken der Beine, mit
  con.

urination, after[11]
uriner, après
Urinieren, nach
  eug., iod., plat.

vomiting, with[16]
vomissement, avec
Erbrechen, mit
  sulph.

walking, when[11]
marchant, en
Gehen, beim
  arn.

after[11]/après la marche/nach dem
  meny.

waterbrash, with[16]
renvoi rempli d'eau
wäßrigen Aufstoßen, Zusammen-
  laufen im Mund, mit
  sil.

wine, drinking[1']
vin, en buvant du
Weintrinken, beim
  cina

yawning, when
bâillement, avec
Gähnen, beim
    cast.[11], **cina,** hydr.[4], ip.[16], laur.[16],
    mag-m.[16], nux-v.[16], olnd., sars.[16]

SIDE, symptoms on **one**
CÔTÉ, symptômes **unilatéraux**
SEITE, einseitige Symptome
    aesc., **agar.,** agn., **ALUM.,**
    ALUMN.[2], am-c., am-m., **ambr.,**
    ANAC., ang.[2, 3], ant-c., ant-t.,
    aphis, **apis**[2], **arg-m., arg-n.,** arn.,
    ars., **ASAF.,** asar., aur., **bar-c.,**
    bar-m., bell., bism., bor., **bov.**[2, 3],
    BRY., calc., camph., cann-s., **canth.,**
    caps., carb-ac.[11], carb-an., carb-v.,
    caust., cham., chel., chin., **chin-s.**[6],
    cic., **cina,** clem., **coc-c.**[2], cocc., coff.,
    colch., coloc., con., croc., cupr.,
    cycl., dig., dros., **dulc.,** euph.,
    euphr., ferr., ferr-s.[11], graph., **guaj.,**
    hell., hep., hura[11], hyos., ign., iod.,
    iris, **KALI-C.,** kali-m.[1'], kali-n.,
    KALI-P., KREOS., LACH., laur.,
    led., **LYC., LYSS.,** mag-c., mag-m.,
    mang., meny., merc., **mez.,** mosch.,
    mur-ac., nat-c., nat-m., nit-ac.[1],
    nux-m., nux-v., oena.[11], **olnd.,**
    orig.[11], **par.,** petr., **PH-AC., phos.,**
    PLAT., plb., puls., rad-br.[3], ran-b.,
    ran-s., rheum, rhod., rhus-t., ruta,
    sabad., sabin., samb., **SARS.,** sel.,
    seneg., sep., sil., **spig.,** spong., squil.,
    stann., **staph., stront-c., SUL-AC.,**
    sul-i.[1'], sulph., tarax., **tarent.**[2],
    tell.[11], teucr., thala.[14], thuj., valer.,
    verat., **VERB.,** viol-o., viol-t., vip.[6],
    xan.[11], **zinc.,** zinc-p.[1']

alternating sides
alternants, côtés
abwechselnde Seiten
    agar., ant-c., cimic., cina[3], **COCC.**[3],
    iris, **LAC-C.,** mang.[6], merc., onos.,
    phos., plat., puls., rad-br.[3], sep.

crosswise, left uper and right lower
croisés, en haut à gauche et en bas à
    droite
kreuzweise links oben und rechts
    unten

AGAR., alum., anac., ant-t.[8], **arn.,**
ars., asc-t.[7], bar-c., bell., **both.**[7],
brom., camph., caps., **carb-an.,**
cham., chel., chin., coff., con.,
cycl., euphr., **fl-ac.,** hep., hyper.,
kali-c., kali-n., lach., laur., **LED.,**
mag-m., meny., merc., mill.,
mur-ac., nat-m., nit-ac., nux-m.,
nux-v., olnd., op., par., ph-ac.,
puls.[1], ran-s., rhod., **RHUS-T.,**
sabad., sabin., samb., sars., sec.,
seneg., spong., **squil., stann.,**
staph., stram., sulph., **TARAX.,**
teucr., **thuj.,** valer., **verat., verb.,**
viol-t.

right upper and left lower
en haut à droite et en bas à gauche
rechts oben und links unten
    acon., **agar.**[6], agn., am-c., am-m.,
    AMBR., ant-c., ant-t., arg-m.,
    ars-i., asar., asc-t.[7], bism., **bor.,**
    both.[7], **bov.,** brom.[8], bry., calad.,
    calc., cann-s., carb-v., **caust.,**
    chel., cic., cina, colch., coloc.,
    croc., cupr., dig., dulc., euph.,
    euphr.[1], **ferr.,** graph., hell., hyos.,
    ign., iod., ip., kali-n.[16], **lyc.,**
    mag-c., mang., med.[8], **merc-i-f.,**
    mez., mur-ac., **nat-c.,** nux-v.,
    perh.[14], **PHOS.,** plat., **plb.,** ran-b.,
    rheum, rhus-t., ruta, sel., **sil.,**
    spig., **SUL-AC.,** viol-o.

left
gauche
linke
    achy.[14], acon., adon.[6],
    agar.[2, 3, 8], agn.[3], **all-c.,** aloe,
    alumn.[2], **am-br.,** am-c.[2, 3],
    am-m.[2, 3], **ambr.**[2, 3], **anac.,**
    ang.[2, 3], ange-s.[14], **ant-c., ant-t.,**
    apis, arg-m., ARG-N., arn.,
    ars.[2, 3, 6], ars-i.[3, 6], **art-v.**[2],
    arum-t., **ASAF., ASAR.,** asc-t.,
    aster., atra-r.[14], **aur.**[2, 3],
    aur-m-n., bapt.[2], bar-c.[2, 3],
    bar-m., bell.[2, 3, 11], **bell-p.**[2, 7],
    benz-ac.[11], **berb.,** bism., bor.[2, 3],
    bov.[2, 3], **brom., bry.,** buni-o.[14],
    calc., calc-ar.[1'], calc-f.[3, 10, 14],

camph.², ³, cann-s., canth.,
CAPS, carb-v.², ³, ⁶, caust.,
cean.⁸, **cedr.**³, ⁶, **cham.**, **chel.**,
chin., chin-s.³, **cic.**², ³, **cimic.**,
CINA, cinnb.³, ¹¹, **CLEM.**,
cocc., coff-t.¹¹, **colch.**, **coloc.**,
con.², ³, cortiso.¹⁴, **CROC.**,
crot-c.¹¹, crot-h.¹¹, **crot-t.**,
cupr., **cycl.**², ³, cyt-l.⁹, ¹⁰, ¹⁴,
daph.⁴, ¹¹, dig.², ³, dros.², ³,
dulc., elat.¹¹, erig.⁸, euon.¹¹,
eup-pur.¹¹, **EUPH.**, **euphr.**,
ferr., ferr-p., ferr-s.¹¹, flav.¹⁴,
flor-p.¹⁴, gels., **GRAPH.**, grat.¹',
guaj., halo.¹⁴, hecla¹⁴,
hed.⁹, ¹⁰, hell.², ³, **hep.**,
hir.¹⁴, hist.¹⁴, hydroph.¹⁴,
hyos.², ³, ign., ind.¹¹, **iod.**², ³,
ip., iris, kali-bi.³, kali-c.², ³, ¹⁴,
kali-chl., **kali-m.**¹', kali-n.², ³,
kalm.¹¹, **KREOS.**, lac-ac.²,
LACH., lat-m.¹⁴, laur.², ³,
led.², ³, lepi.⁸, ¹¹, **lil-t.**³, ⁸, ¹¹,
lith-c., **lyc.**², ³, lycps.¹¹,
mag-c.², ³, mag-m., mag-s.³,
mang., meny., meph.¹⁴,
merc., **merc-c.**, merc-i-f.¹¹,
merc-i-r., **MEZ.**, mosch.,
mur-ac., naja, nat-ar.¹¹,
nat-c.², ³, nat-f.¹⁰, ¹⁴, nat-m.², ³,
nat-s., nid.¹⁴, **nit-ac.**, nux-m.,
nux-v.², ³, oena.¹¹, ol-j.¹¹,
OLND., onop.¹⁴, **onos.**, op.¹¹,
osm., ox-ac., **par.**, paro-i.¹⁴,
perh.¹⁴, **petr.**², ³, ph-ac.², ³,
PHOS., phys., pic-ac.¹¹, plan.¹¹,
plat.², ³, ¹¹, plb., **podo.**², puls.², ³,
puls-n.¹¹, pulx.⁸, ran-b., **ran-s.**,
rheum², ⁷, **rhod.**, rhus-t.², ³,
rumx.⁸, sabad.², ³, **sabin.**,
sal-ac., samb.², ³, sapo.⁸,
sars.², ³, **SEL.**, seneg.², ³, **SEP.**,
sieg.¹⁰, **sil.**, **spig.**, spong.², ³,
SQUIL., **STANN.**, staph.,
stront-c., stroph-s.¹⁴, sul-ac.,
sulfa.¹⁴, sulfonam.¹⁴, **SULPH.**,
tab., **tarax.**, tell.¹⁴, teucr.,
thala.¹⁴, ther., **thuj.**, ust.,
v-a-b.¹⁴, valer.², ³, **verat.**², ³,
verb.², ³, vesp., viol-o., **viol-t.**,
vip-a.¹⁴, xan., **zinc.**², ³, ⁶

coldness of¹¹
froid du
Kälte der linken
    bry., carb-v.³, caust., lyc.,
    rhus-t.³, sapin., sulph.³

heat of ¹¹
chaleur du
Hitze der linken
    bell., lac-ac., rhus-t.

then right
puis droite
zur rechten S. wechselnd
    acon., all-c.¹', ³, ⁷, aloe, arg-n.³,
    ars.³, benz-ac.⁷, brom.³, calc.³, ⁷,
    calc-p., **colch.**, dulc., elaps,
    ferr.³, ⁷, **form.**³, ⁶, form-ac.⁶,
    hed.⁹, ¹⁰, ¹⁴, **iod.**⁷, ip.⁷, kali-c.,
    kreos., lac-c.⁸, **LACH.**, merc-i-r.³,
    naja, nit-m-ac., nux-v.³, phyt.,
    puls.³, rhus-t., sabad.³, ⁶, ⁷,
    stann.³, tarax.³

right
droite
rechte

    abies-c., **acon.**, adlu.¹⁴, **aesc.**,
    agar.², ³, ⁸, **agn.**, **alum.**, **alumn.**²,
    am-c., **am-m.**², ³, ⁴, ⁶, ambr.⁷,
    anac.², ³, ⁸, **ang.**², ³, ant-t.², ³,
    APIS, **ARG-M.**, arist-m.¹¹, **arn.**,
    ARS., ars-i., ars-s-f.¹', art-v.²,
    arum-t.², asaf.², ³, aster.²,
    AUR., aur-ar.¹', **aur-i.**¹',
    aur-s.¹', aza.¹⁴, **BAPT.**,
    bar-c.², ³, **bar-s.**¹', **BELL.**, bism.,
    BOR., **both.**³, ⁷, ⁸, **bov.**², ³,
    cimic.¹⁴, cina², ³, cinnb.⁸,
    clem.², ³, **cocc.**, **coff.**², ³, **colch.**,
    COLOC., **CON.**, corn.², croc.²,
    CROT-C., **CROT-H.**, culx.¹',
    cur.⁷, ⁸, cycl.², ³, cyn-d.¹⁴,
    dicha.¹⁴, **dig.**², ³, dol.⁸, **dros.**,
    dulc., **elaps**³, ⁶, **elat.**², equis.⁸,
    euph.², ³, ⁶, euphr., fl-ac.¹¹,
    form., gels.³, gink-b.¹⁴, gins.⁴,
    glon.¹¹, graph.², ³, guaj., guat.¹⁴,
    harp.¹⁴, hell.², ³, **hep.**,
    hip-ac.⁹, ¹⁴, hyos.², ³, hypoth.¹⁴,
    ign., **indg.**³, iod.², ³, ⁸, **ip.**, **iris**,

kali-bi.[3], kali-c.[2, 3, 8], kali-m.[1'],
kali-n.[2, 3], kalm., kreos.,
laur.[2, 3], led.[2, 3], lil-t., lith-c.,
LYC., lycpr.[8], LYSS., mag-c.[2, 3],
mag-m., mag-p.[3, 6, 8],
mand.[10, 14], mang., meny.,
merc., merc-i-f., methys.[14],
mez., mim-p.[14], moly-met.[14],
mosch., mur-ac., murx.[3, 6],
naja[3], nat-ar., nat-c., nat-m.[2, 3],
nat-s.[7], nit-ac., nux-m.,
NUX-V., oci-s.[9, 14], oena.[11],
olnd.[2, 3], op., pall., par.,
penic.[13], petr., ph-ac.[2, 3], phel.[7],
phos.[2, 3], phyt., pic-ac.[11],
plat.[2, 3], plb., podo., prun.,
psil.[14], PULS., ran-b., RAN-S.,
RAT., rheum[2, 3], rhod.,
rhus-t.[2, 3, 8], rumx.[3], ruta[2, 3, 6],
sabad., sabin., sang., SARS.,
SEC., sel.[14], seneg.[2, 3], sep.[2, 3],
sil., spig., spong.[2, 3], squil.[2, 3],
stann.[2, 3, 14], staph., stront-c.,
SUL-AC., sul-i.[1'], sulph., tarax.,
tarent.[3, 8, 11], tell., teucr.,
thiop.[14], thuj., thyr.[14], tub.[7],
valer.[2, 3], ven-m.[14], verb.[2, 3],
viol-o., viol-t., wye.[11], yuc.[11],
zinc.

coldness of[11]
froid de la
Kälte der rechten
    ars., bar-c.[3], par., rhus-t.,
    sabin.[3]

heat of[11]
chaleur de la
Wärme der rechten
    op.

then left
puis le c. gauche
zur linken S. wechselnd
    acet-ac., acon., am-c.[3, 7],
    ambr.[3, 7], anac.[7], apis[1', 3, 7], ars.[11],
    ars-met. (non: ars-n.), aspar.,
    bar-c.[7], bell., benz-ac.[3, 6], bry.[3],
    calc-p.[3], canth.[3, 6], caust.[7], chel.[3],
    cupr.[3], lil-t.[3, 7], LYC., merc-i-f.[3, 7],
    mez., ox-ac.[3, 6], phos.[3, 7],
    ptel.[11], rheum[7], rumx.[3, 7],

SABAD.[3, 4, 6, 7, 11], sang.,
    saroth.[11], spong., sul-ac.[3, 7],
    sulph., syph.[3], thiop.[14],
    verat.[3, 7]

SILICA, from over use of
SILICA, par l'usage exagéré ou trop
    prolongé de
SILICEA, Folgen des Mißbrauchs von
    camph.[2], FL-AC., hep.[2], merc.[2],
    sulph.[2]

SITTING agg., while
ASSIS agg., étant
SITZEN agg., im
    acon., AGAR., agn., aloe, alum.,
    alumn.[2], am-c., AM-M., ambr.,
    anac., ang.[2, 3, 6], ant-c., ant-t.,
    apis[3], arg-m., arn., ARS., ars-s-f.[1'],
    asaf., asar., aur., aur-i.[1'], aur-m.,
    aur-m-n., bar-c., bar-m., bell.,
    bism., bor., bov., bry., cact., calad.,
    calc., camph., cann-s., canth.,
    CAPS., carb-an., carb-v., caust.,
    cham., chel., chin., cic., cimic.[14],
    cina, clem., cob., cocc., coff.,
    colch., coloc., CON., croc., cupr.,
    CYCL., dicha.[10], dig.[2, 3, 8], dios.[8],
    dros., DULC., equis.[8], EUPH.,
    euphr., ferr., ferr-a.[6], ferr-ar.[1'],
    fl-ac., gamb., graph., grat.[4], guaj.,
    hecla[14], hell., hep., hydrc.[8], hyos.,
    ign., indg.[8], iod., ip., kali-bi., kali-c.,
    kali-m.[1'], kali-n., kali-p., kali-s.,
    kreos., lach., laur., led., LYC.,
    mag-c., mag-m., mang., meny.,
    meph.[14], merc., mez., mosch.,
    mur-ac., nat-c., nat-m., nat-p.,
    nit-ac., nux-m., nux-v., olnd., op.,
    par., petr., ph-ac., phel.[4], PHOS.,
    phyt.[8], PLAT., plb., pneu.[14], prun.,
    psor.[1'], PULS., pyrog.[1'], ran-b.,
    ran-s.[1], rheum, rhod.[1], RHUS-T.,
    ruta, sabad., sabin., samb., sars.,
    sec., sel., seneg., SEP., sil., spig.,
    spong., squil., stann., staph., stram.,
    stront-c., sul-ac., sul-i.[1'], SULPH.,
    tarax., teucr., thuj., tong.[4], tub.[1'],
    VALER., verat., VERB., viol-o.,
    vip-a.[14], VIOL-T., ZINC.,
    ZINC-P.[1']

am.
acon., agar., agn., alum., **alumn.**[2],
am-c., am-m., **anac., ang.**[2, 3]**, ant-t.,**
aral.[3, 6], arg-m.[2], arn., ars., asaf.,
asar.[3], aur., bar-c., bell., bor., **BRY.,**
cadm-s., **calad.,** calc., camph.,
cann-s., canth., caps., carb-an.,
carb-v., caust., cham., chel., chin.,
chion., cic., cina, clem., cocc.,
coff., COLCH., coloc., con., croc.,
cupr., cycl., **DIG.**[2, 3]**, dulc.**[2]**,** ferr.,
gels. **glon., graph.**[3, 7], graph., guaj.,
hell., hep., hyos., ign., iod., ip.,
kali-c., kali-n., kreos., laur., led.,
mag-c., mag-m., mang., meny.,
merc., mez., mosch., nat-ar., nat-c.[3],
nat-m., nit-ac., nux-m., **NUX-V.,**
op., par., petr., ph-ac., phos., plb.,
puls., ran-b., ran-s., **rheum, rhod.**[2]**,**
rhus-t.[2, 3, 4], sabad.[3], sabin., samb.,
sars., sec., sel., **sep.**[2]**, sil.,** spig.,
spong., **squil.,** stann., staph., stram.,
sul-ac., sulph., sumb., tarax., thuj.,
valer., verat., verb.[2], zinc.

aversion to sit[11]
aversion d'être assis
Abneigung zu sitzen
iod., lach.

bent agg.[2, 3]
courbé agg., en se tenant
Gekrümmtsitzen agg.
acon., agn.[3], alum.[3]**, alumn.**[2]**,**
am-m., ang., **ANT-T.,** arg-m.,
ars., asaf., bar-c., bor., bov., **bry.,**
caps., carb-v., caust., cham.,
chel., **chin., cic., DIG., dulc.,**
ferr., **hyos.,** ign.[3], meny., nat-m.[3]**,**
nux-v., phos., plb., **puls., rhod.,**
rhus-t., sabin., samb., sep., spig.,
spong., **squil.,** stann., **sulph.,**
verb., viol-t.[3]

am.[2]
anac., **ang.,** ars., bar-c., **bell.,**
bor., bry., calad., **carb-v.,** caust.,
cham., chel., chin., cina, **colch.,**
coloc., con., dig., **ign., KALI-C.,**
lyc., mang., **merc., mez.,** mosch.,
nux-m., nux-v., op., puls., **rheum,**

rhus-t., **sabad.,** sars., **spig.,**
spong., stann., sulph., tarax.,
verat., verb.

cold seat agg., on a[8]
siège froid agg., sur un
Sitzen auf kalter Unterlage agg.
chim., dulc.[3]**, nux-v.**

down agg., on first
s'asseyant agg., en
Sichniedersetzen agg., beim
agn., alum., **AM-M., ant-t.,**
arg-m., aur., bar-c., bov., bry.,
caust., **chel.,** chin., **coff.,** croc.,
cycl., graph., **hell., ip.,** iris,
kali-c., lyc., **mag-c.,** mang.,
merc., murx., nat-s.[6], nit-ac.,
ph-ac., phos., puls., rhus-t.[3]**,**
ruta, sabin., **samb.,** sars., **SPIG.,**
spong., squil., sulph.[6], thuj.,
valer., verat., viol-t.

am.
acon., ambr., anac., ang.[3], ant-c.,
ant-t., arn., ars., asar., aur.,
bar-c., bell., bov., bry., calc.,
cann-s., canth. **CAPS.,** carb-an.,
carb-v., caust., cham., chin.,
cic., cocc., **CON.,** croc., dig.,
dros., **euph., ferr.,** ferr-ar[1]**'**,
graph., kali-c., kali-n., lach.,
laur., led., lyc., mang., merc.,
mur-ac., nat-c., nat-m., nit-ac.,
nux-v., olnd., petr., ph-ac., **phos.,**
plat., puls., ran-b., rhod., **rhus-t.,**
ruta, sabad., **sep.,** sil., **spig.,**
staph., stram., stront-c., **sulph.,**
thuj., **verat.**

erect agg.[2, 3]
se tenant droit agg., en
Geradesitzen agg.
anac., **ang.,** ars., aur-s.[1]', bar-c.,
bar-s.[1]', **bell.,** bor., bry., calad.,
carb-v., caust., **cham., chel.,** chin.,
cina, **colch., COLOC.,** con., dig.,
ign., KALI-C., kreos., **lyc.,** mang.,
merc., mez., mosch., nat-m.[3]**,**
nux-m., nux-v., op., puls., rheum,
rhus-t., **sabad.,** sars., **spig.,**
spong., staph., sulph., tarax.,
verat., verb., viol-t.[3]

am.²

acon.², **alumn.**, **am-m.**, ang.,
ant-t.², ³, ⁶, ⁸, apis⁸, arg-m.,
ars.², ³, ⁶, asaf., bar-c.², ⁶, bell.⁸,
bor., bov., **bry.**, caps., carb-v.,
caust., cham., chel., **chin.**, **cic.**,
DIG.², ³, **dulc.**, ferr., **hyos.**², ³,
kali-bi.³, ⁶, meny., nat-m.³,
nux-v., **phos.**, plb., **puls.**, **rhod.**,
rhus-t., **sabin.**, **samb.**, **sep.**, spig.,
spong., squil., stann., **sulph.**,
verb.

inability to sit erect¹¹
incapacité de se tenir asis droit
Unfähigkeit geradezusitzen
   lyc., stram.

must sit up in bed with knees drawn
   up, rests her head and arms upon
   knees
doit se mettre au lit, genoux repliés
   en reposant tête et bras sur ses
   genoux
muß sich im Bett mit angezogenen
   Knien aufsetzen, legt ihren Kopf
   und die Arme auf die Knie
   ARS., glon.¹¹

impulse to sit³
désir de s'asseoir, impulsion à
Verlangen, sich zu setzen
   acon.³, ⁴, **agar.**, alum.³, ⁴, am-c.,
   am-m., ambr.⁶, anac.³, ⁴, ant-c.,
   arg-m., arn.³, ¹¹, **ars.**³, ⁶, asar.,
   bar-a.⁶, bar-c., **bell.**, bor., bry.³, ⁴, ⁶,
   calc.³, ⁶, camph., **cann-s.**, canth.,
   caps.³, **carb-v.**³, ⁶, caust.³, ⁶,
   cham.⁴, ¹¹, **chel.**, **CHIN.**³, ⁴, ⁶, ¹¹,
   cocc.³, ⁶, cod.¹¹, colch.³, ⁶, **CON.**³, ⁶,
   croc.³, ⁴, cupr., cycl., dulc.³, ⁴, ⁶,
   euphr., **GRAPH.**³, ⁶, **guaj.**³, ⁶,
   hell.³, ¹¹, hep., hyos., ign., **iod.**, ip.,
   jac-c.¹¹, kali-c., lach., lact.⁴, laur.,
   led.⁶, lil-t., lyc., m-aust.⁴, mag-c.,
   mag-m., **merc.**³, ⁶, mez., mur-ac.³, ⁴,
   nat-ar.¹¹, nat-c., **nat-m.**³, ⁶, nat-s.⁶,
   nit-ac.³, ⁶, **NUX-V.**³, ⁴, ⁶, ¹¹,

olnd.³, ⁴, ⁶, op., petr., **ph-ac.**³, ⁶,
PHOS.³, ⁶, pic-ac.¹¹, plb.,
puls.³, ⁴, ⁶, ¹⁶, ran-b., ran-s., rheum,
rhod., rhus-t.³, ⁴, ruta, sabin.⁴, **sec.**,
sep., sil., **spong.**, **SQUIL.**,
stann.³, ⁴, ⁶, staph.⁴, stront-c.³, ⁶,
sulph.³, ⁴, **tarax.**³, ⁴, teucr.,
verat.⁴, ⁶, verb., viol-t., **zinc.**

Vol. I: *sit/s'asseoir/Sitzen*

wet ground, ailments from s. on³
sol humide, troubles par être a. sur le
nassem Boden, Beschwerden durch
   S. auf
   ars., calc., caust., **dulc.**³, ⁶, **nux-v.**³, ⁶,
   rhod., **rhus-t.**¹', ³, ⁶, sil.

SLEEP agg., **before**
SOMMEIL agg., **avant** le
SCHLAF agg., **vor** dem
   acon., agar., **agn.**, alum., am-c.,
   am-m., ambr., anac., ant-c., arn.,
   ARS., ars-s-f.¹', asar., aur., aur-ar.¹',
   bar-c., **bell.**, bism., bor., **BRY.**,
   calad., **CALC.**, camph., canth.,
   caps., **carb-an.**, **CARB-V.**, **caust.**,
   cham., chel., **chin.**, clem., cocc.,
   coff., coloc., con., cycl., dig., dulc.,
   euph., euphr., **graph.**, guaj., **hep.**,
   ign., ip., **kali-c.**, kali-n., **kreos.**,
   lach., laur., led., **lyc.**, mag-c.,
   mag-m., mang., **MERC.**, mez.,
   mosch., mur-ac., nat-ar., nat-c.,
   nat-m., nit-ac., nux-m., nux-v., par.,
   petr., **ph-ac.**, **PHOS.**, plat., plb.,
   PULS., ran-b., rheum, rhod.,
   RHUS-T., sabad., sabin., samb.,
   sars., sel., seneg., **SEP.**, **sil.**, spig.,
   spong., stann., staph., stront-c.,
   sul-ac., **SULPH.**, tarax., teucr.,
   thuj., verat., verb., viol-t., zinc.

at beginning of s. agg.
au debut agg.
am Anfang des Schlafes agg.
   agar., agn., am-c.³, am-m., aral.,
   arg-m., **arg-n.**, arn., **ARS.**, ars-s-f.¹',
   arum-t.³, aur., bapt., bar-c., **BELL.**,
   bor., **BRY.**, calad., **calc.**, camph.³,
   caps., **carb-an.**, **carb-v.**, caust.,
   cench.¹, **cham.**², chin., cocc., coff.,

con., **CROT-H.**, dulc., **graph., grin.,**
guaj., hep., ign., ip., **kali-ar.,**
KALI-C., kreos., **lac-c., LACH.,**
laur., **lyc.,** mag-c., mag-m., **merc.,**
merc-pr-r.[3], mur-ac., nat-c., nat-m.,
nit-ac.[3], nux-v., **op.,** ph-ac., **phos.,**
PULS., ran-b., **rhus-t.,** sabad.[3],
sabin., samb.[6], sars., sel., **SEP.,** sil.,
spong., stann.[3], staph., stront-c.,
sulph., tarax., teucr., thuj., **valer.,**
verat.

during s. agg.
pendant le s. agg.
während des Schlafes agg.
    acon., aesc.[1'], agn., alum., am-c.,
    am-m., ambr., anac., ant-c.,
    ant-t., apis, arg-n., ARN., ARS.,
    ars-s-f.[1'], aur., aur-ar.[1'], **bar-c.,**
    bar-m., **BELL.,** bism., **BOR.,**
    brom., **BRY., calad.,** calc.,
    camph., **cann-i.,** cann-s., canth.,
    caps., carb-ac., carb-an., carb-v.,
    carbn-s., caust., **CHAM., chel.,**
    chin., chin-ar., cic., cina, clem.,
    cocc., coff., colch., coloc., **con.,**
    croc., cupr., cycl., dig., dros.,
    dulc., euph., ferr., ferr-ar.,
    graph., guaj., hell., **HEP., HYOS.,**
    ign., ip., **kali-ar.,** kali-br., **kali-c.,**
    kali-n., kali-p., kreos., **lach.,**
    laur., led., **lyc.,** mag-c., mag-m.,
    mang., meny., **MERC.,** merc-c.[3],
    mez., mosch., **mur-ac.,** nat-ar.,
    nat-c., **nat-m., nit-ac., nux-m.,**
    nux-v., **OP.,** par., petr., **ph-ac.,**
    phos., plat., plb., **PULS.,** ran-b.,
    ran-s., **rheum,** rhod., rhus-t.,
    ruta, sabin., **samb.,** sars., sel.,
    seneg., **sep., SIL.,** spig., spong.,
    squil., stann., staph., **STRAM.,**
    stront-c., sul-ac., **SULPH.,** syph.[7],
    teucr.[3], thuj., valer., verat.,
    verb., viol-t., **ZINC.,** zinc-p.[1']

am.
    am-m., calad., hell., phos., samb.

after s. agg.
après le s. agg.
nach dem Sch. agg.
    acon., aesc., ail.[2], am-c.[3, 6], am-m.,

ambr.[1], anac., **apis,** arg-m.[1', 3, 6],
arn., ars., ars-s-f.[1'], asaf.,
aur-ar.[1'], bar-m.[3], bell., bor., bov.,
bry., bufo[2, 8], cadm-s., calad.[3],
calc., calc-f.[10], **camph., carb-v.,**
carbn-s., caust., cham., **chel.,**
chin., cina, cob-n.[10], coc-c.[3, 8],
cocc., coff., **con.,** crat.[8], **CROT-C.,**
crot-h.[1'-3, 6], **crot-t.**[1], dig., **dios.**[2],
epiph.[8], **euphr., ferr.,** ferr-ar.,
graph., **hep.,** hom.[8], hyos., ign.,
kali-ar., kali-bi.[3], kali-c., kali-i.[3],
kali-n.[3, 6], kali-p., kreos., lac-c.,
LACH., lob.[3], **lyc.,** mag-c.,
mag-f.[10, 14], merc-c.[8], morph.[8],
mur-ac., myric.[2], naja, nat-ar.,
nat-sil.[1'], nux-m., nux-v., olnd.,
op., paeon., parth.[8], **ph-ac.,**
phos., phyt., pic-ac.[8], **puls.,**
rheum, rhus-t., **sabad.,** samb.,
SEL., sep., spig., **SPONG.,** squil.[3],
stann., **staph., STRAM., SULPH.,**
syph.[8], thuj., tub.[8], uran-n.[3, 6],
valer.[2, 8], **verat.,** ziz.[8]

morning on waking agg.[7]
le matin au réveil agg.
morgens beim Erwachen agg.
    AM-M., AMBR., arn., **ARS.,**
    bell-p.[10], cadm-met.[9, 10], **CALC.,**
    carb-v., CAUST., chel., chin.,
    cob-n.[10], **cocc., con., dig.,**
    ferr-ar.[1'], flav.[14], **graph., HEP.,**
    hyos., ign., kali-ar., kali-c.,
    LACH., lyc., mag-c.[10], **NUX-V.,**
    PHOS., phyt., prot.[14], **PULS.,**
    RHUS-T., samb., **SEP., staph.,**
    SULPH.

afternoon, agg
après le sieste agg.
nach dem Mittagsschlaf agg.
    anac., bar-c.[16], bell.[7], **bry.,**
    caust.[3], chin., con.[16], **graph.**[3],
    lach., mag-c.[10], mag-f.[10, 14],
    nat-m.[16], phos., **puls., SEL.**[3],
    spong., **STAPH.,** sulph.

am.[3]
    fl-ac., kali-bi., meph., nux-m.,
    nux-v.[14], ph-ac., pneu.[14], senec.

am.
    acon., agar., am-c.³, am-m.,
    ambr., apis, **ars.**, bry., **calad.**,
    calc., caps.³, cham., chin., cocc.,
    colch., con., crot-t.³, ⁶, **cupr.**³,
    epiph.³, ferr., **fl-ac.**³, glon.¹', hell.,
    ign., ip., iris³, ⁶, kali-bi.³, kali-p.³,
    kreos., lach., lob.³, **med.**³, ⁶,
    meph.³, ⁶, **merc.**, mygal.⁸, myric.⁸,
    nat-c., nid.¹⁴, **nux-v.**, oxyt.,
    PH-AC., PHOS., puls., ran-b.³, ⁶,
    ruta, sabin., samb., sang., sel.,
    sep., spig., thuj.

falling asleep am., on
s'endormant am., en
Einschlafen am., beim
    merc.

half asleep am., when
demi-sommeil am.
Halbschlaf am., im
    hell.³, **sel.**

long s. agg.
long agg.
langer Sch. agg.
    ambr., anac., arn., ars., asaf., bell.,
    bor., bry., **calc.**, camph., carb-v.,
    caust., cham., cocc., **con.**, dig.,
    euphr., ferr., **graph., hep.**, hyos.,
    ign., kali-c., kreos., **LACH.**, lyc.,
    mag-c., **nux-v.**, ph-ac., puls.,
    rhus-t., spig., **stram., SULPH.**,
    verat.

loss of, from
manque de, par
Schlafmangel, durch
    ambr., ars.⁶, bry., carb-v.², ³, **caust.**,
    chin., **cimic., COCC., coff.**², ³, **colch.**,
    cupr., ip., kreos.³, **lac-d.**¹, laur.,
    merc.³, nat-m., **nit-ac., NUX-V.**,
    ol-j.², olnd., op., pall.³, ph-ac.,
    PHOS.³, pic-ac.¹', puls., ruta, sabin.,
    sang.³, **sel.**, sep., **sulph.**, zinc.,
    zinc-a.⁷, ¹², zinc-o.⁷

short s. am.³
de peu de durée am.
kurzer Sch. am.
    carc.⁹, fl-ac.³, ⁷, kali-bi., med.⁶,

meph.³, ⁶, ¹⁴, nux-m., nux-v.,
    ph-ac.⁶, senec.

slow–broken bones see injuries–bones

SLUGGISHNESS of the body
ENGOURDISSEMENT corporel
TRÄGHEIT, körperliche
    acon.⁴, agar.⁴, ¹¹, alum.⁴, **alumn.**¹',
    am-m., ammc.⁴, anac., **ant-t.**⁴, ¹¹,
    arn., ars., **ASAR.**¹¹, bar-c.⁴, bell.⁴,
    bor.⁴, bruc.⁴, bry.¹', ⁴, cact.¹',
    calad.⁴, calc., calc-p.⁴, camph.,
    cann-s.⁴, canth.¹¹, **caps.**, carb-an.,
    carb-v., carl.¹¹, casc.⁴, **chel.**, chin.⁴,
    cinnb., cocc., **con.**, croc.⁴, cur.,
    cycl.¹², dig.⁴, dirc.¹¹, dulc., ferr-m.¹¹,
    gels., graph.⁴, grat.⁴, guaj., hell.⁴,
    hep.⁴, hera.⁴, hyos.¹¹, ign.⁴, indg.⁴,
    iod., ip., kali-c., kali-m.¹', kali-p.,
    kali-s.¹', lach.⁴, ¹¹, laur., lil-t.¹¹, lyc.,
    m-aust.⁴, mag-c.⁴, mag-m., merc.,
    mez., mur-ac., nat-c., nat-m.,
    nit-ac., nux-v., ol-an.⁴, olnd., **op.**,
    petr., ph-ac., phel.⁴, phos., phys.¹¹,
    plb., puls., rheum⁴, rhod., ruta⁴,
    sabin.⁴, sars.¹', ⁴, ¹¹, **sec.**, sel.⁴, **sep.**,
    sil.⁴, stann., stram., stront-c.⁴,
    sul-i.¹', **sulph.**, thea¹¹, thuj.⁴, verb.,
    zinc.⁴, zinc-p.¹'

lassitude/Mattigkeit
weakness/faiblesse/Schwäche

morning/matin/morgens
    carb-an., chel., nat-c., nat-m.,
    verb.

sitting, while
assis, étant
Sitzen, im
    chel.

forenoon¹¹/matinée/vormittags
    sars.

rising, on¹¹
se levant, en
Aufstehen, beim
    ammc.

SMALLER, sensation
ÉTROITESSE, de petitesse, sensation d'
KLEINERSEINS, Gefühl des
   acon., agar., **calc.,** cact.[3], croc.,
   euphr., **glon.,** graph.[3], kreos., naja[3],
   nux-m.[3], nux-v.[3], sabad., sulph.[3],
   tarent., zinc.[3]

   Vol. I: *delusions – diminished,*
   smaller/imaginations – diminué,
   plus petit/Wahnideen – verkleinert,
   kleiner

SMOKE agg., smoke inhalation
FUMÉE agg., inhalation de
RAUCH agg. Rauchvergiftung
   ars.[3], brom.[3], calc., caust., chin.[3],
   euphr., kali-bi.[3], lyc.[3], naja[3], nat-m.,
   nux-v., olnd., puls.[3], **sep., SPIG.,**
   sulph.

SNOW, ailments from bright[12]
NEIGE brillante, troubles à la suite de
SCHNEE, Beschwerden durch
   blendenden
   glon.

SNOW-AIR agg.
NEIGE agg., temps de
SCHNEEWETTER agg.
   asar.[14], **calc., calc-p.,** caust., cic.,
   CON., fl-ac.[3], **form.**[3, 8], lach.[3], **lyc.,**
   mag-m., merc., nat-c., nux-v.[1],
   ph-ac., phos., puls., rhod., **rhus-t.,**
   SEP., sil., sulph., urt-u., vib.[3]

   ailments from[12]
   troubles à la suite de
   Beschwerden infolge von
   con., sep.

SOFTENING bones
OSTÉOMALACIE
KNOCHENERWEICHUNG, Osteomalazie
   am-c., **ASAF., bell., CALC.,** calc-f.,
   calc-i.[8], calc-p., cic., con.[2], ferr.,
   ferr-i.[2], ferr-m.[2], **ferr-p.**[2], guaj.[8],
   hecla[2], **hep.,** iod., ip., **kali-i.**[2], **lac-c.**[2],

lyc., **MERC.,** merc-c.[3], mez., **nit-ac.,**
nux-m.[2], **ol-j.**[2], parathyr.[14], petr.,
ph-ac., **phos.,** plb., **psor.**[2], **puls.,** rhod.,
ruta, **sep., SIL.,** staph., **sulph.,** syph.[1'],
ther., thuj.[2]

brittle bones/os fragiles/brüchige
   Knochen
caries of bone/carie osseuse/
   Knochenkaries
necrosis bone/nécrose des os/
   Knochennekrose

x-ray, from[9]
rayons X, par les
Röntgenstrahlen, durch
   cadm-met., cortico., cortiso.

spring see seasons

STAGNATED, sensation as if blood
STAGNATION du sang, sensation de
STAGNIERT, als ob das Blut
   acon., bar-c., bell., bry., **carb-v.,**
   caust., croc., crot-t., dig., gels., hep.,
   ign., **lyc.,** nat-m.[4], nit-ac.[16], nux-v.,
   olnd., **pic-ac.,** puls., rhod., **sabad.,**
   seneg., sep., sulph., sumb., zinc.

STANDING agg.
DEBOUT agg., étant
STEHEN agg.
   acon., aesc.[8], **agar.,** agn., aloe,
   alum., alum-p.[1'], alum-sil.[1'],
   alumn.[2], am-c., **am-m.,** ambr.,
   arg-m., arn., ars., ars-s-f.[1'], asaf.,
   asar., atra-r.[14], aur-s.[1'], bar-c.,
   bar-m., bar-s.[1'], **bell., berb.,** bism.,
   bor., **bov.**[2, 3], **bry.,** cact., **calc.,**
   calc-s., calc-sil.[1'], camph.[1], cann-s.,
   canth., caps., carb-an., carb-v.,
   carbn-s., caust., cham., chel., **chin.,**
   chin-ar., cic., cina, **COCC.,** coff.,
   coloc.[2, 3], com.[3], **CON.,** cortico.[14],
   croc., cupr., **CYCL.,** dicha.[10, 14], **dig.,**
   dros., dulc., **euph., euphr., ferr.,**
   ferr-ar., ferr-p., **fl-ac.,** graph., guaj.,
   hell., hep., ign., **kali-bi.,** kali-c.,
   kali-n., kali-p., lach., laur., led.,
   LIL-T., lyc.[2, 3], mag-c., mag-m.,
   mand.[10], mang., meny., merc., mez.,

mosch., mur-ac., **murx.**, nat-c.,
nat-m., nat-s.[3], **nit-ac.**, nux-m.,
nux-v., olnd., op., par., petr.,
ph-ac., phel.[4], phos., **plat.**, plb.,
PULS., **ran-b.**, **rheum**, rhod., **rhus-t.**,
ruta, **sabad.**, **sabin.**, **samb.**,
sarcol-ac.[14], sars.[2, 3], sec.[3], **SEP.**,
sieg.[10], **sil.**, spig., spong., stann.,
staph., stram., stront-c., stroph-s.[14],
sul-ac., **SULPH.**, **tarax.**, teucr.,
thlas.[3], thuj., **tub.**, **VALER.**, **verat.**,
verb., viol-t., **zinc.**, **zinc-p.**[1']

weakness – standing/faiblesse –
debout/Schwäche – Stehen

am.
    agar., agn., am-c., anac., **ang.**[2, 3],
    ant-t., arn., **ARS.**, **asar.**, bar-c.,
    BELL., bor., **bov.**[2], bry., **calad.**,
    calc., camph., **cann-s.**, canth.,
    carb-an., carb-v., chel., chin.,
    cic., cina, cocc., coff., **colch.**,
    coloc.[2, 3], croc., cupr., dig., dios.,
    euph., graph., guaj., hell., hep.,
    ign., **iod.**, ip., kreos., **led.**, mang.,
    meny., merc., merc-c.[3], mez.,
    mur-ac., naja, nat-m., nit-ac.[2, 3],
    nux-m., **nux-v.**, par., petr., **phos.**,
    plb., **ran-b.**, rheum, rhus-t.[2, 3],
    ruta, sars., sec., **sel.**, **spig.**,
    spong., **squil.**, stann., staph.,
    stram., sul-ac., sul-i.[1'], tarax.,
    tarent., thuj., vip-a.[14]

erect[8]
se tenir droit
Geradestehen
    ars., bell., **dios.**, kali-p.

impossible[11]
unmöglich
    acon., acon-f., ant-t., calc-p.,
    canth., cocc.[4, 6], con.[4, 6], cupr.[4, 6],
    cupr-s.[4], dulc., hep.[4, 6], hydrc.,
    hyos., iod., **kali-br.**[2, 11], lach.[4, 6]
    merc., merc-ns., nat-m.[4, 6],
    nit-ac.[4, 6], nux-v.[4, 6], op., phys.,
    plb., sabad.[4], sec.[4, 6, 11], stann.[6],
    staph.[4, 6], stram.[4, 6, 11], sul-ac.[4],
    tarent.

till afternoon[11]
jusqu'après-midi
bis nachmittags
    bell.

STARVING with exhaustion,
    sensation of
MOURIR DE FAIM avec prostration,
    sensation de
VERHUNGERN mit Erschöpfung,
    Gefühl von
    ign.

STIFFENING OUT of body[3]
RAIDISSEMENT du corps
STEIFMACHEN des Körpers
    ang., camph., cham., **cina**[16], cupr.,
    ign., **ip.**, just.[15], phos.[16], stram.

    cough, before[15]
    toux, avant la
    Husten, vor dem
        cina, led.

    touch, from (children)[15]
    attouchement, par (chez les enfants)
    Berührung, durch (bei Kindern)
        apis

STONE-CUTTERS, for; silicosis
TAILLEURS DE PIERRE, pour les;
    silicose
STEINSTAUB, Folgen der Einatmung
    von; Silikose
    agar-t.[14], ars.[3, 6], brom.[3], **CALC.**,
    ictod.[6], ip., **lyc.**, mag-m.[14], nat-c.,
    nat-ar.[3], nit-ac., penic.[14], ph-ac., **puls.**,
    SIL., sulph.

mining/mineurs/Bergleuten

STOOL agg., **before**[3]
SELLE agg., **avant** la
STUHLGANG agg., **vor**
    acon., **ALOE**, am-c., am-m., ant-t.,
    ARG-N., ars., asar., bar-c., bor.,
    bry., calad., calc., canth., caps.,
    carb-an., carb-v., caust., cham.,

chin., cocc., colch., dig., **DIOS.,**
dulc., ferr., **GAMB.,** kali-c., lach.,
MAG-C., mang., **MERC.,** merc-c.,
mez., nat-c., nat-s., nux-v., op.,
petr., phos., psor., puls., **RHEUM,**
rhod., rhus-t., sabad., sep., spig.,
staph., stront-c., sulph., **THUJ.,**
VERAT.

during st. agg.[3]
pendant la s. agg.
während St. agg.
    acon., agar., alum., am-c., am-m.,
anac., ang., ant-c., apis, **ARS.,**
bar-c., bor., bry., calad., calc.,
canth., caps., carb-an., carb-v.,
caust., **CHAM.,** chin., coloc., con.,
dulc., euph., ferr., graph., hell.,
hep., ign., ip., **IRIS, KALI-BI.,**
kali-c., lach., lyc., **MERC.,** merc-c.,
mur-ac., nat-c., nat-m., nit-ac.,
nux-m., nux-v., olnd., phos., **PULS.,**
rheum, rhus-t., sabin., sars., sel.,
sep., sil., spig., spong., staph.,
stront-c., sul-ac., **SULPH.,** verat.,
zinc.

after st. agg.[3]
après la s. agg.
nach St. agg.
    aesc.[8], aeth., aloe, **ALUM.,** am-c.,
am-m., ambr., apoc., ars., bor.,
calc., calc-p., canth., caps.,
carb-an., carb-v., **CAUST.**[3, 7],
chin.[3, 7], cocc., coloc., con., fl-ac.,
GAMB., graph., hell., hep., hir.[14],
hydr., **IGN.,** iod., **IRIS,** kali-bi.,
kali-c., kali-n., lach., lept., lyc.,
mag-m., merc., **MERC-C.,** mez.,
mur-ac., nat-c., nat-m., nit-ac.,
nux-m., **NUX-V.,** petr., **PHOS.**[3, 7],
plat., podo., puls., rat., rheum[3, 7],
rhus-t., ruta, **SEL.,** seneg., sep.,
sil., stann., staph., stront-c.,
sulph., tell., teucr., verat.[3, 7]

    am.[3]
    acon., agar., aloe, alum., **am-m.,**
ant-c., ant-t., ars-i.[3, 6], asaf., aur.,
bar-c., bism., **bor.,** bov., **BRY.**[3, 7],
calc-p., canth., caps., caust.,

cham., cina, coff., **COLCH.,**
coloc., **con.,** croc., cycl.,
cyt-l.[10, 14], dig., dulc., ferr.,
fl-ac., GAMB., glon., guaj., hell.,
hep., ip., kali-bi.[3, 7], mag-c.,
mand.[7], mang., meny., **merc.**[7],
mur-ac., nat-c., **nat-m.**[3, 6],
NUX-V.[3, 7], op., ox-ac.[3, 6, 7], par.,
ph-ac., plb., psor., **puls.,** rauw.[14],
rheum, **RHUS-T.,** sabad., **sang.,**
seneg., sep., **SPIG.,** squil., **sulph.,**
thuj., verat.

STOOP shouldered
VOUTÉES, épaules
GEBEUGTE Haltung
    arg-n.[3], **calc.**[5, 7], **carb-v.**[3], cocc.[3],
coff.[7, 12], coloc.[3], **lyc.**[5, 7], **mang.**[3],
med.[7], nat-c.[7], nux-v.[7], op.[7],
PHOS.[3, 6, 7, 12], sil.[5, 7], **SULPH.,** ter.[6, 7],
tub., verat.[3]

STOOPING agg.[3]
SE PENCHER en avant **agg.**
BÜCKEN agg.
    am-c., bell., **BRY., calc.,** caust., lyc.,
mang., nux-v., puls., sep., sil., **spig.,**
sulph., valer.

    am.[3]
    colch., hyos., iris

STREAMING of blood, sensation
CIRCULE, sensation de sang qui
STRÖMEN des Blutes, Gefühl vom
    ox-ac.

STRENGTH, sensation of
PUISSANCE, de force, sensation de
KRAFTGEFÜHL, vermehrtes
    agar., alco.[11], anh.[10], ars.[6], bell.[11],
bov.[11], bry.[11], **bufo,** calc-f.[9], carbn-o.[11],
chin-s.[11], clem.[11], cob.[11], **coca**[6, 11],
coff., corn.[11], cot.[11], elae.[11], erech.[11],
ferr.[11], **fl-ac.,** gast.[11], gels.[11], gins.[11],
helon.[11], kola[6], lach.[3, 6], lil-t.[11],
meny.[11], **nat-p.**[3, 6], nep.[10, 13, 14],
ol-j.[11], **OP.,** ped.[11], phos.[11], pic-ac.[6],

pip-m.[6, 11], plat.[11], sars.[11], stram.,
vanad.[14], wies.[11], zinc.[3, 6]

anger, after[11]
colère, à la suite de
Zorn, infolge von
 carbn-s.

coition, after[11]
coït, après le
Koitus, nach
 merc-c.

muscular[11]
force musculaire
Muskelkräfte
 agar.[6], alco., anh.[6], ars.[6], camph.,
 coca, cod., **fl-ac.**[6, 11], gels.,
 keroso, kola[6], **nat-p.**[6], nitro-o.,
 phos., tab., thea, zinc.[6]

perspiration, during[11]
transpiration, pendant la
Schweiß, bei
 op., pilo., stach.

walking, while[11]
marchant, en
Gehen, beim
 bapt., chin.

STRETCHING
S'ÉTIRER, besoin de
SICHZUSTRECKEN, Bedürfnis
 acon., **aesc.**, agar., all-c.[8], **alum.**[3, 6, 16],
 alumn.[2], **am-c.**, ambr., aml-ns.[7, 8],
 ang., ant-t., apis, arn., **ARS.**, art-v.[2],
 arum-t., asar.[8], bar-a.[11], bar-c.,
 bell., bol-la.[11], bor.[3, 16], bov., brach.,
 brom., bry.[2, 3, 4], caj., calad., **calc.**,
 calc-p., calc-s.[2], camph., cann-s.,
 canth., caps., **carb-ac.**[2], carb-an.,
 carb-v., cast.[8], **CAUST., CHAM.**,
 chel., chin., chin-s.[4], chlf., cimic.,
 cimx., cina, cit-v.[2], clem.[3], cocc.[3, 4],
 colch., croc.[3], cur.[2], cycl., daph.,
 dig., dios., dros., dulc.[4], elat.[3, 8],
 ferr., form., gins., gran., **graph.**,
 guaj., haem., hell.[3, 4, 16], hep.,
 hydrc.[11], hyos., ign.[3, 8], ind., ip.[3],
 kali-bi., kalm., kreos., lach., lact.[4],
 laur., led., lil-t., lim.[11], lob., lyc.[3],

mag-c., mang.[4, 11], **menis.**[11], meph.,
merc., merc-c., merc-i-r., **mez.**,
mur-ac.[3], nat-c., **nat-m.**, nat-s.,
nit-ac.[3], **NUX-V.**, olnd.[3, 6, 16],
onis.[4, 11], op., ox-ac., petr., ph-ac.,
phel., **phos.**, plan., **plat.**, plb.,
podo.[2], polyp-p.[11], prun., **PULS.**,
ran-b.[1], raph., rhod.[4], **RHUS-T.**,
rhus-v., ruta[3, 4, 6, 16], **sabad.**,
sabin.[2, 3], **sec.**[3, 4, 7, 8], sel., senec.[6],
seneg.[3], **sep.**, sil., spong., squil.,
stann., staph., stram.[3], sul-ac.[3],
sulph., tab.[4], tarent., tart-ac.[4, 11],
teucr., tong.[4, 11], tub-r.[13], valer.,
verat.[3, 4], verb., vinc.[2], viol-o.,
wildb., zinc.

daytime/journée, pendant la/
 tagsüber
 mang.

morning/matin/morgens
 ars., **calc., carb-v.**, cedr.[11], ferr.,
 hell.[4, 11], graph.[4], lyc., nux-v.,
 phos., puls.[4], rhod.[4, 11], sep.[4, 11],
 sulph.[4, 16], tab., tarent., verat.

 6 h
 sep.

 7 h
 cedr.

 8–11 h[2]
 nat-m.

 am.[7]
 sec.

 bed, in
 lit, au
 Bett, im
 graph.[4], hell., meph.[4], merc.[4],
 petr., phos.[4], puls.[4], rhod., sep.,
 sulph.[4]

 of arms[16]
 des bras
 der Arme
  petr.

desire to[7]
désir de
Verlangen
   aml-ns., plb., sec.

stupefied, as if
stupéfié, comme
betäubt, wie
   meph.

waking, on
réveil, au
Erwachen, beim
   dulc., sep.

forenoon/matinée/vormittags
   aloe, ant-t., bov., mag-c., mez.,
   mill., mur-ac., nat-m.

11 h
   mit.

noon/midi/mittags
   am-c., menis.[11]

afternoon/après-midi/nachmittags
   arum-t., cina[11], form.[11], jug-r.,
   nux-v., plat., rhus-t.

13 h
   form.

16 h
   cina, plan.

17–21 h[16]: bell.

sleeping, after
sommeil, après le
Schlaf, nach dem
   verat.

evening/soir/abends
   bell.[4], cann-s., chin.[4], graph.,
   nat-c., rhus-t., sumb., tab., verat.

chill, during
frissons, pendant les
Fieberfrost, während
   tab.

night/nuit/nachts
   CAUST., cocc.[11], nat-c., sulph.

bed, in
lit, au
Bett, im
   cocc.

sleep, in
sommeil, pendant le
Schlaf, im
   nat-m.

waking, when
réveil, au
Erwachen, beim
   merc.

agg.[3]
   am-c.[3, 6], calc., colch., iod., med.[7, 8],
   meph.[14], merc-c., PLAT., PULS.,
   rad-br., RHEUM, RAN-B.[3, 6],
   rhus-t.[3, 6, 8], sep., staph.[3], sulph.,
   thuj.

air am., in open
air am., en plein
Freien am., im
   ol-an.

always[4]
toujours
immer
   puls, rhod., sabad., staph., tab.

am.[3, 6]
   alet.[3], alum.[3], aml-ns.[8], ANT-T.,
   arn.[3], bell., berb.[6], calc.[3, 7], carb-v.[16],
   dios., graph.[3], guaj., halo.[14], hep.,
   ign.[3], lyc.[3], mand.[10], nat-f.[14], nux-v.[3],
   perh.[14], phos.[6], plat.[3, 6, 16], plb.[8],
   podo., puls.[3, 16], pyrog.[3], rhus-t.[3, 8],
   sabad., sabin., sec.[3, 7, 8], teucr.[8],
   tub-r.[14], v-a-b.[14]

bending–backward am./plier en
   arrière am./Rückwärtsbeugen am.

anguish with impending menses
angoisse avant la menstruation, avec
qualvoller Angst bei bevorstehender
   Menses, mit
   carl.

anxiety, from
anxiété, par
Angst, aus
   nat-c.

arms, the[4]
bras, les
Arme, die
   spong., squil., stann., tab.

backward
en arrière
rückwärts
   glon., hydr.

   am.[16]: bor.

breakfast, after
petit déjeuner, après le
Frühstück, nach dem
   lach.

chill, before
frissons, avant les
Fieberfrost, vor
   aesc., ant-t., aran.[2], arn., **ars.,**
   bry.[1], **eup-per.,** ign., ip., **nat-m.,**
   nux-v., plan., rhus-t.

   during/pendant les/während
   alum., alumn.[2], ars., bry., caps.,
   coff., daph., elat., **eup-per.,**
   ferr-p.[3], ip., **kreos.,** laur., mur-ac.,
   nat-s., nit-ac., nux-v., petr.,
   rhus-t., ruta, tab., teucr.

coldness, during internal
froid intérieur, par sensation de
Kältegefühl, bei innerem
   bol-la.[2], nat-s.

continually[4]
continuellement
anhaltend
   puls., rhod., sabad., staph., tab.

   violently/véhémence/heftig

colic, during
coliques, pendant les
Koliken, bei
   haem.

convulsive, paroxysmal
convulsivement, par accès
krampfartig, anfallsweise
   ang.[4], bell., camph.[4], carbn-h.,
   chin., cic.[4, 6], cimic.[6], cina, hydr-ac.,
   ip.[4], lach.[4], lyc., merc.[4], nux-v.[4, 16],
   op.[6], sabad.[4], sec.[4, 6], sil.[4], stram.[4, 6],
   sulph.[4], thuj.[4], verat.[4]

cough, after
toux, après la
Husten, nach
   merc.[16], sang.

dinner, after
déjeuner, après le
Mittagessen, nach dem
   mag-c.

eating, after
mangé, après avoir
Essen, nach
   ip.

fever, during
fièvre, pendant la
Fieber, im
   alum.[3], **ars.**[2], bell.[3], **bor.**[3], bry.[3],
   CALC.[3, 16], **calc-p.**[2], caust.[3], cham.[3],
   eup-per.[2], nat-m.[3], **nux-v.**[3],
   RHUS-T.[2, 3], **SABAD.**[3], sep.[3],
   spong.[3], sulph.[3], thuj.

high up to reach things[16]
en haut pour atteindre quelque chose
sich hochrecken, um Dinge zu
   erreichen
   rhus-t.

house, in the
maison, dans la
Haus, im
   ruta

impossible
unmöglich
   acon., phos.

by pains[16]
par douleurs
durch Schmerzen
  bell.

lying down, after[2]
étendu, après s'être
Hinlegen, nach dem
  COCC.

menses, before
menstruation, avant la
Menses, vor den
  PULS.[1]

  during/pendant la/während der
   carb-an.

  after[6]/après la/nach den
   carb-an.

out affected parts agg.[3]
étendre les parties affectées agg.
Ausstrecken der befallenen Teile
  agg.
    alum., am-c., am-m., anac., ang.,
    ant-c., arg-m., arn., aur., bar-c.,
    bell., bov., bry., CALC., cann-s.,
    caps., carb-v., caust., cham.,
    chin., cina, clem., colch., coloc.,
    con., croc., dig., dros., dulc.,
    ferr., fl-ac., graph., guaj., hep.,
    ign., IOD., kali-c., laur., lyc.,
    mag-m., mang., meny., merc.,
    merc-c., mur-ac., nat-m., nux-v.,
    petr., phos., plat., plb., psor.,
    puls., rheum, rhus-t., ruta,
    sabin., sel., SEP., spig., spong.,
    stann., staph., SULPH., THUJ.,
    valer., verat.

  am.[3]
    agar., alum., am-m., anac., ant-t.,
    asar., bell., berb., bor., carb-an.,
    carb-v., cham., chel., chin., coff.,
    cupr., dig., dros., dios., dulc.,
    ferr., guaj., hep., ign., kali-c.,
    mag-c., mez., mur-ac., nat-m.,
    nat-s., nux-m., nux-v., olnd.,
    ox-ac., par., petr., phos., plat.,
    puls., rheum., rhod., RHUS-T.,

    sabad., sabin., SEC., stann.,
    staph., thuj., verb., zinc.

painful
douleureux
schmerzhaft
  sec.

perspiration, during[3]
transpiration, pendant la
Schwitzen, beim
  alum., bel., BOR., bry., CALC.,
  caust, cham., NAT-M., nux-v.,
  RHUS-T., sabad., sep., spong.,
  sulph.

shuddering, during
frissonnement, pendant le
Schaudern, Frösteln, beim
  ars., puls.

sitting, while[16]
assis, étant
Sitzen, beim
  alum.

sitting and reading, while
assis et en lisant, étant
Sitzen und Lesen, beim
  euphr.

sleep, during[11]
sommeil, pendant le
Schlaf, im
  nat-m.

sleepiness with[4]
somnolence avec
Schläfrigkeit mit
  ant-t., bell., chin., lach., meph.,
  sabad.

sleeplessness, during[4]
insomnie, pendant l'
Schlaflosigkeit, bei
  dulc.

  after/après l'/nach
   sulph.

slept enough, as if he had not
dormi, comme s'il n'avait pas assez
geschlafen, als hätte er nicht ge-
gend
am-c., mill.

supper, after
souper, après le
Abendessen, nach dem
nit-ac.

tossing about, with[4]
se tourne et retourne
Herumwerfen, mit
rhod.

unsatisfactory
peu satisfaisant
unbefriedigend
graph.

urination, before
uriner, avant
Urinieren, vor
PULS.

violently for hours[8]
véhémence des heures entières, avec
heftig, stundenlang
aml-ns., plb.

*continually/continuellement/
anhaltend*

waking, on[4]
réveil, au
Erwachen, beim
bell.[16], dulc.[4, 11], hell., ign.[2], meph.,
nit-ac.[16], merc.[4, 11], phos., sulph.

walking in open air am.
marcher en plein air. am.
Gehen im Freien am.
ox-ac., plan.

yawning, with[3, 4]
bâillements, avec
Gähnen, mit
acon.[3, 4, 8], aesc.[2], agar.[2-4, 8],
all-c.[8], alum.[3], am-c.[3], ambr.[3],
ang., ant-t.[3, 4, 8], arn.[3, 8],
ARS.[3, 4, 6], asar.[8], bar-c., bell.,

bor.[3], bov.[3], bry.[2-4], calc.[3, 8],
cann-s.[3], canth., caps., carb-v.,
cast.[8], caust., CHAM.[3, 6],
chin.[3, 4, 8], chin-s.[4], cocc., cur.[2],
dig.[4], dros., elat.[3, 8], ferr., form.[3, 6],
gran.[4], graph.[3], guaj.[2-4], hell.,
hep.[3, 8], ign.[3, 8], ip.[3], kreos.,
lach.[2, 4], lact.[4], laur., led.[3], mag-c.,
mang.[4], meph.[4], merc.[3], merc-c.[3],
mez., mur-ac.[3], nat-m.[4], nit-ac.[3],
NUX-V.[2-4, 6, 8], olnd.[3, 6], onis.[4],
petr., ph-ac., phos., plat.[3],
plb.[3, 4, 8], puls.[3, 4, 6], ran-b.[3],
rhod.[4], RHUS-T.[3, 6, 8], ruta,
sabad., sec.[3, 4, 8], senec.[6], seneg.[3],
sep., sil.[3, 8], spong., squil.[3, 4, 6],
stann., staph.[2-4, 7], sulph.[3, 4, 8],
tab.[4], tart-ac.[4], tong.[4], valer.,
verat., verb.[3], viol-o.[2], zinc.

forenoon[4]
matinée
vormittags
ant-t.

without sleepiness[2]
sans somnolence
ohne Schläfrigkeit
viol-o.

SUDDEN manifestation[7]
SUBITS, symptômes
PLÖTZLICH auftretende Symptome
ACON., BELL.

SULPHUR, abuse of
SULPHUR, abus de
SCHWEFEL, Folgen des Mißbrauches
von
acon.[2, 3], ars., calc., camph.[2, 3],
cham.[2, 3], chin., iod.[2], merc., nit-ac.[2],
PULS., rhus-t.[2, 3], sep., thuj.[12]

summer see seasons

SUN, from exposure to
SOLEIL, suites d'exposition au
SONNE, Folgen von Sonnenbestrah-
lung
acon.[3, 6, 12], adlu.[14], aeth.[3, 6], agar.,

aloe[3], aml-ns.[3, 6], anh.[9], **ANT-C.,**
arg-m., arn.[3], **ars.**[2, 7], **bar-c.,**
BELL.[1, 7], brom., **bry.,** cact.[7, 8, 12],
cadm-s., calc., calc-f.[10, 14], **camph.,**
carb-v., cina[3, 6], clem., cocc.[7, 12],
crot-h.[12], **euphr.,** fago.[8], **gels.**[1, 7],
GLON., graph., ign., iod., ip., **kalm.,**
LACH.[1, 7], lappa[3], **lyss.,** mag-m.,
med.[7], merc-c.[3], mur-ac.[12], **NAT-C.,**
NAT-M., nat-n.[3], **nux-v., op.,**
prot.[14], prun.[12], **psor., PULS., sel.,**
stann., stram.[2, 3, 7, 12], sul-i.[1'], sulph.,
syph.[12], ther.[3, 7], thuj.[7], **valer.,**
verat-v.[12], zinc.

ailments from[12]
troubles à la suite de
Beschwerden infolge von
acon., agar., ant-c., bell., cact.,
cadm-s., cocc., crot-h., gels.,
glon., kalm., lach., mur-ac., op.,
prun., stram., sulph., syph.,
verat-v.

chronic[12]/chroniques/chronische
nat-c.

am.[3, 7]
anac.[6], con.[3, 6], crot-h.[3], iod.[3],
kali-c.[7], kali-m.[3], pic-ac.[3], **plat.**[3, 6],
rhod.[7], rhus-t.[3], **stram.**[3, 6, 7],
STRONT-C.[3, 6], tarent.[3], **thuj.**[6]

exertion in
exercice au
Anstrengung in der
ANT-C.

sunburn[3]
hâle, brûlure solaire
Sonnenbrand
acon.[2, 3], agar., ant-c., **BELL.**[2, 3],
bry., **camph.**[2, 3], clem.[2, 3], cortiso.[14],
cyl-l.[14], euphr., **hyos.**[2, 3], lach., lyc.,
mur-ac.[2], nat-c., op., **PULS., sel.,**
sulph., **valer.**

sunstroke
coup de soleil, insolation
Sonnenstich
acon.[2, 3, 6-8], agar.[2, 7],
AML-NS.[2, 7, 12], **ant-c.**[2, 7, 8, 12],

apis[6, 10], arg-m., **arn.**[2, 7], **ars.**[2, 7],
bell., bry.[8], **cact.**[2, 7, 8, 12],
camph.[1, 7], **carb-v.**[2, 7], cit-l.[2, 7, 12],
crot-h.[12], cyt-l.[10, 14], euph-pi.[12],
gels.[2, 6-8, 10, 12], **GLON.,**
hydr-ac.[8, 10, 12], hyos.[3, 6], kalm.[2, 7],
lach.[8, 10], lyc.[12], lyss.[12],
nat-c.[1', 2, 3, 7, 8], nat-m.[12],
nux-v.[3], **op.**[2, 7, 8, 10, 12], pop-c.[12],
rhus-t.[12], stram., syph.[12], **ther.,**
thuj.[12], usn.[8], valer.[12], **verat.**[2, 7],
verat-v.[1, 7]

ailments from[12]
troubles à la suite de
Beschwerden infolge von
arg-m., camph., **LACH.**[2, 7],
NAT-C.[2, 7, 10, 12], thuj.

SUPPRESSED condylomata[1']*
SUPRIMÉS, condylomes
UNTERDRÜCKTE Kondylome
merc., nit-ac., staph., **thuj.**

abscesses – pus/abcès – pus /
Abszesse – Eiter
coryza/Schnupfen
gonorrhoea/gonorrhée/Gonorrhoe
mucous secretions – suppressed/
muqueuse, hypersécrétion –
supprimée/Schleimhautabsonde-
rungen – unterdrückte
perspiration – suppression/transpira-
tion – supprimée/Schweiß – unter-
drücktem
Vol. III: *leucorrhoea – suppressed/*
leucorrhées – supprimés/
Fluor – unterdrückter
lochia – suppressed/lochies –
supprimées/Lochien – unter-
drückte
menses – suppressed/menstrua-
tions – supprimées/Menses –
unterdrückte

eruptions*
éruptions supprimées
Hautausschläge
acon., **ail.**[3], alum., am-c., ambr.,
anac.[12], ant-c.[12], ant-t.[3],
apis[3, 6, 8, 12], **ARS.**[1, 7], ars-i.,
ars-s-f.[1'], asaf.[8, 12], bad.[2], bar-c.[1'],
bell., BRY., calad., calc.,

camph.[3, 8, 12], caps.[3], carb-an.,
carb-v., **caust., cham.**, chin.[3],
cic.[8], clem.[6], con., **cupr.**, cupr-a.[12],
cupr-ar.[12], **DULC., gels., graph.,**
hell.[6, 8,] **hep.**, hyos.[6], iod.[3], **IP.,**
KALI-BI.[3], kali-c., **kali-s.,**
kreos.[3], lach., laur.[6], **lyc.,**
mag-c.[3], mag-s.[8], merc., **mez.,**
nat-c., nit-ac., **nux-m., NUX-V.**[3],
op., **PETR., PH-AC.**, phos., plb.[12],
PSOR., ptel.[12], **puls., rhus-t.,**
sars., sel., senec.[3], **sep.**, sil.,
staph., STRAM., sul-ac.,
SULPH., thuj., **tub., tub-k.**[12],
verat., verat-v.[6], **viol-t.**, x-ray[9],
ZINC.

fail to break out, when
qui ne « sortent » pas
kommen nicht heraus
ail., am-c., ant-t., **stram., sulph.,**
zinc.

exanthemata[12]*
exanthèmes
Exantheme
ail.[6], hell., verat.

mother milk*
sécrétion de lait supprimée
Milchsekretion
acon.[6, 8], agar., **agn.**, aur., aur-i.[1'],
aur-s.[1'], **bell.**[8], **BRY.**, calc.,
calc-sil.[1'], camph-br.[8], **carb-v.,**
CAUST., cham., chim., cimic.[1'],
cycl.[6], dulc., frag.[11], **hyos.**, ign.[11],
iod., lac-d., **lach., merc.**, mill.[12],
phyt.[8], **PULS., rhus-t., sec.,**
senec.[6], **sil.**, sul-i.[1'], **sulph., urt-u.,**
verat., zinc.[6, 8, 12]

convulions–suppressed/
convulions–supprimés/
Konvulionen–Unterdrückung

anger, from
colère, par
Zorn, durch
cham.

haemorrhoids
hémorrhoïdes supprimées
Haemorrhoiden
aloe[7], am-m.[7], apis[7], ars., **calc.,**

caps.[1, 7], carb-v., **coll.**[2, 6, 7], cupr.,
ign.[2], lycps.[12], **mill.**[2, 7], **NAT-M.**[2, 7],
NUX-V., OP.[2, 7], phos., puls.,
ran-b.[7], **SULPH.**

suppuration see abscess

SWELLING in **general**
TUMÉFACTION en **général**
SCHWELLUNG, allgemeine
acon., agar., agn., all-s.[11], aloe[3, 11],
alum., am-c., am-m., ambr., anac.,
ant-c., anthraco.[4], **APIS**, arg-m.,
arg-n.[3], **arn., ARS.**, ars-i., ars-s-f.[1'],
asaf., asar.[3, 4], aur., aur-m.[4],
bar-c., bar-m.[4], **BELL.**, bell-p.[9],
bism., bor., bov., **BRY.**, bufo,
buth-a.[9], calad., **calc.**, calc-i.[3],
calc-sil.[1'], camph., cann-s., **canth.,**
caps., carb-an., carb-v., **carbn-s.,**
caust., celt.[11], **cham.**, chel., **chin.,**
chin-s.[4], cic., cina[4], clem., cocc.,
coff., colch., coloc., com., con.,
conch.[11], cop., cortiso.[9], croc.,
crot-h. crot-t.[4], cupr., cycl., **daph.**[4],
dig., dor.[11], dros., **dulc.**, eucal.[2, 11],
euph., euphr., **ferr.**, frag.[11], graph.,
guaj., hell., **hep.**, hip-ac.[9], hydr.[3],
hyos., ign., iod., **kali-ar., KALI-BI.,**
kali-c., kali-i.[4], kali-n., kreos.,
lach., laur., led., **lyc., m-arct.**[4],
mag-c., mag-m., mang., **MERC.,**
merc-c.[4], mez., mosch., mur-ac.,
naja, narcin.[11], **nat-c.**, nat-m.,
nit-ac., nux-m., **NUX-V.**, olnd.,
op., par., ped.[11], petr., **ph-ac., phos.**,
phyt.[3], plat.[4], **plb., PULS.**, ran-b.,
ran-s.[4], raph.[11], rauw.[9], rhod.,
RHUS-T., rhus-v.[11], ruta, sabad.,
sabin., samb., sang.[3], saroth.[9], sars.,
sec., seneg., **sep., sil., spig.**, spong.,
squil., stann., staph., **stram.,**
stront-c., sul-ac., **sulph.**, tarent.[11],
ter.[4], teucr.[3], thal.[14], **thuj.**, urea[11],
urt-u.[11], valer., verat., **vip.**, zinc.,
ziz.[11]

right side, on[16]
droit, du côté
rechten Seite, der
ars.

affected parts, of
affectées, des parties
befallenen Teile, der
ACON., ACT-SP., agn., alum.,
alum-sil.[1]', ant-c., ant-s-aur., apis,
arn., ars., ars-i., asaf., aur., aur-s.[1]',
bar-c., bar-i.[1]', BELL., bov., BRY.,
calc., calc-i.[1]', calc-sil.[1]', cann-s.,
canth., carb-an., carb-v., caust.,
cedr., cham., chin., cic., clem., cocc.,
colch., coll., con., CROT-H.,
crot-t., cub., cupr., dig., dulc.,
euph., EUPHR., ferr., ferr-ar.[1]',
ferr-p., fl-ac., GELS., graph., guaj.,
guare.[2], hell., hep., hippoz.[2], hydr.,
ign., iod., KALI-C.[3], kali-bi.,
kali-i., kali-m.[1]', lach., led., lyc.,
mag-c., mang., MERC., MERC-C.,
mur-ac., nat-c., nat-m., nit-ac.,
nux-v., ox-ac., petr., ph-ac., phos.,
phyt., plb., psor., PULS., ran-b.,
RHOD., RHUS-T., ruta, sabin.,
samb., sang., sars., sec., SEP., SIL.,
spig., SPONG., stann., staph.[3],
stram., SULPH., thuj., valer., zinc.

inflammatory
inflammataire
entzündliche
ACON., agn., alum., am-c., ant-c.,
ant-t.[3], apis, arn., ARS., ars-i.,
ars-s-f.[1]', asaf., aur.[4], bar-c.,
BELL., bor.[4], bry., CALC.,
calc-sil.[1]', cann-s., CANTH.,
carb-an., carb-v., caust., chin.,
cocc., colch., con., crot-h.[4], cupr.,
euph., gran.[4], graph., guaj., hep.,
hyos.[4], iod., kali-ar., KALI-BI.,
KALI-C., kali-i., kali-n.[4], led., lyc.,
mag-c., mang.[4], MERC., mez.[4],
mur-ac.[4], nat-c., nat-m., nit-ac.,
nux-v., petr., ph-ac.[4], phos., phyt.,
plb., puls., rhus-t., sabin., samb.,
sars., sec., seneg.[4], SEP., sil.,
spong., stann., stram.[4], SULPH.,
thuj., zinc.

painful[16]
douloureuse
schmerzhafte
dig.

puffy, edematous
bouffie, oedémateuse
aufgedunsen, ödematös
acon., agar., am-c., am-m., ANT-C.,
APIS, apoc., arn., ARS., ars-s-f.[1]',
asaf., aur., aur-m., bar-c., bell.,
bry., CALC., calc-sil.[1]', CAPS.,
carbn-s., cedr., cham., chin.,
cina, cocc., colch., coloc., con.,
CUPR., DIG., dros., dulc., FERR.,
GRAPH., guaj., HELL., hyos., iod.,
ip., kali-c., kreos., lach., laur., led.,
lith-c.[2], lyc., mag-c., merc., mez.,
mosch., nat-c., nat-m.[2], nit-ac.,
nux-m., nux-v.[3], OLND., op., phos.,
phyt., plb., puls., rheum, rhust-t.,
samb., sars., seneg., sep., sil., spig.,
spong., SQUIL., staph., stram.,
sulph., teucr., verat., verb., zinc.,
ziz.[2]

bones, of
os, des
Knochen, der
am-c., ambr.[4], ang.[3], ant-c.[4],
arg-m.[3], ASAF., aur., bell., bry.,
bufo[3], CALC., calc-f.[3], calc-p.,
carb-an., clem., coloc., con.,
conch.[11], daph.[2, 4], dig., dulc., euph.,
ferr., fl-ac., guaj., hep., iod., kali-i.,
kreos., lac-ac.[1], lach., led.[4] lyc.,
mang., merc., mez., nat-c., nat-m.,
nit-ac., petr., PH-AC., PHOS.,
phyt.[2], plb., PULS., rhod., rhus-t.,
ruta, sabin., sep., SIL., spig.,
STAPH., stront-c.[3], SULPH., thuj.,
verat.

sensation of sw.[16]
sensation de t.
Gefühl von Schw.
ars.

cartilages, of
cartilages, des
Knorpel, der
ARG-M., calc.[2], sil.[2]

glands, of
glandes, des
Drüsen, der
acon., acon-l.[8, 12], aesc., agn.,

ail.[3, 6, 8], aln.[8, 12], alum.,
alum-sil.[1'], **alumn.[2]**, am-c., **am-m.**,
ambr. **anthraci.**, ant-c., ant-t.,
apis[2, 3, 8], aq-mar.[6, 8], arg-m., arn.,
ars.[1], ars-br.[8], **ARS-I.**, ars-s-f.[1'],
arum-t., asaf., astac.[2, 8, 12], aur.,
aur-ar.[1'], aur-i.[1'], **aur-m.[2, 8]**,
aur-s.[1'], **bad.[2, 3, 6, 8, 10]**, bapt.,
BAR-C., BAR-I., BAR-M., bar-s.[1'],
BELL., berb.[1], bor., bov., **BROM.**,
bry., bufo, calad., **calc.**, calc-ar.[6],
calc-f.[3, 6, 8, 10], calc-hp.[6], **CALC-I.**,
calc-m.[12], calc-p., **CALC-S.**,
calc-sil.[1'], calen.[8, 12], camph.,
cann-s., **canth.**, caps., **CARB-AN.**,
CARB-V., carbn-s., caust., **cham.**,
chim.[12], chin., cic., cinnb.[4], **CIST.**,
CLEM., coc-c.[11], cocc., coloc.,
CON., cor-r.[3, 4, 6], cory.[6, 8], croc.,
crot-h., cupr., cycl., dig., dros.[7],
DULC., eucal.[2, 11], euph., euphr.[12],
eupi.[12], **FERR.[1]**, ferr-ar., ferr-i.,
fil.[8], fl-ac.[3, 6], fuc.[6, 10], **GRAPH.**,
hall[12], ham[3, 6], **hecla[2]**, hed.[10], hell.,
HEP., hippoz.[2], hydrc.[6], hyos., ign.,
IOD., iris[2, 3], **kali-ar., kali-bi.[2]**,
kali-br.[2], **kali-c., kali-chl.,**
kali-bi.[2], kali-br.[2], **kali-chl.,**
kali-i., kali-m.[1', 3, 6, 12], kreos.[4],
lach., **lap-a.[6, 8, 12]**, led., **lith-c.[2, 12]**,
LYC., mag-c., mag-m., mang.,
med., **MERC., MER-C.**, merc-cy.[8],
merc-d., **merc-i-f., merc-i-r.,**
mez., mur-ac., **nat-c.**, nat-m.,
nat-p.[2], nat-s.[3, 6], **NIT-AC.,**
nux-v., ol-j.[6], petr., **ph-ac.,**
PHOS., phyt., plb., psor., **puls.,**
RHUS-T., rumx.[8], ruta, sabad.,
sabin., samb., sars., scir.[8, 12],
scroph-n.[8, 12], sec.[2, 12], **sep., SIL.,**
sil-mar.[8, 12], sol-a.[12], sol-o.[12],
spig., **SPONG.**, squil., **stann.,**
staph., stict.[12], stram., stront-c.,
sul-ac., sul-i.[1', 3, 6], SULPH.,
symph.[12], **syph.[1', 2]**, tab.[12], tax.[8],
ter.[4], teucr., ther.[1'], thiosin.[8, 12],
THUJ., tub.[3, 6, 8], uran-n.[2], **verat.,**
viol-o., viol-t.[2], zinc.

bluish/bleuâtre/bläuliche
  arn., ars., aur., **carb-an.**, carb-v.,

con., ferr-i., hep., **lach.**, mang.,
merc., merc-i-f., puls., sil., sul-ac.

cold/froide/kalte
  ars., asaf., bell., **cocc., CON.,**
  cycl., dulc., lach., **merc.[3]**, rhod.,
  spig., **sulph.[3]**, thuj.[2]

emaciation, with[2]
amaigrissement, avec
Abmagerung, mit
  ars., ars-i., bar-c., calc., calc-i.,
  calc-p., carb-v., caust., **cist., con.,**
  graph., mag-c., mag-m., nat-m.,
  nit-ac., **ol-j.**, petr., ph-ac., phos.,
  psor., **sil.**, staph., sul-ac., sulph.

eruption, with[16]
éruption, avec
Hautausschlag, mit
  dulc.

hard/dure/harte
  agn., alumn.[1'], ant-c., arn., ars.,
  ars-i.[1'], asaf., **bad.[2]**, bar-c.[1', 3],
  bar-m.[3], bell.[3], brom.[1'], **bry.,**
  calc-f.[7], calc-sil.[1'], **carb-an.,**
  caust., chin., **CON.**, dig., graph.,
  hep.[1', 3], **IOD., kali-i.**, lach., led.,
  merc., mez., nux-v., **phos.,**
  phyt.[1', 3], **puls., RHUS-T.**, sabin.,
  samb., sil.[3], **spong.**, staph.[1'],
  stront-c., sul-i.[1'], **sulph., tarent.[3]**

hot/chaude/heiße
  acon., am-c., ant-c., ant-t.[3], arn.,
  asaf., **BELL., BRY.**, bufo[3], **calc.,**
  canth., **carb-an.**, carb-v., **cham.[2]**,
  chin., clem., cocc., euph., **hep.,**
  kali-c., led., **MERC.**, nux-v.,
  petr., **PHOS., phyt.**, puls.,
  rhus-t., sars., sil., **sulph.**

inflammatory/inflammatoire/
entzündliche
  acon., agn., am-c., ant-c., **arn.,**
  ars., asaf., **bad., bar-c.**, bar-m.[1'],
  BELL., bor., **bry.**, calc., **carb-an.,**
  carb-v., caust., **cham.[2]**, cinnb.,
  clem., cocc., **CON.**, dros.[7], **hep.,**
  hyos., **kali-i., lyc.**, mang.,
  MERC., mez., mur-ac., nat-c.,

knotted cords, like
corde à nœuds, comme une
perlschnurartig
BAR-M., calc., cist., con., **dulc.,**
hep., **iod.,** lyc., rhus-t., **sil.,**
sul-i.[1]', tub.

menses, during
mestruation, pendant la
Menses, während der
kali-c., lac-c.

nodes, like
nœuds, comme des
Knoten, wie
bry., iod.[1]', nit-ac.

painful
douloureuse
schmerzhafte
acon., am-c.[2], anan.[2], ant-c.,
anthraco.[2], arn., ars.[2], aur.,
aur-i.[1]', **bar-c.[2], BAR-M., BELL.,**
calc., **calc-p.[2],** canth., **caps.[2],**
carb-an., carb-v.[2, 6], caust.[2],
cham.[2], chin., clem., **CON.[2, 6],**
cop.[2], cor-r., crot-t.[2], cupr.[2],
graph.[3], **hep.,** ign.[2], **iod.,** kali-c.[2, 6],
kali-i., lyc.[3], **merc.[2],** mosch.[3],
nat-m.[2], **nit-ac.,** nux-v., phos.[3],
phyt., psor.[2], **puls.,** rhus-t., **sil.,**
spig., stann., staph., sulph.[2]

painless
indolore
schmerzlose
ars., asaf., **CALC.,** cocc.[1], **con.,**
cycl., dulc., **ign.,** lach., merc.[3],
nit-ac., ph-ac., plb., **sep.,** sil.,
staph., sulph., thuj., **tub.[7]**

scarlet fever, after
scarlatine, après
Scharlach, nach
am-c.[15], **BAR-C., lac-c.[2]**

scarlet fever/scarlatine/Scharlach

joints, of
articulations, des
Gelenke, der
abrot., acon., **ACT-SP.,** agn., anag.,

ant-c.[3], **ant-t., apis,** apoc., **arn., ars.,**
asc-t., aur., **aur-m., BELL.,** berb.,
bov.[6], **BRY.,** bufo, **calc.,** calc-f.,
canth.[6], caust.[1]', cedr.[6], chin.,
chin-s.[6], **cimic.,** clem., **cocc.,**
COLCH., coloc.[3], con., dulc.[1]',
ferr-p., guaj., ham., HEP., hip-ac.[9],
iod.[3, 6], kali-ar.[1]', **kali-bi.[1]', kali-chl.,**
kali-i., kali-m.[6], **kalm.,** kreos.[3],
lac-ac., lac-c.[1]', **lach., LED., lyc.,**
mang., med., **merc.,** nat-m., nux-v.,
puls.[3], **ran-b.[6], rhod., rhus-t.,** sabin.,
sal-ac., samb.[6], sil., sol-t-ae., stict.,
SULPH., tarent., **ter.,** thuj., **verat-v.**

mucous membranes, of[3]
muqueuses, des
Schleimhäute, der
arg-n., ars-i., hydr.

periosteum, of
périoste, du
Periost, des
acon.[3], ant-c., **ASAF., aur.,** bell.,
bry., chin., **kali-i.,** mang., **merc.,**
mez., **nit-ac., PH-AC., puls,** rhod.,
rhus-t., ruta, sabin., sil., staph.,
sulph.[3]

wounds see wounds–swelling

SWOLLEN sensation
ENFLÉ, sensation d'être
SCHWELLUNG, Gefühl von
acon., aesc.[6], agar., aloe, alum.,
am-c.[4], am-m., ambr., **aml-ns.[3],**
anac., ant-c., ant-t., apis, **aran.,**
arg-m., **arg-n.,** arn., ars., asaf.,
asar., aur., bapt., bar-c., **bell.,**
berb.[3], **bism.,** bov., bry., caj.,
calad., calc., **calc-p.,** cann-i.,
cann-s.[3], canth., **caps.,** carb-ac.,
carb-an.[4], carb-v., carbn-s., caust.,
cedr., cench.[7], cham., chin., cic.[3],
cimic., cina, **coc-c., cocc.,** colch.,
coloc., com., con., **cor-r.,** crot-h.,
crot-t., **cupr.,** cycl., dig., dulc.,
euph., **euphr.,** gels.[3], **glon.,** graph.[4],
GUAJ., ham.[6], hell., hep., hyos.,
ign., ip., kali-c., kali-n., kreos.,
LACH., laur., led., lyc., mag-c.,
mang., **MERC., MERC-I-F.,** mez.,

mosch., nit-ac., nux-m., nux-v.,
olnd., **op., PAEON., PAR.,** petr.,
ph-ac., phos., plat., plb., **PULS.,**
ran-b.[1], ran-s., rhod., **RHUS-T.,**
sabad., sabin., samb., **sang.,** sars.,
seneg., sep., sil., **SPIG.,** spong.,
stann., staph., stram., sul-ac.,
sulph., tarax., thuj., valer., verat.,
zinc.

bones, of
os, des
Knochen, der
ant-c., bell., chel., guaj., **puls.,**
rhus-t., spig.

glands, of
glandes, des
Drüsen, der
ant-c., aur., **bell.,** bry., carb-v.,
chin., clem., con., dulc., hep.,
ign., kali-n., lach., m-arct.[4], merc.,
nat-m.[4], nit-ac., nux-m., nux-v.,
PULS., rhus-t., sabin., spig., **spong.,**
staph., sulph.[4], zinc.

internal parts, of[3]
parties internes, des
innerer Teile
anac., ant-t., arn., ars., **asar.,** aur.,
BELL., bism., bov., bry., calad.,
caps., carb-v., cina, cocc., con.,
euph., guaj., hyos., **IGN.,** kali-c.,
laur., merc., nux-m., olnd., op.,
par., petr., plat., ran-b., ran-s.,
rhod., sars., **sep., spig., stann.,**
tarax., **verat.,** zinc.

SYCOSIS
SYKOSE
adlu.[14], aesc.[7], **agar.,** agn.[6], alum.,
alumn., am-c.[7], am-m.[7], anac.,
anan.[2, 7, 12], ang.[7], ant-c., ant-t.,
anthraco.[2, 11], apis, aran., **ARG-M.,**
ARG-N., arn.[2], **ars.**[2, 3, 7], asaf.[2, 7],
asar.[7, 14], asim.[7], aspar.[7], **aster.,** aur.,
aur-m., aur-m-n.[12], **bar-c.,**
benz-ac.[1, 7, 12], berb.[2, 7], berb-a.[14],
bor.[1, 7], bov.[7], bry., bufo[7], calad.[7],
calc., cann-i.[7], cann-s.[7], canth.[7],
caps.[6, 7], carb-ac.[7], carb-an., carb-v.,

carbn-s., cast.[12], caul.[7], **caust.,** cedr.[7],
cham., chim.[7], chin.[7], cic.[7, 14], cimic.[7],
cinnb., clem.[1, 6, 7], cob-n.[14], coc-c.[7],
coch.[7], colch.[6, 7], coloc.[7], con., cop.[7],
croc.[7], crot-h.[7], crot-t.[7], cub.[7],
cupr-a.[7], cycl.[7], cyna.[14], dig.[7], dor.[7],
dulc., epig.[7], erech.[7], erig.[7], ery-a.[6, 7],
eup-pur.[7], euph.[7], euph-pi.[7], euphr.,
fago.[7], **ferr., fl-ac.,** flav.[14], gamb.[7],
gels.[7], gnaph.[7], **graph.,** guaj.[6], guat.[14],
helon.[7], hep.[7], hydr.[6, 7], influ.[7], **iod.,**
kali-bi.[2, 6, 7, 12], kali-c., **kali-i.**[3, 6, 7],
kali-m.[7, 12], kali-n.[7], **KALI-S.,**
kalm.[1, 3, 6, 7], kreos.[2], kres.[14], lac-c.[7],
lach., lil-t.[7], lith-c.[7], **lyc.,** mag-c.[2, 7],
mang., MED., merc., **merc-c.**[2],
merc-d.[7], **merc-sul.**[2], **mez.,** mill.[12],
mosch.[7], murx.[7], nat-c.[2, 7], **nat-m.**[2, 6, 7],
nat-p.[2], **NAT-S., NIT-AC.,** nux-v.[7],
ol-j.[7], orig-v.[7], pall.[7], pareir.[7],
penic.[13, 14], petr., petros.[6, 7],
ph-ac.[2, 3, 6, 7, 12], phos.[7], **phyt.,**
pic-ac.[12], pip-n.[7], plat.[7], plb.[7], pneu.[14],
prun.[7], psor.[6, 7], puls.[7], rat.[7], rauw.[14],
rhus-t.[7], sabad.[3, 6, 7], sabin., sacch-l.[7],
sanic.[7], sarr.[7], **sars., sec., sel.,** senec.[7],
seneg.[7], **SEP., sil.,** spig.[7], **STAPH.,**
still.[7], stram.[7], **sulph.,** tab.[7], tell.[14],
ter.[7], <u>**THUJ.**</u>[1, 1'], thyr.[14], uran-n.[7],
ven-m.[14], vib.[7], zing.[6]

SYNALGIA[3]
SYNALGIE
apis, tarent.

SYPHILIS ✳
aethi-a.[12], agn.[6], ail.[12], allox.[14],
aln.[12], am-c.[3], anag.[2, 12], **anan.**[2, 12],
ang.[2], ant-c.[6], **ant-t.**[2], apis[2, 12],
arg-i.[12], arg-m., arg-n.[6, 12], arn.[2],
ars., ARS-I., ars-met.[8, 12], **ars-s-f.,**
asaf., asar.[14], asc-t.[2, 12], astra-e.[14],
AUR., aur-ar.[1', 12], aur-i.[1', 12],
AUR-M., AUR-M-N., aur-s.[1'], bad.,
bell.[7], benz-ac., berb.[2], berb-a.[12],
buni-o.[14], cadm-met.[9], **calc-f.**[3, 6, 12, 14],
calc-i., calc-s., calo.[8, 12], **carb-an.,**
carb-v., **caust.**[2, 7, 12], **cean.**[2],
chim.[2, 12], chin-ar.[12], chr-o.[12], **cinnb.,**
clem., cob-n.[14], **colch.**[6, 7], **con.,**

convo-s.[14], cop.[6], cor-r., cory.[6, 8, 12], crot-h., cund.[2, 12], cupr.[6], cupr-s.[12], echi.[12], ery-a.[6], eryth.[12], eucal.[12], euph.[2, 6, 12], ferr.[7, 12], ferr-i.[2, 6], fl-ac., franc.[12], **graph.**[12], guaj., ham.[6], hecla[2, 12], **hep.**, hip-ac.[14], **hippoz.**[2, 12], hir.[14], hydr.[6, 12], hydrc.[12], hyoth.[14], iber.[14], **iod., iris**[2], **jac.**[2, 7, 12], jac-c.[12], jatr.[3], jug-r.[12], **kali-ar., kali-bi.,** kali-br.[12], kali-c.[7], **kali-chl., KALI-I., kali-m.**[2], **KALI-S.,** kalm.[2, 3, 6, 7], **kreos.**[2, 6, 12], lac-c.[2, 7, 12], lac-d.[7], **lach., LAUR.**[2], **led.,** lith-c.[12], lyc.[1', 2, 7], maland.[12], MERC.[i, 1'], merc-aur.[6], **MERC-C., merc-d.**[2, 7], **MERC-I-F., MERC-I-R., mez.,** mill.[7], nep.[14], **NIT-AC.,** nux-v.[6], ol-sant.[6], osm.[12], penic.[14], perh.[14], petr., petros.[6], **ph-ac., phos., PHYT.,** pilo.[12], pitu.[14], plat-m.[8], psor.[12], reser.[14], rhod.[6], sabad.[6], **sang.**[2, 6, 12], **sars.,** sec.[7], sel.[12], **sep.**[2], **SIL.,** spong.[6], **staph.,** stict.[12], **STILL.,** strych-g.[12], **sul-i., sulph., SYPH.,** ter.[6], thala.[14], thiop.[14], **thuj.,** thymol.[14], **thyr.**[7, 12], ulm.[12], vac.[12], **viol-t.**[2, 12], xan.[6]

congenital[8]
congénitale, syphilis
angeborene Syphilis
    aethi-m., ars-i., ars-met., **aur.,** calc-f., **calc-i.,** cor-r., kali-i., kreos.[8, 12], **merc., merc-d., nit-ac.,** pilo.[12], psor., syph.[8, 12]

serologie, with irreducible[14]
sérologie irréductible, à
Seroreaktionen, mit irreponiblen
    astra-e.

TALKING agg.[3]
PARLER agg.
REDEN agg.
    acon., agar., alum.[3, 4], am-c.[3, 4], am-m., ambr.[3, 4], **ANAC.,** arg-m.[3, 14], arg-n., **arn.**[3, 4], ars., arum-t., aur., bar-c., **bell.**[1', 3], bor.[3, 4], **bry.,** **CALC.**[3, 4], **CANN-S.,** canth., caps., **carb-v.,** caust., **cham., CHIN.,** cic., **COCC.**[3, 4], coff., con., croc., dig.,

dros., **dulc.,** euphr., ferr., ferr-p., fl-ac., **graph.,** hell., **hep.,** hyos., ign., **iod.,** ip., kali-c., led., lyc., mag-c., **mag-m., MANG.,** merc., merc-c., merc-cy., mez., mur-ac., **NAT-C., NAT-M.,** nux-m., nux-v., par., petr., **PH-AC., phos.,** phyt., plat., plb., puls., raja-s.[14], ran-b., **RHUS-T.,** sars., **SEL., sep.,** sil., **spig.,** spong., squil., **STANN.**[3, 4], staph., stram., stront-c., sul-ac., **SULPH.**[3, 4], **verat.**

Vol. I: *conversation/Unterhaltung talking/parler/Reden*

am.[3]
    ferr., rhus-t., sel.

TEETH together agg., biting[3]
DENTS, agg. en serrant les
ZÄHNE agg., Zusammenbeißen der
    alum., **AM-C.,** anac., bell., bry., carb-an., caust., chin., coff., colch., dig., graph., **guaj.,** hell., **hep., hyos., ip.,** lach., mang., merc., petr., puls., **rhus-t.,** sars., **sep.,** sil., spong., staph., **sul-ac.,** sulph., **verb.**

am.[3]
    ars., chin., cocc., coff., euph., mag-m., **staph.**

brushing, cleaning the, agg.[3]
se brossant les, agg. en
Zähneputzen agg.
    carb-v., coc-c.[3, 8], lyc., ruta, **staph.**[3, 8]

TENSION externally
TENSION externe
SPANNUNG, äußerliche
    acon., agar., agn., aloe, **alum.,** alum-p.[1'], alum-sil.[1'], **alumn.**[2], am-c., **am-m.,** ambr., anac., ang.[3, 4], ant-c., ant-t., apis[3, 6], arg-m., **arg-n., arn.,** ars., **asaf.,** asar., **aur.,** aur-s.[1'], **BAR-C.,** bar-i.[1'], bar-m., bar-s.[1'], **bell.,** berb., bism., bor., bov., **BRY.,**

calc., camph., cann-s., canth.,
caps., **carb-an.,** carb-v., **CAUST.,**
cham., **chel.,** chin., chin-s.[4], cic.,
clem., cocc., colch., **COLOC.,**
CON., croc., crot-h., **cupr.,**
dig., dros., euph., euphr.,
ferr., glon., graph., guaj.,
hell., hep., hyos., ign., iod., ip.,
kali-ar., **kali-c.,** kali-n., kreos.,
lach., laur., **led.,** lyc., **m-arct.[4],**
mag-c., mag-m., mang., med.[2],
meny., **merc., mez., mosch.,**
mur-ac., **nat-c.,** nat-m., nat-p.,
nit-ac., nux-m., **nux-v.,** olnd., op.,
par., **petr.,** ph-ac., **PHOS., PLAT.,**
plb., **PULS.,** ran-b., **rheum,** rhod.,
RHUS-T., ruta, sabad., **sabin.,**
samb., sars., **sec.,** seneg., **sep.,**
sil., **spig., spong.,** squil., stann.,
staph., stram., **STRONT-C.,**
sul-ac., sul-i.[1'], **SULPH.,** tarax.,
teucr., **thuj.,** valer., verat.,
VERB., viol-o., viol-t., x-ray[9],
zinc.

prevents motion[7]
l'empêche de se mouvoir
verhindert Bewegung
  apis

internally
interne
innerliche
  acon., aesc., agar., agn., alum.,
  am-m., ambr., anac., ang.[3], ant-c.,
  ant-t., apis[3], arg-m., arn., **ars.,**
  ASAF., asar., **aur.,** bar-c., bar-i.[1'],
  bar-s.[1'], **BELL., berb.,** bov., bry.,
  calc., camph., cann-s., **caps.,**
  carb-ac., carb-an., carb-v.,
  caust., cham., chel., chin., **cic.,**
  clem., coc-c., cocc., coff., colch.,
  coloc., com., con., croc., crot-t.,
  cupr., cycl., dig., dros., **dulc.,**
  euph., euphr., ferr., gels., **glon.,**
  graph., guaj.[16], hell., hep., hydr-ac.,
  hyos., **hyper.,** ign., iod., ip., kali-c.,
  kali-n., kreos., lach., lact.[3], laur.,
  led., lob., **LYC.,** mag-c., mag-m.,
  mang., meny., **merc.,** mez., **mosch.,**
  mur-ac., naja, nat-c., nat-m.,
  nit-ac., nux-m., **NUX-V.,** olnd., **op.,**

osm., **PAR.,** petr., ph-ac., **PHOS.,**
plat., plb., **PULS., RAN-B.,** ran-s.,
rauw.[9], **rheum,** rhod., **rhus-t.,** ruta,
sabad., sabin., samb., sec., seneg.,
SEP., sil., **spig.,** spong., squil.,
stann., staph., stram., STRONT-C.,
sul-ac., sul-i.[1'], **SULPH.,** tab., tarax.,
teucr., thuj., valer., **verat.,** verb.,
zinc.

arteries, of[11]
artères, des
Arterien, der
  chlor., **coff.**[7, 11], gels.

bones, of
os, des
Knochen, der
  agar., ang.[4], arg-m.[11], **asaf.**[1], bar-c.[2],
  BELL., bry., **chin.**[2, 11], cimic., cocc.,
  con., crot-h., dig., dulc., kali-bi.,
  mang.[4], merc., nit-ac., rhod., **ruta,**
  sulph., valer., zinc.

glands, of
glandes, des
Drüsen, der
  alum., am-c.[4], ambr., ang.[3, 4],
  arg-m., arn., aur., **bar-c.,** bell.,
  bov., **bry.,** calc., carb-an., **caust.,**
  clem., coloc., **con.,** dulc., graph.,
  kali-c., lyc., m-arct.[4], merc.,
  mur-ac., nux-v., **PHOS., puls.,**
  rhus-t., sabad., sabin., sep., sil.,
  spong., staph., stront-c., **sulph.,**
  thuj.

joints, of[3]
articulations, des
Gelenke, der
  am-c.[4], anac., ant-t., **ARG-M.,**
  arn., ars., asaf., bell., **bov.,**
  BRY.[3, 11], calc., calth.[11], caps.,
  carb-an., carb-v., **carl.**[11], **CAUST.,**
  cham., clem.[11], colch., coloc., con.,
  croc., dig., dros., euph., euphr.,
  graph., hell., hep., iod., **kali-c.,**
  kali-n., kreos., lach., laur., **LED.**[2, 3],
  LYC., mag-c., manc.[11], **mang.,**
  merc., **mez.,** mur-ac., **NAT-M.,**
  nit-ac., nux-v., par., petr., phos.,
  plat., **PULS.**[2, 3], rheum, **rhod.,**

rhus-t.[3, 4], ruta, samb., **seneg.**[3, 4, 11],
SEP., sil., spig., spong., **stann.**,
sul-ac., **SULPH.**, **teucr.**, verat.,
verb., zinc.

muscles, of
muscles, des
Muskeln, der
   ACON., am-c.[4], am-m., anac.,
   ang.[3, 16], ant-c., arn., ars., bell.,
   berb.[3], bufo[3], cann-i., cann-s., canth.,
   caps.[3], carb-v., caust., chin., dulc.,
   graph., **guaj.**, kali-ar.[1'], kali-c.,
   lach., led., **mosch.**, **nat-c.**, **nat-m.**,
   nat-p.[1'], **NIT-AC.**, **NUX-V.**, olnd.,
   ph-ac., **PHOS.**[3], **PHYS.**, phyt., **plat.**,
   plb., **puls.**, **rhus-t.**, **SEP.**, **sil.**, stann.,
   staph., sulph., verb., wies.[11], zinc.,
   zinc-p.[1']

tremulous[16]
tremblante
zittrige
   petr.

TETANUS, prophylaxis of[7]
TÉTANOS, prophylaxie du
TETANUS-Prophylaxe
   ARN., **HYPER.**, **LED.**, tetox., thuj.

THIRST for **large** quantities
SOIF de **grandes** quantités
DURST auf **große** Mengen
   acet-ac.[7], **acon.**, **ARS.**, bad.,
   BRY., calen.[2], camph., carbn-s.,
   chin., coc-c., **cocc.**, cop., **eup-per.**,
   ferr-p., ham., jatr.[2], lac-c.[3], lac-d.,
   lil-t.[3], **lycps.**, merc-c., **NAT-M.**,
   PHOS., pic-ac., **podo.**[2], sol-n.,
   stram., **SULPH.**, **VERAT.**, vip.[6]

   often/souvant/oft
   acon.[2], arn.[2], ars.[16], **bell.**[2], **BRY.**,
   cop., **eup-p.**[2], lac-c., **lac-d.**[2],
   lil-t.[2, 3], **nat-m.**, ruta[16], samb.[2],
   syph.[2], **tarent.**[2]

   at long intervals
   à intervalles éloignés
   mit langen Pausen
   BRY., hell.[8], podo.[8], **sulph.**[8],
   verat.[8]

small quantities, for
petites quantités, de
kleine Mengen, auf
   anac.[3], ant-t., apis, **ARS.**,
   arum-t., bell., bry.[3], cact., calc.[3],
   caps.[3], carb-v.[3], **chin.**, cimic.[7],
   cupr., cupr-ar., gast.[11], **hell.**,
   hep.[3], hyos., lac-c., **lach.**, laur.[3],
   LYC., merc-i-r., nat-m.[3], nux-v.[3],
   phos., **rhus-t.**, sanic.[7], squil.,
   sulph., tab.

   often/souvent/oft
   acon., ant-t., apis, **ARS.**, arum-t.,
   bell., cact., **chin.**, **coloc.**, **corn.**,
   eup-per., hyos., kali-n.[6], lac-c.,
   lyc., **nat-ar.**, puls., rhus-t., sanic.[7],
   sulph., verat.

THIRSTLESS during heat
ABSENCE DE SOIF pendant la fièvre
DURSTLOS im Fieber
   acet-ac.[7], aesc.[2], **aeth.**, agar., **AGN.**[3],
   all-c.[3], **alum.**, alum-p.[1'], alum-sil.[1'],
   am-m.[3, 6], anac.[3], ang.[3], **ant-c.**, **ant-t.**,
   APIS, arg-m., arn.[3], **ars.**[3, 16], ars-h.,
   asaf., bar-c., bell.[3, 16], bov., brom.[3],
   bry.[3], **calad.**[2], **calc.**, calc-p.[3], camph.,
   canth.[3], carb-an., **carb-v.**, **caust.**,
   cham.[3, 6, 16], **CHEL.**[3], chin., chin-m.[2],
   chin-s.[6], **cimx.**, **CINA**, cocc., **coff.**[3, 6],
   coloc.[3], **con.**[3, 16], cycl., dig., **dros.**,
   DULC.[3, 6], euph.[3, 16], **ferr.**, **GELS.**,
   gran.[11], graph.[3], guaj.[3, 16], hell.,
   hep.[3, 16], hydr-ac.[2], hyos.[2], **ign.**, **ip.**,
   kali-c., kali-n.[3, 16], kreos.[3], **lach.**[3],
   laur.[3], lec., **led.**, lyc., mag-c.[3], mang.[3],
   med., meny., **merc.**[3, 6], **mur-ac.**,
   nat-c.[3], nat-m.[3], **nit-ac.**, **nux-m.**,
   olnd.[3], op., **ph-ac.**, phos.[3, 16], plb.[3],
   puls., rheum[3, 16], **rhod.**[3, 11], rhus-t.,
   RUTA[3, 16], **SABAD.**, sabin.[3], **samb.**,
   SEP., sil.[16], spig., spong.[3, 16], squil.[3, 16],
   stann.[16], staph.[3, 16], stram.[2, 3, 16],
   sulph., tarax.[3, 6, 16], thuj.[3], valer.[3],
   verat.[3, 16], **viol-t.**[3]

THREADS, sensation of
FILS, sensation de
FÄDEN, Gefühl von
bry., coc-c., ign., lach., **osm.,** par.,
plat., VALER.

pain–drawing–bones–thread/
douleurs–tiraillantes–os–linéaires/
Schmerzen–ziehende–Knochen–
Faden

THROMBOSIS
THROMBOSE
acetan.[12], **ars.**[1, 7], **apis**[2, 7], **both.**[7, 8],
calc-ar.[12], carb-v.[3, 16], cortico[9],
kali-m.[2, 3, 6, 7, 12], kres.[13], lach.[8],
nat-s.[7], sec.[12], **vip.**[3, 6]

inflammation – phlebitis/
inflammations – phlébite/
Entzündungen – Phlebitis

albuminuria, in[7]
albuminurie, au cours d'
Albuminurie, bei
calc-ar.

pneumonia, in[7]
pneumonie, au cours de
Pneumonie, bei
am-c.

wet agg.[7]
humidité agg.
Nässe agg.
nat-s.

TICKLISH
CHATOUILLEUX
KITZLIG
KALI-C.[7], solin.[12], zinc.[11]

TOBACCO agg.*
TABAC agg.
TABAK agg.
abies-n.[3, 8, 12], acon., act-sp.[2],
agar., **alum., alumn.**[2], ambr.,
anac.[3], ang.[2, 3], **ant-c.,** arg-m.,
arg-n., **ARS.,** aur-m-n.[6], bell.,
bor.[8], brom.[1', 3], **bry.,** cact.[3],

calad., calc., calc-caust.[6], calc-p.[8],
camph., cann-i.[8], carb-an.,
carbn-s., caust.[3], cham.[3], chel.,
chin., chin-ar.[8, 12], chin-m.[12], cic.,
clem., coca, coc-c., **cocc., coff.**[3, 6],
coloc., con., conv.[3], cupr.[3], **cycl.,**
dig., dor.[2], **euphr.,** ferr., **gels.,**
hell., hep., hydr., **IGN.,** iod.,
ip., kali-bi.[3, 8], kali-br.[3],
kalm.[3, 6, 8, 12], lac-ac., **lach.,**
lob.[8, 12], **lyc., mag-c.,** mag-m.[14],
mand.[10], **meny.,** merc.[3], mur-ac.[8],
naja[3], nat-c.[3], **nat-m.,** nicot.[12],
NUX-V., okou.[14], olnd.[3], osm.,
par., petr., **phos., PLAN.,** plb.[8],
psil.[14], **PULS.,** ran-b., rhus-t.,
ruta, sabad., sabin., sars., scut.[12],
sec.[8], **sel.,** sep., sil., sol-m.[12],
SPIG., SPONG., STAPH., stel.[8],
stront-c.[3], stroph-h.[6, 12], sul-ac.,
sulph., tab.[3, 8], **tarax., thuj.,**
verat.

chewing agg.
chiquer agg.
Kauen von T. agg.
ARS., carb-v., ign.[8], lyc., nux-v.,
plan., sel.[8], tab.[2], **verat.**

nicotinism[10]*
nicotinisme
Nikotinvergiftung
ign., okou.[14], nux-v., tab.

smoking, when breaking off
fumer, suites d'arrêt de
Rauchen, beim Aufhören mit
calad.

ailments from[12]
troubles à la suite de
Beschwerden infolge von
abies-n., arg-n., ars., chin-ar., lob.,
lyc., phos., scut., sep., spig., staph.,
stroph-h., thuj., verat.

am.
aran., aran-ix.[10], arn.[6], bor.,
carb-ac., coloc., **hep.,** levo.[14], merc.,
naja[3], nat-c., **sep.,** spig., stront-c.[3],
tarent.[3, 6], tarent-c.[3, 8]

aversion to
aversion de
Abneigung gegen
  acon., acon-l.[11], alum.[6], ant-t.,
  arg-n.[7], arn., bov., brom., bry.,
  CALC., camph., canth.,
  carb-an., chlor., cimic., clem.[11],
  cocc., con., grat.[6], **ign.,** jug-r.[11],
  lach., led.[7], **lob.**[3, 4, 6, 8], **lyc.,**
  mag-s., mand.[9], meph.,
  nat-ar.[11], **nat-m., NUX-V.,**
  op., phos., phyt.[7], plan.[6-8],
  psor., **puls.,** spig., staph.[6],
  stry.[7], **sulph.,** tarax., thuj., til.,
  v-a-b.[14], valer., zing.

  morning/matin/morgens
    meph.

  sensitive to smell of
  sensible à l'odeur de
  empfindlich gegen Geruch von
    agar.[11], ars-h.[2], **asc-t.**[2], **bell.,**
    casc.[2, 8], chin., **ign., lob.**[2, 8], **lyc.**[2],
    lyss., **nux-v.,** phos., **puls.,** sol-n.[11],
    tab.[11]

  smoking (his accustomed cigar)
  fumer son cigare accoutumé, pour
  seine gewohnte Zigarre
    alum., alum-p.[1'], ant-t.[2, 3],
    arg-m., **arn.,** asar., bell.[3], bor.,
    brom., bry., **calc.,** calc-p.,
    camph., canth.[3], carb-an.,
    casc.[2], chin.[3], clem., coc-c.,
    cocc.[3], coff., con.[16], euphr.,
    ferr.[1'], ferr-i.[11], grat., **IGN.,** ip.[3],
    jug-r.[11], kali-bi., kali-n., lach.,
    led.[3, 16], lob.[3], **lyc.,** mag-s.,
    meph.[3], mez.[3], nat-ar., nat-m.,
    nat-s., nicc., nux-m.[3], **nux-v.**[2, 3],
    olnd., op., ox-ac., par.[3], phos.,
    plat.[3, 16], psor., **puls.,** rhus-t.[3],
    sars.[3, 16], sep., spig., stann.[3],
    staph.[3], **sulph.,** tarax., tell.,
    thuj.[3]

  morning/matin/morgens
    ox-ac.

  forenoon/matinée/vormittags
    kali-bi.

  afternoon[1]/après-midi/nach-
    mittags
    ign.

  evening[2]/soir/abends
    arg-n.

  breakfast, after[11]
  petit déjeuner, après le
  Frühstück, nach dem
    psor.

  in spite of[14]
  fume autant, mais
  raucht trotzdem
    thiop.

desire for t.
désir de t.
Verlangen nach T.
  aran-ix.[9, 10, 14], **ars.**[12], **asar.**[8], bell.,
  calad.[1'], **calc-p.**[3, 6, 12], **camph.**[12],
  carb-ac., carb-v.[8], **chin.**[12], chlor.[11],
  coca[2, 8], coff.[3], con.[11], daph.,
  eug., glon.[3, 6], kreos., manc.,
  med.[1', 7], narz.[11], (non[16]: nat-c.),
  nicot.[7], nux-v., ox-ac., **phos.**[12],
  plan.[12], plat., plb., rhus-t.[3], **spig.**[12],
  staph., TAB., ther., thuj.

  evening[11]/soir/abends
    ox-ac.

  dinner, after[11]
  déjeuner, après le
  Mittagessen, nach dem
    nat-c.

  smoking
  fumer, de
  rauchen, zu
    calad., carb-an., card-m.,
    cast-eq.[2], coff.[3], daph.[3], eug.,
    glon., ham., led., lyc., med.[3],
    nat-c.[3, 16], nux-v.[3], staph.[3], ther.

  snuff
  tabac à priser
  Schnupftabak
    bell.

disgust for t., remedies to [3, 5, 7]
dégoûter du t., remèdes pour
Widerwillen gegen T. zu erregen;
   Mittel, um
   arg-n.[7], ars.[7], calad., calc., camph.[5],
   caust., con.[5], ign., lach., nep.[13, 14],
   nicot.[7], nux-v., petr., plan.[3, 5-7],
   STAPH., stry.[7], sulph., tab.[7], v-a-b.[13]

TORPOR of the left side of the body
TORPEUR du côté gauche du corps
ERSTARRUNG der linken Körperseite
   acon.

TOUCH agg.
ATTOUCHEMENT agg.
BERÜHRUNG agg.
   acon., aesc., **AGAR., agn.**, aloe,
   am-c., am-m., ambr., anac.,
   ANG.[2, 3, 8], ange-s.[14], **ant-c.,**
   ant-t., APIS, ARG-M., arg-n.[7],
   arn., ars., ASAF., asar., aur.,
   aur-ar.[1'], **aur-s.**[1'], bar-c., bar-i.[1'],
   BELL., bor., bov., **BRY.**, bufo[1'],
   cact., calad., calc., calc-f.[10, 14],
   calc-p., calc-sil.[1'], camph., **cann-s.,**
   canth., caps., carb-an., **carb-v.,**
   cast.[3], caust., **CHAM., chel.,**
   CHIN., chin-ar., **CHIN-S.**, cic.,
   cimic.[6], **cina, cinnb.**, clem., **COCC.,**
   COFF., COLCH., coloc., com.[8],
   con., croc., **CROT-C.**, crot-h.,
   CUPR., cupr-a.[8], cycl., dig., dros.,
   dulc., equis.[8], eup-per.[6], **euph.,**
   euph-l.[8], euphr., ferr., ferr-i.,
   ferr-p.[3, 8], fl-ac.[3], foll.[14], graph.,
   GUAJ., HAM., hell, helon.[8], **HEP.,**
   HYOS., ign., iod., ip., **KALI-AR.,**
   kali-bi., KALI-C., kali-i.,
   kali-m.[1'], **kali-n., kali-p.**, kali-s.,
   kali-sil.[1'], **kreos.**, lac-c.[3], lac-d.[1'],
   LACH., laur., **led., lil-t.**[8], lob.[8],
   LYC., mag-c., mag-m., MAG-P.,
   mand.[14], **MANG., med.**, meny.,
   meph.[4, 14], **merc., merc-c., mez.,**
   mosch., mur-ac., **murx.**[3, 6, 8],
   nat-c., **nat-m.**, nat-s.[1', 3, 7],
   nat-sil.[1'], **NIT-AC.**, nux-m.,
   NUX-V., olnd., **op.**, osm.,

   ox-ac.[8], **par.**, petr., **ph-ac., phos.,**
   plat., plb., **puls., RAN-B.**, ran-s.,
   RHOD., RHUS-T., ruta, sabad.,
   SABIN., sal-ac., **sang.**, sanic.[3],
   sars., **sec., seneg., SEP.**, sieg.[10],
   SIL., SPIG.[1], **spong.**, squil.,
   stann., **STAPH., stram., stront-c.,**
   stry.[8], sul-ac., sul-i.[1'], **SULPH.,**
   syph.[1', 3, 7], **tarax., tarent., tell.,**
   teucr.[2, 3], thal.[14], **ther.**[8], **thuj.,**
   urt-u.[8], valer., **verat.**, verb.,
   viol-o., viol-t., vip-a.[14], **zinc.,**
   ziz.[6]

   cannot bear limbs touch each other
      at night[7]
   ne supporte pas que ses jambes se
      touchent la nuit
   kann nachts nicht die gegenseitige
      Berührung der Glieder vertragen
      psor.

   children, in
   enfants, chez les
   Kindern, bei
      ant-t.[4], apis[2], **cina**[2, 4]

   feet, of
   pieds, des
   Füße, der
      KALI-C.[2, 3], nux-v.[3]

   slight
   leger
   leichte
      ACON.[3], **APIS**[3], ars., **BELL.,**
      CHIN., coff., **colch.**, ign., **LACH.,**
      lyss.[2], mag-m., **MERC.**, merc-c.[3],
      mez., nit-ac.[3], **NUX-V.**, ph-ac.,
      phos., stann.

   throat agg., of[2, 3]
   gorge agg., de la
   Halses agg., des
      bell., **LACH.**

am.
   agar., alum., **alumn.**[2], am-c., am-m.,
   anac., ant-c., arn., **ars.,**
   ASAF.[2, 3, 6, 8], bell., bell-p.[7], **bism.,**
   bry., CALC., calc-a.[6], canth.,
   cast.[3, 6], caust., **chel.**, chin., **coloc.,**

con., **CYCL.**, dros., euph., euphr., **grat.**[3, 4, 6], hep.[2, 3], kali-c.[2, 3], petr., ph-ac., **phos.**, plb., sang.[3], sep., spig.[3], spong., staph.[3], sulph., tarax., **THUJ.**, viol-t., zinc.[3]

illusions of being touched
illusions d'être touché
Sinnestäuschung, berührt zu werden
acon., **alum.**, anac., ant-t., arn., ars., **asaf.**, asar., bar-c., **bell.**, bism., bor., bov., bry., **calc.**, cann-s., canth., caps., caust., chel., coc-c., cocc., coloc., con., **croc.**, dros., dulc., glon., graph., guaj., hell., hep., hyos., **ign.**, indg., iod., kali-c., kali-n., kreos., **lach.**, laur., lyc., mag-c., mag-m., meny., merc., mosch., nat-c., nat-m., nux-v., olnd., op., **par.**, ph-ac., phos., plat., **plb.**, **puls.**, ran-b., ran-s., rheum, rhod., **RHUS-T.**, ruta, sabad., samb., seneg., sep., sil., **spig.**, spong., squil., staph., **stram.**, sul-ac., **sulph.**[1], tarax., thuj., valer., verat., verb.

pain vanishes on t. and appears elsewhere
douleur disparaît et apparaît ailleurs, au toucher la
Schmerz verschwindet bei B. und erscheint an anderer Stelle
ant-t.[2], asaf., sang., staph.[3]

TOUCHING anything agg.
TOUCHER qc. agg.
BERÜHREN agg., **etwas**
acon., am-c., am-m., arg-m., arn., bell., bor., **bry.**, **calc.**, **cann-s.**, **carb-v.**, **caust.**, **CHAM.**, chin., dros., kali-c., kali-n., led., lyc., merc., nat-c., phos., plat., **puls.**, sec., **sil.**, spig., verat.

cold things agg.
froides agg., des choses
kalter Gegenstände agg.
calc., **HEP.**, **lac-d.**, merc., **nat-m.**, pyrog., **RHUS-T.**, **SIL.**, thuj., zinc.

warm things agg.
chaudes agg., des choses
warmer Gegenstände agg.
sulph.

TRAVELLING, ailments from[12]
VOYAGES, troubles à la suite de
REISEN, Beschwerden infolge von
cocc., con.

TREMBLING externally
TREMBLEMENT externe
ZITTERN, äußerliches
aur., aur-ar.[1'], aur-i.[1'], aur-s.[1'], **bapt.**[1', 3, 6, 11], **bar-c.**, bar-i.[1'], bar-m., bar-s.[1'], **bell.**, ben-n.[11], benz-ac.[11], berb.[4], bism., **bor.**, both.[7], bov., brom., bruc.[4], **bry.**, bufo, buth-a.[9, 10], cadm-met.[10], cadm-s., caj.[11], **calad.**, **calc.**, calc-caust.[4, 11, 12], calc-f.[10, 14], **calc-i.**[1'], calc-m.[11], **calc-p.**, calc-sil.[1'], calth.[11], **camph.**, canch.[11], cann-i., cann-s., canth., caps., **carb-ac.**, carb-an.[4], **carb-v.**, carbn-h.[11], carbn-o.[11], **carbn-s.**, cast.[2], **caust.**, **cedr.**, cham., **chel.**, chin., **chin-ar.**, **chin-s.**, chlorpr.[14], **CIC.**, cic-m.[11], **CIMIC.**, **cina**, cinch.[11], cinnm.[2], **cit-v.**[2, 11], clem., **coca**[2], **COCC.**, cod., **coff.**, coff-t.[2, 7, 11], coffin.[11], **colch.**, coloc., **CON.**, cop.[2], cortico.[9, 10], cortiso.[10], croc., **crot-h.**, crot-t., **cupr.**, cupr-a.[4], cupr-ar.[6], cupr-s.[2], dig., digin.[11], dios., dros., dubo-h.[11], **dulc.**, echit.[11], esp-g.[13], euph.[3], euphr., fagu.[11], **ferr.**, ferr-ar.[4], ferr-ma.[4, 11], ferr-p., fl-ac.[1'], **GELS.**, gins.[6, 11], glon., gran.[3, 4, 6, 11], **graph.**, guaj., **hell.**, helo., hep., hydr-ac.[4, 11], **hyos.**, **hyper.**[2], iber.[11, 14], **ign.**, inul.[11], **iod.**, ip., **iris**[2], jab.[6], kali-a.[11], **kali-ar.**, kali-bi.[11], **kali-br.**, **kali-c.**, kali-cy.[11], **kali-fcy.**, kali-i.[11], kali-n.[11, 16], kali-p., kali-s., kali-sil.[1'], **kalm.**, kiss.[11], kreos., lac-ac., lach., lat-m.[9], lath.[3, 6], laur., **lec.**, **led.**, lil-t.[1', 2, 11],

lob.[3, 4, 6, 11], **lol.**[3, 10-12], lon-x.[11],
lyc., lycps.[2], **lyss.**, m-arct.[4],
m-aust.[4], mag-c., mag-m., mag-p.,
mag-s., manc.[3, 11], mang., meny.,
meph., **MERC., merc-c.**, merc-d.[11],
merc-i-f.[11], merc-ns.[11],
merc-pr-r.[11], **mez.**, morph.[11],
mosch., mur-ac., mygal., naja[1'],
NAT-AR., nat-c.[1], nat-hchls.[11],
nat-m., nat-s., nat-sil.[1'],
nicc.[4, 6, 11], nicot.[11], **nit-ac.**,
nux-m., **nux-v.**, oena.[11], ol-an.[4],
olnd., OP., ox-ac., pall., par.,
ped.[11], petr., **ph-ac., phel.**[2, 4],
phos., phys.[2, 3, 6, 11], **phyt., pic-ac.**,
pip-n.[3], plan., **PLAT., plb.**,
polyg-h., prun.[4, 11], psil.[14], **psor.**,
PULS., ran-a.[11], ran-b., ran-s.,
rauw.[9, 14], reser.[14], rheum, rhod.,
RHUS-T., russ.[11], ruta, **sabad.**,
sabin., sal-ac.[6], sang., sars.,
scut.[11], **sec.**, sel., senec.[11], **seneg.**,
sep., sieg.[10], **sil.**, spig., spig-m.[11],
sol-n.[11], spong., squil.[3, 6], **stann.**,
staph., **STRAM.**, stront-c., **stry.**,
sul-ac., sul-h.[11], sul-i.[1'], **SULPH.**,
tab., tanac., tarax., **tarent.**, tax.[11],
teucr., thal.[11, 14], thea, **THER.**,
thuj., thyreotr.[14], til.[11], valer.,
vanad.[7], **verat.**, verat-v.[11], verb.,
verin.[11], vesp.[2, 11], viol-o.,
vip.[3, 4, 6], **vise.**, wies.[11], x-ray[9],
ZINC., zinc-cy.[11], zinc-o.[4],
zinc-p.[1'], zinc-s.[11]

weakness – tremulous/faiblesse –
tremblante/Schwäche – zittrige

right side, of[11]
droit, de le côté
rechten Seite, der
    merc.

internally
interne
innerliches
    abrot.[3, 6, 7], ambr., ang.[3], **ant-t.**,
    aran-ix.[10, 14], **arg-n.**, asaf., bell.,
    bell-p.[9], **brach.**, bry., calad.,
    CALC., calc-sil.[1'], **camph.**, caps.,
    carb-v., carbn-s., **caul., caust.**,
    chin-s.[11], cina, **clem.**, cocc., colch.,

con., **crot-h.**, cycl., dicha.[14],
esp-g.[13], **eup-per.**, gels.[7], glon.[3],
GRAPH., hep.[3, 16], hura[11], **IOD.**,
kali-c., kali-n., kali-sil.[1'], kreos.,
lach.[3, 6], **lec.**, lil-t., **lyc.**, meph.,
merc., mosch., nat-ar., **nat-c.**,
nat-m., nep.[10, 13, 14], nit-ac.,
nux-m., **nux-v.**, par., petr., **phos.**,
plat., puls., RHUS-T., ruta,
sabad., sabin., samb., **seneg.**,
sep., sil., **spig., STANN., STAPH.**,
stront-c., SUL-AC., sul-i.[1'], **sulph.**,
teucr., ther.[3, 6], thuj.[3], valer.,
x-ray[9], zinc.

night[16]/nuit/nachts
    nat-m., plat.

climacteric period, during[7]
ménopause, pendant la
Klimakterium, im
    caul., sul-ac.

whole body, in[2]
tout le corps, de
ganzen Körper, am
    alum-sil.[1'], ant-t., **arg-n.**, ars.,
    ars-s-f.[1', 2], ars-s-r., bell., calc.[16],
    carbn-s., **chel., cimic.**[3], **cocc., ferr.**,
    GELS., inul., iod.[3], **kali-br.**,
    kali-sil.[1'], **nat-m., nat-s., phos.**[2, 3],
    sep., stram., sul-ac., sulph.[16], ther.[3],
    verat.

morning/matin/morgens
    alumn., **arg-m., arg-n.**, ars.,
    bar-c., calc., carb-v.[2], cimic.,
    con., dulc., gran.[11], graph., lyc.,
    mag-c., nat-m., nicc.[6], **nit-ac.**[2],
    nux-v., petr., phos., sil., sulph.

breakfast, before
petit déjeuner, avant le
Frühstück, vor dem
    calc., con., nat-m., nux-v., staph.

rising, on[4, 11, 16]
levant, en se
Aufstehen, beim
    bar-c.[4, 11], dulc.[11], petr.

    am.[16]: mag-c.

waking, on
réveil, au
Erwachen, beim
   arg-m., bar-c.[4], calc.[4, 16], carb-v.[4],
   caust., **dulc.,** euphr.[4], hyper.,
   mag-c., nit-ac., phos., tarent.,
   verat.[3]

forenoon/matinée/vormittags
   ars., carb-v.[11], carbn-o., lyc.,
   nat-m., ol-an.[4, 11], **plat.,** sars.,
   sulph.[4]

9.30 h[11]
   phys.

10 h
   bor.

exertion, on
exercice physique, par l'
Anstrengung, durch
   gels.

noon[4]/midi/mittags
   sulph.

after sleep
après la sieste
nach dem Mittagsschlaf
   nat-m.

afternoon/après-midi/nachmittags
   ant-t.[4], carb-v., **gels.,** lyc., lyss.,
   pic-ac.

13 h[11]
   verat-v.

15 h[2]
   asaf., **nux-v.**

17 h[11]
   ped.

evening/soir/abends
   bruc.[6], caust.[6], chel., iber.[11],
   lach.[6], lyc., mez., mygal., nat-m.,
   nit-ac.[6, 16], nux-v.[6], pic-ac.[1], plb.,
   sil.[6], stront-c., sulph.

19 h[11]
   phys.

bed, in
lit, au
Bett, im
   anag.[11], eupi., lyc., nux-v., samb.

sleep, after
sommeil, après le
Schlaf, nach
   carb-v.

walking, after
marche, après la
Gehen, nach
   sil.

night/nuit/nachts
   bell., hyos., lyc., merc.[1', 6], **op.**[2],
   phos., rat.[4]

half awake, while[16]
moitié éveillé, à
halbwach
   sulph.

3 h
   rhus-t.

dreaming, after
rêve, après un
Träumen, nach
   calc.[11], nicc.[11], phos., sil.

sleep, after
sommeil, après le
Schlaf, nach
   sil.

affected parts, of[3]
affectées, des parties
leidender Teile
   caust.

air, in open
air, en plein
Freien, im
   calc., kali-c., laur., **plat.**

   am.
      clem.

alternating with convulsions[11]
alternant avec convulsions
abwechselnd mit Konvulsionen
    merc.

convulsive movements of limbs[11]
mouvements convulsifs des
    membres
krampfartigen Bewegungen der
    Glieder
    arn.

weakness[11]/faiblesse/Schwäche
    ferr.

alone, am. when[11]
seul, am. étant
allein, am. wenn
    ambr.

anger, from
colère, par
Zorn, durch
    acon., alum.[7], ambr., arg-n., aur.,
    cham.[3, 6], chel., cop., daph., ferr-p.[7],
    lyc., m-austr.[4], merc., nit-ac.,
    nux-v.[3, 6], pall.[1], petr.[3], phos., plat.[2],
    ran-b., sep., staph., zinc.

    with/avec/mit
    acon., alum.[7], ambr., arg-n.,
    aur., cham.[3, 6], chel., cop., daph.,
    ferr-p., lyc., m-aust.[4], merc.,
    nit-ac., nux-v.[3, 6], pall., petr.,
    phos., plat.[2], ran-b., sep., staph.,
    zinc.

anxiety, from
anxiété, par
Angst, aus
    abrot.[6], aeth.[2], ambr., ARS., aur.,
    bell., bor., calc., canth., carb-v.,
    caust., cham., chel., coff., con., croc.,
    cupr., euph.[16], ferr.[11], graph., lach.,
    lyc., mag-c., mez., mosch., nat-c.,
    nit-ac., nux-m., phos., plat., psor.,
    puls., rhus-t., samb., sars., sep.,
    sulph.[16], valer.

with[6]/avec/mit
    abrot., acon., agar.[16], ant-c., aur.,
    bell., cina, croc., petr.[16], puls.,
    ther., verat.

ascending, on
montant, en
Steigen, beim
    merc.

attacks, before[3]
crises, avant les
Anfällen, vor
    absin.

bed, in[11]
lit, au
Bett, im
    merc-ns.

breakfast, after
petit déjeuner, après le
Frühstück, nach dem
    arg-n.

    am.
    calc., con., nat-m., nux-v., staph.

caressing, while
caresses, par des
Zärtlichkeiten, bei
    caps.

climacteric period, during
ménopause, pendant la
Klimakterium, im
    kali-br.[2, 7], ther.[6]

coffee, from smell of[11]
café, par odeur de
Kaffeegeruch, durch
    sul-ac.

coition, after[6]
coït, après le
Koitus, nach
    calc.

cold drinks am.
froides am., boissons
kalte Getränke am.
    phos.

coldness, during
froid, pendant le
Kälte, bei
  bor.

with coldness[2]
avec froid
mit Kälte
  bufo, hyos.[6], **merc., mosch.,**
  nux-m., op.[2, 6], plat.[6]

company agg.
société agg.
Gesellschaft agg.
  ambr., lyc.

conversation, from
conversation, par
Unterhaltung, durch
  ambr., bor.

convulsive[3]
convulsif
konvulsives
  am-c.[11], ang., ars.[11], bar-m.[2, 3],
  bism., canth.[11], ign., lol.[11], merc.[11],
  nux-v., op., plb., sabad., tab.[11]

spasmodic/spasmodique/
  spastisches

coughing, from
toux, par
Husten, durch
  am-c.[16], ant-t.[3], bell., **cupr., phos.,**
  seneg.[16]

dinner, during
déjeuner, pendant le
Mittagessen, beim
  mag-m.

dipsomania with[2]
dipsomanie avec
Trunksucht mit
  ant-t., **ars.**[2, 3, 6]**, crot-h., lach.,**
  mag-p., nux-v.[2, 3, 6], sul-ac.[3, 6],
  sulph.[3, 6]

dreams, during[4]
rêves, pendant les
Träumen, während
  calc., m-arct.

after[4]/après/nach
  ferr-ma., nicc.

drinking, after excessive
bu, après avoir trop
Trinken, nach übermäßigem
  plb.

eating, after
mangé, après avoir
Essen, nach dem
  alum., ant-c., caust.[4], lyc.[3, 4, 16],
  mag-m.[4], olnd.[3], phel.[4], tab.[4], zinc.[4]

emotions, after
émotions, après
Gemütsbewegungen, nach
  arg-n., **COCC.,** coff.[6], cycl.[7], ferr.,
  hep., merc., nat-c., nat-m., petr.[2],
  phys.[2], **plb., psor., STAPH.,** stram.,
  thyreotr.[14], **zinc.**

exercise, from[11]
exercices physiques, par
Körperübungen, durch
  merc., plan., polyg-h.

exertion, on[6]
efforts, au cours des
Anstrengung, bei
  alco.[11], am-caust.[6, 11], anac.,
  ant-t., **arn.,** ars., chin-s.,
  COCC.[2, 6], iod., merc.[11], nat-c.,
  nat-m., rhus-t., sec.[6, 11], **sil.**[2, 6]

agg.[3]
  anac., ant-t., arn., ars., chin-s.,
  cocc., iod., nat-c., nat-m., rhus-t.,
  sec., sil.

on slight
au moindre effort
bei geringer
  bor., **cocc.,** ferr., **merc.,** phos.,
  plat., plb., polyg-h., **rhus-t.,** sec.,
  stann., zinc.

eyes agg., closing[11]
yeux agg., en fermant les
Augenschließen agg.
  merc.

faintness, during[7]
évanouissement, pendant l'
Ohnmacht, in der
  asaf.[11], **lach.**[2], nux-v., petr.,

fatigue, after
fatigue, par
Übermüdung, durch
  plb.

fear, from[2]
peur, par
Furcht, aus
  calc.

feet, on washing[11]
pieds, en se lavant les
Fußwäsche, bei der
  merc.

fever, during
fièvre, pendant la
Fieber, im
  acon.[6], ars., calc., camph., cann-i.[6],
  caps.[6], cist., eup-per., kali-c., lach.,
  mag-c., mygal., sep.

fright, from
frayeur, par
Schreck, durch
  acon.[2, 3, 6], arg-n., **aur.,** calc.[3, 6],
  coff., glon., hura, ign., mag-c.,
  merc., nicc., **op., plat.**[2], puls.,
  ran-b.[2], rat., rhus-t., sep., **stram.**[2],
  tarent.[2], zinc.[3, 6]

headache, during[3]
maux de tête, pendant les
Kopfschmerzen, bei
  arg-n.

  with chill[16]
  avec frissons
  mit Fieberfrost
    carb-v.

hungry, when
faim, par la
Hunger, bei
  alum., crot-h., olnd., stann., **sulph.,**
  zinc.

intention tremor[3]
intentionel, t.
Intentionstremor
  anac., arg-n., bell., cic., **cocc.,** gels.,
  iod., merc., phos., phyt., rhus-t.,
  samb., **sec.,** zinc.

joy, from
joie, par
Freude, vor
  acon., aur., cimic.[2], coff., cycl.[2],
  merc., valer.

looking down, on
regardant en bas, en
Abwärtssehen, beim
  kali-c.

lying, while
couché, étant
Liegen, im
  clem.

  on left side agg., on back am.[2]
  sur le côté gauche agg., sur le dos
    am.
  auf der linken Seite agg., auf dem
    Rücken am.
    kalm.

meeting friends
rencontrant des amis, en
Treffen von Freunden, bei
  tarent.

menses, before
menstruation, avant la
Menses, vor den
  alum., hyos.[2, 3], kali-c.[2, 3], lyc.[2, 3],
  nat-m.[2, 3], sep.[3], stann.[2, 3, 6]

  during/pendant la/während der
  agar.[3], arg-n., calc-p., caul.[3],
  caust.[3], cina[2], **graph., hyos.,**
  kali-c.[3], **lec.,** mag-c.[4], merl.,

nat-m.[2, 3], nicc.[6], **nit-ac.**, plat.[2, 3],
puls.[6], **stram.**[2, 3, 6], wies.[11]

after/après la/nach den
chin.

mental exertion, from
intellectuel, par travail
geistige Anstrengung, durch
aur., bor.[1], **CALC.**[2], **plb.**[1], vinc.

motion, on
mouvement, au
Bewegung, bei
anac., arg-n., canth.[4], iod.,
kali-ar.[1'], phyt., puls.[4], sulph.[16],
zinc.

hands and feet, of[11]
mains et des pieds, des
Händen und Füßen· von
cann-i.

am.
merc., plat.

music, from
musique, par la
Musik, durch
aloe[2, 7], **AMBR.,** thuj.[7]

nausea, with[2]
nausée, avec
Übelkeit, mit
ars.[11], **calc.,** carb-v.[11], chel.,
cimic.[11], eup-per., plat., tab.[11],
vesp.[2, 11]

noise, from
bruits, par
Geräusche, durch
aloe[2], bar-c., caust., **cocc.,** hura,
kali-ar., mosch., tab.

nursing infant, after
allaitement, après
Stillen, nach dem
olnd.

old age, in[3, 6]
personnes âgées, chez les
Alter, im
alum.[7], ambr.[7], aur.[7], bar-c., calc.,
con., kali-c.[7], merc.[7], op.[7], phos.[7],
plb.[3], plb-a.[6], sil., stront-c., sulph.,
zinc.[7]

pains, with the
douleurs, pendant les
Schmerzen, bei
bism.[7], **cocc., NAT-C.,** nit-ac.[3],
plat., puls., sul-ac.[3], zinc.[3]

after[11]/après les/nach
bry.

palpitation, with[2]
palpitation, avec
Herzklopfen, mit
acon., benz-ac., calc-ar.

paroxysmal
paroxysmes, en
anfallsweise
anthraci.[2], arg-n.[3], crot-h.[3, 6],
ferr.[3, 6], lyc.[3, 6, 16], **merc.**

periodical
périodique
periodisches
ARG-N.

perspiration, with[2]
transpiration, avec
Schweiß, mit
ars.[16], merc.[3, 6], mosch.[6], rhus-t.

cold[3]/froide/kaltem
merc., mosch., **puls.**[2]

after[2]/après/nach
apis

playing the piano, while
jouant du piano, en
Klavierspielen, beim
nat-c.

rest, during[11]
repos, pendant le
Ruhe, in der
   eupi.

   am.
      merc.[11], nep.[10]

rising, on[3]
levant, en se
Aufstehen, beim
   ambr.[7], nat-m., rhus-t.

   from sitting in affected parts
   d'un siège dans les parties affectées
   vom Sitzen in den befallenen Teilen
   CAUST.

sexual excess, t. after[2]
sexuel, t. après excès
sexueller Ausschweifung, Z. nach
   phos.

   excitement, t. during
   excitation sexuelle, t. pendant
   Erregung, Z. während sexueller
   graph.

side lain on
côté où on est couché, sur le
Seite, auf der man liegt, der
   clem.

sleep, before
sommeil, avant le
Schlaf, vor dem
   carb-an.[4], nat-m., petr.[4], sep.[4, 16]

   during/pendant le/im
      apis[2], **chlf.**[2], con., kali-c.[16], rheum[2]

   starting from[16]
   tressaille au cours du
   Auffahren aus dem
      petr.

smoking, from
fumer, par
Rauchen, durch
   hep., nat-m., **nux-v.**[2], sil., sulph.

sneezing, on[7]
éternuant, en
Niesen, beim
   BOR.

something is to be done, when
quelque chose doit être fait, si
etwas getan werden muß, wenn
   KALI-BR.

spasmodic[3, 6]
spasmodique
spastisches
   ang., bar-m., bism., **ign., nux-v.,**
   op., plb., **sabad.**

   convulsive/convulsif/konvulsives

standing, while
debout, étant
Stehen, beim
   merc.

stitching in ear, from[16]
piqûres dans les oreilles, par
Stiche im Ohr, durch
   thuj.

stool, before
selle, avant la
Stuhlgang, vor
   hydr., merc., sumb.

   during/pendant la/während
      carbn-s.

   after/après la/nach
      ars., carb-v., caust., **CON.,** lil-t.,
      merc.[2]

supper, after
souper, après le
Abendessen, nach dem
   alum., caust.

surprise, agg. from[11]
surprise, agg. par
Überraschung, agg. durch
   merc.

thunderstorm
orage et un éclair, pendant un
Gewitter, bei
   agar., **morph.,** nat-p., **phos.**

touch, unexpected
attouchement inattendu, par
Berührung, durch unerwartete
  cocc.

urination, during[11]
uriner, pendant
Urinieren, beim
  gels.

  after[16]/après/nach
  ars.

vertigo with
vertige avec
Schwindel mit
  am-c., ars., bell., **camph.,** carb-v.,
  crot-h., **dig., dulc., glon.,** nat-m.,
  puls.

vexation, from
contrariété, par
Ärger, durch
  acon., **aur.,** cham.[6], coff.[1'], lyc.,
  nit-ac., nux-v.[6], petr.[6, 16], ran-b.

voluptuous
voluptueux
wollüstiges
  calc.

vomiting, while[11]
vomissement, pendant le
Erbrechen, beim
  colch., eup-per.[2], gran.

  after[11]/après le/nach
  ars.

waking, on
réveil, au
Erwachen, beim
  abrot., bar-c.[4], calc., carb-v.[2, 4],
  caust.[4], **cina, dulc.**[2], euphr.[4],
  ferr-ma.[4], **ign.**[2], lach., m-arct.[4],
  merc., nicc.[4], nit-ac., orig.[11], **petr.**[4],
  phos.[3', 4], rat., samb.[4, 16], sil.[4],
  stront-c.[4], sulph.[4], tarent., verat.[3]

walking, while
marchant, en
Gehen, beim
  am-c., cupr-ar.[6], lac-ac., merc.,
  nux-v., stry.[11]

  after/après la marche/nach dem
  cupr.[16], ust.

weakness, from[6]
faiblesse, par
Schwäche, aus
  agar., **anac.,** ant-t., **bapt.,** bell., bry.,
  caust., **chin.**[3, 6], cocc., con., kali-c.,
  mang., **nat-m.**[3, 6], **stann.**[3, 6], ther.,
  verat., zinc.

wine, from
vin, par le
Wein, durch
  con.

worm affections, in[1']
vers, par
Würmer, durch
  sabad.

writing, while
écrivant, en
Schreiben, beim
  lyss.[10], **phos., sil.**

TRICKLING sensation, like drops
S'ÉGOUTTENT, sensation de gouttes
  qui
TROPFEN fielen, als
  agar.[3], ambr., arg-n.[3], arn., bell.,
  berb.[3], **CANN-S.,** caust.[3], cot.[3],
  croc.[3], glon.[3], graph.[3], kali-bi.[3],
  mag-m.[3], nat-m.[3], nux-m.[3], petros.[3],
  phos.[3], rhus-t.[3], sep., spig., stann.[3],
  tarent.[3], thuj., vario.[3], verat.

hot drops[3]
gouttes chaudes
heiße Tropfen
  stann., sulph.

TUBERCULOSIS, prophylaxis of[7]
ANTITUBERCULEUSE, prophylaxie
TUBERKULOSE-Prophylaxe
bac., sulph., tub.[7]

lupus vulgar
lupus vulgaris
Lupus vulgaris
abr.[8, 12], agar., alum., alum-sil.[1'],
alumn., am-ar.[8], ant-c., apis[8],
arg-n., **ARS.**, **ars-i.**, ars-s-f.[1'],
aur-ar.[8, 12], aur-i[8], aur-m., **bar-c.**,
bell.[1], calc., calc-ar.[2], calc-i.[8],
calc-p.[2], calc-s.[8], calc-sil.[1'],
calo.[12], **carb-ac.**, **carb-v.**, **carbn-s.**,
caust., chr-o.[12], cic.[1], **cist.**,
cund.[2, 8], ferr-pic.[8, 12], form.[8],
form-ac.[8], graph., guar.[8], guare.[12],
hep., hippoz.[12], **hydr.**[2, 8, 12],
hydrc., irid.[8], kali-ar., **kali-bi.**,
kali-c., **kali-chl.**, **kali-i.**[8],
kali-m.[2], kali-s., **kreos.**, lach.,
LYC., m-arct.[1], merc-i-r.[1], **nit-ac.**,
ol-j.[1], **phyt.**, **psor.**, ran-b.[1'],
rhus-t.[1], sabin.[1], sep., **sil.**, spong.,
staph., sulph., thiosin.[8, 12],
THUJ., **tub.**[8], **tub-k.**[12], urea[8],
x-ray[8]

in rings/annulaire/ringförmig
sep.

TUMORS, benign
TUMEURS bénignes
TUMOREN, benigne

polypus/polypes/Polypen

angioma, fungus haematodes,
hemangioma
angiome, hémangiome
Haemangiom
abrot.[8], ant-t., **ARS.**, bell., **calc.**,
CARB-AN., **carb-v.**, clem., **kreos.**,
LACH., lyc., manc.[8], **merc.**, **nat-m.**,
nit-ac., nux-v., **PHOS.**, **puls.**,
rhus-t., sep., **SIL.**, staph., **sulph.**,
THUJ.

atheroma, steatoma
athérome, kystes, sébacés
Atherom
agar., ant-c.[4], anthraci.[2], **bar-c.**,
bell.[2], benz-ac.[6, 8, 12], brom.[6], **calc.**,
caust[2], clem[2], **con.**[2, 6, 8, 12], daph[8],
GRAPH., **guare.**[2, 11], **hep.**, kali-br.[2, 6],
kali-c., kali-i.[6, 12], lac-ac.[2], lach.[7, 12],
lob., lyc., m-arct.[4], mez.[6, 8], nat-c.,
nit-ac.[2, 4, 6, 12], **ph-ac.**[2, 12], **phyt.**[2, 6, 12],
rhus-t.[2, 12], **sabin.**[4, 6], sil., spong.[4],
staph.[12], **sulph.**[2, 4, 6], thuj.[2], vanad.[12]

reappearing every 4 weeks
récidive toutes les 4 semaines, avec
kommt alle 4 Wochen wieder
calc.

suppurating/suppurant/eiternd
calc., **carb-v.**, **sulph.**[4]

cheloid see keloid

colloid[2]
colloïdes
kolloide
carb-ac., hydr., phos.

cystic
kystiques
zystische
agar., **apis**[1, 7], apoc.[2, 6], ars.[2, 3],
aur.[1', 3, 6], **BAR-C.**, benz-ac.[6], bov.[12],
brom., **CALC.**[1, 7], calc-f.[6], calc-p.[8],
calc-s., caust.[3], **con.**[3, 6], form-ac.[6],
GRAPH., **hep.**[1, 7], hydr.[3], **iod.**[3, 6, 8],
kali-br.[7, 8], kali-c.[3], **lyc.**[3, 6], **med.**[7],
merc-d.[6], nit-ac., **PHOS.**[3], platan.[8],
sabin.[3], sil., spong.[3], staph.[8, 12],
sulph., **thuj.**[3, 6]

bones, of
os, des
Knochen, der
mez.

encephaloma
encéphalome
Hirntumor
acet-ac., arn.[2], **ars., ars-i.,** art-v.[2],
bell.[2], **calc.,** carb-ac., **carb-an.,**
caust., **croc.**[2], hydr.[2], kali-i., **kreos.,**
lach., nit-ac., nux-v.[2], **PHOS.,**
plb.[12], **sil.,** sulph., **thuj.**

enchondroma[8]
enchondrome
Knorpelgeschwulst
calc.[2], calc-f., conch.[12], lap-a.,
sil.[1', 2, 6, 8, 12]

erectile
érectiles
erektile
lyc., **nit-ac., phos.,** staph.

fibroid
fibrome
Fibrom
arb.[7], bell.[2], bry.[2], **calc., CALC-F.,**
calc-i.[7, 8], **calc-s.,** chol.[7], chr-s.[8],
con., fl-ac.[7, 10], frax.[7], graph.[3, 8],
hydr.[7], **hydrin-m.**[8, 12], **kali-br.**[7],
kali-i.[8, 12], **lap-a.**[2, 7, 8, 12], led.[2],
lil-t.[12], lyc.[12], **PHOS.,** phyt.[7],
sec.[8, 12], **SIL.,** tarent.[12], ter.[12],
teucr.[12], thiosin.[8], thlas.[12],
thyr.[8, 12], tril.[3, 8], ust.[7, 12], xan.[12]

haemorrhage, with[8, 12]
hémorrhagie, avec
Blutung, mit
calc.[3], **hydrin-m.,** lap-a.[8], nit-ac.[3],
phos.[3], sabin.[8], sul-ac.[3], thlas.,
tril., ust.

ganglion
Ganglion
am-c., arn., aur-m., **benz-ac.**[2, 3, 8, 12],
bov.[12], calc-f.[6], **carb-v.,** ferr-ma.[12]
iod.[6], kali-m.[8], ph-ac., **phos.,** plb.,
rhus-t., **ruta,** sil., sulph., thuj.[6, 12],
zinc.

keloid, cheloid
chéloïde
Narbenkeloid
ars.[7], **bad.**[3], **bell-p.**[6, 7], calc.[7],

calc-f.[6, 10], carb-v.[7], caust.[6, 7],
crot-h.[7], cupre-l.[12], **FL-AC.**[7, 8],
gast.[7], **GRAPH.**[6, 7], hyper.[7], **iod.**[6, 7],
junc-e.[7], kali-bi.[3], **lach.**[7], maland.[12],
merc.[7], **NIT-AC.**[6-8, 12], nux-v.[7],
phos.[7], phyt.[7], psor.[7], rhus-t.[7],
sabin.[7, 8], **SIL.**[1, 7], sul-ac.[7], sulph.[7, 12],
thiosin.[7], tub.[7], vac.[7, 12], vip.[7]

lipoma[2, 8]
lipome
Lipom
agar.[2, 12], **am-m.**[2], **BAR-C.**[2, 6, 8],
BELL.[2], **calc.,** calc-ar.[8], croc.[2],
graph.[2], **kali-br.**[7], **lap-a.**[2, 7, 8], phos.[2],
phyt., thuj.[8, 12], ur-ac.[8, 12]

naevus
Naevus, Muttermal
abrot.[3, 6, 10], **ACET-AC.,** arn.[3],
ars.[3], bell-p.[10], **calc.,** calc-f.[3, 6],
carb-an.[3], **carb-v.,** con.[3], cund.[2, 8],
ferr-p.[2, 3, 6, 10, 12], **FL-AC., graph.**[3, 4],
ham.[3, 6], lach.[3], **lyc.,** med.[7],
nit-ac.[3, 4], nux-v., **petr.**[3, 4], **ph-ac.**[3, 4],
PHOS., rad.[3], rad-br.[6, 8],
rumx.[3, 6], **sep.**[3], **sil.**[3, 4], sul-ac.[3, 4],
sulph.[3, 4], **thuj.,** ust.[3], vac.

neuroma
neurogliome
Neurom
all-c.[8], calc., calen.[8], staph.

noma
Noma
alum., alumn., **ars.,** bapt.[8], calc.,
carb-v., **con.,** elat., **guare.**[2], hydr.[8],
kali-chl.[8], **kali-p.,** kreos.[8], **lach.**[8],
merc., **merc-c.**[8], **mur-ac.**[8], sec.[8],
sil., sol-t-ae.[12], sul-ac.[8], sulph.,
tarent-c.[3]

osteoma[2, 12]
ostéome
Osteoma
mez.

papillomata[8]
papillomes
Papillome
ant-c., **calc.**[1', 2], nit-ac., staph.,
thuj.

TURNING around agg.
RETOURNANT agg., en se
SICH HERUMDREHEN agg.
  agar., aloe, calc., cham., **ip.**, kali-c.,
  merc., nat-m., par., **phos.**, sil.

bed, in
lit, au
Bett, im
  acon., agar., am-m., anac., ars.,
  asar., **bor.**, **brom.**[3], **bry.**, calc.,
  cann-s., **caps.**, **carb-v.**, caust., chin.,
  cina, cocc., **con.**, cupr., dros., **euph.**,
  ferr., graph., **hep.**, kali-c., kreos.,
  lach., led., **lyc.**, mag-c., merc.,
  nat-m., nit-ac., **nux-v.**, petr., phos.,
  plat., plb., **PULS.**, ran-b., rhod.,
  rhus-t., ruta, sabad., sabin., samb.,
  sars., **sil.**, **staph.**, **sulph.**, thuj.,
  valer.

head
tête, en tournant la
Kopfes, Drehen des
  am-m., anac., **arn.**, ant-c., ars.[3],
  asar., bar-c., **bell.**, bov., **bry.**,
  CALC., camph., cann-s., canth.,
  carb-an., carb-v., caust., cham.,
  chin., **CIC.**, cocc., coff., coloc., con.[3],
  cupr., dros., dulc., glon., **HEP.**,
  hyos., **ign.**, ip., kali-c., lach., lil-t.[3],
  lyc., mag-c., mez., **nat-c.**, **nat-m.**,
  nit-ac., **nux-v.**, par., petr., ph-ac.,
  phos., plat., **puls.**, **rhus-t.**, sabad.,
  sabin., samb., **sang.**, sars., **sel.**, **sep.**,
  spig., **SPONG.**, stann., staph.,
  sulph., thuj., verat., viol-t., zinc.

left agg., right to[3]
gauche agg., en se tournant de
  droite à
links agg., sich drehen von rechts
  nach
  sulph.

right am., left to[3]
droite am., en se tournant à
rechts am., sich drehen nach
  lach., phos.,

twisting involuntarily, t. and[16]
tordant le corps involontairement,
  en tournant et
windet sich unwillkürlich, dreht und
  lyc.

TWITCHING
SOUBRESAUT
ZUCKEN
  abies-c.[11], acon., acon-c.[11], **AGAR.**,
  agn., alum., alum-p.[1'], alum-sil.[1'],
  alumn.[2, 11], am-c., am-m., **ambr.**,
  ant-c., **ant-t.**, apis, aran.[2], **arg-m.**,
  arg-n., arn.[2, 3, 11], **ars.**, **ars-i.**,
  ars-s-f.[1', 11], ars-s-r.[11], arund.[2, 11],
  ASAF., asc-t.[2], aster., atro., **bar-c.**,
  bar-i.[1'], bar-m., **bell.**, bism.[3], bor.,
  brom., bruc.[11], **bry.**, bufo, **CACT.**,
  cadm-s.[2, 11], calc., calc-i.[1'] calc-p.[11],
  calc-s., calc-sil.[1'], **camph.**, cann-i.,
  cann-s.[3, 11], **canth.**, caps., carb-ac.,
  carb-v., **carbn-s.**, carc.[9], **caust.**,
  cedr.[2], cerv.[11], cham., **chel.**, **chin.**,
  chin-s., chlf.[2], chlor., **cic.**, cic-m.[11],
  cimic., cina, **clem.**, **cocc.**, **cod.**,
  coff.[1', 2], coff-t.[11], colch., coloc.,
  con., croc., crot-h., **cupr.**,
  cupr-s.[2, 11], cypr.[2], cyt-l.[11], dig.,
  dol.[2, 11], dor.[2], dros., dulc.[3, 11],
  ferr.[1'], form.[3], **gels.**[2], **glon.**[2, 3, 6],
  graph., guaj., hedeo.[11], **hell.**, hep.[3],
  hydr-ac.[3, 11], **HYOS.**, **IGN.**, **IOD.**,
  ip., juni.[11], **kali-ar.**, kali-br., **KALI-C.**,
  kali-i.[2], kali-m.[1'], kali-n.[11, 16],
  kali-p., kali-s., kali-sil.[1'], kreos.,
  lach., lact.[11], laur., lipp.[11], lon-x.[11],
  lyc., **lyss.**, mag-c.[3], mag-m., mag-p.,
  meny., **merc.**, **merc-c.**, **MEZ.**,
  morph.[11], **mosch.**[2], **mur-ac.**, mygal.,
  nat-ar., **NAT-C.**, nat-f.[9], **nat-m.**,
  nat-p., nat-s.[1'], nat-sil.[1'], **nit-ac.**,
  nitro-o.[11], **nux-m.**[2, 6, 11], **nux-v.**,
  par., petr., **ph-ac.**, **phos.**, phys.[2, 3, 11],
  phyt.[1'] pic-ac.[11], plat., **plb.**, **podo.**[6],
  psor., puls., **ran-b.**[2, 3], rat.[3, 11], rhod.,
  rhus-t., **rhus-v.**[11], ruta, sabad.[2, 3],
  sabin., salin.[11], sarcol-ac.[9], scut.[11],
  sec., sel., senec-j.[11], seneg., **sep.**,
  sil., sol-n.[11], **spig.**, spong., squil.[3],
  stann., staph.[3, 11], **STRAM.**,

stront-c., **stry.**, sul-ac., sul-i.[1]',
sulph., tab.[11], tanac., tarax.,
tarent.[3], ter.[2], thuj., valer.,
verat.[2, 3], **verat-v.**[2, 3], viol-t.,
vip.[3, 11], **visc.**, x-ray[9], **ZINC.**,
zinc-m.[11]- **zinc-p.**[1]'

daytime[2]/journée, pendant la/
tagsüber
bar-c., lyss

morning[11, 16]/matin/morgens
rheum

waking, on
réveil, au
Erwachen, beim
chel.[2], menth-pu.[11]

noon[11]/midi/mittags
petr., **ZINC.**

evening[11]/soir/abends
aether

bed, in[11]
lit, au
Bett, im
ped., petr., ran-b., sil.

night[11]/nuit/nachts
ambr., cupr.-a., op., staph., tab.

sleep, during[11]
sommeil, pendant le
Schlaf, im
graph., nat-c., petr., sel., **ZINC.**

chill, during[2, 11]
frissons, pendant les
Fieberfrost, im
stram.

dentition, during[2]
dentition, pendant la
Zahnen, beim
cham., ter., zinc.

dipsomania, in[2]
dipsomanie avec
Trunksucht, bei
crot-h., phos.

electricity, as from[11]
électrique, comme par un courant
Elektrizität, wie durch
acon., arn., clem., **daph.**, dulc.,
plb., sec.

fever with[2]
fièvre avec
Fieber mit
bell., nit-s-d., rhus-t.[11], **spong.**

typhoid[2]
typhoïde
typhoidem
CALC., cham., **colch.**, crot-h.,
**cypr., gels., HYOS., lyc., ter.,
zinc.**

fright, after
frayeur, par
Schreck, durch
op., stram.

haemorrhage with[2]
hémorrhagie avec
Blutung mit
chin.

here and there
çà et là
hier und dort
alum.[16], agar., ant-c.[3], chel.[3], **cocc.**,
colch., **kali-c.**, kali-n., lyc., mez.,
nat-c.[16], nat-m., ph-ac., phos., rhod.,
sep., **stry.**, sulph., **ZINC.**

internally
interne
innerliches
atro., bov., **cann-s.**, cic.[11], seneg.

leucorrhoea with[3]
leucorrhée avec
Fluor mit
alum.

menses, during[3]
menstruation, pendant la
Menses, während der
bell., calc-s.[2], chin., cocc., coff.,
kali-c., plat., sec., sulph.

after[3]/après la/nach den
chin., cupr., kreos., **nat-m.**[2, 3],
puls.

one-sided[15]
côté, d'un
einseitiges
apis

paralysed part, of
paralysée de la partie
gelähmten Teiles, des
apis, **arg-n.**, merc., nux-v., phos.,
sec., stram., stry.

parturition, during[2]
accouchement, pendant l'
Entbindung, während der
cinnm.

labor ceases, t. beginns when[2]
douleurs cessent, s. commence
quand les
Wehen, Z. beginnt beim Aufhören
der
sec.

rest, during[1']
repos, pendant le
Ruhe, in der
valer.

right side
à côté droite
rechtsseitig
caust., tarent.[3]

single parts, of[3]
isolées, de parties
einzelner Teile
agar., alum., chin., **cocc.**, nux-v.,
puls., zinc.

sleep, during
sommeil, pendant le
Schlaf, im
alum.[1], **ant-t.**[2], anac., **ars.**, **bar-c.**[2],
bell., brom.[11], caust., **cham.**[2, 6],
chlf.[2], cina[6], cinnb., **colch.**[2], con.,
cupr., dulc., graph.[16], **hell.**[2],
HYOS.[2], hyper.[2], ign.[6], **kali-c.**,
kiss.[11], **lyc.**[2, 6, 16], mag-c., merc.[16],

mez., nat-c., nat-m., op.[11], petr.[16],
ph-ac., phos., puls.[11], rheum[2],
seneg., **sep.**[2], sil., stann., **stram.**[2],
stront-c., sul-ac., **sulph.**, tep.[11],
thuj., **ZINC.**

on going to
en s'endormant
Einschlafen, vor dem
acon., **agar.**, all-s.[2], aloe[2], alum.,
arg-m., **ARS.**, **BELL.**[3], calc.[3],
carb-v.[1'], **cham.**[3], cob., hyper.,
ign., iodof.[2], **KALI-C.**, mag-m.[11],
phys., puls.[3], **sel.**, sep.[3], **stront-c.**,
stry., sul-ac., sulph., zinc.

subsultus tendinum
soubresauts des tendons
Sehnenhüpfen
agar., am-c., ambr., **ars.**, **asaf.**,
bell., **calc.**, **camph.**, **canth.**, **chel.**,
chlor., cupr.[6], **HYOS.**, **IOD.**, kali-c.[6],
kali-i., lyc., mez., **mur-ac.**, **ph-ac.**,
phos., rhus-t., **sec.**, squil.[6], **stry.**,
sul-ac.[16], **ZINC.**

touch, on[11]
touché, étant
Berührung, bei
morph., phos., stry.

agg.
stry.

upper part of body on lying down[16]
moitié supérieure du corps en
s'étendant, de la
Oberkörpers beim Sichhinlegen, des
nat-m.

waking, on[4]
réveil, au
Erwachen, beim
ars., bell., **camph.**[2], carc.[9], cham.[6],
chel.[2], **cod.**[2], **hyos.**[6], laur.[2], lyc.,
mag-m., op.[11], sang.[11], stront-c.

worm affections, in
vermineuses, au cours d'affections
Wurmbefall, bei
cina, sabad.[1', 2]

ULCERS, glands
ULCÈRES des glandes
GESCHWÜRE der Drüsen
  ambr., ant-c., arn., **ARS.,** asaf., aur.,
  aur-ar.[1]', **bell.,** calc., **canth.,** carb-an.,
  carb-v., caust., clem., coloc., **con.,**
  cupr., dulc., **hep.,** hyos., ign., kali-c.,
  kali-p., kreos., **lach.,** lyc., merc.,
  nit-ac., **ol-j.**[2], ph-ac., **PHOS., phyt.,**
  rhus-t., **rhus-v.**[2], sars., sep., **SIL.,**
  spong., squil., sul-ac., **sulph.,** thuj.,
  zinc.

cancerous see cancerous–ulcers
cartilages see cartilages–ulcers

UNCLEANLINESS agg.
MALPROPRETÉ agg.
UNSAUBERKEIT agg.
  CAPS., chin., psor., puls., **sulph.**
  all-c.[3], **CAPS., chin., psor.,** puls.,
  sulph.

UNCOVERING agg.
SE DÉCOUVRIR agg.
ABDECKEN agg., sich
  acon., acon-f., **agar., am-c.,**
  ant-c., arg-m., **arg-n.,** arn., **ARS.,**
  asar., **atro.,** aur., aur-ar.[1]', **bell.,**
  benz-ac., bor., **bry.,** calc-sil.[1]',
  camph., cann-s.[3], canth., **caps.,**
  carb-an., caust.[3, 6], **cham., chin.,**
  cic., clem., cocc., coff., colch.,
  con., dios., dros.[8], **dulc., graph.,**
  hell., **HEP.,** hyos., **ign.,**
  KALI-AR., kali-bi., KALI-C.,
  kali-i., **kali-sil.**[1]', kalm.[12], kreos.,
  lach., led.[2, 3], **LYC., lycps.,**
  mag-c., mag-m., MAG-P.,
  mang.[16], meny., **merc.,** mur-ac.,
  nat-c., nat-m., NUX-M.,
  NUX-V., ph-ac., **phos.,** psor.[3, 6],
  puls., rheum, **RHOD., RHUS-T.,**
  rumx., sabad., **SAMB.,** sang-n.[12],
  sep., **SIL., SQUIL.,** staph., stram.,
  STRONT-C., sulph.[3], thuj.,
  ZINC., zinc-p.[1]'

least[3]
si peu que ce soit
geringste, das
  hep., nux-v., rhus-t., **sil.**

single part agg.
isolée agg., d'une partie
einzelnen Teiles agg., eines
  bry., **HEP., ip.**[2], **nat-m.,**
  RHUS-T., SIL., squil., stront-c.,
  thuj.

cold becoming/froid – attraper/
Kälte – Kaltwerden

feet, of[8]
pieds, les
Füße, der
  calc., cupr., nux-m., sil.

ailments from[12]
troubles à la suite de
Beschwerden infolge von
  kalm., sang-n.

am.[3]
  acon., alum., apis[1', 3, 8], ars.,
  asar.[3, 6], aur., **bor.**[3, 6], bry., **calc.**[3, 6],
  camph.[3, 8], cann-s., carb-v., cham.,
  chin., coff., **ferr.,** ign., **IOD.**[3, 6],
  kali-i., kali-s., lach., led.[3, 6],
  LYC.[3, 8], merc., mosch., mur-ac.,
  nit-ac., nux-v., onos.[8], op., phos.,
  plat., **PULS.**[3, 6], rhus-t., **sec.**[1', 3, 8],
  seneg., sep., **spig.**[3, 6], staph.,
  sulph.[3, 6], **tab.**[8], **verat.**[3, 6]

aversion to[6]
aversion de
Abneigung gegen
  arg-n.[7], **ars.**[3, 6], aur.[1', 6], **bell.**[3, 6],
  calc-s.[1]', clem., colch., hep., mag-c.,
  nat-m., nux-m., **nux-v.**[3, 6], samb.,
  sil., **squil.**[3, 6], **stront-c.**[3, 6]

desire for[6]
désir de
Verlangen, sich abzudecken
  acon.[3, 7], **aloe**[1', 6], **apis,** ars-i.[1]',
  asar., calc.[6, 7], calc-s.[1]',
  camph.[1', 3, 6], ferr., **iod.**[3, 6],
  kali-i.[1]', led.[1]', manc.[11], merc.[1]',

mosch.[1'], op.[1', 6], **puls.**[3, 6],
sec.[1', 3, 6, 7], spig., stram.,
sulph.[3, 6]

morning[11]/matin/morgens
fl-ac.

sleep, on going to[11]
s'endormant, en
Einschlafen, vor dem
op.

waking, on[11]
réveil, au
Erwachen, beim
plat.

kicks the covers off[6]
repousse ses couvertures
schleudert die Decken weg
BRY.[7], camph., **cham.**, iod.

in coldest weather[7]
par temps très froid
bei größter Kälte
hep., sanic., sulph.

UNDRESSING agg., after
DÉSHABILLÉ agg., après s'être
AUSZIEHEN der Kleidung agg.,
nach dem
am-m., **ARS.**, calc., carc.[9], **cocc.**,
crot-t.[3], **DROS., dulc.**[3], hep., mag-c.,
merc.[3], mez., mur-ac., nat-s.,
NUX-V., olnd., plat., **puls.,**
RHUS-T., rumx.[3], sep., **sil., spong.,**
stann.,sul-ac.[3], tub.[3]

air, in open
air, en plein
Freien, im
phos.

URAEMIA[3]
URÉMIE
URAMIE
apis, ars., bapt., bell., **canth., hyos.,**
op., sulfa.[14], **stram., verat-v.**

URIC ACID diathese, lithaemia[3]
URIQUE, diathèse; uricémie
HARNSAURE Diathese, Anlage zur
Steinbildung
berb., chin-s., coc-c., **lyc.,** nat-s., sep.,
urt-u.

URINATION, am. after[3, 7, 8]
MICTION, am. après la
URINIEREN, am. nach dem
benz-ac.[1'], bor.[3], bry.[7], chin-s.[3], cyt-l.[9],
eug.[7], **GELS., ign., LYC.**[3], **ph-ac.,**
sang.[3], sil.[3, 7, 8], **tab.**[7], ter.[3], verat.[3]

VACCINATION, after *
VACCINATION, après
POCKENIMPFUNG, Folgen von
acon.[8, 12], **ant-t.**[3, 6-8], **apis**[1, 7], **ars.,**
bell.[6, 8, 12], bufo[7], crot-h.[8, 12], echi.,
graph.[12], hep., kali-chl.,
kali-m.[2, 3, 6-8, 12], lac-v.[12], **MALAND.,**
merc.[3, 6, 8, 10, 12], **MEZ.**[7, 8, 12], **ped.**[7],
phos.[12], **psor.**[7], rhus-t.[3], sabin.[2, 7],
SARS.[7, 8], sep.[8], **SIL.**[1, 7], skook.[12],
SULPH.[1, 7], **THUJ.**[1, 7], tub.[2, 7],
VAC.[6, 7, 12], **vario.**[3, 6, 7, 10, 12]

prophylactic[3, 7]
prophylactique
prophylaktische
sulph., thuj., vario.[3]

VARICOSE veins
VARICES
KRAMPFADERN
alum.[4], alum-sil.[1'], **alumn., am-c.**[4],
ambr., ang.[4], **ant-t.,** apis[12],
arist-cl.[10], **ARN., arg-n., ars.,**
ars-s-f.[1'], asaf., **bar-c.**[4], **bell.,**
bell-p.[6, 12], **berb.**[1], brom.[1'], **bry.**[4],
CALC., calc-f., calc-p., calc-s.[1'],
calen.[12], camph.[4], **carb-an.,**
CARB-V., carbn-s.[1'], card-b.[12],
card-m.[6, 10, 12], **caust.,** chel.[4],
chin.[4, 12], chin-s.[12], cic.[4], clem.,
coll.[10], coloc., con.[4], **croc.**[4], **crot-h.,**
cycl.[4], **ferr.,** ferr-ar., **ferr-p.**[6], **FL-AC.,**
form-ac.[6], **graph., HAM.,** hecla[14],
hep., hyos.[4], kali-ar.[12], kali-n.[4],
kreos., lac-c.[12], lach., **lyc., LYCPS.,**

m-aust.[4, 12], mag-c., mag-f.[10],
mand.[10], meli.[10], meny.[4], merc-cy.[12],
mez.[6], mill., mosch.[4], **mur-ac.**[4, 12],
nat-m., nux-v., olnd.[4], op.[4],
paeon., petr.[12], ph-ac.[4, 12], **phos.**[4, 6],
plb., PULS., pyrog.[12], **ran-s.**[2, 12],
rhod.[4], **rhus-t.**[4], ruta[10], sabin., sars.[4],
scir.[12], sec.[3], **sep.**, sil., sol-n.[12], **spig.**,
spong.[4, 12], staph.[4], stront-br.[12],
stront-c.[4, 12], sul-ac., **sulph.**, thuj.,
vip., zinc.

inflammation – blood vessels –
phlebitis/inflammations –
vaisseaux sanguins – phlébite/
Entzündungen – Blutgefäße –
Phlebitis

blue
bleue
blaue
    carb-v., lycps., **mur-ac.**[4], **PULS.**[2]

burning
brûlantes
brennende
    apis, **ARS., calc.**

    night/nuit/nachts
    ARS.

bursting, as if[7]
éclatant, comme
berstend, wie
    vip.

constricting sensation[2]
constriction, sensation de
Zusammenschnüren, Gefühl von
    ang.

dipsomania, from[2]
dipsomanie, par
Trunksucht, durch
    crot-h.

inflamed see inflammation–blood
vessels–phlebitis

itching
démangeantes
juckende
    ant-t.[4], berb.[4], bruc.[4], **caps.**[4],
    carb-v.[4], caust.[4], **graph.**, lach.[4],
    m-aust.[4], nux-v.[4], plb.[4], puls.[4],
    sep.[4], sil.[4], sul-ac.[4], **sulph.**[4]

net work in skin
varicosités cutanées
Besenreiservarizen
    berb., **calc., carb-v., caust.**, clem.,
    crot-h., lach., lyc., nat-m., ox-ac.,
    plat., sabad., thuj.

painful
douloureuses
schmerzhafte
    brom., **caust., ham., lyc., mill.**,
    petr.[2], **PULS.**, sang., thuj.[3], vip.[7],
    zinc.[3]

pimples, covered with
boutons, couvertes de
Pickeln, bedeckt mit
    graph.

pregnancy, during
grossesse, pendant la
Schwangerschaft, während der
    FERR., lyc., **lycps., mill., nux-v.**[2],
    PULS., zinc.

soreness
meurtries, comme
wund, wie
    am-c.[4], ang.[4], bar-c.[4], **caust.**[4],
    graph., grat.[4], **HAM.**[1], hep.[4],
    ign.[4], **kali-c.**[4], kali-n.[4], m-arct.[4],
    merc,[4], mur-ac.[4], nat-m.[4], **nux-v.**[4],
    phos.[4], puls., rhus-t.[4], sil.[4], sul-ac.[4],
    sulph.[4], vip.[7]

stinging
piquantes, cuisantes
Stechen, feines
    apis, graph., ham., **PULS.**

stitching
piquantes
stechende
    alum.[4], **ant-t.**[2, 4], ars.[4], bar-c.[4],

caust.[4], grat.[4], kali-c., **kali-n.**[4], lyc.,
merc.[4], nat-m.[4], nux-v.[4], phos.[4],
sil.[4], sul-ac[4], **sulph.**[4]

ulceration
ulcère
Geschwür
aesc., alumn.[1'], anac., ant-t.,
arist-cl.[14], arn.[14], ars., calc., calc-f.[14],
carb-v., card-m., CAUST., cecr.[14],
cham.[4], cinnb., crot-h., crot-t.[6],
des-ac.[14], **fl-ac., graph.,** grin., **ham.,**
hydr., hydr-ac., kali-s., kreos.,
LACH., LYC., merc., mez., **nat-m.,**
parath.[14], **PULS.,** pyrog., raja-s.[14],
rhus-t., rib-ac.[14], sars., sec., **sil.,**
sul-ac., **sulph.,** syph., thuj., **zinc.**

swollen
tuméfiées
geschwollene
apis, berb.[1], puls.

young persons, in[7]
jeunes gens, chez les
jungen Menschen, bei
ferr-p.

VALUTS, cellars agg.
CAVE, souterrains agg.
KELLER, Gewölbe agg.
aran.[3], **ARS., bry.,** calc., **carb-an.,**
caust., dulc.[3], **kali-c.**[3], lyc., merc-i-f.[3],
NAT-S.[3], **PULS.,** sep., stram.

VEINS swollen evening[16]
VEINES gonflées le soir
VENEN, abends Schwellungen der
carb-v.

VENESECTION, ailments from[12]
PHLÉBOTOMIE, troubles à la suite de
VENAESECTIO, Beschwerden infolge
von
senec., squil.

inflammation – blood vessels –
phlebitis/inflammations –
vaisseaux sanguins – phlébite/
Entzündungen – Blutgefäße –
Phlebitis

VENOUS pulsations[1]
VEINEUSES, pulsations
VENEN, Pulsationen in den
asaf.

VIGOR, decreased[3, 6]
VIGUEUR diminuée
KRÄFTE, Abnahme der
ars-i.[1'], carb-an.[1', 3, 6], carb-v., cocc.,
ferr-p.[1'], laur., mag-m., op., ph-ac.[7],
phos.[1'], sulph., tub.[1', 7], verat.[3],
vinc.

VIOLENT EFFECTS[3]
VIOLENTS EFFETS
HEFTIGER KRANKHEITSVERLAUF
acon., alum., anac., **ars., BELL.,** bry.,
canth., carb-v., **CHAM.,** cupr., glon.,
hep., **hyos.,** ign., iod., **lach.,** merc.,
NUX-V., STRAM., sulph., **tarent.,**
verat.

VOMITING agg.
VOMISSEMENT agg.
ERBRECHEN agg.
acon., **AETH.**[3, 8], **ant-t.,** arn., **ARS.,**
asar., bell., **bry., calc.,** caps., cham.,
chin., cina, cocc., **colch.,** coloc.,
con., **CUPR.,** dig., **dros.,** ferr.,
graph., **hyos.,** iod., **IP.,** lach., **lyc.,**
mez., mosch., nat-m., **nux-v.,** op.,
phos., plb., PULS., ran-s., ruta,
sabin., **sars.,** sec., **sep.,** sil., stann.,
SULPH., verat.

am.
acon., agar., anac.[15], ant-t.[3], ars.,
asar.[14], carbn-s., **coc-c.,** colch., **dig.,**
eup-per.[3], helia.[8], hell.[3], hyos.,
kali-bi.[3], lat-m.[9], nux-v., op., plb.[3],
puls., **sang., sec., tab.**[3]

WAKING, on
RÉVEIL, au
ERWACHEN, Beschwerden beim
acon., agar., agn., alum., alum-sil.[1'],
alumn.[2], **am-c., AM-M., AMBR.,**
anac., **ant-c.,** ant-t., apis[3], arg-n.[7],
arn., ARS., aur., bapt.[6], bar-c., bell.,
benz-ac., bism., bor., bov., bry.,
bufo., cact., cadm-s., calad., **CALC.,**

calc-p., calc-s., cann-s., canth.,
caps., carb-an., carb-v., CAUST.,
cench., cham., **chel., chin.,** cic.,
cina, clem., coc-c., **cocc.,** coff.,
colch., **con.,** corn., croc., **crot-h.,**
crot-t., cupr., cycl., **dig.,** dros.,
dulc., euph., euphr.[3], ferr., ferr-ar.[1'],
fl-ac.[3], form., **graph.,** guaj., **HEP.,**
hydr., **HYOS., ign., ip., kali-ar.,**
KALI-BI., kali-c., kali-i., kali-n.,
kali-s., kreos., **LACH.,** laur., led.,
lyc., lycps.[3], mag-c., mag-m., mang.,
meny., **merc.,** merc-c.[3], **merc-i-f.,**
mez., mosch., mur-ac., naja, nat-c.,
nat-m., NIT-AC., nux-m., **NUX-V.,**
op., **ONOS.,** palo.[14], par.[3], petr.,
ph-ac., **PHOS., phyt.,** plat., psor.,
PULS., ran-b., ran-s., rauw.[14],
rheum, rhod., **rhus-t.,** ruta, sabad.,
sabin., **samb., sang.,** sars., sel.,
seneg., **SEP., sil.,** spig., spong.,
squil., stann.[3], **staph.,** stram.,
stront-c., sul-ac., **SULPH.,** tarax.,
teucr.[3], thuj., trios.[14], tub.[3],
VALER., ven-m.[14], verat., viol-o.,
viol-t., **zinc.**

sleep–after–morning/sommeil–
après–matin/Schlaf–nach–
morgens

agg. on w. at night[3]
agg. au r. la nuit
agg. beim E. nachts
    ambr., bry.[3, 4], carb-v., chin.,
    COCC., colch., ip., lach.[4], nat-c.,
    nat-m., **NUX-V.,** ph-ac., **puls.,**
    ruta, sabin., **sel.,** sep.

siesta, from[3]
sieste, d'une
Mittagsschlaf, aus dem
    caust.

am.
    am-m., ambr., **ars.,** bry., **calad.,**
    calc., cham., chin., cocc., **colch.,**
    hell., ign., ip., kreos., lach., meph.[4],
    nat-c., **nux-v., onos.,** ph-ac., **PHOS.,**
    puls., ruta, sabin., samb., sel., **SEP.,**
    spig., thuj., vip.[4]

WALK, late learning to
MARCHE, retard d'apprentissage
GEHEN, lernt spät
    agar., **bar-c.,** bell., **CALC.,**
    CALC-P., CAUST., lyc.[6], merc.[6],
    NAT-M., nux-v., **ph-ac.[6], phos.[6],**
    pin-s.[6], **sanic., sil.,** sulph.

    tardy development of bones[8]
    retard du développement osseux
    späte Knochenentwicklung
    calc.[1', 8], calc-f., **calc-p.,** sil.

WALKING agg.
MARCHER agg.
GEHEN agg.
    acon., **AESC., agar., agn.,** aloe,
    alum., alum-p.[1'], am-c., **am-m.,**
    ambr., anac., ang.[3], ant-c., **ant-t.,**
    apis, arg-m., arg-n.[3], **arn., ars.,**
    ars-i., asaf., **asar.,** atra-r.[14], **atro.,**
    aur., aur-ar.[1'], aur-m.[1'], **bapt.,**
    bar-c., bar-i.[1'], bar-s.[1'], **BELL., berb.,**
    bor.[3], **bov., BRY., cact.,**
    cadm-met.[14], cadm-s., **calad.,**
    CALC., CALC-S., camph., cann-s.,
    canth., caps., **carb-ac., carb-an.,**
    carb-v., **carbn-s., CAUST.,** cham.,
    chel., CHIN., chion., cic., cina,
    clem., **COCC., coff., COLCH.,**
    coloc., **CON.,** conv., cortico.[14],
    croc., cupr., cycl., dicha.[14], **dig.,**
    dros., dulc., euph., euphr., **ferr.,**
    ferr-ar.[1'], ferr-i., ferr-p.[1'], **FL-AC.[3],**
    form., gels., **glon., gran., graph.,**
    guaj., **hell., hep.,** hyos., ign., **iod.,**
    ip., kali-c., kali-n., kali-p., kali-sil.[1'],
    kreos., **lach.,** laur., **LED., lil-t.,** lyc.,
    mag-c., mag-m., **mag-p.,** mang.,
    meny., **merc.,** merc-c.[3], methys.[14],
    mez., mosch., mur-ac., **murx.,** nat-c.,
    nat-m., nat-p., nat-s., nat-sil.[1'],
    NIT-AC., nux-m., **NUX-V.,** olnd.,
    op., paeon., par., **petr., ph-ac.,**
    PHOS., phyt., plat., plb., **psor.,**
    puls., **ran-b.,** ran-s., **rheum,** rhod.,
    RHUS-T., ruta, sabad., **sabin.,**
    samb., **sars.,** sec., **sel.,** seneg., **SEP.,**
    sil., SPIG., spong., **squil., STANN.,**
    staph., stram., stront-c., sul-ac.,
    sul-i.[1'], **SULPH.,** tab.[3], **tarax.,**

tarent., teucr., thiop.[14], thuj., tub., valer., verat., **verat-v.**, verb., viol-o., viol-t., **zinc.**

am.

acon., agar., agn., alum., alumn., am-c., **am-m.**, ambr., anac., ang.[3], ant-c., ant-t., apis, apoc., aran-ix.[14], arg-m., arg-n.[3], arn., **ars.**, ars-s-f.[1'], asaf., asar., **AUR.**, aur-m.[3], aur-s.[1'], bar-c., bell., bism., bov., **brom.**, **bry.**, buni-o.[14], calc.[3], calen.[4], canth., **caps.**, carb-v., caust., cham., chin., cic., cina, cocc., coloc., **CON.**[3], cortiso.[14], crot-h., cupr., **CYCL.**, **dios.**, **dros.**, **DULC.**, **EUPH.**, euphr., **FERR.**, ferr-ar., **fl-ac.**, glon., graph., guaj., halo.[14], hep., hyos., ign., indg., iod., kali-bi., kali-c., **KALI-I.**, kali-n., kali-p., **kali-s.**, kreos., lach., laur., **lyc.**, lycps.[3], **mag-c.**, **mag-m.**, mag-p.[3], mang., **meli.**, **meny.**, meph.[14], **merc.**, mez., **mosch.**, mur-ac., nat-c., **nat-m.**, nat-s.[1'], nid.[14], nit-ac., nux-m.[1], olnd., op., palo.[14], par., petr., **ph-ac.**, phos.[3], **plat.**, plb., **PULS.**, pyrog., **ran-b.**, raph., **rhod.**, **RHUS-T.**, ruta, **SABAD.**, sabin., **SAMB.**, sars., sel., seneg., **sep.**, sil., spig., spong.[3], stann., staph., stront-c., sul-ac., **SULPH.**, **TARAX.**, tere-ch.[14], teucr., thal.[14], thuj., tub.[1', 7], **VALER.**, **verat.**, **verb.**, **viol-t.**, vip-a.[14], **zinc.**

after w. agg.[3]
après la marche agg.
nach dem G. agg.
 kali-bi., **kali-c.**, lyc., ruta, stann. stram., sulph.,

ailments from[12]
troubles à la suite de
Beschwerden infolge von
 sel.

air agg., in open
air agg., en plein
Freien agg., im
 acon., **agar.**, agn., alum., alum-p.[1'], **am-c.**, am-m., ambr.,

anac., ang.[3], ant-c., arg-m., arn., **ARS.**, ars-s-f.[1'], asar., aur., aur-ar.[1'], aur-s.[1'], bar-c., **bell.**, bor., bov., **bry.**, calad., **calc.**, calc-sil.[1'], **camph.**, cann-s., canth., caps., **carb-ac.**, **carb-an.**, **carb-v.**, carbn-s.[1'], **CAUST.**, cham., **chel.**, chin., chin-ar., cic., **cina**, clem., **COCC.**, **coff.**, **colch.**, coloc., **con.**, croc., dig., dros., dulc., euph., **euphr.**, ferr., ferr-ar.[1'], **FL-AC.**[3], graph., **guaj.**, hell., **hep.**, hyos., ign., iod., ip., **kali-c.**, kali-n., **kali-p.**, kreos., lach., laur., **led.**, lyc., mag-c., mag-m., **MAG-P.**, mag-s.[4], mang., meny., **merc.**, merc-c., mez., mosch., mur-ac., nat-ar., nat-c., nat-m., nit-ac., **nux-m.**, **NUX-V.**, olnd., op., par., petr., ph-ac., **phos.**, **plan.**, plat., plb., **psor.**, **puls.**, ran-b., **ran-s.**, rheum, rhod., **rhus-t.**, ruta, sabad., sabin., sars., **SEL.**, **seneg.**, **sep.**, **sil.**, **SPIG.**, spong., **stann.**, staph., **stram.**, stront-c., sul-ac., **SULPH.**, tarax., teucr., thuj., valer., verat., **verb.**, viol-t.[1], zinc.

am.

acon., aesc.[6], agar., aloe, **ALUM.**, am-c.[3], am-m., ambr., anac., ang.[3], ant-c., ant-t.[4], aran.[6, 14], arg-m., **ARG-N.**, arn., ars.[3], asaf., **asar.**, **aur.**, bapt., bar-c., bar-s.[1'], bell., bism., bor., bov., **brom.**, **bry.**, calc., calc-s., caps., carb-ac., carb-v., carbn-s., caust., cic., cimic.[14], cina, **con.**, croc.[4], dios.[6], **dulc.**, **FL-AC.**, gamb., **graph.**, hed.[10], hep.[3], hyos., ign., iod.[6, 10], ip.[4], kali-c., **KALI-I.**, kali-n., **KALI-S.**, lach.[6], laur., **lil-t.**, **LYC.**, **mag-c.**, mag-f.[10, 14], **mag-m.**, mag-s.[4, 10, 14], mand.[10], mang., meny., merc., **merc-i-r.**, mez., mosch., mur-ac., **naja**, nat-ar., nat-c., nat-m., nat-s.[1', 7], nicc.[4], nit-ac., op., ox-ac., par., petr., **ph-ac.**, phel.[4], phos., pip-n.[3], plat., plb., **PULS.**, rauw.[14], rhod., **RHUS-T.**, ruta[3],

sabin., **sang.**, sars., sel., **seneg.**,
sep., spig., spong.[3], **stann.**, staph.,
stront-c., sul-ac., **sulph., tarax.**,
tarent.[1',7], **teucr., thuj.**, verat.,
verb., vinc.[4], viol-t., zinc.

aversion to[11]
aversion pour la marche
Abneigung gegen
agar., aza.[14], cham., clem., fago.,
kali-bi., nit-ac.

backward impossible[3]
aller en arrière impossible
Rückwärtsgehen unmöglich
cocc., mang.

beginning of w. agg
au début de la marche, agg.
Beginn des Gehens agg., am
acon., **agar.**, am-c., ambr., anac.,
ang.[3,6], ant-c., ant-t., arn., ars.,
asar., aur., bar-c., bell., bov., **bry.**,
cact., calc., cann-s., canth., **CAPS.**,
carb-an., **carb-v., caust.**, cham.,
chin., cic., cina, cocc., **CON.**, croc.,
cupr., cycl., dig., dros., **EUPH.**,
FERR., graph., kali-c., kali-n., lach.,
laur., led., **LYC.**, mag-c., mang.,
merc., mur-ac., nat-c., nat-m.,
nit-ac., nux-v., olnd., petr., ph-ac.,
phos., phyt.[6], plat., plb., **PULS.**,
ran-b., rhod., **RHUS-T., ruta,**
sabad., sabin., **samb.**, sars., sep.,
sil., spig., staph., stram., stront-c.,
sulph., **thuj.**, valer., verat., **zinc.**

bent, agg.[3]
courbé agg.
gebücktes G. agg.
bry.

am.[3]
arn., **CON., hyos., lyc.**, nux-v.,
phos., rhus-t., sabin., sulph.,
viol-t.

bridge agg., on a narrow[3]
pont étroit agg., sur un
Brücke agg., über eine schmale
bar-c., ferr., sulph.

circle, in a[16]
cercle, en
Kreis, in einem
bell.

desire for[3,6]
désir de marche
Verlangen zu gehen
acon.[3], arg-m.[1',6], arg-n., **ars.**[3,11],
aur., bism.[6], caj.[11], calc.[3,16],
chlor.[11], cod.[11], fl-ac.[3], gins.[11],
iod., lepi.[11], lil-t.[3], lyc.[3], mag-c.[3],
merc., mosch.[6], naja[3,11], **op.**,
paeon.[3], paull.[11], phos.[3], ruta[3],
sep., spirae.[11], **stront-c.**, tarent.[3],
thlasp.[3], thuj.[3], valer.[8], zinc-a.[11]

night[6]/nuit/nachts
iod., merc.[11], **op.**

air, in open[4]
air, en plein
Freien, im
asaf.[11], clem., crot-t., fla-ac.[7],
lach., lact., lyc., mez.[11], phos.[4,11],
puls., teucr.

down stairs agg.[1']
descendre un escalier agg.
Treppen Herabgehen agg.
bor.

descending/descente/Abwärts-
bewegung

easily
facilement
leichtes, müheloses
thuj.[16], zinc.[6]

fast agg.
vite agg.
schnelles agg.
alum., alum-sil.[1'], **ang.**[3], arg-m.,
apis, arn., ARS., ars-i., ars-s-f.[1'],
aur., aur-ar.[1'], aur-i.[1'], **aur-m.**,
aur-s.[1'], **BELL.**, bor.[3], **BRY., cact.,**
calc., calc-s., calc-sil.[1'], **cann-s.,**
caust., chel., chin., cina, cocc.,
coff., **CON.**, croc., **cupr.**, dros.,
ferr., ferr-ar., hep., hyos., **ign.,**
iod., ip., **kali-ar., kali-c.**, kali-p.,

kali-sil.[1'], laur., **led., lyc., merc.,**
mez., nat-ar., nat-c., **nat-m.,**
nit-ac., nux-m., **nux-v., olnd.,**
PHOS., plb., PULS., rheum,
rhod., rhus-t., ruta, sabin.,
seneg., sep., **SIL., spig.,** spong.,
squil., staph., sul-ac., **SULPH.,**
verat., zinc.

running/courir/Laufen

am.
ant-t.[3], arg-n., ars.[1'], **aur-m.[3],**
brom.[1'], canth., carb-ac., **ign.,**
mag-c.[3], mag-m.[3], nat-m., petr.,
rhus-t.[3, 7], sabin.[3], SEP., sil.,
stann., sul-ac., TUB.

level agg., on a[3]
à plat agg.
ebenem Weg agg., auf
ran-b., verat.

rough ground agg., over[3]
irrégulier et dur agg., sur un terrain
unebenem Boden agg., auf
clem., lil-t., phos., podo.

running water agg., over[3]
eau courante agg., au dessus d'une
fließendes Wasser agg., über
ang., bar-c., brom., **ferr.,** hyos.,
sulph.

slowly am.
lentement am.
langsames G. am.
agar., **AUR.,** aur-i.[1'], **AUR-M.,**
cact., calc-s., **FERR.,** ferr-ar., iris,
kali-p., lyc.[7], **PULS.,** sep., **tarent.**

stone pavement agg., on[3]
chemin pavé agg., sur un
Steinpflaster agg., auf
aloe, ant-c., ars., **con., hep.,** nux-v.,
sep.

wind agg., in the
vent agg., au
Wind agg., im
acon., **agar., ars., asar.,** aur.,
aur-ar.[1'], **BELL., calc.,** carb-v.,

cham., chin., con., euphr., **graph.,**
lach., **lyc.,** mur-ac., nat-c., nux-m.,
NUX-V., phos., plat., **puls.,** rhus-t.,
SEP., spig., **stann.,** thuj.

WARM agg.
CHALEUR agg.
WÄRME agg.
acon., adlu.[14], **aesc.[7],** aeth.[8], **agar.,**
agn., **all-c.,** aloe[1', 7], **ALUM.,**
alumn.[2], ambr., **anac.[2, 3, 8], ant-c.,**
ant-t., APIS, aq-mar.[14], **ARG-N.[1, 7],**
arn., **ARS-I.,** asaf.[6-8], **asar.[2, 3],**
aster.[14], aur., **auri.[1', 7], aur-m.,**
bar-c., bar-i.[1'], **bell.,** beryl.[14],
bism., bor., brom.[1'], **bry.,**
calad.[1, 7], calc.[2, 3, 5, 8], calc-i.[1', 7],
calc-s.[7], camph., cann-s., canth.,
carb-v., **carbn-s.,** caust., cench.[1'],
cham., chin.[2, 3, 8], cimic.[14], cina,
clem.[8], **coc-c.[1],** cocc., coff.[1], colch.,
coloc., **com.[8],** conv.[8], cortico.[9],
cortiso.[9, 14], **croc.[1, 7], crot-h.[3],** dig.,
dros., dulc., euph., euphr., ferr.[2, 3, 8],
ferr-i., **FL-AC.[1', 3, 6-8],** flav.[14], foll.[14],
gels., **glon., graph., grat.[7], guaj.,**
ham.[7], hed.[10], helio.[8], hell., hep.[3],
hip-ac.[14], hist.[14], hydroph.[14],
hyos.[3, 8], iber.[8, 14], ign., **ind., IOD.,**
ip., jug-c.[8], just.[8], kali-br.,
kali-c.[2, 3, 14], **KALI-I.[3, 7, 8], kali-m.[8],**
KALI-S.[1, 7], lac-c., lach., laur.,
LED., lil-t.[3, 6, 7], lyc., mag-c.[10],
med.[7, 8], **merc., mez.,** mur-ac.,
nat-c., **NAT-M.[1, 7], NAT-S.[1, 7],**
nit-ac.[2, 3, 8], nux-m.[2, 3, 8], nux-v.[2, 3],
op., ph-ac., phenob.[13, 14], **phos.,**
phyt.[1'], pic-ac.[1'], pitu.[14], **PLAT.[1, 7],**
prot.[14], **PULS.,** rauw.[9, 14], rhus-t.[2, 3, 4],
sabad., **sabin.[1, 7], SEC.,** sel., **seneg.,**
sep.[2, 3], sil.[2, 3], spig., **spong.[1, 7],**
staph., stel.[8], sul-ac.[8], **sul-i.[1', 7],**
SULPH.[1, 7], tab., teucr., **thuj.[1, 7],**
trios.[14], **tub.[7],** verat., **vesp.[7],** visc.[14],
zinc.

heat, sensation – vital, lack/
  chaleur, sensation – vitale,
  manque/Hitzegefühl – Lebens-
  wärme

ailments from[12]
troubles à la suite de
Beschwerden infolge von
  acon., gels., nat-c.

am.[2]
  acon., agar.[1',2], alum-sil.[1'], alumn.,
  am-c.[2], anac., ant-c.[1',2,6,7],
  arg-m.[2,6], arist-cl.[9,10], arn.[2],
  ARS.[1',2,4,6-8], asar., aur.[2,8], bad.[8],
  bar-c.[2,6], bell.[1',2,8], bell-p.[10,14],
  bor., bov., bry.[1',2,8], calc.,
  calc-f.[1',7,8,10,14], calc-p.[1'], calc-s.[1'],
  CAMPH.[2,8], canth., caps.[2,6,8],
  carb-an., carb-v., cast.[6],
  CAUST[1',2,4,8], cench.[1'],
  cham.[1',2,4,6,7], chel.[1'], chin.[2,6],
  cic.[2,14], cimic.[8], clem., cocc.,
  coff.[2,7,8], colch.[1',2,6,14], coll.[8],
  coloc.[1',2,6,8,10], con.[2,6], cor-r.[8],
  cupr-a.[8], cycl.[6,8], cyn-d.[14], dig.,
  DULC.[2,6,8], ferr.[1',2], flor-p.[14], form.[8],
  gink-b[14], graph., gymno.[2,8], hell.,
  HEP.[2,3,6,8], hyos.[2], ign.[2,3,8], ip.,
  kali-ar.[1'], kali-bi.[1',8], KALI-C.[2,6,14],
  kali-p.[8], kreos.[2,6,8], lac-d.[1'],
  lach.[2,8], laur., led., levo.[14], lob.[8],
  lyc.[1',2,4,8], lycpr.[8], mag-c.[2,3,10],
  mag-m.[2,14], mag-p.[1',8], mand.[9,10],
  mang., med.[1'], meny., merc., mez.,
  moly-met.[14], MOSCH., mur-ac.,
  nat-c., nat-m.[2], nid.[14], nit-ac.,
  nux-m.[2,6,8], NUX-V.[2,6,8], onop.[14],
  ph-ac.[2,6,8], petr., phos.[1',2], phyt.[8],
  psor.[8], puls., pyrog.[1',6], ran-b.,
  rheum[2], rhod.[2,8], RHUS-T.[1',2,3,6,8],
  rumx.[8], ruta, SABAD.[1',2,4,8],
  samb., sars.[1',2], seneg., sep.[2,4,8],
  sil.[2,3,6,8], spig.[1',2], spong.[2,6],
  squil., staph.[2,8], stram.[2,3,8],
  STRONT-C.[2,4], sul-ac.[2,8], sulph.[2,4],
  syph.[1'], thea[8], ther.[1'], thuj.[2,6],
  tub.[1',7], verat.[2,8], verb., viol-t.,
  xero.[8], zinc.

air agg.
air chaud agg.
Luft agg., warme
  agn., aloe, ambr., anac.[2,3], ant-c.,
  ant-t., arg-n., arsi-i., asar.[2,3,6],
  aur., aur-i.[1'], aur-m., bry., calad.,

calc., calc-i.[1'], calc-s., cann-s.,
carb-v., cham., cina, coc-c.[2], cocc.,
colch., croc., dros., euph., fl-ac.,
GLON., ign., ind., IOD., ip.,
kali-bi., KALI-S., LACH., led.,
lyc., MERC., mez., nat-m., nat-s.,
nit-ac.[2,3], nux-m., nux-v., op.,
ph-ac.[3], phenob.[13,14], phos.,
pic-ac., plat., podo., PULS.,
rhus-t.[2,3], sabin., sars., sec., sel.,
seneg., sep.[2,3], sul-i.[1'], sulph.,
teucr., thuj., xan.

am.[2]
  acon., agar., alumn., am-c., anac.,
  ant-c., arn., ARS.[2,6], asar.,
  AUR.[2,8], bar-c.[2,6], bell., bor.,
  bov., bry., calc.[2,8], CAMPH.,
  canth., caps.[2,6], carb-an., carb-v.,
  CAUST.[2,6,8], cham., chin., cic.,
  cina, coc-c., coff., colch.[2,6],
  coloc.[2,6], con., dig., DULC.[2,6],
  ferr., graph., HELL., HEP.[2,6],
  hyos., ign., ip., KALI-C.[2,6],
  kreos., lach., laur., led.[8], lyc.,
  mag-c.[2,8], mag-m., mag-p.[6],
  mang., meny., merc.[2,8], mez.,
  MOSCH., mur-ac., nat-ar.[1'],
  nat-c., nat-m., nat-s.[6], nit-ac.,
  NUX-M., NUX-V., par., petr.[2,8],
  ph-ac.[2,6], phos., psor., ran-b.,
  rhod.[2,6], RHUS-T.[2,6,8], ruta,
  SABAD., samb., sars., sel.,
  seneg., sep., sil.[2,6], spig.,
  spong.[2,6], squil., staph., stram.,
  STRONT-C.[2,6], sul-ac., sulph.,
  thuj.[2,6], verat., verb., viol-t.,
  zinc.

becoming warm agg.[2,3]
s'échauffant agg., en
Erwärmung agg.
  acon.[2,3,8], am-c., ANT-C.[2,3,8],
  bar-i.[1'], bell.[2,3,8], bor.[3],
  brom.[3,7,8], BRY.[2,3,8], calc.[3,8],
  caps., carb-v.[2,3,8], coff., dig.,
  gels.[2], glon., hep., ign., ip.,
  KALI-C., lach.[1'], lyc.[3,8], mez.,
  nat-m., nux-m.[2,3,8],
  nux-v.[2,3,8], olnd., op., sep.,
  sil., staph., thuj., zinc.

air agg., in open
air agg., en plein
Freien agg., im
    acon., agn., alum., alumn.[2],
    ambr., anac.[2], **ant-c.**, asar.[2],
    aur., aur-i.[1]', **aur-m.**, bar-c.,
    bell., bor., bov., **BRY.**, calad.,
    calc., cann-s., **carb-v.**, caust.,
    cham., chin., cina, cocc., coff.,
    colch., coloc., croc., dros.,
    dulc., euph., **GELS.**[2], **glon.**,
    graph., ign., **IOD.**, ip., kali-c.,
    lach., led., **LYC.**, mang., **merc.**,
    mez., nat-c., nat-m., **nat-s.**,
    nit-ac., nux-m.[2], nux-v.[2], olnd.,
    op., petr., ph-ac., **phos.**, plat.,
    PULS., rhus-t.[2], **sabad.**, sabin.,
    sec., sel., **seneg.**, sep., **sil.**,
    spig., spong., staph., **sulph.**,
    teucr., thuj., **verat.**

am.[2]
    acon., agar., am-c., ant-c., **arn.**,
    ARS., asar., **aur., bar-c., bell.**,
    bor., bov., **bry., calc., camph.**,
    canth., **caps.**, carb-an., carb-v.,
    caust., cham., chin., cic., clem.,
    coc-c., colch.[1]', **con.**, dig., **dulc.**,
    ferr., **GRAPH., hell., hep., hyos.**,
    ign., KALI-C., kreos., lach., **lyc.**,
    mag-c., mag-m., **mang.**, meny.,
    merc., mez., **MOSCH.**, mur-ac.,
    nat-c., nat-m., **nit-ac., nux-m.**,
    NUX-V., petr., **ph-ac.**[1]', [2], **phos.**,
    ran-b., rhod., **RHUS-T.**, ruta,
    SABAD., samb., **sars.**, sel., **sep.**,
    sil., spig., **spong.**, staph., stram.,
    verat., verb., viol-t., zinc.

bed agg.
lit chaud agg.
Bettwärme agg.
    aeth., agn., **alum.**, alumn.[2],
    ambr., anac.[2], [3]. **ant-c., ant-t.**,
    APIS, arg-n., arn., ars-i., **asaf.**,
    asar.[2], [3], aur., aur-i.[1]', **aur-m.**,
    aur-s.[1]', bar-c., bell-p.[8], bov.,
    bry., calad., calc., calc-f.[10],
    calc-i.[1]', **calc-s., camph.**,
    cann-s., **carb-v.**, carbn-s.[1]', [7],
    caust.[2], [3], cedr., **CHAM.**, chin.,

cina, cinnb.[1]', **clem., coc-c.**,
cocc., colch., coloc.[3], croc.,
daph., **DROS.**, dulc., **euph.**,
fl-ac., glon., goss., **graph.**,
hell., hyos., ign., **iod., ip.**,
kali-c.[2], [3], **kali-chl.**, kali-m.[1]',
kali-s., lac-c., lach., LED., lyc.,
mag-c., med.[7], **MERC., mez.**,
mur-ac., nat-c., **nat-m.**, nit-ac.,
nux-m.[2], [3], **nux-v.**[2], [3], **OP.**,
ph-ac., phenob.[13], [14], phos.,
phyt., **plat.**, psor., **PULS.**,
rhod.[3], [4], [6], **rhus-t.**[2], [3], [4], [6], sabad.,
SABIN., sars., **SEC.**, sel.,
seneg., sep.[2], [3], **sil.**[3], [6], spig.,
spong., staph., stram.,
stront-c.[3], **sul-i.**[1]', **SULPH.**,
teucr., **thuj., verat.**, visc.[8],
x-ray[9]

cold extremities, with
froides, avec extrémités
kalten Extremitäten, bei
    CAMPH., LED., mag-c., med.,
    SEC.

am.
    agar., **am-c.**, arn., **ARS.**, ars-s-f.[1]',
    aur., bapt.[3], bar-c., bell., **BRY.**,
    calc-p., camph., canth., **caust.**,
    cic., cocc., **coloc.**, con., **dulc.**,
    graph., HEP., hyos., **kali-bi.**,
    KALI-C., kali-i., kali-p., lach.,
    LYC., mag-p., mosch., nit-ac.,
    NUX-M., NUX-V., petr., ph-ac.,
    phos., RHUS-T., rumx., sabad.,
    sep., **SIL.**, spong., squil., **stann.**,
    staph., stram., stront-c., sul-ac.[3], [6],
    sulph., **tarent.**, thuj.[6], **TUB.**,
    verat.[2], [3]

room agg.
chambre chaude agg.
Zimmerwärme agg.
    acon., aeth.[6], **agn., all-c.**[1]', [8],
    alum., alum-sil.[1]', **alumn.**[2],
    am-c.[3], ambr., **anac.**[2], [3], [6], **ant-c.**,
    ant-t., **APIS**, aran-ix.[10], aran-sc.[8],
    arg-n., ars-i., arn., **asaf.**,
    asar.[2], [3], [6], aur., aur-i.[1]', **aur-m.**,
    aur-s.[1]', bapt.[3], [8], bar-c., bar-i.[1]',
    bell., bor., **brom., bry.**, bufo,

calad., calc., calc-i.[1'], calc-p.,
CALC-S., cann-s., **carb-ac.,
carb-v., CARBN-S.,** caust., cina,
coc-c., cocc., colch., crat.[8],
CROC., culx.[1'], **dros.,** dulc.,
euphr.[8], **fl-ac., glon., GRAPH.,**
hell., hep.[2, 3], hip-ac.[9, 14], hyos.,
hyper.[8], ign., **ind., IOD., ip.,**
kali-c., **KALI-I., KALI-S.,** lach.[1'],
laur., **led., lil-t.,** luf-op.[14], **LYC.,
mag-m.**[1], med.[7], **merc., merc-i-f.,**
mez., mosch., mur-ac., nat-ar.,
nat-c., nat-m., **nat-s.,** nit-ac.,
nux-v.[2, 3, 8], **op.,** oxyt., ph-ac.,
phos., **pic-ac.,** plat., pneu.[14], **ptel.,
PULS.,** ran-b., rhus-t.[2, 3, 8],
SABIN., sanic., SEC., sel.,
SENEG., sep.[2, 3, 6, 8], spig.,
spong., staph., **sul-i.**[1'], **SULPH.,
tab., thuj., til., tub., verat.,** vib.[8]

am.[6]
    aur-ar.[1'], carb-v., **caust.,** cham.,
    chel., chin., chin-ar.[1'], cocc.,
    cycl.[1'], guaj., **hep.**[1, 6], mag-p.[1'],
    mang., merc., nux-m., nux-v.,
    plat., rhus-t.[1'], **rumx., sil.**

stove agg.
poêle agg., du
Ofenwärme agg.
    ant-c., apis, arg-n., ars.[3], **bry.,**
    bufo, **cimic.**[3], **cocc., con.,**
    cupr.[3], **euph., iod., GLON.,**
    kali-i., laur., mag-m., **merc.,**
    nat-m., nux-v.[3], **op.,** psor.[3],
    puls., SEC., thiop.[14], **zinc.**[2, 3]

    he is cold and stiff on approach-
      ing
    devient raide et froid en
      s'approchant d'un poél ou
      d'un radiateur chaud
    ist kalt und steif, wenn er sich
      dem Ofen nähert
    laur.

ailments from[12]
troubles à la suite de
Beschwerden infolge von
    glon.

am.
    acon., agar., am-c., **ARS.,** aur.,
    bar-c., bell., bor., bov.[3], camph.,
    canth., caps., caust., cic., cocc.,
    con., conv., **dulc.,** graph.[3], hell.,
    HEP., hyos., **IGN.,** kali-c., lach.[3],
    mag-c., **MAG-P.,** mang., meny.[2, 3],
    mosch., **nux-m., NUX-V.,** petr.,
    ran-b., rhod., **RHUS-T.,** sabad.,
    SIL., stront-c., sulph., tub.[1']

wraps agg.
couvertures, enveloppes chaudes agg.
Umhüllung agg., warme
    acon., ant-c.[1'], ant-t.[1', 6], **APIS,
    arg-m., arg-n.,** arn.[3], **ars-i.,
    asar.**[2, 3], aur., aur-i.[1'], **aur-m.,**
    aur-s.[1'], **bor.,** brom.[1'], **bry., calc.,**
    calc-i.[1'], calc-s., **camph.,** carb-v.,
    carbn-s., **cham.,** chin., **coc-c.,**
    coff., **crot-h.**[3], cupr.[3], **ferr., ferr-i.,
    fl-ac.,** glon., ign., **IOD., ip.**[3],
    kali-bi.[3], kali-i.[3], **KALI-S.,
    lac-c.,** lach., **LED., LYC.,
    MAG-P.**[3], merc., mosch., mur-ac.,
    nit-ac., nux-v., op., phos., plat.,
    PULS., rhus-t., sabin.[1', 3], **SEC.,
    seneg.,** sep., **spig.,** staph., **sul-i.**[1'],
    SULPH., tab., thuj., **verat.**

am.[2]
    ars.[1'], colch.[1'], **HEP.,** psor.[2, 3],
    rhod.[1'], rhus-t.[15], sabad.[3], **SIL.**

desire for warm bed[11]
désir de lit chaud
Verlangen nach Bettwärme
    spig.

clothing[1']
habits chauds
Kleidung, warmer
    alum., ars., **bar-c.**[6], bell., calc.[1'],
    caul., graph., hep., kali-c.,
    nat-c., nat-s., plb., psor.[6],
    sabad.[6], sil.

    Vol. I: *fur/fourrures/Pelze*

afternoon[11]/après-midi/nach-
    mittags
    nux-v.

in spite of sensation of heat[14]
malgré la sensation de chaleur
trotz Hitzegefühles
    achy.

stove[11]
poêle, chaleur du
Ofenwärme
    bar-c.[6], cic., ptel., **sil.**[6], tub.[1']

warmth[3, 6]
chaleur
Wärme
    alum., am-br.[6], arg-m., **ars.,**
    bar-c.[3], calc.[1'], caps., **caust.,**
    colch., con., **hep., kali-c.**[3, 6, 14],
    moly-met.[14], ph-ac., psor., **sabad.,**
    sil., thuj.[3], tub.

WASHING clothes, laundry, ailments
from[12]
**BLANCHISSAGE, lessive troubles à la
suite de**
WASCHEN der Wäsche, Beschwerden
infolge von
    phos., sep., ther.

WATER, dashing against inner parts,
sensation of
**EAU qui gicle contre des parties
internes, sensation d'**
WASSER gegen innere Organe spritzt,
Gefühl als ob
    ars.[3], bell., carb-ac.[3], carb-an.[3],
    chin.[3], cina, **crot-h.**[3], **CROT-T.,** dig.,
    ferr., glon.[3], hell., **hep.**[3], **hyos.**[3],
    jatr.[3], kali-c.[3], kali-m.[1'], laur.,
    nat-m.[3], ph-ac., **rhod., rhus-t.**[3],
    spig.

heat–warm water–dashed/
    chaleur–eau chaude–l'aspergeait/
    Hitzewallungen–warmem
    Wasser–bespritzt

seeing or hearing of running w. agg.[3]
voir ou entendre de l'e. courante
agg.
Sehen oder Hören von fließendem
W. agg.
    ang., apis, arg-m., bell.[3, 6], brom.,

canth., **LYSS.**[3, 6, 8, 10], nit-ac.,
stram.[3, 6], sulph.[3, 6], ter.

Vol. I: *hydrophobia/hydrophobie/*
    Tollwut

pouring out of w. agg.[10]
versant de l'e. agg., en
Wasserausschütten agg.
    lyss.

wading in, ailments from
patauger dans l'e., troubles à la suite
de
Waten im, Beschwerden infolge von
    ars., dulc., mag-p.

working in w. agg.[3, 6, 8]
travailler dans l'e. agg.
Arbeiten im W. agg.
    calc., calc-p.[3, 6], mag-c.

ailments from[12]
troubles à la suite de
Beschwerden infolge von
    calc.

hands in cold w. agg., with[3]
mains dans l'e. froide, avec ses
Händen im kalten W. agg., mit
    lac-d., mag-p., phos.

am.[3]
    jatr.

WAVELIKE sensations
VAGUES, sensation de
WELLEN, Gefühl von
    acon.[3], am-c., aml-ns.[3], anac.[3], ant-t.[3],
    arn.[3], asaf.[3], **BELL., bism.,** caps.,
    caust., chin.[3], clem., cocc.[3], coff.[3, 6],
    con., dig., dulc.[3], ferr-p.[3], fl-ac.[3],
    glon.[3], hyos.[3, 6], iod., kali-c., kali-n.,
    lach.[3], lyc., mag-c., mez.[3], **nit-ac.,**
    nux-v., olnd.[3], par.[3, 6], petr., plat.[3],
    rhod.[3], sars., senec.[3], **sep.,** sil., spig.[3],
    stann., stict.[3, 6], stront-c., **SULPH.,**
    teucr.[3], verb., viol-t.[3]

WEAKNESS, enervation
FAIBLESSE, asthénie
SCHWÄCHE

abies-c., abies-n., abrot., absin.,
acet-ac., achy.[14], **acon.,** acon-c.[11],
acon-f.[11], adlu.[14], adox.[11],
adren.[7, 8, 12], aesc., aesc-g.[2, 11],
aeth., aether[11], agar., agar-cpn.[11],
agar-em.[11], agar-pa.[11], **agar-ph.**[11],
agar-pr.[11], agar-st.[11], agav-t.[14], **agn.,**
ail., alco.[11], **alet.**[1', 2, 6, 8, 12], alf.[7, 8],
all-c., all-s., **aloe,** alst.[8, 12], alst-s.[11],
alum., alum-p.[1'], alum-sil.[1'], alumn.,
AM-C., am-caust.[11], am-m., **ambr.,**
aml-ns.[2, 11], ammc.[4, 11], amor-r.[14],
amph.[11], amyg.[11], **ANAC., anag.**[2],
anan.[2], **ang.**[2, 3, 4, 7, 11, 16], anil.[11],
ant-ar.[2, 6, 11], **ant-c.,** ant-m.[2, 11],
ant-o.[11], **ANT-T.,** anth.[11], anthraci.,
anthraco.[2, 11], **antip.**[8], aphis[4, 11],
APIS, apoc., apoc-a.[11], apom.[11],
aq-m.[14], aq-pet.[11], aral.[11], **aran.,**
aran-sc.[11, 12], arg-cy.[11], **ARG-M.,**
arg-n., arist-cl.[10], **ARN., ARS.,** ars-h.,
ARS-I., ars-m., ars-s-f., ars-s-r.[2],
arum-d.[2, 11], arum-i.[11], arum-m.,
arum-t., asaf., asar., asc-t., asim.[11],
aspar.[2], astac.[11], aster., atha.[4, 11],
atra-r.[14], atro.[11], **aur.,** aur-ar.[1'],
aur-fu.[4, 11], **aur-m.**[2, 8, 11], aur-m-n.[11],
aur-s.[1'], **aven.**[7, 8, 12], **bals-p.**[8], **BAPT.,**
bar-a.[6, 11], **BAR-C.,** bar-i.[1'], **bar-m.,**
bart.[11], bell., bell-p.[8, 9, 14], ben.,
ben-n.[11], **benz-ac.,** berb., berbin.[11],
beryl.[10], **bism., bol-la.,** bol-s.[11], bor.,
both.[11], bov., brach., **BROM.,**
bruc.[4], brucin.[11], **bry.,** bufo,
buth-a.[9, 10, 14], buni-o.[14], **cact.,**
cadm-met.[10, 14], cadm-s.[6, 7], cain.,
caj.[11], calad., **CALC.,** calc-ar.[1'],
calc-caust.[6, 11], calc-hp.[8], **CALC-I.**[1, 1'],
calc-m.[11], **calc-p.,** calc-s., calc-sil.[1'],
camph., cann-i., cann-s., **canth.,**
caps., **CARB-AC., carb-an., carb-v.,**
carbn-chl.[11], carbn-h., carbn-o.[11],
carbn-s., card-m., **carl.**[11, 12], casc.[4],
cass.[11], cast.[6, 11], cast-v., **caul.,**
caust., cedr., cench.[1', 11], cent.[11],
cere-b.[11], cerv.[11], **cham., CHEL.,**
chelo.[12], **chim., CHIN.,** chin-ar.,
CHIN-S., chion., chlf., chlol.,

chloram.[14], chlorpr.[14], chr-ac.[2, 11],
cic., cich.[11], cimic., cimx., **cina,**
chinch.[11], cinnb., cinnm.[2], cist.[12],
cit-l.[2, 11], cit-v.[11], **clem.,** cob.,
cob-n.[9, 10, 14], coc-c.,
COCA[2, 6, 8, 11, 12], **cocc.,** coch.[2],
cod.[11], **coff., COLCH.,** colchin.[11, 12],
coll.[11], coloc., colocin.[11, 12], com.,
CON., conin.[11,] conin-br.[12], conv.[7],
cop., cor-r.[6], corn.[2, 11], cortico.[9],
cot.[11], crat.[6, 8], croc., **crot-c., crot-h.,**
crot-t., cub., culx.[1'], **cupr.,**
cupr-a.[4, 11], **cupr-ar.,** cupr-s., cur.,
cycl., cyn-d.[14], cyt-l.[10, 11], **daph.**[4, 11],
der.[11], dicha.[10, 14], **DIG., digin.**[11],
digox.[11], dios., dip.[8], diph.[8], dirc.[11, 12],
dor., **dros.,** dubo-m.[11], **dulc.,**
echi.[3, 6, 8], elat., equis.[11], erig.[11],
ery-a.[11], ery-m.[12], eryt-j.[11], eucal.[2, 11],
eug., eup-per., eup-pur., euph.,
euph-a.[12], euph-c.[11], euph-hy.[11],
euph-ip.[11], euphr., eupi.[11], fago.,
fagu.[11], **FERR.,** ferr-ar., ferr-cit.[8],
FERR-I., FERR-M., ferr-ma.[4, 11],
ferr-p., fic.[10], fil.[12], **fl-ac.,** flor-p.[14],
form., frag.[11], franz.[11, 12], gad.[11],
gal-ac.[11, 12], galeg.[12], galin.[14],
gamb.[2], gast.[11, 12], **GELS.,** gent-l.,
gent-q.[12], get.[11], gink-b.[14],
gins.[4, 6, 11, 12], glon., goss., gran.,
GRAPH., grat., guaj., guan.[11],
guar.[2], guare., haem.[6], hall[11], **ham.,**
hed.[14], hedeo.[11], **hell.,** hell-o.[11],
helon., **HEP.,** hera.[11, 12], hip-ac.[14],
hipp., hir.[14], hist.[9, 14], home.[11],
hydr., hydr-ac., hydrc.[11], **HYOS.,**
hyosin.[11], **hyper.,** hura, iber.[2, 11, 14],
ign., ind., indg., **IOD., ip., irid.**[8, 12],
iris, jab., jal.[11], jasm.[11], jatr.,
jug-c.[11], jug-r., juni.[11], **KALI-AR.,**
kali-bi., kali-br., **KALI-C.,** kali-chl.,
kali-cy.[11], **KALI-FCY., kali-i.,**
kali-m.[1'], kali-n., kali-ox.[11],
KALI-P., kali-perm.[11], kali-s.,
kali-sil.[1'], kali-t.[11], **KALM.,** kino[11],
kiss.[11], kou.[11], kreos., kres.[10, 13, 14],
lac-ac., **lac-c., lac-d.**[1', 2, 7], **LACH.,**
lachn., lact.[4, 11], lam.[4], lapa.[11],
lat-k.[11], lat-m.[9, 14], **LAUR., LEC.,**
led., lepi., lept., lil-s.[11], lil-t., lim.[11],
lina.[11], linu-c.[11], lipp.[11], lith-c.[8],

lith-m.[8], lob., lob-c.[11, 12], lob-p.[8],
lob-s., **lol.**[11], luf-op.[10, 14], **lyc.,**
lycps., lyss., m-arct.[4], m-aust.[4],
marco.[11], mag-c., mag-f.[10, 14],
mag-m., **mag-p.**[2, 8], mag-s., manc.,
mand.[10, 11, 14], mang.[1', 3, 4, 6],
mang-o.[11], **MED.,** mela.[11], meli.,
menis.[11], meny., meph., **MERC.,**
merc-br.[11], **MERC-C., MERC-CY.,**
merc-d.[11], merc-i-f., merc-i-r.,
merc-meth.[11], merc-ns.[11],
merc-sul.[2, 11], merl.[2, 11], methys.[14],
mez., mill., mit.[11], moly-met.[14],
mom-b.[11], morph., mosch., murx.,
MUR-AC., mygal., **myric.**[2, 11],
nabal.[11], naja, napht.[11], narcin.[11],
narz.[11], nat-ar., **nat-c.,** nat-f.[9],
NAT-HCHLS., nat-lac.[11], **NAT-M.,**
nat-n., **NAT-P., NAT-S., nat-sal.**[8, 12],
nat-sil.[1'], nat-sula.[11], nep.[10, 13, 14],
nicc., nicot.[11], nid.[14], **NIT-AC.,**
nit-m-ac.[11], nit-s-d.[4, 11], nitro-o.[11],
nuph., **nux-m., nux-v.,** oena.,
okou.[14], ol-an., **ol-j., OLND.,**
onos.[12], **op.,** opun-v.[11], orch.[12],
orig.[11], orni.[11], osm., ost.[11],
ox-ac., oxyg.[11], paeon., pall.,
palo.[14], pana.[11], par., parathyr.[14],
parth.[12], paull.[11], ped., penic.[13, 14],
perh.[14], **petr., PH-AC.,** phal.[11],
phel., **PHOS., phys., phyt., PIC-AC.,**
pilo.[11], pimp.[11], pip-m.[11], pitu.[9],
pix.[11], plan., **plat., PLB.,** plb-chr.[11],
plect.[11], plumbg.[11], podo., polyg-h.,
polyp-p.[11], prun-p.[11], **PSOR.,** ptel.[1],
(non: petl.), **puls.,** puls-n.[11],
pyrog.[3, 6], pyrus[11], ran-a.[4], **RAN-B.,**
ran-s., **raph.,** rat., rham-f.[11], rheum,
rhod., rhus-g.[11, 12], **RHUS-T.,**
rhus-v.[2, 11], ric.[11], **rob.**[2, 11], **rumx.,**
rumx-a.[11], ruta, **sabad.,** sabin.[11],
salin.[11], samb., samb-c.[11], **sang.,**
sanic., santin.[11], sapin.[11],
sarcol-ac.[8, 9, 14], saroth.[14], sarr.,
sars., scor.[11], scorph-n.[11], scut.[11, 12],
SEC., SEL., senec., **seneg.,**
senn.[11, 12], **SEP.,** sieg.[10], **SIL.,**
silphu.[12], sin-n., sium[11], sol-m.[11],
sol-n., sol-t.[11], sol-t-ae., solid.[3, 8],
solin.[11], sphing.[11], spig., spira.[11],
spirae.[11], **spong., SQUIL., STANN.,**

STAPH., stict., still., stram.,
stront-c., stroph-h.[8], stry., stry-p.[7],
SUL-AC., sul-h.[11], sul-i., sulfa.[9, 14],
sulfon.[8], sulfonam.[14], **SULPH.,**
sumb., syph., **TAB.,** tanac.[8, 11],
tang.[11], tann-ac.[11], tarax.,
TARENT., tarent-c.[6], tart-ac.[11],
tax.[4, 11], **tell., TER.,** tere-ch.[14],
teucr., thal.[11], thea[8, 11], **ther.,**
thiop.[14], **thuj.,** thymol.[9, 14], thyr.[3],
til., tox-th.[11], trach.[11], tril., trom.,
TUB., tub-r.[13, 14], tus-p.[11], upa.[11],
uran.[6], uran-n.[6-8, 11], urea[10], ust.,
uva[2], v-a-b.[13, 14], vac.[11], valer.,
ven-m.[14], **VERAT.,** verat-v., verb.,
verin.[11], vesp., vib.[3, 6], vip-a.[14],
vichy[11], vinc., viol-o.[2], viol-t., vip.,
visc.[9], voes.[11], wies.[11], wildb.[11],
wye.[11, 12], x-ray[14], xan., **zinc.,**
zinc-ar.[8], zinc-m.[11], zinc-o.[4, 12],
zinc-p.[1'], **zinc-pic.**[8, 12], zinc-s.[11],
zing., ziz.[11]

convalescence/Rekonvaleszenz
flabby feeling/mollesse, sensation/
  Erschlaffung, Gefühl
heaviness/lourdeur/Schweregefühl
lassitude/Mattigkeit
lie down/s'étendre/sich hinzulegen
relaxation/relâchement/
  Erschlaffung
weariness/fatigue/Müdigkeit

daytime
journée, pendant la
tagsüber

    agar., **am-c.,** cench.[1'], cob-n.[9],
    corn., graph., iod., indg., lyc.,
    lyss.[2], mag-c., mosch., nat-ar.,
    nat-c., **nat-m.,** nit-ac., op., ph-ac.,
    phos., phys., pip-m., plan., **stann.,**
    sulph., tarent., ter., uran-n.[2]

heat of day, during
chaleur du jour, pendant la
Tageshitze, in der
    sel.

    w.-heat/f.-chaleur/Sch.-Hitze

walking am.
marcher am.
Gehen am.
    ph-ac.

*w.-walking/f.-marcher/Sch.-
    Gehen*

morning/matin/morgens
    acon-l.[11], agar., alum.[4], am-c.,
    am-m., **ambr.**, amph.[11], ant-c.,
    ant-s-aur., apoc., aran.[6], **arg-m.,
    ARS., ars-i.,** ars-s-f.[1'], asc-t.,
    atra-r.[14], atro., aur., aur-ar.[1'],
    aur-i.[1'], **bell.**, bism.[6], bor., bruc.[4],
    bry., bufo, caj.[11], **calc.,** calc-i.[1'],
    calc-s., canth.[4], caps., carb-an.,
    carb-v., carbn-s., celt.[11], cham.,
    chel., chin-s., cimic., cinnb.,
    clem., coc-c., colch., **con.,** corn.[11],
    croc., crot-h., cycl., dig., digin.[11],
    dios., dros., erig., euphr., eupi.,
    fago., flor-p.[14], form., **gels.,**
    gnaph., **graph.,** ham., hyper.,
    hom.[7], **iod.,** jal., kali-bi., kali-c.,
    kali-m.[1'], kali-n., kali-p., lac-c.,
    lac-ac., **LACH.,** lact.[4], levo.[14],
    LYC., mag-c., mag-m., meli.,
    merc., merc-c., merl.[11], morph.,
    mur-ac., naja, **nat-ar., nat-c.,
    nat-m., nat-p., nat-s.,** nat-sil.[1'],
    nit-ac., nux-v., op., osm., ox-ac.,
    ped., perh.[14], **petr., PH-AC.,
    phos.,** pic-ac., plat., prun.,
    pulm-a.[13], **puls.,** ran-b., **rhus-v.,**
    rob., ruta, sabad., sang., **SEP.,
    sil., spig.,** stach.[11], **stann., staph.,
    stront-c.,** stry.[11], sul-ac.[16], **sulph.,**
    sumb., syph., tab., ther., thuj.,
    til., valer., **verat.,** viol-t., zinc.,
    zinc-p.[1']

bed, in
lit, au
Bett, im
    ambr., arn., **carb-v.,** caust.,
    chin., cinch.[11], **con.,** ham.[12],
    hell., hep., hom.[7], lach., mag-c.,
    nat-m., phos., **PULS., sil.,
    staph.,** stront-c.

while sitting up in
en se dressant sur son séant
beim Aufsitzen im
    nat-m.

fasting
jeûnant, en
Fasten, beim
    con.

ideas at night, after copious
    flow of
pensées diverses, après une nuit
    surchargée de
Gedankenflucht, nach nächtlicher
    tab.

lying
couché, étant
Liegen, im
    PULS.

w.-lying/f.-couché/Sch.-Liegen

rising, on
se levant, en
Aufstehen, beim
    alum., asc-t., aur-m-n., bov.,
    BRY., calc-caust.[11], carbn.[11],
    caust., chin., cina, colch.,
    corn., crot-t., dig., dios.,
    dulc., eupi., **ferr.,** ham., hep.,
    ign., iris, lac-ac., **LACH.,**
    lyc., mez., nat-m.[4, 16], nux-v.,
    op., petr., **PH-AC.,** phos.,
    plb., puls.[4], puls-n., rhus-v.,
    scut.[11], **sep., sil., stann.,**
    sulph., thuj., ust.

am.
    acon., carb-v., caust., con.,
    kali-c., mag-c., nat-c.,
    nat-m., phos., **puls.**

after
après s'être levé
nach dem
    alumn., **arg-m., arg-n.,** bry.,
    carb-an., hep., kali-n., **lach.,
    nit-ac., nux-v.,** peti.[11],
    PH-AC., rhod., til.

waking, on
réveil, au
Erwachen, beim
    acon., agar., alum., alum-p.[1'],
am-c.[6], ambr., ant-c., **arg-m.,**
arn.[4], aur., bell.[4], berb., **bry.,**
calc., calc-sil.[1'], cann-s.,
carb-an., carb-v., cast.,
cast-v.[11], cham., chel., chin.,
clem., coca, colch., coloc., con.,
corn., crot-t., cycl., dros. **dulc.,**
euph.[4], fago., gels., gnaph.,
graph., grat., hep., hyper., ign.,
iod.[4], jab., kali-c., kali-sil.[1'],
lach., lyc., mag-c., mag-s.[4],
mang.[16], nat-m., **nux-v.**[1], **phos.,**
pic-ac., plb.[4], podo., rhus-t.,
sabad., **sang., sep., sil., spig.,**
staph., stram., **syph.**[1', 7], tab.,
ter., thuj.[4], verat., xan., zinc.

5 h[11]
    napht.

6 h
    pic-ac.

6.30 h
    ham.

7 h
    cham., elat., graph.

8 h
    dios., phys.

8.30
    fago.

10 h, until/jusqu'à/bis
    nit-ac.

forenoon
matinée
vormittags
    abrot.[11], acon., alum., am-c.,
ambr., ang., ant-t., bart.[11], bruc.[4],
BRY., calc.[16], carb-an., carb-v.,
corn., fago., fl-ac., graph., grat.,
hell., indg., kali-cy., kali-n., lach.,

lyc., mag-m., mang., nat-m.,
nux-m., ox-ac., **ph-ac.,** phel.,
phys., **plat.,** ptel., ran-b., sabad.,
sars., scroph-n.[11], sep., staph.[3],
tab., tarent.

agg.[8]
    acal., bar-m., bry., calc., con.,
corn., lac-c., lach., lyc., **nat-m.,**
nit-ac., phos., psor., sep., stann.,
sulph., tub.

9 h
    chin-s., cocc., merl., nat-s.,
ox-ac., ped., perh.[14], peti.,
phys., ptel., sep.

    am.
      tarent.

9–11 h
    tarent.

10 h
    aq-mar.[14], bor.[6], cast., cench.[1'],
equis., gels., lycps., merc-d.,
phys.

    am.
      gels.

10–12 h
    calc-s.

11 h
    arg-m., **lach.**[2], nat-c.[6], phos.[3, 11],
ptel., sep.[3], **sulph.,** thuj., zinc.

noon
midi
mittags
    bov., carb-v., caust., clem., con.,
cycl., fago., helon., hyper.,
nat-m., nit-ac., ox-ac.[11], ph-ac.[4],
phos., phys.[11], phyt., ptel., sil.,
sulph., teucr., thuj., zinc.[4]

12.30 h
    gels., sol-t-ae.

15 h, until/jus'à/bis
    hyos.

18 h, until/jusqu'à/bis
phyt.[11], ptel.

am.
    hyper.

sleep, after[11]
sommeil, après le
Schlaf, nach dem
    bor., con., cycl., nat-m.

    w.-afternoon-sleep/f.-après-midi-
    sommeil/Sch.-nachmittags-
    Schlaf

afternoon
après-midi
nachmittags
    acon., aeth., **alet.**, am-c., amyg.,
    anac., apis, aq-pet.[11], arg-n., aur.,
    bar-c.[16], bell., bor.[16], brom., **bry.**,
    cast., carb-an.[16], carbn.[11], cinch.,
    coc-c., coca, colch.[14], con.[16],
    coloc., com., digin.[11], erig., fago.,
    ferr., **gels.**, glon., ham., helon.,
    hydr-ac., hyos., ign., iod.[16], iris,
    kali-c.[2, 4], kali-n.[4, 16], lyc., lycps.,
    mag-c., merl., mez., mur-ac.,
    nat-c.[4], nat-m., nat-p., nat-s.,
    nit-ac., nux-v., ol-an.[4], phys.,
    phyt., plb.[4], ptel., ran-b.[4], rhus-t.,
    ruta, sang., sep.[16], **sil.**, spirae.[11],
    staph., stram., stry., **SULPH.**,
    thuj., zinc., zing.

13 h
    astac.[11], ferr-p., phys., pic-ac.,
    verat-v.

13.30 h
    lyc.

14 h
    chel., gels., nux-v., sulph.

14–15 h
    guan.[11], plb-chr.[11], sulph.

14–16 h
    ign.

15 h
    ham., lyss.[2], mag-c., nat-s.,
    nep.[13, 14]

15–16 h[14]: reser.

16 h
    caust., gad.[11], hydr., iris, lyc.,
    mang., merc-i-f., phys.

17 h
    coff., coloc., **lac-d.**[2], lyc., merc.[16]

17 h, until/jusqu'à/bis
    tarent.

17–23 h[14]: perh.

17.30 h
    stram.

18 h[16]: merc.

18 h, until/jusqu'à/bis
    merc.

sleep, after
sommeil, après le
Schlaf, nach dem
    bor.[16], chin-s., ferr., gels.,
    kali-c.[16], nat-m.[16]

    w.-noon-sleep/f.-midi-sommeil/
    Sch.-mittags-Schlaf

walking, while
marchant, en
Gehen, beim
    caust.[16], lyc., mag-c., pic-ac.,
    ran-b.

    am.[11]
        nat-s.

    after/après la marche/nach dem
        ery-a., euph., hyper.

evening
soir
abends
    acon., aloe, alum.[4], **am-c.**,
    am-m.[16], aphis[4, 11], apis, apoc.,

ars., asaf., asar.[4, 16], bapt.,
bell.[4, 16], berb., bor., bov.,
brom., bruc.[4], bry., calc.,
calc-p., **calc-s.**, carb-v., carl.,
caust., chin.[4], clem., cob., coc-c.,
coca, coloc., colocin.[11], con.,
croc., cycl., dios., dirc., erig.[11],
ery-m.[11], euphr., eupi., fago.,
ferr., ferr-ar.[1'], form., **graph.**,
grat., haem., helon., hep., hydr.,
hydr-ac., **ign.**, indg., iris, itu[11],
jac., jac-c.[11], **kali-bi.**, kali-c.,
kali-m.[1'], kali-n.[16], kali-sil.[1'],
kalm., **lach.**, laur.[4], lim.[11], lob.,
lyc., lycps., mag-c., merc.,
merl., mez., mur-ac., murx.,
naja, **NAT-M.**, nat-n., nicc.[2],
nit-ac., nux-v., ox-ac., pall.,
petr., phos., plat., plb., psor.,
puls-n., rat.[4], rhus-g., rhus-t.,
rumx., ruta, senec., **sep.**, sil.,
spig.[4], stront-c., sulfonam.[14],
sulph., sumb., tab., **tart-ac.**[11],
thuj., tub.[1'], upa., valer., zinc.,
zinc-p.[1']

18 h
   helon., lyc.

19 h
   gins., mag-c., nat-m., phys.,
   pic-ac., sep., verat-v.

20 h
   astac.[11], bar-c., mang., pana.[11],
   phys., sep.

20.30 h
   pip-m.

21 h
   dirc., mag-s., op., phys., pic-ac.

   am.
   phos.

21.30 h
   lyc., sep.

   am.
      asc-t., calc-s., colch., nit-ac.

in open air[11]
en plein air
im Freien
   chel., **CON.**, grat., naja,
   nat-m., pic-ac., sabad.

bed, in
lit, au
Bett, im
   lyc.

eating, after
mangé, après avoir
Essen, nach dem
   bov.[11], **croc.**

   *w.-supper/f.-dîner/Sch.-Abend-
   essen*

night
nuit
nachts
   acon-l.[11], am-c.[4], ambr., ant-c.,
   anthraci., anthroco.[11], calc.,
   canth., carb-an., carb-v., chel.,
   coca, crot-t.[4], ferr-i., gnaph.,
   hell., hyper., kreos., mur-ac.[11, 16],
   naja, nat-m., nux-v., rhus-t.,
   sep.[16], **sil.**, sulph., tab., thuj.

22 h
   elat., fago., phys.

23 h
   nat-m.

midnight
minuit
Mitternacht
   ambr., op., **rhus-t.**

after/après/nach
   nat-m., rhus-t.

2 h[16]: sep.

3 h
   nat-m., **sec.**[2], zing.[11]

4 h
   sulph.

abortion, after[11]
avortement, après l'
Fehlgeburt, nach
   ruta

from w.[8]
par f.
infolge von Sch.
   alet., caul., chin., chin-s., **helon.,**
   sec., **sep.**[6], sil.[6]

acute diseases, with[3]
maladies aiguës, avec
akuten Krankheiten, bei
   aeth., ail.[3, 7], ant-t., apis, ars.,
   calc-p.[7], gels., guar.[7], kali-m.[1'],
   merc-cy., mur-ac., psor.[7], verat.

w.–sudden/f.–subite/Schw.–
*   plötzliche*

Addison's disease, in[2]
maladie bronzée, dans la
Addison' Syndrom, bei
   calc., iod.

air, in open
air, en plein
Freien, im
   am-c., am-m., ambr., **atro.**[11],
   bry., calc., chin., clem., coff.,
   coloc., con., ferr., grat., kali-c.,
   mag-c., merc., merc-c.[11], mur-ac.,
   nux-v., **plat.,** sang., **spig.,** verat.

am.
   chel., colch., **CON.,** croc., gels.,
   grat., hed.[10, 14], naja, nat-m.,
   pic-ac., sabad.

w.-evening-am./f.-soir-am./Sch.-
*   abends-am.*

for want of
par manque d'
aus Mangel an frischer Luft
   meli.

fresh air am.
grand air am.
frische Luft am.
   calc.

albuminuria, in[2]
albuminurie, dans l'
Albuminurie, bei
   ars., calc-ar., dig., iod., merc-c.,
   nat-c., ter.

alcoholic drinks am.
spiritueux am.
alkolische Getränke am.
   canth., nit-s-d.[11], thea[11]

alternating with sensation of
   strength[4]
alternant avec sensation de puissance, de force
abwechselnd mit Kraftgefühl
   ars., chin., colch.[14]

trembling/tremblement/Zittern
   ferr., plb.[7]

anaemia, in[2]
anémie, par
Anämie, durch
   chin., **FERR.**[2, 3, 6], **KALI-C.,** nat-c.,
   nat-m.[2, 6], **PHOS.**

anaemia/anémie/Anämie

anger, after
colère, après
Zorn, nach
   mur-ac.[6], zinc.

anxiety, with[16]
anxiété, avec
Angst, mit
   am-c., aur., calc., caust., rhus-t.

appetite, w. increases with[3]
appétit augmenté avec
Appetit, Schw. wächst mit dem
   ail.

apoplexy, from[7]
apoplexie, à la suite de
Apoplexie, infolge von
   bar-c.

apoplexy/apoplexie/Apoplexie

ascending stairs, from
monter l'escalier, par
Treppensteigen, durch
 alum-sil.[1'], **anac.,** ars., ars-i.,
 ars-s-f.[1'], bar-m.[1'], blatta-a.[11],
 CALC., calc-p., calc-sil.[1'],
 carbn-s.[1'], coff., colch., croc.[7],
 fago., **IOD.,** kali-ar.[1'], **lyc.,** m-arct.[4],
 mag-c.[16], nat-m., nat-n.[11], nux-v.[4],
 ox-ac., ph-ac., phys., pic-ac., puls.,
 sarcol-ac.[8], spig., **stann.,** sulph.,
 zinc-a.[11]

ascites, from[15]
ascite, par
Aszites, durch
 LYC.

bed, on going to
s'endormir, avant de
Einschlafen, vor dem
 arn., cinnb., lycps., mur-ac., rumx.,
 ter.

beer, after
bière, après avoir bu de la
Bier, nach
 coc-c.

 am.
  thea

breakfast time, about
petit déjeuner, au moment du
Frühstückszeit, um die
 sep.

 after/après le/nach dem Frühstück
 arg-n., brom., carb-v., cham.[16],
 con.[16], dig., lach., nux-v.,
 ph-ac., sil., still.[11], thea, verat.

 am.
  calc., con., nat-m., nux-v.,
  staph.

businessman, worn out[11]
homme d'aiffaires épuisé
Geschäftsmann, erschöpfter
 clem., lyc.

 Vol. I: *business–man/affaires–*
  hommes/Geschäften–
  Geschäftsmann

children, in
enfants, chez les
Kindern, bei
 bar-c., bell., calc., carb-v.[12], cham.[4],
 cina[4], kali-c.[4], lach., **lyc.,** nux-v.,
 sil., **sulph.**

chill, before
frissons, avant les
Fieberfrost, vor
 ars., chin., nat-m., thuj.

 during/pendant les/im
  agar.[2], aran., ars., asar.[16], astac.[2],
  chin., coc-c., ip., lach., **nat-m.,**
  petr.[16], **phos.,** psor.

 after[2]/après les/nach
  apis, sulph.[16]

chilliness, with[16]
frissonnement, avec
Frösteln, mit
 sep.

climacteric period, during[7]
ménopause, pendant la
Klimakterium, im
 CHIN.[2, 3, 6, 7], chin-ar.[6], cocc.,
 con.[6, 7], crot-h.[2, 7], dig.[8], helon.[2, 3, 6, 8],
 kali-p.[2, 7], lach.[3, 6, 8], magn-gl.,
 phos.[3, 6], sabin.[1'], sep.[3, 6, 8], sul-ac.,
 tab.[3, 6]

cloudy, damp weather, in
nuageux, par temps
wolkigem, feuchtem Wetter, bei
 sang.

coffee am.[11]
café am.
Kaffee am.
 eug.

 from odor of
 par odeur de
 durch Kaffeegeruch
 sul-ac.

coition, after
coït, après le
Koitus, nach
   agar., ambr.[6], berb., **CALC.,**
   carb-an.[4], chin., clem., **con., dig.,**
   graph., kali-c., kali-p., lil-t., lyc.,
   mosch., nat-c.[8], **nat-m.,** nit-ac.,
   nuph.[2], petr., **ph-ac., phos.,** plat.[6],
   SEL., sep., sil., staph., tarent.,
   tax.[11], vichy[11], **ziz.**[2]

cold, after exposure to[11]
refroidissement, après
Abkühlung, nach
   ars.

cold weather, in
froid, par temps
kaltes Wetter, durch
   apis, lach.

coldness, during
froid, pendant le
Kälte, bei
     aeth., apis, atha.[11], con., guare.,
     nat-m., thuj.

   from[2]/par/durch
     ars., CARB-V., VERAT.

colic with[3]
colique avec
Kolik mit
   cast., tab.

company, in[16]
société, en
Gesellschaft, in
   sep.

conversation, from[16]
conversation, par
Unterhaltung, durch
   sil.

convulsions, after
convulsions, après
Konvulsionen, nach
     acon., agar.[16], **alm-ns.**[2], ars.,
     art-v.[2], carbn.[11], **cupr.**[2], **ip.**[2],
     merc-c., **oena.**[2], sec., stram.[16],
     stry., sulph.[16], tab.

epileptic/épileptiques/epilepti-
schen
   aster.[2], camph., **plb.**[2], **sulph.**[2]

hysterical/hsystériques/hysteri-
schen
   ars.

coryza, during[16]
coryza, pendant le
Schnupfen, beim
   calc., graph.

cough, after[3]
toux, après la
Husten, nach
   cor-r., verat.

   from[16]/par/durch
   ars.

dampness, from exposure to
humidité, par
Naßwerden, durch
   ars.

death, as of approaching
mort, comme à l'approche de la
Sterben, wie zum
   ars., con.[4], dig.[4], mag-m[4]., nat-c.[4],
   olnd., op.[4], sec.[4], spig.[4], **vinc.**[4, 7]

dentition, in[2]
dentition, pendant la
Zahnen, beim
   calc., calc-p., **ip.**

descending steps
descendant l'escalier
Treppenherabgehen, beim
   stann.

diabetes mellitus, in[2]
diabète sucré, par
Diabetes mellitus, durch
   arg-m., ars., lac-ac.

diarrhoea, from
diarrhée, par
Diarrhoe, durch
   acet-ac.[7], **alum.,** alum-p.[1'], **alumn.**[2],

ambr., ant-c.², ant-t.²⁶, **apis,
ARS.,** bar-m.², **bor.,** both., bry.,
carb-v., **CHIN.,** chin-ar.¹′, coloc.,
con., **corn.²,** crot-t.², **dulc.,**
euph-a.², **ferr.,** gast.¹¹, gnaph.,
graph., hura, hydr., hyos.¹⁶,
iod., ip., iris, kali-c., kali-chl.,
kali-m.², kali-p.², lil-t., mag-c.,
merc., merc-cy., **NAT-S.,
NIT-AC.,** nuph.², **NUX-M.²,**
nux-v., **OLND.,** op., ox-ac., petr.,
PHOS., phyt., **PIC-AC., PODO.,**
ric.¹¹, **rhus-t.¹⁴,** sec., senec., sep.,
**SIL., sul-ac., tab., tarent.,
tart-ac.², VERAT., zinc.**

does not weaken³′
n'affaiblit pas
schwächt nicht
ph-ac.

dinner, before
déjeuner, avant le
Mittagessen, vor dem
nat-m., sabin.¹¹, sil.¹⁶, thuj.

during/pendant le/beim
am-c.¹⁶, bov., nat-ar.¹¹, nat-s.,
teucr.

after/après le/nach dem
alum.¹⁶, am-c., am-m., ant-c., ars.,
ars-h.², asar., bapt., bov., cain.,
calc., carb-v., cast., chel., **chin.,**
cob., cycl., dig., euph-a.¹¹, graph.,
grat., ign., indg., iod., **lach.²,** lyc.,
mag-c., mur-ac.¹⁶, nat-m., nat-p.,
nit-ac.¹⁶, ol-an., ox-ac., perh.¹⁴,
phel., **ph-ac.,** phos., plat., plect.,
sars., sep.¹⁶, **sil.,** squil., **sulph.,
thuj.,** zinc.

am.
ambr., sars.¹⁶

diphtheria, in²
diphtérie, dans la
Diphtherie, bei
ail., alum-sil., apis, brom., **canth.,
chin-ar., crot-h.,** diph.⁸, **ign.;
kali-bi., kali-perm.,** lac-c., **LACH.,
MERC-CY., merc-i-f.,** mur-ac.,

nat-ar., nux-v., **PHYT.,** sal-ac., sec.,
sulph.

dipsomania, in²
dipsomanie, dans la
Trunksucht, bei
ars., carbn.-s.¹′⁷, **kali-br., nat-s.²¹²,**
phos., ran-b.⁷, **sel.**

drawing and jerking in limbs, after
tiraillantes et secousses dans ses
membres, après douleurs
Ziehen und Rucken in den Gliedern,
nach
sulph.

dream, after a
rêve, après un
Traum, nach einem
calc-s., op., teucr.

drinking, after¹⁶
bu, après avoir
Trinken, nach dem
nat-m.

dropsy, in²
hydropisie, dans l'
Wassersucht, bei
APIS, ars., eup-pur, hell., seneg.

eating, before
manger, avant
Essen, vor dem
cinnb.

while/en mangeant/beim
am-c.², bufo, mag-c., ptel., sulph.⁴

after/après avoir mangé/nach dem
act-sp., alum.³, **anac., ant-c.³¹⁶,
ARS.,** ars-s-f.¹′, asar.³, bar-a.¹¹,
BAR-C., bar-s.¹′, brom., calc.³⁶,
calc-p., cann-s., carb-an., **chin.,**
cina³, clem., **con., croc.,** crot-c.,
cycl., dig., ferr.⁶, ferr-ma., hep.,
hyper., kali-c., kali-sil.¹′, lach.³⁴,
lyc.¹, mag-c., mag-m.³, meph.,
merc-c., mur-ac., **nat-c.³⁶,**
nat-m., **nit-ac.³,** nux-m.³, nux-v.,
ox-ac.², **PH-AC.,** phos., rhod.,

rhus-t., ruta, sang., sars.², sel.,
sep.⁶, ¹⁶, **sil., staph.,** sul-ac.,
sulph., tell., teucr., thea, thuj.,
uran-n.³

am.
   aster., **hep.², IOD.²,** nat-c.¹⁶, petr.,
   sapin.¹¹, sil.

emissions, after
pertes séminales, après
Samenverlusten, nach
   acet-ac., agar., aur., **bar-c., calad.²,**
   calc., calc-p.⁸, canth., carb-an.,
   carl., **chin.,** chin-b.², **cob.³, ⁶, ⁸,**
   coff.², con., cupr., **cypr.²,** dam.⁸,
   dig., **dios.³, ⁶, ⁸,** ery-a.⁸, ferr.³,
   form.⁸, **gels.,** ham.², **hydr.,** iod.,
   KALI-BR.², kali-c., lach.³, ⁴, **LYC.,**
   med.², ⁸, naja, **nat-m.,** nat-p., **nuph.²,**
   NUX-V., op.², **PH-AC., PHOS.,**
   pic-ac., plb., puls., **sabad.³,** sars.,
   sel., sep., SIL., stann., STAPH.,
   sul-ac.³, **sulph.², ⁸,** ust., zinc.⁸

erections, from
érections, par
Erektionen, durch
   aur., aur-m.¹¹, carbn-s.

excess, after any
excès, par quelque
Exzeß, durch irgendeinen
   agar.ˣ, **anac.⁸, calc-p.⁸, carb-v.⁸,**
   caust.ˣ, **chin.⁸,** chin-ar.⁸, corn-f.⁸,
   cur.ˣ, gins.⁸, kali-c.⁸, nat-m.⁸,
   ph-ac.⁸, phos.⁸, plb., sel.⁸, stroph-h.⁸

excessive³
übermäßige
   ars., bapt., chin., ferr., **ferr-pic.⁷,**
   gels., ph-ac., tab.

excitement, after
excitation, après
Erregung, nach
   con., phos.⁶, stry., thea

exertion, from⁷
exercises physiques, par
Anstrengung, durch
   acon., **alum-p.¹',** ambr., **arn.,**

ars-s-f.¹', aur-ar.¹', aur-m.¹', bry.,
calc., chin., cocc., coff.,
ferr-ar.¹', ferr-i.¹', kali-ar.¹',
kalm.¹¹, macro.¹¹, mag-c., merc.,
nit-m-ac.¹¹, nit-s-d.¹¹, rhod.¹',
rhus-t.¹', ⁷, sil., sul-i.¹', verat.

from slight
par les moindres
durch die geringste
   acon., **agar.,** ail., apis, **ARS.,**
   ars-i., ars-s-f.¹', alum., **am-c.,**
   anac., bapt., berb., **BRY.,**
   CALC., calc-sil.¹', **carb-v.,**
   carbn-s.¹', cham., clem., **cocc.,**
   colch., CON., CROT-H., dor.,
   ferr., ferr-i., **gels.,** ham.⁷, ign.,
   jatr., kali-c., kali-n., kalm.,
   lac-d.¹', **LACH., lyc., mag-m.,**
   merc., merc-c., nat-ar., NAT-C.,
   nat-m., nat-p., nux-m., petr.,
   PH-AC., PHOS., PIC-AC., plb.,
   psor., ptel., **RHUS-T., SEL.,**
   sep., sol-n., **spig., SPONG.,**
   stann., staph., stram., sul-i.¹',
   sulph., sumb., ther., thuj.,
   TUB.¹⁵, verat., ziz.

   w.-motion – least/faiblesse-
     mouvement – moindre/Sch.-
     Bewegung – geringste

am.
   ferr., kali-n.

exhilaration, as after
exaltation, comme après une grande
Heiterkeit, wie nach großer
   cinnb.

faintlike⁴
défaillance, comme une
ohnmachtsähnliche
   ant-t., **ars.²,** bar-c., berb.⁴, ¹¹,
   carb-v.², ⁴, ¹¹, CAUST.², ³, ⁴, ¹¹,
   cham.³, **coca²,** cocc.³, croc.³,
   cupr-c., **dig.²,** digin.¹¹, dulc.,
   EUP-PER.², ferr., **goss.²,** ign.,
   kali-c., kali-i.¹¹, lyc.¹¹, mez.¹¹,
   mosch., **NUX-V.², ³,** olnd., **petr.², ⁴,**
   sep., sil., spong.³, sulph., upa.¹¹,
   verat.², ³, zing.², ¹¹

febrile[11]
fébrile
fiebrige
  ang., cham., kali-n., nit-ac.

feet, while washing the
lavant les pieds, en se
Füßewaschen, beim
  merc.

fever, during
fièvre, pendant la
Fieber, im
  acon., alum.[16], am-m.[11], ant-t.,
  anthraci.[2], **apis**[2, 11], aran., **ARS.,**
  bapt., bry., calc.[11, 16], carb-v.,
  crot-h.[11], **eup-per.**[2], eup-pur.,
  ferr., **ign.,** lyc., morph.[11], **mur-ac.,**
  nat-c., **nat-m.,** nicc.[11], nit-ac.,
  petr.[16], **ph-ac., PHOS., puls., rob.,**
  rhus-t., sarr., sep.[11, 16], sul-ac.[11],
  sulph., thuj.[11]

  after/après la/nach dem
    apis[11], **aran.,** gent-l.[11], morph.[11],
    sal-ac.[2], sulph.[11], syph.[2]

  following prolonged fever
  après des fièvres prolongées
  nach langem Fieber
    colch.[7], **psor.**[7], **SEL.**

    convalescence/Rekonvaleszenz

food, from sour
aliments acides, par des
Speisen, durch saure
  aloe

fright, from
frayeur, par
Schreck, durch
  coff., merc., op.

grief, from
chagrin, par
Kummer, durch
  caust., ign., ph-ac., pic-ac.[2]

growing fast, after[7]
croissance trop rapide, suite de
Wachstum, nach schnellem
  hipp., ph-ac.

haemorrhage, in[2]
hémorrhagie, dans l'
Blutungen, bei
  carb-v., CHIN., chin-s., ferr.,
  hyper., ign., rat.

headache, from
maux de tête, par des
Kopfschmerzen, durch
  ars-h., bufo, calc.[16], cob., fago.,
  glon., kali-c.[16], lac-d.[7], naja, sil.[16]

  during[2]/pendant les/bei
    ANT-C., aran., ars-h.[11], bism.,
    bufo[11], calc-ar., carb-v., chin.,
    chin-s., cob.[11], fago.[11], glon.[11],
    lil-s.[11], naja[11], **sil., thuj.,** thymol.[9],
    verat.

heartburn, from[16]
pyrosis, par
Sodbrennen, durch
  lyc.

heat, from
chaleur, par
Hitze, durch
  aster., **carbn-s.,** coc-c., **lach.,**
  nat-c., nat-p., **puls., puls-n.**[11],
  rhod., **SEL., sulph.,** tab., vesp.

  bed, of
  lit, du
  Bettwärme
    aster.

  room, in hot
  chambre très chaude, dans une
  Zimmer, im heißen
    cinnb., **puls.**

    entering, from bed
    en allant du lit
    beim Betreten eines heißen Zim-
      mers aus dem Bett
      aloe

summer, of
été, en
Sommerhitze
    alum., **ant-c.**[8], **ars.**[2], **carbn-s.**[1', 7],
    corn., GELS.[2, 8], **IOD., lach.,**
    NAT-C., nat-m., **SEL.**

sun, of the
soleil, au
Sonnenhitze
    ars.[2], **GELS.**[2], **NAT-C., SEL.**

    w.-walking – heat/f.-marcher –
    chaleur/Sch.-Gehen – Sonnen-
    hitze

thrills of heat, from
poussées fébriles, par
Überlaufen von Hitze, durch
    cocc.

walk and rapid cooling, after
    heated
promenade échauffante suivie de
    refroidissement rapide, après
    une
Gehen und danach schneller Ab-
    kühlung, nach Erhitzung beim
    bry.[11], **rhus-t.**

heat, after flushes of
chaleur, après bouffées de
Hitzewallungen, nach
    dig.[12], nat-c.[16], **SEP.**[2, 7], **SULPH.**[2],
    xan.[7]

hunger, from
faim, par
Hunger, durch
    alum., crot-h.[2], **IOD.,** nat-c.[16], **phos.,**
    spig.[1, 16], sul-i.[1'], **SULPH.,** ter.[2], **zinc.**

hysteric[16]
hystérique
hysterische
    phos.

injuries, from[8]
traumatismes, par
Verletzungen, durch
    acet-ac.[2, 7, 8], **arn.**[6, 8], calen.,
    camph.[2], carb-v., dig.[2], **sul-ac.**[7, 8]

intermittent
intermittente
zeitweilig aussetzende
    apis, nat-ar.[1] (non: nat-c., nat-s.)

jaundice, from[8]
ictère, par
Ikterus, durch
    ferr-pic., pic-ac., tarax.

joints, of
articulations, des
Gelenke, der
    acon., aesc., agar.[3], agn.[3], **aloe,**
    alum.[3], am-c.[3], anac.[3], ang.[3], **ant-t.**[3],
    arg-m., ARN., ars., asar.[3], aur.,
    bar-c.[3], bell.[3], bor., bov., **bry.,**
    CALC., calc-p.[3, 6], cann-s.[3], canth.[3],
    carb-an., carb-v., carbn-s., **caust.,**
    cham., chel., **chin.,** chin-ar., cimic.,
    clem., cocc.[3], colch.[3], coloc., **CON.,**
    cupr.[3], cycl.[3], dig.[3], dros.[3], dulc.[3],
    euph., **ferr.,** ferr-ar., ferr-p.[3], graph.,
    hep.[3], hyos.[3], ign.[3], **KALI-C.,**
    kali-n.[3], **kali-s.,** kreos.[3], **lach., led.,**
    LYC., mang., **MERC.,** merc-c., mez.,
    morph., mosch.[3], murx., **nat-c.**[3],
    nat-m., nit-ac., nux-m.[3], **nux-v.,**
    olnd.[3], par.[3], **petr., ph-ac.**[3], **phos.,**
    plat.[3], plb., podo., **PSOR., puls.,**
    ran-b.[3], raph., rheum[3], rhod.,
    RHUS-T., ruta[3], sabad.[3], sars.[3],
    SEP., sil., spong.[3], stann.[3], **staph.,**
    stront-c.[3], sul-ac.[3], **SULPH.,** tarax.[3],
    thuj., valer.[3], **verat.,** viol-o.[3], zinc.[3],
    zing.

leaning towards left during menses
    am.
pencher à gauche pendant la
    menstration am.
Neigen nach links während der
    Menses am.
    phel.

leucorrhoea with[2]
leucorrhées avec
Fluor mit
    aesc., alet.[2, 8], alum.[3, 8], arg-n.,
    bar-c.[3, 4], berb.[2, 6], **CALC.**[2, 8], calc-p.,
    calen., carb-an.[8], **caul.**[2, 8], **caust.**[2, 8],
    CHIN.[3, 6, 8], **cocc.**[6, 8], coll.[6], con.[2, 6, 8],

frax.[6], **GRAPH.**, gua.[8], **ham.**, helin.[8],
helon.[2, 8], hydr.[2, 8], **iod., kali-bi.**[3],
kali-c.[6], **KREOS.**[2, 3, 4, 8, 11], **lyc., lyss.,**
nabal.[1], **NAT-M.**, nicc.[6], onos.[8],
petr., ph-ac., phos.[8], **phys., psor.**[8],
puls.[8], rob., **senec.**[6], sep.[8],
STANN.[2, 8], sul-ac., tarent.[2, 11], tril.,
vinc.[6], zinc.

from[16]/par/durch
  con.

lifting, from
soulever, par
Heben, durch
  CARB-AN., kali-sil.[1'], nat-c.[16]

looking down, on
regardant en bas, en
Herabsehen, beim
  kali-c.

loss of fluids, from[2]
perte de fluides vitaux, par
Verlust von Körpersäften, durch
  calc., **CHIN.**[2, 6], **cur.**, ferr.[1'],
  ferr-ar.[1'], ham.[7], hydr.[7], lachn.,
  nat-m., nuph., PH-AC.[1', 2], **phos.,**
  psor., sec., **sep.**

loss of sleep, from
manque de sommeil, par
Schlafmangel, durch
  COCC., colch.[8], cupr., glon.[2],
  hydr.[2], **ip.**[2], **nat-m.**[2, 11], nux-v.[8],
  osm.[11], **puls.**[11]

love, from unfortunate
chagrin d'amour, par
Liebeskummer, durch
  ph-ac.

  Vol. I: *ailments–love*

lying agg.
être couché agg.
Liegen agg.
  agar., alum., bar-c., bry., carb-v.,
  carl., coca, cycl., gels., nat-c.,
  nat-m., nit-ac., nux-v., petr.,
  phys., pip-m., **puls.**, rhus-g.[11],
  spig., zinc-m.

am.
  acon-f., ars., bry.[4], hedeo.[7],
  lach., mag-c., nat-m.[4], nit-ac.[4],
  ph-ac.[16], **psor.**, sabad.[4], **sep.**

  on back
  sur le dos
  auf dem Rücken
    cast.

  shower, before
  averse, avant une
  Regenschauer vor einem
    gels.

masturbation, from[6]/par/durch
  aven., bell-p.[9], **nat-m.**, phos.[2, 6]

meeting am., in interesting
réunion intéressante, à la suite d'une
Begegnung am., bei interessanter
  pip-m.

menses, before
menstruation, avant la
Menses, vor den
  alum.[3, 8, 16], **am-c.**[8], aur-s., **bell.,**
  brom., calc.[3, 3'], carb-ac.,
  carb-an[8], carb-v.[3], **chin.**[8], cimic.,
  cinnb.[2, 3], **cocc.**, ferr., glyc.[8],
  graph.[8], **haem.**[8], **helon.**[8], ign.[3, 8],
  iod., kali-p.[3], **mag-c.**, merc.[3],
  nat-m., nicc.[8], nux-m., phel.,
  phos.[3], puls.[8], sec.[3], **verat.**[8], zinc.

  at beginning
  au début de la
  am Beginn der
    brom.[3], cocc.[3], ferr.[3], mag-m.[3],
    phel.

  appearance of m. am.
  à l'arrivée de la m. am.
  Eintreten der M. am.
    cycl., mag-m.

  during/pendant la/während der
    agar., aloe, alum., alum-p.[1'],
    am-c., am-m., **ars.**, ars-i.,
    ars-s-f.[1'], bar-c., bar-i.[1'], bar-s.[1'],
    bell., berb., bor., bov., brom.[7],
    bufo, cact., calc., calc-i.[1'],

calc-p., **calc-s.**, cann-s.[3],
CARB-AN., carb-v., carbn-s.,
caul., **caust.**, cimic., **cinnb.,**
cocc., eupi., ferr., ferr-i.,
graph., helon., ign., **iod.**, ip.,
kali-c., kali-n.[16], **kali-s., lach.,**
lil-t., lyc., **mag-c., mag-m.,**
mag-s.[9], mosch., **murx.**, nat-ar.,
nat-c., nat-m., **nicc., nit-ac.,**
nux-m., **nux-v.**, ol-an.[3], **petr.,**
phel., **phos., sabin., sec.,**
senec., **SEP.**, stann., **sulph.,**
tarent., thuj., tril., **tub.**[1], uran.,
verat., vinc., wies.[11], zinc.[3],
zinc-p.[1']

am.
   sep.[1]

can scarcely breathe, must lie
   down
respiration pénible
   difficultueuse, doit s'étendre
kann kaum atmen, muß sich
   hinlegen
   nit-ac.

desire to lie down, with
désir de s'étendre, avec le
Verlangen sich hinzulegen,
   mit dem
   bell., ip., **nit-ac.**

end of/fin de la/Ende der
   bov., iod.

going up stairs, when
montant l'escalier, en
Treppensteigen, beim
   iod.

   w.-ascending/f.-monter/Sch.-
      Treppensteigen

painful/douloureuse/schmerz-
   hafter
   bell., bufo

stool, after
selle, après la
Stuhlgang, nach
   nux-v.

w.-stool/f.-selle/Sch.-Stuhlgang

talk, can scarcely
parler, peut à peine
reden, kann kaum
   carb-an., cocc.[2], **stann.**

after/après la/nach den
   agar.[3], **alum., alumn.**[2], am-c.[8],
   am-m.[8], aran.[3], **ars.**[3, 6, 8],
   bell.[3, 3'], benz-ac., berb., cact.[3],
   calc.[3, 8], calc-p., carb-ac.[3],
   carb-an., carb-v.[6, 8], cast.[3],
   chin., chin-s.[2], **cimic.**,
   cocc.[3, 6, 8], ferr.[3, 6, 8], ferr-pic.[6],
   glyc.[6], graph.[3, 8], **helon.**[2, 3, 6],
   iod., **IP.**, kali-c.[3, 8], kali-p.[3, 6],
   mag-c.[8], nat-m., nit-ac.[3],
   nux-v.[3], **phos.**, pic-ac.[6], plat.,
   sapin.[11], sec., sep.[3], stann.[3],
   sulph., thlas.[8], thuj., tril.[8],
   verat.[8], vinc.[8]

disproportionate to loss of blood
disproportionné avec la perte de
   sang
in keinem Verhältnis zum
   Blutverlust
   ham.[2], **ip.**

mental exertion, from
travail intellectuel, par
geistige Anstrengung, durch
   aloe, anag.[2], apis, arn., ars., aur.,
   aur-ar.[1'], bar-a.[6], **bell., CALC.,**
   calc-sil.[1'], cham., **chin.**[2], cocc.,
   CUPR., FERR-PIC., ign., **kali-c.,**
   kali-n., kali-p.[7], **LACH., LEC.,**
   lil-s.[11], **lyc.**, mag-c.[7], **NAT-C.,**
   nat-m., **nux-v.**[7], okou.[14], **par.**[2],
   ph-ac., pic-ac.[2], **PSOR., PULS.,**
   sabad., **SEL.**, sep., sil., spong.,
   sulfonam.[14], **sulph.**, thuj.

occupation am.
Beschäftigung am.
   croc.

milk, after[16]
lait, après ingestion de
Milch, nach dem Trinken von
   sul-ac.

mortification, after
mortification, par
Kränkung, nach
  ign.

motion, from
mouvement, par
Bewegung, durch
  agar., ammc., apoc., **arg-m.,**
  ARS., asaf., bry., cann-s., cocc.,
  hydr-ac., kali-bi., kali-n., lach.,
  mang-o.[11], merc., merl., mur-ac.[4],
  narcin.[11], nat-m.[4], nit-ac.[16],
  nux-v., phel., **phos.,** plb., sep.[4],
  spig.[4, 16], **SPONG.,** stann.[16],
  staph., sulph., tab.

am.
  cham.[16], colch., coloc., cycl., gels.,
  kreos., **lyc.,** mosch., pip-m., **plat.,**
  plb., **rhod.,** stann.[4]

gentle m. am.
doux de m. am.
leichte B. am.
  kali-n.

least m., on[3']
le moindre m., par
geringsten B., bei der
  anac., lyc., nux-m., spig., verat.

  w.-exertion/f.-exercices physi-
  ques/Sch.-Anstrengung

when moved from horizontal
  position
quand il est soulevé de la position
  couchée
wenn er aus dem Liegen auf-
  gehoben wird
  rob.

moving arms, on
mouvant les bras, en
Bewegen der Arme, beim
  nat-m.

muscular[3]
muscles, des
Muskelschwäche
  acon., agar., alum.[3, 8], alumn.[1'],

am-c., am-m., anac., ant-c., arn.,
ars.[3, 8], asaf., aur., **BAR-C.,**
bar-m.[2, 3], bell., berb., bry.[3, 8],
calc.[2, 3, 8], cann-s., canth., **carb-ac.,**
carb-v.[3, 8], caust.[3, 8], cham.,
chin., chlol.[2], cimic.[3], cocc.[1', 3],
colch.[3, 8], **con.**[3, 8], cortico.[9], **croc.,**
dig., dros., **dulc.,** euphr., **ferr.,**
ferr-m.[2], ferr-p., **GELS.**[2, 3, 8], graph.,
hyos., iod., kali-bi., kali-c.[3, 8],
kali-n., **kali-p.**[3, 8], laur., **lyc.,**
macro.[11, 12], mag-c., mag-m.,
mag-p.[3, 8], mang., meny., merc.[3, 8],
mez., mur-ac.[1'], **nat-c., NAT-M.**[3, 6],
NIT-AC., nux-v.[3, 8], olnd., **op.**[2],
petr., ph-ac.[1', 3], phos., phys.[3, 12],
PIC-AC.[1', 2], **plat., plb.**[2, 3, 6], puls.,
rad-br.[3], rheum, **rhod.,**
sabad.[3, 8, 11, 12], sarcol-ac.[9], sec.,
sep., sil.[3, 8], sin-n.[2], spig., stann.,
stram., stront-c., sul-ac.[3], **sulph.,**
ter.[2], thuj., **verat.**[2, 3], verat-v.[3],
zinc.[3, 8]

paralytic[1']
paralysie, par
Lähmung, durch
  alumn.

music, from[7]
musique, par la
Musik, durch
  lyc.

nausea, with[11]
nausée, avec
Übelkeit, mit
  aeth., **agar.**[2], alumn.[2], ang.[2],
  calc.[2, 11], **camph.**[2], cimic., cob.,
  crot-t., gran., hell., sabad., sang.,
  sep., stront-c.[11], **verat.**

nervous
nerveuse
Neurasthenie
  acon., aesc.[2], **agar.**[2], **agn.**[2, 3, 11],
  alet.[2], **alum.,** alum-p.[1'], alumn.[2],
  am-c., am-m.[2], ambr., **anac.**[2, 8],
  ang.[3], **aran.**[2], **arg-n.**[2, 3, 6], arn.,
  ars., asaf.[2, 3, 6], **asar.,** aur.,
  aven.[6, 10], bar-c., bar-i.[1'], **bell.,**
  bry., **calc.,** calc-p., calc-sil.[1'],

calen.[11], camph., carb-an.,
carb-v., carbn-s., cast.[3, 6, 10],
caust.[3, 6], cham., **CHIN.**, chin-ar.[6],
chin-s.[2], cic.[1], **cimic.**[2, 3], **COCA**[2],
COCC., coff., colch., **con.**, croc.,
cupr., cur., cycl.[2], cypr.[12],
dig., dios.[2], **fl-ac.**[3, 6], **form.**[3],
GELS.[2, 8], graph., **guaj.**, hedeo.[11],
helon.[2], hell., hep., hydr-ac.[4],
hydrc.[2], hyos., **ign., iod.**, kali-br.[8],
kali-n., **KALI-P.**, lac-c.[2], lach.,
lact., laur., **LEC.**, led., **lil-t.**[3],
lyc., mag-m.[3], meph.[6], **merc.**,
mosch., mur-ac., **NAT-C.**, nat-m.,
NAT-P., nat-s.[2], **NAT-SIL.**[1'],
NIT-AC., nux-m., **NUX-V.**, op.,
petr., **PH-AC.**[1], **PHOS.**, phys.[2],
PIC-AC., pip-m.[6], **plat., plb.,**
PULS., rhus-t., sabin., sars.,
scroph-n.[11], sec., **SEL.**[1], **SEP., SIL.**,
spig., spong., squil., **STANN.**,
STAPH., stram., stry-n.[10], stry-p.[6],
sul-ac., **sulph.**, sumb.[2], tab.[6],
tarent.[2, 3, 11], **teucr., ther.**[2, 3],
valer., verat., vib.[3], **viol-o.**, zinc.,
zinc-m., **ZINC-P.**[1', 10],
zinc-pic.[3, 6, 10]

afternoon/après-midi/nachmittags
cimic.

walk, after a
marche, après une
Gehen, nach dem
petr.

nursing the sick, from
soins donnés aux malades, par
Krankenpflege, durch
cimic., **COCC., nit-ac.**, olnd.,
zinc., **zinc-a.**[7]

sit up with sick person[7]
veiller quelque
Wachen bei Kranken
carb-v., cocc., **nux-v.**, puls.

nursing women, in
lactation, par
Stillen, durch
calc.[2], **calc-p.**[2], **carb-an., CARB-V.**[2],

CHIN., lyc.[2], olnd., **PH-AC.**, phos.[2],
phyt.[2], **sil.**[2], **sulph.**[2]

nursing agg./allaiter agg./Stillen
agg.

old people, of
personnes âgées, chez les
alter Menschen
ambr., aur., **BAR-C.**, carb-v.[8], **con.**,
cur., eup-per.[8], glyc.[8], nit-ac.[8, 12],
nux-m., op., **phos.**, sec., **sel., sul-ac.**

w.-sudden – eruption/f.-subite –
éruption/Sch.-plötzliche – Haut-
ausschlag

operation, from
opération, par
Operation, durch
acet-ac.[7, 8], carb-v.[1'], hyper.[8]

injuries – operation/traumatismes –
opération/Verletzungen –
Operation

pain, from
douleurs, par
Schmerzen, durch
arg-m., ARS., carb-v., cham.[16],
hep.[1'], hura, kali-p., kalm.[1'],
pic-ac.[3], plb., **rhus-t.**

sacrum, in
sacrodynie
Kreuzbein, im
sep.

palpitation, with[16]
palpitations, avec
Herzklopfen, mit
aur., caust., sang., sul-i.[1']

paralytic
paralytique
lähmungsartige
agar.[1'], **alum.**, alum-p.[1'],
alumn.[1', 7], am-m., ambr.[1'], anac.[1'],
ang.[3, 4], **arg-m., ARS.**, art-v.[2],
bapt.[1'], **bar-c., bar-m.**, bell., **bism.**,
bry., **calc.**, calc-ar.[1'], camph.,
cann-i.[1'], canth., caps.[4], carb-v.,

caust., **cham.,** chel., **chin.,**
cimic.[1'], cina, **COCC., colch.,**
con., crot-h., cupr.[7], dig., dros.,
euph., **ferr.,** ferr-ar., ferr-ma.[4],
GELS., HELL., hyos., ign.[1'], ind.,
kali-n., lach., laur., **merc.,** mez.,
mosch., **MUR-AC.,** nat-c., nat-m.[4],
nat-p., **nit-ac.,** nux-m.[1'], nux-v.,
olnd., PH-AC., PHOS., plat.[1'],
plb., psor.[1'], **puls., rhod., rhus-t.,**
sabad., sarcol-ac.[14], sil., **stann.,**
stront-c., sulph.[3], valer., **VERAT.,**
zinc.[1', 4]

morning after rising[16]
matin après s'être levé
morgens nach dem Aufstehen
phos.

motion, on
mouvement, au
Bewegung, bei
aeth., arg-m.

pain, with
douleurs, avec
Schmerzen, mit
arg-m., verat.

painful parts, in
parties douloureuses, dans les
schmerzhaften Teilen, in den
cham., **verat.**

sliding down in bed
glisse au fond de son lit
rutscht im Bett hinunter
ant-t.[2], **apis,** arn.[6], **ars.,** arum-t.,
bapt.[2, 3, 6], **bell.**[2], carb-v., chin.[2, 3],
colch.[1',3], croth-h.[1'], **hell.,** hyos.[1', 6],
lyc.[2], mosch., **MUR-AC.,** nux-m.,
nit-ac., PH-AC., PHOS., rhus-t.,
zinc.[2, 3, 16]

parturition, in[3]
accouchement, pendant l'
Entbindung, während der
arn., asaf., **BELL.,** bor., bry., calc.,
camph., carb-an., carb-v., **caul.**[2, 3],
caust., **cham.,** chin., cimic., cocc.,
coff., **con.**[2], **gels.,** graph., hyos.,
ign., **KALI-C.**[3, 16], **KALI-P.,** kreos.,

lyc., mag-c., mag-m., merc., mosch.,
nat-c., **nat-m.,** nux-m., **nux-v., OP.,**
phos., plat., **PULS.,** rhus-t., ruta,
sabad., **SEC., sep.,** stann., sul-ac.,
sulph., thuj., zinc.

periodical
périodique
periodische
ARG-N., hep.[2]

every other morning
tous les 2 matins
jeden 2. Morgen
nit-ac.

perspiration, from
transpiration, par
Schweiß, durch
acon., agar., am-c., ambr.,
aml-ns., ant-c., **ant-t.**[3], ant-o.[11],
anthraci., apis, **ARN.**[3], **ars.,**
ars-i.[6], ars-s-f.[1'], bar-c., ben.,
BRY., bov., caj.[11], **calad., calc.,**
CAMPH., canth.[3, 6], **CARB-AN.,**
carb-v., carl.[11], cast.[6], **CAUST.**[3],
CHIN., chin-ar., CHIN-S., coca[11],
cocc., croc., dig., **FERR., ferr-ar.,**
ferr-i., ferr-p., gels.[11], graph.,
hep.[6], hist.[9], hura[11], hyos., ign.,
IOD., jatr.[11], kali-bi., kali-n.,
lac-c., lyc., mag-c.[7], **MERC.,**
morph.[11], nat-c.[11], **nat-m.**[1], **nit-ac.,**
nux-v.[3], op., **ph-ac., PHOS.,**
PSOR., puls., **pyrog.,** ran-s.[11],
rhod., **SAMB., sec.,** senec.[6], **SEP.,**
sil., stann., sulph., tarax.,
tarent.[11], **TUB., verat., verat-v.**

night/nuit/nachts
ars., bar-c., bry., **carb-an., chin.,**
eupi., ferr., hall[11], **merc.,** nat-c.[11],
ph-ac.[11], **phos.**[2], **samb.,** stann.,
tarax., **TUB.**

parturition. after[7]
accouchement, après
Entbindung, nach der
samb.

suppressed foot sweat, from[2]
supprimée des pieds, par
unterdrückten Fußschweiß, durch
   sil.

while awake; dry, burning heat
   while sleeping
étant réveillé, chaleur sèche et
   brûlante en dormant
beim Erwachen; trockene,
   brennende Hitze im Schlaf
   SAMB.

with perspiration, w.[2]
avec transpiration, f.
mit Schweiß, Sch.
   ALOE, calc., chin., chin-m.,
   dig., jab., lyc., ph-ac., sal-ac.,
   sul-ac., **tarent.**

with cold[2]
avec t. froide
mit kaltem
   camph., carb-v., cupr., **merc.,**
   ph-ac., ter., VERAT.

playing piano, from[1']
jouer du piano, par
Klavierspielen, durch
   anac.

pleasant[11]
agréable
angenehme
   cann-s., morph.

pleasure, from
joie, par
Freude, durch
   crot-c.

pregnancy, in[2]
grossesse, pendant la
Schwangerschaft, in der
   alet.[1'], alum., alumn., calc-p.,
   helon., murx., **sulph., verat.**

progressive[2]
fortschreitende
   acon., ars.[3], caust.[3], cupr-ar., **dig.,**
   kreos.[3], **ol-j., phos., plb.,** verat.[3]

quinine, from abuse of[1']
quinine, abus de
Chinin-Mißbrauch, durch
   ars-s-f.

rapid
rapide
schnell zunehmende
   ARS., laur., **sep., VERAT.**

   w.-sudden/f.-subite/Sch.-plötzliche

reaction, with lack of[2]
réaction, avec manque de
Reaktionsmangel, mit
   am-c., laur., **OP., sulph., valer.**

   reaction, lack/réaction, manque/
   Reaktionsmangel

fat people, in[2]
adipeux, chez les gens
Adipöser
   CAPS.

reading, from
lecture, par
Lesen, durch
   anac., **aur.,** ph-ac., plb., **sumb.**

   aloud
   haute voix, à
   lautes
      stann.

rest, during[11]
repos, au
Ruhe, in der
   coloc., con., kreos., lyc.[2, 11, 16],
   rhod.[1']

   w.-lying/f.-coucher/Sch.-Liegen
   w.-sitting/f.-assis/Sch.-Sitzen

   am.[11]
      bry.

resting head on something and
clothing eyes am.
reposant sur un appui et les yeux
clos am., la tête
Kopfanlehnen und Augenschließen
am.
anac.

restlessness, with[2]
agitation, avec
Ruhelosigkeit, mit
ARS.[2, 3], **bism., colch.,** lycps., lyss.,
ph-ac., RHUS-T.[2, 3], zinc.[3]

riding, from
aller en voiture ou à cheval
Reiten oder Fahren, durch
cere-b.[11], cocc., petr., **psor.**[1], sep.,
sulph., tet.[1] (non: ter.)

in open air am.
en plein air am.
im Freien am.
cinnb.

rising, on
se levant, en
Aufstehen, beim
acon-c., ammc., arn., **ARS.,** atro.,
BRY., clem., coca, fago., ham.,
hydr., hyper., jab., lyc., mag-c.,
nat-ar., **nat-m.,** olnd., osm., phyt.,
pic-ac., ptel., rhus-g.[11], **rhus-t.,**
sol-t-ae., teucr., thuj., uran.

*w.-morning – rising/f.-matin –
se levant/Sch.-morgens – Aufstehen*

after/après s'être levé/nach dem
am-c., coc-c., hydr., mag-c.

seat, from a
siège, d'un
Sitz, vom
chin.

room, in[14]
chambre, dans une
Zimmer, im
asar.

agg. from closed[14]
agg. dans une ch. fermée
agg. durch ein geschlossenes
asar.

sea-bath, after
bain de mer, après un
Meer, nach Baden im
mag-m.

sedentary habit, from[7]
sédentaires, par habitudes
sitzende Lebensweise, durch
nux-v., sulph.

sexual excesses, after[2]
sexuels, par excès
sexuellen Ausschweifungen, nach
ars., aven.[6], chin.[6], coca, con.[6], **dig.,**
gins.[6], kali-c.[6], **nat-m.**[2, 6], **ph-ac.**[6],
phos., ust.

side, of left[2]
côté gauche, du
Seite, der linken
arg-n., lach.

sit down, desire to[6]
s'asseoir, désir de
sich hinzusetzen, Bedürfnis
alum.[4], ambr., anac.[4], ars., bry.[4, 6],
calc., caust., cham.[4], chin., **cocc.**[4, 6],
colch., croc.[4], dulc., kali-n., led.,
lil-t., m-aust.[4], **merc.,** mur-ac.[4],
nat-m., nat-s., nux-v.[4, 6], ol-an.[4],
olnd., ph-ac., rhus-t.[4], sabin.[4],
stann., staph.[4], stront-c., sulph.[4],
tarax.[4], verat.

sitting
assis, étant
Sitzen, im
agar., anac., arg-m.[4], **ars.,** aur.,
bry., carl., caust.[4], chel., chin.,
cocc., colch., fago., graph.,
kali-n., led.[4], **lyc.,** m-aust.[4],
mag-c., mang., merc.[4, 6], merc-i-f.,
mur-ac.[4], **nat-m.,** nit-ac., nux-v.[4],
phos.[4], **plat.,** plb., ptel., ran-b.[4],
RHUS-T., ruta, sabad., staph.,
stront-c.[4], **sulph.,** thuj.[4]

w.-rest/f.-repos/Sch.-Ruhe

am.
  bry., euph-a.[11], glon., nux-v.,
  sapin.[11]

walk, after a
marche, après la
Gehen, nach dem
  RUTA

sleep, during
sommeil, pendant le
Schlaf, im
  bufo

  after/après le/nach dem
    agar., ambr.[2], bor., bor-ac.,
    camph., carl., chel., chin-s., coca,
    colch., con., cycl., dor., ferr.,
    gels., gent-l., **kali-n.**[6], **lach.**, lyc.,
    mez., nat-n., sec., sep., sil.,
    sin-n.[2], zinc.

  am.
    alum.[16], mez., **ph-ac., phos.**

  loss of, from
  manque de, par
  Schlafmangel, durch
    COCC., colch.[8], cupr.[1], glon.[2],
    hydr.[2], **ip.**[2], **nat-m.**[2, 11], nux-v.[8],
    osm.[11], **puls.**[11]

    as from[16]
    comme par
    wie durch
      plat.

sleepiness, from
somnolence, par
Schläfrigkeit, durch
  coff., chlol.[2], gran., hep.[11], nit-ac.,
  rhus-t.[11]

  as from/comme par/ wie durch
    aeth.[2], chen-v.[2], cimic., dig.,
    kali-n., merc-sul.[2], peti.[11], petr.,
    phel., plat., **rhus-t.,** thuj.

  morning/matin/morgens
    verat.

afternoon, walking am.
après-midi, marcher am.
nachmittags, Gehen am.
  ruta

sleeplessness, from
insomnie, par
Schlaflosigkeit, durch
  cypr.[2, 11], **kreos.**[2]

smoking, from
fumer, par
Rauchen, durch
  asc-t., clem.[3], **hep.**

  *w.-walking – smoking/f.-marcher –
  fumé/Sch.-Gehen – Rauchen*

somnambulism, after
somnambulisme, après
Schlafwandeln, nach
  sulph.

sporting[7]
sportive
Sport, durch
  arn., ars., coca, fl-ac., rhus-t.

spring, in
printemps, au
Frühling, im
  apis, **BRY.**[2]

standing, on
debout, étant
Stehen, im
  acon.[2], acon-c.[11], agn., **apis**[2], asaf.,
  aster.[2], berb., **cic.,** cocc.[4], crot-h.,
  cupr.[4], cur., ham.[11], hep.[4], **kali-c.**[2],
  kali-n.[4], lach.[4], led.[4], merc.,
  MERC-CY.[2, 11], mur-ac., nat-m.,
  nit-ac.[4], nux-v.[4], ol-an.[4], ped.[11],
  plat.[4], ran-b., spig., staph.[4],
  sul-ac.[1, 4, 6], **sulph.,** ther.[4], zing.

stimulants am.
Stimulantien am.
  phos.

  *w.-coffee/f.-café/Sch.-Kaffee
  w.-tea/f.-thé/Sch.-Tee*

stomach, in[2]
estomac, à l'
Magen, im
  calc-p., calc-s., crot-t., HYDR.,
  podo.

as from[16]
comme de l'
wie vom M. aus
  mag-c.

pain in, from
douleurs à l', par
Magenschmerz, durch
  nux-v.[2]**, podo.**

and back
et dorsale
und Rückenschmerzen
  sep.

stool, before
selle, avant la
Stuhlgang, vor
  hydr., mez., nat-hchls., **rhus-t.,**
  verat.

during/pendant la/während
  aesc., apis, atro., bell., **bor.,**
  carbn-s., cob., colch., crot-h.,
  crot-t.[2], **cupr-a.**[2], kali-i., lact.,
  nit-ac.[2], pic-ac., plan., **PLAT.,**
  sec., **verat.**

after/après la/nach dem
  aeth., **aloe,** ant-t., apis, apoc.,
  arn., **ARS., ARS-MET.,** ars-s-f.[1'],
  bapt.[2], bism., bov., **calc.,**
  carb-an.[16], **carb-v., carbn-s.,**
  cast-v.[11], caust., chin., **chin-s.,**
  clem., cocc.[3], coch.[3], colch.,
  coloc., com., **CON.,** cop., crot-h.,
  crot-t., dios., **dulc.,** eupi., ferr-ma.,
  graph., ign., **iod.,** ip., **jatr.**[2]**, lach.,**
  lil-t., lipp.[11], **lyc.,** mag-c., **med.,**
  MERC., mez., nat-m., **NAT-S.,**
  NIT-AC., nux-m.[2]**, nux-v., petr.,**
  phos., phys., **PIC-AC.,** plan.,
  PODO., pyre-p.[11], rham-f.[11],
  sabad., sacch., **SEC., sep., sil.**[2]**,**
  sulph., ter., thuj., trio.[1] (non: tril.),
  trom., tub.[3], **VERAT.,** vinc.

stooping, on
baissant, en se
Bücken, beim
  graph.

storm, before and during a
tempête, avant et pendant une
Sturm, vor und während
  sil.

thunderstorm, during
orage, pendant un éclair et un
Gewitter, bei
  caust., nat-c., nat-p., nit-ac.,
  petr., rhod., sil.

sudden
subite
plötzliche
  acon., act-sp., **aeth.**[6], ail.[3],
  am-c.[3, 6], am-m.[4], ambr.[3, 4],
  ant-ar.[6], ant-c.[1', 6], **ant-t.**[3, 6]**, apis,**
  apoc.[6], **arg-m.,** arg-n.[3], arn.[3, 6],
  ARS., ars-h., **ars-i.**[6]**, bapt.**[3, 6],
  bell.[2, 3, 16], bry.[3, 6], calc., camph.,
  cann-s.[4], carb-ac.[6], **carb-v.,**
  caust.[3, 6, 16], cham., colch., con.,
  CROT-H., cupr.[3], cupr-ar.,
  dig.[3, 6, 16], dulc.[4], fl-ac.[3], **gels.**[3, 6],
  glon.[3], **GRAPH., hell.**[3, 6]**, hep.,**
  hydr-ac.[3, 6]**, ip.,** jatr.[6], kali-br.[6],
  kali-c.[16], kali-cy.[7], kalm.[3], lach.,
  laur., lith-c.[3, 6], lyc., mag-c.[3],
  merc-c.[3], merc-cy.[3], naja[3],
  nit-ac.[3], **nux-v.,** petr.[4, 16], **phos.,**
  ran-b., rhus-t.[3, 6], sabad.[3, 6], sec.,
  sel., SEP., sil.[3], spong., stann.,
  stram., **sulph.**[3, 6]**, tab.**[3, 6], tarent.,
  tax., thuj.[3], **verat., verat-v.**[3, 6],
  vip.[4], zinc.[3, 6, 16]

collapse/collapsus/Kollaps

daily/tous les jours/täglich
  hep.

afternoon/après-midi/nachmittags
  lyc., ran-b.

13.30 h
  iodof.

walking, after
marche, après la
Gehen, nach dem
   graph.

evening/soir/abends
   fl-ac.

chilliness, during
frilosité, pendant la
Frösteln, bei
   sep.

diarrhoea, with[2]
diarrhée, avec
Diarrhoe, mit
   crot-t.

dressing after rising, while
s'habillant après s'être levé, en
Anziehen nach dem Aufstehen,
   beim
   stann.

eruption comes out, after the
éruption, après l'apparition d'une
Hautausschlag herausgekommen
ist, nachdem
   ars.

old people, in[7]
personnes âgées, chez les
alten Menschen, bei
   kali-cy.

sitting, while
assis, étant
Sitzen, im
   cham., lyc., ran-b.

w.-sitting/f.-assis/Sch.-Sitzen

vanish, as if senses would
s'évanouir, comme si elle allait
Sinne schwinden, als ob die
   ran-b.

walking, from
marche, par la
Gehen, durch
   carb-v.[16], con.[16], sabad., wildb.

w.-walking/f.-marcher/Sch.-
Gehen

sunstroke, from[2]
coup de soleil, par
Sonnenstich, durch
   glon., verat-v.

supper, after
dîner, après le
Abendessen, nach dem
   alum., bov., chin., lach., mag-c., sil.

w.-evening – eating/f.-soir –
mangé/Sch.-abends – Essen

suppressed eruptions, from[1']
supprimées, par éruptions
unterdrückte Hautausschläge, durch
   ars-s-f.

syphilis, in[2]/au cours de
Syphilis, bei
   kali-i., lyc., staph.

talking, from
parler, par
Reden, durch
   act-sp., **ALUM.,** am-c.,
   am-caust.[11], ambr., arn.[7], **calc.,**
   cocc., dor., **ferr.,** hydrc.[11], **hyos.,**
   iod., jac-c.[11], **nat-m., ph-ac.,**
   psor., sep., sil., **STANN., SULPH.,**
   ust.[2], wies[11]

of peoples, from the
autres, par conversation des
anderer, durch das
   alum., am-c., ars., verat.

Vol. I: *talk – others/parler –*
autres/Reden – anderer

tea am.[11]
thé am.
Tee am.
   dig.

tobacco, from[4]
tabac, par
Tabak, durch
   clem., hep.

w.-smoking/f.-fumer/Sch.-Rauchen
w.-walking – smoking/f.-marcher –
fumé/Sch.-Gehen – Rauchen

toothache, after[16]
maux des dents, après
Zahnschmerzen, nach
nat-c.

with[16]/avec/mit
mang.

tremulous
tremblante
zittrige
agar., **alum.,** anac., anag.[2],
ant-t.[3, 6], **apis, ARG-N., ars.,**
bapt., bell.[3, 6], berb.[3, 6], bor.[4],
bry.[3, 6], calc-ar.[1'], caps.[4], carb-v.,
caul., caust.[3, 4, 6, 16], **chin.**[2, 3, 4, 6],
chin-s.[4], clem., **cocc., CON.,**
crot-h., cupr.[16], **gels.,** graph.[4],
hep., hyos.[4], kali-c.[3, 4, 6, 16],
kali-n., **kalm., LACH.**[2], lyc.,
lycps.[2], mang.[3, 6], med.[1'],
nat-m.[3, 16], **nit-ac.,** ol-an.[4], olnd.[4],
ox-ac., petr.[7, 16], **phos., plat.,**
plb.[4], **puls.,** rhus-t.[16], **sep.,** spig.[4],
STANN., ther., thuj.[3], verat.[3, 6],
vip.[3], zinc.[6]

night, on waking
la nuit au réveil
nachts beim Erwachen
brom.

dinner, after
déjeuner, après le
Mittagessen, nach dem
ant-c.

w.-dinner/f.-déjeuner/Sch.-
Mittagessen

stool, after
selle, après la
Stuhlgang, nach
ARS., carb-v., caust., **CON.**

w.-stool/f.-selle/Sch.-Stuhlgang

urination, after
uriner, après
Urinieren, nach
cimic., **lyss., phos., pic-ac.**[2]

after copious
après une miction abondante
nach reichlichem
caust., gels., med.

vertigo, with[2]
vertige, avec
Schwindel, mit
acet-ac., crot-t.[11], **cupr-s.,** dulc.[7],
graph.[11], hell.[11], **sil.,** uran-n.

vexation, after
contrariété, après
Ärger, nach
ars., calc-p., lyc., **nat-m.,** nux-v.,
petr., sep.[16], verat.

vomiting, with[11]
vomissement, avec
Erbrechen, mit
aeth., ars., bol-s., **calc.**[2], crot-t.,
gran., kali-c.[11, 16], phos.[16],
SANG.[2, 11], sulph.[16], tab.

after[11]/après/nach
aloe, ant-c.[2], ant-t., apom.,
ars.[11, 16], bar-c.[2, 11], cadm-s.[2, 11],
colch.[2], der., gran., mag-c.[11, 16],
nat-s., op., phyt., sel.,
verat.[2, 11, 16], zinc.[16]

waking, on
réveil, au
Erwachen, beim
aeth., alco.[11], aloe, ambr.,
aq-pet.[11], arg-m., ars-h., bell.,
bism., bry., carbn-s., card-m.,
cham., chel., chin., clem., **cycl.,**
dig., dios., **dulc.**[2], echi.[3, 6], equis.,
erig., erio.[11], euphr.[4], ferr.,
ferr-p., form., hipp., hura, ign.[6],
lac-ac.[1] (non: lac-c.), lyc., mang.,
myrig., nabal.[11], nat-ar., nat-m.,
nat-p., nux-m., nux-v.[6], op.,
ph-ac., podo., ptel., **PULS.,**
puls-n.[11], rhod., rhus-t., sang.,
sec.[6], sel.[6], **sep.,** sulph., sumb.,

syph.[3], tab., teucr., thuj., upa., xan.

w.-dream/f.-rêve/Sch.-Traum

morning[16]/matin/morgens
mag-c.

dream, from a
rêve, par un
Traum, durch einen
  calc-s.[1], op., teucr.

after/après/nach dem
  arg-m., calc-s., cedr., cycl., iod., wildb.

walking, from
marche, par la
Gehen, durch
  acon., acon-f.[11], aesc., agar.,
  ALUM., ALUM-P.[1]', alum-sil.[1]',
  am-c.[4], ambr.[4], **anac.,** ang.[11],
  arg-m.[1', 4], arn., **ARS., ars-i.,**
  aur-ar.[1]', aur-m.[1]', aur-s.[1]', bar-c.,
  bar-i.[1]', bar-m., bar-s.[1]', **berb.,**
  bov., brom., **BRY., CALC.,**
  CANN-I., carb-an., carb-v.,
  carbn-s., caust.[8, 16], cench.[1]',
  cham., chel., **chin.,** chin-ar.,
  clem.[16], coca, cocc., **coloc., CON.,**
  cupr., **cupr-ar.,** cycl.[8], digin.[11],
  ery-a.[11], ery-m.[11], euph.,
  euph-a.[11], fago.[11], **FERR.,** ferr-ar.,
  ferr-i., ferr-ma., **fl-ac.,** franz.[11],
  gins., graph.[4], ham., helon., hep.,
  hyper., ind., indg., **iod.,** kali-ar.[1]',
  kali-c., kali-m.[1]', kali-p.,
  kali-sil.[1]', **lac-d., LACH.,** led.[4],
  lyc., lyss.[11], mag-c., mag-m.,
  mag-s.[4], **med.,** meny., merc.,
  merl., mez., morph.[11], **MUR-AC.,**
  narcin.[11], **nat-ar., nat-c.,**
  nat-hchls., **nat-m.,** nat-n.[11], **nat-s.,**
  nat-sil.[1]', nicot.[11], **NIT-AC.,**
  nux-m., nux-v.[4], pall., petr.,
  PH-AC., PHOS., phys., phyt.,
  PIC-AC., plb., polyg-h., **PSOR.,**
  puls., puls-n., ran-b.[4, 11], rheum,
  rhod., rhus-d.[8], **RHUS-T.,** ruta,
  sabin., sarcol-ac.[8], **SEP., sil.,**
  spig.[1], **SQUIL.,** stann., **staph.,**

stram., stront-c.[4], sul-i.[1]', **SULPH.,**
sumb., tarent., tell., thea[4], thuj.,
til., tril., tub.[1]', **verat.,** wies.[11],
wildb.[11], **zinc.,** zinc-p.[1]'

*w.-afternoon – walking/f.-après-
  midi – marcher/Sch.-nach-
  mittags – Gehen*

am.
  ambr.[16], anac., bry.[16], calc.[11, 16],
  coloc., merc., nat-m., **RHUS-T.,**
  ruta, SULPH.

*w.-daytime – walking/f.-journée –
  marcher/Sch.-tagsüber – Gehen*

air, in open
air, en plein
Freien, im
  act-sp., agar., **ALUM.,** alumn.[2],
  am-c., ambr., ang.[16], arg-m.,
  ars-s-f.[1]', berb.[4], bry., **calc.,**
  calc-sil.[1]', carb-v., caust.,
  chin.[4], coff., chel., **cocc.**[1], **coll.,**
  coloc.[4, 16], **con.,** euph.[4, 16], ferr.,
  graph., grat.[4], hep., hyos.,
  kali-bi., kali-c., lact., lyc.[4, 16],
  m-arct.[4], m-aust.[4], mag-c.,
  mag-m.[4], merc., nat-m., **nux-v.,**
  ph-ac.[4], puls., rhod., **RHUS-T.,**
  sang., sep., **sil., spig.,** sulph.,
  zinc.

am.
  agar., am-c., asar.[14], caust.,
  chin-s.[4], croc.[4], **fl-ac.,** grat.[4],
  kali-i., ox-ac., sapin.[11], **sulph.**

after w. in open air[16]
après la marche en plein air
nach dem G. im Freien
  graph., sil.

breakfast am., after
petit déjeuner am., après le
Frühstück am., nach dem
  coca

commencing to walk, on
commencement de, au
Beginn des, im
   carb-v.

cough and expectoration, from
toux et expectoration, par
Husten und Auswurf, durch
   nux-v.

dinner, before[11]
déjeuner, avant le
Mittagessen, vor dem
   hyper.

   w.-dinner/f.-déjeuner/Sch.-
   Mittagessen

eating, after[11]
mangé, après avoir
Essen, nach dem
   hep.

   w.-eating/f.-manger/Sch.-Essen

heat of the sun, in
chaleur au soleil, dans la
Sonnenhitze, in der
   lach., nat-c.

   w.-heat – sun/f.-chaleur – soleil/
   Sch.-Hitze – Sonnenhitze

house, in the
maison, dans la
Hause, im
   agar., ferr-ma., sapin.[11], sec.,
   sumb.

menses, during
menstruation, pendant la
Menses, während der
   murx.[2], phel.

rapidly
vite, marche
schnelles
   agar., coc-c., olnd.

   am.
   stann.

riding, after
voiture ou à cheval, après avoir
   été en
Reiten und Fahren, nach
   petr.

   w.-riding/f.-voiture/Sch.-Fahren

short walk, from[2]
courte promenade, par une
kurzen Gang, durch einen
   calc., cann-i., **con.**

   after a[2]/après une/nach einem
   nat-c., ruta, **sulph., ter.,** tub.[1, 7]

slowly am.
lente am., promenade
langsames G. am.
   ferr.

smoking, after
fumé, après avoir
Rauchen, nach
   sulph.

   w.-smoking/f.-fumer/Sch.-
   Rauchen
   w.-tobacco/f.-tabac/Sch.-Tabak

storm, before and during a
tempête, avant et pendant une
Sturm, vor und während
   sil.

warm room, in
chaude, dans une chambre
warmen Zimmer, im
   aloe, ambr., croc., **iod.,** merl.,
   PULS.

   w.-heat – room/f.-chaleur –
   chambre/Sch.-Hitze – Zimmer

weather agg.
temps chaud agg.
Wetter agg., warmes
   ANT-C., camph.[3], **iod.,** lach.[3],
   nat-ar., nat-c.[3], nat-m., nat-p.,
   podo.[3], **sel., SULPH.**[1], vip.[11]

wine agg.[1] (non: am.)
vin agg.
Wein agg.
  ars., lyc., phos., **thuj.**

am.[11]
  ars., **thuj.,** visc.[14]

worms, with[2]
vers, avec
Würmern, bei
  cic., **cina, merc.**

writing, from
écrire, par
Schreiben, durch
  cann-s., ran-b., sil.

yawning, after
bâillement, après
Gähnen, nach
  eug., **nux-v.**

WEARINESS
FATIGUE
MÜDIGKEIT
  acon., adlu.[14], aesc., agar., **ALUM.,**
  alum-p.[1'], **am-c.,** ambr., **anac.,**
  ang.[3, 4], **anh.**[9, 10], **ant-c., ant-t.,**
  aphis[4], aran.[4], aran-ix.[10], arg-m.,
  arg-n., arist-cl.[9, 10], **arn., ars., ars-i.,**
  asaf., asar., aur., aur-ar.[1'], aur-m.,
  aur-s.[1'], **bapt.,** bar-c., bar-m., bell.,
  bell-p.[9, 10], **BENZ-AC.,** berb.,
  beryl.[9], bism., bor.[3, 4], bov., bruc.[4],
  bry., cadm-met.[9, 10], calad.[4], **calc.**[1'],
  calc-f.[9], **CALC-P., calc-sil.**[1'], camph.,
  CANN-S., canth., caps., **carb-ac.,**
  carb-an., **carb-v., CARBN-S.,** carc.[9],
  caust.[1], cecr.[14], cench.[1'], cham.,
  CHEL., chin., cic., cimic., cimx.,
  cina, cist.[4], clem., cob-n.[9, 10],
  coc-c., cocc., coff., colch., coloc.,
  con., cortico.[9], cortiso.[9], **CROC.,**
  crot-c., cupr., cycl., dicha.[10], dig.,
  dros., dulc., erig.[10], esp-g.[10, 13],
  euph., euphr., **FERR.,** ferr-ma.[4],
  ferr-p., **GELS.,** gran.[4], **GRAPH.,**
  grat.[4], guaj.[4], guat.[9], **ham.,** harp.[14],
  hecla[14], hed.[9, 10], hell., helon., **hep.,**
  hist.[9, 10], **hyos.,** ign., iod.[4], **ip.,**

kali-bi.[1', 3], kali-c., kali-chl.[4],
kali-m.[1'], kali-n., **KALI-P.,** kali-s.,
kali-sil.[1'], kalm.[1'], **kreos.,** lac-ac.,
LACH., lact.[4], **laur., LEC.**[1], led.,
luf-op.[10], **LYC.,** m-arct.[3], m-aust.[4],
mag-c., mag-f.[10], mag-m., mand.[9, 10],
mang., med.[7], meny., meph.[4, 14],
MERC., mez., mosch., **mur-ac.,**
murx.[4], naja[14], **nat-c., NAT-M.,**
nat-s., nat-sil.[1'], nep.[10], nit-ac.,
nux-m., NUX-V., ol-an.[4], olnd., op.,
par., petr., PH-AC., phenob.[13],
PHOS., phyt.[3], **PIC-AC., plat.,** plb.,
prun.[4], psil.[14], **psor., PULS.,** ran-b.,
rauw.[9], **rheum, rhod., rhus-t.,**
rib-ac.[14], **RUTA,** sabad., sabin.,
samb., saroth.[9], sars., sec., senec.,
seneg., **SEP.,** sieg.[10], **SIL.,** spig.,
spong., squil., **stann., STAPH.,**
stram., stront-c., **sul-ac.,** sulfa.[9],
SULPH., sumb., **tab.,** teucr., ther.[4],
thiop.[14], thuj., **TUB.,** v-a-b.[13], valer.,
verat., verb., viol-o., visc.[9], x-ray[9],
ZINC., zinc-p.[1']

flabby feeling/mollesse, sensation/
  Erschlaffung, Gefühl
heaviness/loudeur/Schweregefühl
lassitude/Mattigkeit
lie down/s'étendre/sich hinzulegen
relaxation/relâchement/
  Erschlaffung
weakness/faiblesse/Schwäche

morning/matin/morgens
  alum.[4], am-c., ambr., ant-c.[4], **ars.,**
  aur.[4], bar-c.[4], bell.[4], bov.[4], **bry.**[1],
  calad., carb-an.[4], **carb-v.,**
  carbn-s., cast.[6], caust.[4], **cham.,**
  chel.[4], chin.[4], cob-n.[9, 10], con.[4],
  cortiso.[9], croc.[4], dros.[4], erig.[10],
  ferr.[4], hep.[4], kali-c.[4], **kali-chl.,**
  lac-ac., **LACH.,** lact.[4], lyc.[4],
  m-aust.[4], **mag-c.**[1], mag-m.,
  meph.[14], mur-ac.[4], **nat-m.,**
  NUX-V., petr., phos.[4], prun.[4],
  puls.[4], rhus-t.[4], sabad.[4], **SEP.,**
  sil.[4], spig.[4], stann.[4], staph.,
  stront-c.[4], sul-i.[1'], **sulph.,** teucr.[4],
  ther.[4], thuj.[4], valer.[4], zinc.

rising, on[4]
se levant, en
Aufstehen, beim
   bov., ferr., hep., puls., stann.,
   teucr.

waking, on[4]
réveil, au
Erwachen, beim
   alum., am-c., ambr., ant-c., aur.,
   bar-c., bell., bism., **bry., calc.,**
   cann-s., **carb-an., caust.,** chel.,
   chin., cob-n.[9], **con.,** cycl., dros.,
   dulc., hep., kali-c., lact., **lyc.,**   ˙
   m-aust., **mag-m., nat-m., nux-v.,**
   phos., prun., rhus-t., sabad., sep.,
   spig., staph., stront-c., teucr.,
   ther., **thuj.,** valer., **zinc.**

forenoon[4]/matinée/vormittags
   am-c., erig.[10], esp-g.[13, 14], hell.,
   mag-m., nat-s., phel., seneg.

noon[13, 14]/midi/mittags
   esp-g.

afternoon[4]/après-midi/nachmittags
   adlu.[14], am-c., iod., kali-c., mag-c.,
   mag-m., nat-c., ol-an., phos., staph.,
   thuj.

   am.[14]: kali-c.

evening/soir/abends
   berb., carb-v., ign., meph.[14],
   methys.[14], **mur-ac.,** pall., **sulph.**

air, in open
air, en plein
Freien, im
   carb-v.

night[4]/nuit/nachts
   dulc., kreos., merc., sabad., sabin.

agg.[7]
   arn., ars., cann-s., chin., **coff.,**
   RHUS-T., verat.

air am., in open[9, 10]
air am., en plein
Freien am., im
   hed.

ascending stairs, from[1']
monter l'escalier, par
Treppensteigen, durch
   sul-i.

climacteric period, during[8]
ménopause, pendant la
Klimakterium, im
   bell-p., calc.

coition, after[3]
coït, après le
Koitus, nach
   agar., calc., kali-c., lyc., nit-ac., sel.

conversation, from/par
Unterhaltung, durch
   ambr.

diarrhoea, after[1']
diarrhée, après
Diarrhoe, nach
   sul-i.

eating, while
mangeant, en
Essen, beim
   kali-c.

   after/après avoir mangé/nach dem
     ant-c., **ARS., bar-c., carb-an.,**
     card-m., chin., kali-c., **lach.,**
     mur-ac., **nat-m., nux-m., rhus-t.,**
     ruta, sang.

emissions, after[3]
pertes séminales, après
Samenverlusten, nach
   chin., led., plb., puls., sabad., staph.

exertion, from mental
travail intellectuel, par
Anstrengung, durch geistige
   alum., **aur., lach., LEC., PIC-AC.,**
   puls., thuj.

   Vol. I: *work–fatigues/travail–*
     fatigue/Arbeit–ermüdet

physical e. am.[9]
exercice physique am.
körperliche A. am.
 hed.

leucorrhoea with[4]
leucorrhée avec
Fluor mit
 prun.

 after[4]/après/nach
 con.

menses, before
menstruation, avant la
Menses, vor den
 alum., **bell.**, **nat-m.**

 during/pendant la/während der
  am-c., bor., calc-p., **caust.**, **ign.**,
  iod., kali-c., mag-c., **nit-ac.**,
  nux-m., petr., sul-i.[1'], thuj.

 am.[9]
 hed.

 after/après la/nach den
  alumn.[2], bell.[2, 6], carb-an.[2, 6]
  cub.[2], nat-m.[2], nux-v.[6], phos.[6],
  plat.[2, 6], thuj.

playing piano
jouer du piano, par
Klavierspielen, durch
 anac.

reading, from
lire, par
Lesen, durch
 aur.

sexual excitement, from[6]
sexuelle, par excitation
sexuelle Erregung, durch
 sars.

sit down, desire to[4]
s'asseoir, désir de
sich hinzusetzen, Bedürfnis
 dulc., stann., sulph.

sitting, while
assis, étant
Sitzen, im
 bry.[4], chin.[4], led.[4], mag-c.[4], **merc.**,
 ol-an.[4], plat.[4], plb.[4], rhus-t.[4]

standing, when
debout, étant
Stehen, beim
 led.[4], **mur-ac.**, nat-m.[4], plat.[4]

talking, after
parler, par
Reden, durch
 ALUM., **calc-p.**, **sulph.**

 much t.[16]
 beaucoup parlé, après avoir
 vieles R.
  calc.

waking, on[4]
réveil, au
Erwachen, beim
 alum., am-c., ambr., ange-s.[14],
 ant-c., aur., bar-c., bell., bism.,
 bov., **bry.**, **calc.**, cann-s., **carb-an.**,
 caust., chel., **con.**, cycl., dros., dulc.,
 ferr., lact., **lyc.**, m-aust., **mag-m.**,
 nat-m., prun., rib-ac.[14], sep., spig.,
 teucr., **thuj.**, valer., **zinc.**

 am.[14]: thiop.

walking, on[4]
marchant, en
Gehen, beim
 bry., chin., con., ferr., lach., led.,
 mag-c., mag-m., plb., stram.

 air, in open[4]
 air, en plein
 Freien, im
  alum., coff., ferr., m-arct.,
  mag-c., nat-m., rhod., sep.,
  sulph.

 am.[4]
  caust., croc., ruta, sul-ac.

after
après la marche
nach dem
    agar.[4], alum.[4], anac.[14],
    carb-an.[4], caust.[4], clem.[4], coff.[4],
    con.[4], graph.[4], iod.[4], **lac-d.**[1', 7],
    mur-ac., nux-v.[4], ph-ac.[4], plat.[4],
    sabad.[4], sabin.[4], sul-i.[1'], valer.[4]

pregnancy, in[7]
grossesse, pendant la
Schwangerschaft, in der
    calen.

WEATHER
TEMPS
WETTER

change of w. agg.
changement de t. agg.
Wetterwechsel agg.
    abrot., achy.[14], acon.[1'], alum.[1, 3, 6],
    alumn., **am-c.**[1, 7], anh.[14], ant-c.,
    ant-t., apis, aran.[3, 6, 7], ars.,
    asar.[14], bar-c.[1', 3, 6, 7], **bell.**,
    benz-ac., bor., brom., **BRY.**[1, 7],
    calc., calc-f.[1', 7, 8, 10], **calc-p.**,
    carb-v.[7, 12], carbn-s., **caust.**,
    cham.[2, 7, 11], **chel.**, chin.[7, 8], cinnb.[1'],
    colch., crot-c.[7], crot-h.[3, 6], cupr.[3, 11],
    cur.[7], **dig.**, <u>DULC.</u>[1, 7], euph.,
    galph.[14], **gels.**, **graph.**[1, 7], harp.[14],
    hep.[1, 7], hyper., **ip.**[1', 7], kali-bi.,
    kali-c., kali-i.[3, 6, 7], **kalm.**[2, 7], lach.,
    lept.[12], mag-c.[3, 6-8], mand.[14],
    mang., meli., **merc.**[1, 7], merc-i-r.[12],
    mez., mosch.[7], **nat-c.**, nat-m.[7],
    nat-p.[1'], nat-sil.[1'], nit-ac.,
    NUX-M., nux-v., **petr.**, **ph-ac.**,
    PHOS., phys.[3], phyt.[7], **PSOR.**,
    puls., **RAN-B.**, rheum[1, 7], **RHOD.**,
    <u>RHUS-T.</u>[1, 7], **rumx.**, ruta[7, 8],
    sang.[3, 6, 7], sep., **SIL.**, spig.[1', 3, 6, 7],
    stann.[1', 14], stict.[7, 8], stront-c.,
    sulph., tarent.[7, 8], **teucr.**[3],
    thuj.[3, 6, 7], **TUB.**, verat.[1, 7],
    vip.[3, 6, 7, 11]

ailments from[12]
troubles à la suite de
Beschwerden infolge von
    carb-v., merc-i-f., ran-b.

am.[14]: onop.

spring, in[8]
printemps, au
Frühling, im
    all-c., ant-t., gels., kali-s., nat-s.

cold to warm agg.
du froid au chaud agg.
von kalt zu warm agg.
    ant-c.[3, 6], brom.[1'], **BRY.**, carb-v.,
    chel., crot-h.[3, 6], **ferr.**, gels.,
    KALI-S., lach., lyc., nat-c.[3, 6],
    nat-m., **nat-s.**, nux-v.[3, 6], **PSOR.**,
    puls., sep.[3, 6], **SULPH.**, **TUB.**

warm to cold agg.[3, 6]
du chaud au froid agg.
von warm zu kalt agg.
    acon.[3], **ars.**, calc.[1'], calc-p.[1'],
    calc-sil.[1'], carb-v., **caust.**,
    DULC.[1', 3, 6, 15], hep.[1'], **MERC.**[15],
    nat-sil.[1'], nit-ac.[1'], **nux-v.**, puls.,
    ran-b.[1', 3, 6], rhus-t.[15], sabad., **sil.**,
    stront-c., tub.[1'], **VERAT.**[15]

clear w. agg.
beau t. agg.
schönes W. agg.
    acon., aloe[7], asar., **bry.**, **caust.**,
    hep., **nux-v.**, plb., sabad., spong.

cloudy w. agg.
nuageux agg.
wolkiges W. agg.
    aloe[3], am-c., ammc.[3], aran.[3],
    arn.[3], ars.[3], aur.[3], bar-c.[3], ben-n.[3],
    bry., calc., calen.[3, 7], **cham.**, **chin.**,
    dulc., hyper.[3], gels.[3], lach.[1'],
    mang., merc., naja[3], nat-c.[3],
    nat-m.[3], nat-s.[3], **nux-m.**, phys.[3],
    plb., **puls.**, rhod., **RHUS-T.**,
    sabin.[3], sang.[3], **sep.**, stram.[3],
    sulph., verat., viol-o.[3]

am.[3]
caust.

cold dry w. agg.
sec et **froid** agg.
trocken-kaltes W. agg.
 abrot.[8], **ACON.**, aesc.[8], agar.[8],
 alum.[1', 3, 8], alumn.[2], am-c.[4],
 apoc.[8], **ars.**, ars-i.[3], **ASAR.**, aur.[8],
 bac.[8], **bar-c.**[8], bell., bor., **bry.**,
 calc.[1', 4, 8], calc-i.[1'], calc-p.[1'],
 camph.[4, 8], caps.[4, 8], carb-an.,
 carb-v., **CAUST.**, cham., **chin.**[8],
 cist.[8], coc-c.[1'], cocc.[4], coff.[1'],
 crot-h., cupr.[8], cur.[8], daph.[4],
 dulc.[1', 4, 8], euph.[8], ferr-ar.[1'],
 fl-ac.[3], **HEP.**, ign.[8], **ip.**, **KALI-C.**,
 kali-sil.[1'], kreos.[8], lach.[4], lappa[3],
 laur., lyc.[4], mag-c., mag-p.[8],
 med.[3], mez., mur-ac., nat-c.[8],
 nat-s.[3], nit-ac.[1', 3, 4], nit-s-d.[8],
 nux-m.[1', 4], **NUX-V.**, **petr.**[8],
 ph-ac.[4], phos.[1', 4], phys.[3],
 physal.[3], phyt.[1'], plat.[3], plb.[3, 8],
 psor.[1', 8], **puls.**[3], rhod., rhus-t.[4, 8],
 rumx.[8], sabad., sel.[8], sep., **sil.**,
 spig., **spong.**, staph., sulph., tub.[8],
 urt-u.[8], **verat.**[2], viol-o.[8], visc.[8],
 zinc.

 am.
 led.[3, 6], sil.[1']

cold wet w.
froid et **humide** agg.
naßkaltes W. agg.
 abrot.[1'], aesc.[1'], **agar.**,
 all-c.[3, 6, 12], all-s., **AM-C.**,
 ant-c., **ant-t.**[1', 3, 8], **apis**, **aran.**,
 arg-m., **arg-n.**, arn.[8], **ARS.**,
 ars-i., ars-s-f.[1'], asc-t., **aster.**,
 aur., aur-ar.[1'], **aur-m-n.**,
 BAD., **bar-c.**, bar-i.[1'], bar-s.[1'],
 bell., bell-p.[10], bor.[1], bov.,
 bry., **CALC.**, **CALC-P.**, calc-s.,
 calc-sil.[1'], **calen.**[7], canth.,
 caps.[3, 6], carb-an., **carb-v.**,
 carbn-s., cham., chin., **cimic.**[1],
 clem., **COLCH.**, coloc.[3], con.,
 cupr., **DULC.**, elaps[3, 6], erig.[6],
 eucal.[3, 6], **ferr.**, **fl-ac.**, **form.**,
 gels., glon.[3], **graph.**, **guaj.**[8],
 hep., **hyper.**, **iod.**, ip., **kali-bi.**,
 kali-c., kali-i., kali-m.[1'], kali-n.,

kali-p., kali-sil.[1'], **lach.**, **lath.**,
laur., lept.[3, 6], **lyc.**, mag-c.,
mag-p.[1'], **mang.**, **MED.**, **merc.**,
merc-c.[3], merc-i-f., **mez.**,
mur-ac., naja[14], **nat-ar.**, **nat-c.**,
nat-m.[3, 6], **NAT-S.**, **nit-ac.**,
NUX-M., nux-v., onop.[14],
paeon., penic.[13, 14], **petr.**, phos.,
physal.[8], **phyt.**, polyg-h.[7],
psor.[1'], **puls.**, **PYROG.**, ran-b.,
RHOD., **RHUS-T.**, rumx.[3, 6],
ruta, sars., seneg., sep., **SIL.**,
spig., stann., staph., **still.**[3, 6],
stront-c., **sul-ac.**, **sulph.**,
tarent., teucr.[3], thuj., **TUB.**,
urt-u.[8], **verat.**, zinc., zinc-p.[1'],
zing.[3, 6]

night and warm days in autumn
 agg.[8]
nuit et **jours chauds** en automne
 agg.
nachts und **warme Tage** im
 Herbst agg.
 merc.

old people, in[12]
personnes âgées, chez les
Alter, im
 ammc.

ailments from[12]
troubles à la suite de
Beschwerden infolge von
 all-c., dulc., gels., lath., merc-i-f.,
 phyt.

 am.[1']
 aur-m.

dry w. agg.
sec agg.
trockenes W. agg.
 acon.[2], alum., alumn.[2], ars.,
 ASAR., bell.[2], bor.[2], **bry.**,
 carb-an., carb-v., **CAUST.**,
 cham.[2], **HEP.**, ip.[2], **kali-c.**, laur.[2],
 mag-c.[2], mez.[2], mur-ac.[2], **NUX-V.**,
 phos., rhod.[2], sabad., **sep.**, sil.,
 spig.[2], spong., staph., sulph., zinc.

am.²
  agar., **am-c.**²˒ ⁸, **ant-c., aur.,** bar-c.,
  bell., **bor.,** bov., bry., **CALC.**²˒ ⁸,
  canth., **carb-an., carb-v.,** cham.,
  chin., clem., con., **cupr., DULC.,**
  ferr., hep., ip., kali-c.²˒ ⁸, **kali-n.,**
  lach., laur., lyc., mag-c.,
  magn-gr.⁸, **mang., merc.,** merc-c.,
  mez., moly-met.¹⁴, **mur-ac.,**
  nat-c., nit-ac., NUX-M., nux-v.,
  petr.²˒ ⁸, phos., **puls., rhod.,**
  RHUS-T., ruta, sars., seneg.,
  sep., sil., **spig.,** stann., **staph.,**
  still.⁸, **stront-c., sul-ac., sulph.,**
  verat., zinc.

dry warm w. agg.⁶
sec et **chaud** agg.
trocken-warmes W. agg.
  ant-c., carb-v., cocc., lach.

ailments from¹²
troubles à la suite de
Beschwerden infolge von
  ant-c., kali-bi., lach.

am.⁸
  alum., **calc-p.,** nat-s., nux-m.³˒ ⁶˒ ⁸,
  penic.¹³˒ ¹⁴, rhus-t., **sulph.**³˒ ⁶˒ ⁸

foggy w. agg.
brumeux, brouillard agg.
nebliges W. agg.
  abrot.⁶, aloe³, **aran.**³˒ ⁶, ars.³, bapt.⁸,
  bar-c.⁶, bry., calc.³, calen.³, cham.,
  chin., dulc.³˒ ⁶, **gels.**³˒ ⁸, **HYPER.,**
  mang., merc.³, mosch., nat-m.³,
  nat-s.³˒ ⁶, nux-m., plb., **rhod.,**
  RHUS-T., sep., **sil.,** sulph., **thuj.**³˒ ⁶,
  verat.

frosty w., hoarfrost agg.³
glacial, givre agg.
Frost, Rauhreif agg.
  agar., calc., carb-v., caust., **CON.,**
  lyc., mag-m., merc., nat-c., nux-v.,
  ph-ac., phos., **puls.,** rhus-t., **SEP.,**
  sil., sulph., syph.

hot w. agg.⁸
très chaud agg.
heißes W. agg.
  acon.¹˒ ⁸, aeth.¹˒ ⁸, aloe⁶˒ ⁸,
  ant-c.³˒ ⁶˒ ⁸, ant-t.⁶, **apis**⁶, bapt.⁶,

bell., bor., brom.¹′, **bry.**³˒ ⁶˒ ⁸,
carb-v.³, cocc.³, croc., **crot-h.**⁶˒ ⁸,
crot-t., **cupr.**⁶, **gels., glon.,** hep.³,
kali-bi.¹′˒ ⁸, **lach.**³˒ ⁶˒ ⁸, **nat-c.,**
nat-m., nat-s.¹′, nit-ac., **op.**⁶,
phos.³˒ ⁶˒ ⁸, pic-ac., **podo., puls.**³˒ ⁸,
sabin., sel.³˒ ⁶˒ ⁸, syph.

and cold night³
et nuits fraîches
und kalte Nächte
  acon.

ailments from¹²
troubles à la suite de
Beschwerden infolge von
  ant-c., kali-bi., lach.

rain, agg. during³
pluie, agg. pendant la
Regen, agg. während des
  aran., elaps., erig., glon., ham.,
  lac-c., lach.¹′, mag-c., mang.,
  merc.⁸, nat-s.¹′, oci-s.¹⁴, phyt.,
  ran-b.¹′˒ ³, **rhus-t.**¹⁵, sabin., senn.,
  tub.¹′

storm, approach of a
tempête et un orage, troubles avant
  une
Sturm, Gewitter, Beschwerden beim
  Herannahmen von
  agar., arg-m.³, **aur., bell-p.**⁸,
  berb.³, **bry.,** calc.¹′, calc-f.³,
  caust., **cedr.,** dulc.³, **gels.,**
  hep.³˒ ⁶, hyper., **kali-bi., lach.,**
  lyc., mag-p.³, mand.¹⁰, mang.¹′˒ ³,
  med., meli., **nat-c.,** nat-m., nat-p.,
  nat-s.⁸, nit-ac., petr., **phos.,**
  phyt.⁸, **PSOR.,** puls., **ran-b.,**
  RHOD., rhus-t., sep., sil., sul-ac.³,
  sulph., syph., thuj., **tub.,** zinc.³˒ ⁶

during/pendant la/beim＊
  agar., aran.³′, arg-m.⁶, aur.,
  bry., calc.⁷, carb-v., caust.,
  conv.³′, elaps¹′, erig.³′, **gels.,**
  glon.³′, ham.³′, **lach.,** mag-c.³′,
  mand.¹⁴, mang.³′, **med.,**
  morph.²˒ ¹², **NAT-C.,** nat-m.,
  nat-p., nit-ac., nit-s-d.¹², petr.,
  phos., phyt.³′˒ ⁸, prot.¹⁴, psor.,

puls.$^{2,\ 12}$, ran-b.$^{3'}$, **rhod.**,
sabin.$^{3'}$, **sep., sil.**, syph., thuj.,
tub.$^{1'}$

am.^{7}
carc., **sep.**

Vol. I: *cheerful – thunders/*
gai – orage/froh – Blitz

after/après la/nach dem
asar.^{14}, calc-p.^{3}, carc.^{7}, rhus-r.$^{3,\ 6}$,
sep.$^{3,\ 7}$, tub.$^{1'}$

ailments from^{12}
troubles à la suite de
Beschwerden infolge von
crot-h., gels., morph., nat-c.,
nat-p., nit-s-d., phos., psor.,
puls., rhod., syph.

lightning-stroke^{12}
coup de foudre
Blitzschlag
morph., phos.

warm and **wet** w. agg.
chaud et **humide** agg.
feucht-warmes W. agg.
aloe$^{3,\ 6}$, aran-ix.^{10}, bapt.^{8}, bell.^{6},
brom.$^{1',\ 3,\ 6,\ 8}$, bry.^{3}, calc-f.^{10},
CARB-V., carbn-s.$^{1',\ 3,\ 7,\ 8}$, caust.$^{1'}$,
erig.^{10}, **gels.**, ham.$^{3,\ 6-8}$, **iod., ip.**^{3},
kali-bi., LACH., lath.^{12}, lyc.^{3},
mand.^{10}, mang.$^{3,\ 6}$, merc-i-f.^{12},
nat-m.$^{3,\ 6,\ 7}$, **NAT-S.**, phos.^{8},
puls.^{3}, rhus-t.^{3}, sabad.^{3},
SEP.$^{3,\ 6,\ 8,\ 15}$, **sil., SYPH.**$^{7,\ 12}$,
tub.$^{1'}$, **verat.**^{3}, vip-a.^{14}

ailments from^{12}
troubles à la suite de
Beschwerden infolge von
carb-v., gels.

am.^{6}
aloe, bell., brom., **carb-v.**, cham.^{8},
gels., ham., hep., **ip.**, kali-c.^{8},
nat-m., sep., sil.^{8}

wet w. agg.
humide agg.
feuchtes W. agg.
achy.^{14}, agar., alum-sil.$^{1'}$, **AM-C.**,
amph.^{8}, anac.^{7}, ant-c., **ant-t.,**
ARAN.$^{1,\ 7}$, arg-m., **arg-n., ARS.,**
ars-i., ars-s-f.$^{1'}$, aster.^{8}, aur.,
BAD., bar-c., bar-m., bell.,
blatta^{12}, bor., bov., brom., bry.,
CALC., calc-f.$^{1',\ 7}$, **calc-p., calc-s.,**
calc-sil.$^{1'}$, calen.$^{7,\ 8}$, canth.,
carb-an.^{1}, **carb-v.**, caust.$^{1'}$, cham.,
chim.^{8}, chin., chin-s.^{8}, **cist.**, clem.,
colch., con., crot-h.^{8}, cupr.,
cur.$^{7,\ 8}$, **DULC.**, elaps, elat.^{8},
erig.$^{3,\ 3'}$, euphr.^{8}, **ferr.**, form.^{8},
gels.$^{2,\ 8,\ 12}$, **glon.**$^{2,\ 3}$, **graph.**$^{2,\ 3}$,
ham., hep., hyper., **iod.**, ip.,
kali-c., **kali-i.**, kali-m.$^{1'}$, kali-n.,
lac-ac.$^{2,\ 7}$, lac-c.^{3}, lac-d.$^{1'}$, **lach.**,
lath.$^{8,\ 12}$, laur., **lem-m., lyc.**, lyss.^{2},
mag-c., **mag-p.**, magn-gr.^{8}, **mang.**,
meli., **merc.**, mez., mur-ac., **naja,**
nat-ar., nat-c., NAT-HCHLS.,
NAT-S., nit-ac., NUX-M., nux-v.,
oci-s.^{9}, onop.^{14}, paeon., petr.,
phos., **phyt., PULS.**, rad-br.^{8},
ran-b., rauw.^{9}, **RHOD., RHUS-T.,**
ruta, sabin.^{3}, sang., sars., seneg.,
senn.^{3}, **sep., sil.**, sin-n.^{12}, spig.,
stann., staph., stict.^{12}, still.^{8},
stront-c., sul-ac., sul-i.$^{1'}$, **sulph.,**
sumb., syph.^{12}, teucr., **thuj., tub.,**
verat., zinc., zinc-p.$^{1'}$, zing.^{2}

am.$^{2,\ 7}$
acon.^{2}, alum.$^{1',\ 3,\ 6-8}$, alumn.^{2},
ars., ASAR.$^{2,\ 3,\ 7,\ 8}$, aur-m.^{3}, **bell.,**
bor.^{2}, bov.^{7}, **BRY., carb-an.,**
carb-v., CAUST.$^{2,\ 3,\ 6-8}$, **cham.,**
fl-ac., **HEP.**$^{2,\ 3,\ 6-8}$, **ip.**, laur., mang.,
MED.$^{7,\ 8}$, mez., mur-ac.$^{2,\ 7,\ 8}$,
nit-ac., NUX-V.$^{2,\ 3,\ 7,\ 8}$, oci-s.$^{9,\ 14}$,
plat., rhod., **sabad., sep., sil.,**
spig., **spong.**, staph., sulph., zinc.

wind
vent, troubles par
Wind, Beschwerden im
acon., anac.^{4}, **ars.**, ars-i., arum-t.^{8},
asar., **aur.**$^{1,\ 7}$, aur-ar.$^{1'}$, **bell.**, bry.,
bufo, calc., **calc-p.**, canth.^{3},

caps.[3], carb-an.[3], carb-v., caust.,
CHAM., chin., coff.[1', 7], colch.[3],
coloc.[3], con., cupr., elaps, **euphr.,**
graph., **HEP.**[3, 8], hyos.[3], ip.[3, 7],
kali-c.[3], **lach.,** LYC., mag-c.[3, 8],
mag-p.[1'], med.[3], mur-ac., nat-c.,
nit-ac.[3, 16], **nux-m.**[1, 7], **NUX-V.,**
ph-ac.[3], **PHOS.,** plat., **psor.,**
PULS., rheum[3], **RHOD., rhus-t.**[3],
sabad.[3], samb.[3], sel.[3], sep.[3, 4, 6],
sil.[3], spig., **SPONG.**[3], squil.[3],
stram.[3], stront-c.[3], sul-ac., sulph.,
tab.[3], thuj., tub.[3], verb.[3], zinc.

ailments from[12]
troubles à la suite de
Beschwerden infolge von
    kalm.

am.[3, 6]
    arg-n., ferr.[3], iod.[3], nux-m.,
    sec.[3], tub.[3]

cold
froid, bise, mistral
kalten
    acon., all-c.[2], apis[3], arn.[3], **ars.,**
    ars-i., **asar., BELL.,** bell-p.[9],
    bry., cadm-s.[7, 12], calc-p.,
    carb-an., carb-v., **caust.,**
    cham.[1], cupr., ferr-ar., **HEP.,**
    ip., **kali-bi.,** lach.[3, 6],
    mag-p.[1', 3, 12], nit-ac.[4, 7, 11, 16],
    NUX-V., psor., **rhod.**[1', 8],
    RHUS-T.[2, 3], rumx.[3], sabad.,
    sep., sil., SPONG., thlas.[3],
    tub.[7], verat.[2], zinc.[3]

ailments from[12]
troubles à la suite de
Beschwerden infolge von
    acon., bry., cadm-s., hep.,
    mag-p.

riding in, am.
aller en voiture ou à cheval au,
    am.
Fahren oder Reiten im, am.
    arg-n., tub.[1', 7, 15]

ailments from[12]
troubles à la suite d'
Beschwerden infolge von
    sang-n.

cold and wet, ailments from
froid et humide, troubles à la
    suite de
feuchtkaltem, Beschwerden infolge
    von
    all-c.[1', 12], calc.[12]

desire to be in[7]
désir d'être au
Verlangen, im W. zu sein
    tub.

sensation of
sensation comme d'un
Gefühl wie von
    agar.[1'], **camph.**[3], canth., **chel.,**
    chin.[3], **cist.**[6], cor-r., croc.[3],
    graph., lach.[6], **LYSS.,** med.[3],
    mez.[3, 6], **mosch.,** naja[3], nat-m.[3],
    nux-v., olnd., petr.[3], puls.,
    rhus-t., sabin., sep.[3], spig.,
    squil., stram., syph.[3], ther.[3],
    thuj.[6], thyr.[3]

blowing on coverd parts
soufflant sur les parties
    couvertes
bläst, der auf bedeckte Körper-
    teile
    camph.

cold/froid/kaltem
    camph., croc., **lac-d., laur.,**
    LYSS., mosch., rhus-t., samb.

warm, south
chaud, du sud
warmen Südwind
    ars-i., asar.[14], bry.[3, 6],
    carb-v.[3, 6], euphr.[3, 6], **gels.**[2, 7],
    ip., lach.[1'], nat-c.[3], rhod.[3, 6],
    sil.[3, 6]

warm and wet w. agg.[2]
chaud et humide agg.
feuchtwarmer W. agg.
    acon., HEP.

windy and **stormy** weather*
venteux et **gros** temps, troubles par
windiges und **stürmisches** Wetter
  acon., **all-c.**², **am-c.**², arg-m.¹',
  ars., asar., aur., aur-ar.¹', **BAD.**,
  bell., bry., carb-v., caust.³, **cham.**,
  chel.³, **chin.**, chin-ar., con.,
  erig.¹⁰, euphr., gels.³, graph.,
  hep., hyper.², ip.², **KALM.**², **lach.**,
  lyc., mag-c., **mag-p.**, mez.¹',
  mur-ac., nat-c., nat-m.³, nit-s-d.¹²,
  NUX-M., **nux-v.**, petr., **phos.**,
  plat., **psor.**, **puls.**, ran-b.¹', ⁸,
  RHOD., rhus-t., ruta, **sep.**, spig.,
  sul-ac., sulph., tab.³, thuj.

ailments from¹²
troubles à la suite de
Beschwerden infolge von
  nit-s-d., psor., rhod.

WET
HUMIDITÉ
NÄSSE

applications
applications humides, troubles par
Umschläge, Beschwerden durch
feuchte
  AM-C., am-m., **ANT-C.**, bar-c.,
  bell., bor., bov., bry., **CALC.**,
  cann-s.³, **canth.**, carb-v., **CHAM.**,
  CLEM., con., crot-h.⁸, dulc.,
  kali-c., **kali-n.**, lach.³, ⁶, ⁸, laur.,
  lyc., mag-c., **merc.**, mez., mur-ac.,
  nat-c., nit-ac., nux-m., nux-v.,
  phos., puls., **RHUS-T.**, sars., **sep.**,
  sil., **spig.**, stann., staph., **stront-c.**,
  sul-ac., **SULPH.**, zinc.

am.²
  alumn., **am-m.**, ant-t., **ars.**,
  ASAR.², ³, ⁶, ⁸, bor., bry.,
  caust.², ³, ⁶, cham., **chel.**², ³, ⁶,
  euphr.², ³, ⁶, laur., **mag-c.**, mez.,
  mur-ac., **nux-v.**, **PULS.**², ³, ⁶,
  rhod., sabad., sep., **spig.**², ³, ⁶,
  staph., zinc.

cold, wet a. agg.²
froides et humides agg.
naßkalte U. agg.
  AM-C., am-m., **ANT-C.**, apoc.¹',
  ars.⁶, bar-c., **bell.**, **bor.**, bov.,
  bry., cadm-met.¹⁴, **CALC.**,
  canth., **carb-v.**, **cham.**, **CLEM.**,
  con., dulc., graph.⁶, **hep.**⁶,
  kali-c., **kali-n.**, lach.⁶, **laur.**,
  lyc., mag-c., **merc.**, **mez.**,
  mur-ac., nat-c., **nit-ac.**², ⁶,
  nux-m., nux-v., **petr.**², ⁶, ph-ac.⁶,
  phos.¹', ², **puls.**¹', ², **RHUS-T.**,
  ruta⁶, **sars.**, **sep.**, **sil.**², ⁶, **spig.**,
  stann., **staph.**, **stront-c.**, **sul-ac.**,
  SULPH., syph.¹', **zinc.**

am.⁷
  aloe⁷, alum.⁸, aml-ns., anac.¹⁴,
  apis⁷, ⁸, argn-n.⁷, ⁸, arn., aur.,
  asar.⁸, bell.⁸, bry.¹', ⁶, ⁷, ferr-p.⁸,
  fl-ac.⁶, ⁷, glon., iod.⁶, ⁷, kali-m.⁸,
  kali-p., **led.**¹', ⁶, ⁷, lyc.⁸, merc.⁸,
  nat-hchls.¹⁴, phos.⁸, pic-ac.,
  puls.⁶⁻⁸, sabin.⁸, sec.¹', ⁷, spig.⁶

warm, wet a. agg.⁶
chaudes et humides agg.
feuchtwarme U. agg.
  apis, bry., **fl-ac.**, lach.¹', ⁶, ¹⁰,
  led., phyt.¹', **puls.**, **sec.**

am.⁶
  alum-sil.¹', anac.³, ant-c.³, ⁶,
  ars.¹', ³, ⁶⁻⁸, ars-i.³, bry.⁸,
  calc-f.¹', ⁷, ⁸, coloc., fl-ac.⁷,
  hep.³, ⁶, kali-bi.³, ⁶, kali-c.³,
  lach.⁸, **mag-p.**³, ⁷, ⁸, nux-m.⁸,
  paraph.¹⁴, ph-ac., phos.¹',
  pyrog.³, rad-br.³, ⁸, **rhus-t.**³, ⁸,
  ruta, sep.⁸, **sil.**⁶, ⁷, sulfa.¹⁴,
  thiop.¹⁴, thuj., x-ray¹⁴

getting *
se mouiller, troubles par
Durchnässung, Beschwerden von
  acon.³, **ALUM.**³, am-c., ant-c.,
  ant-t.², ³, **apis**, arn.³, ars.,
  bell., bor., **bry.**, **CALC.**,
  calc-p., **calc-s.**, camph., carb-v.,
  CAUST., cham.⁶, chin., **colch.**,
  dulc., euph., fl-ac.³, **hep.**, hyos.³,

ip., kali-bi.³, **kali-c.**³, lach., **lyc.**,
malar.¹², merc-i-r.¹², nat-m.³,
NAT-S.³, ⁶, nit-ac., **nux-m.**,
nux-v.³, phos., phyt.³, **PULS.**,
ran-b.⁶, rhod.¹², **RHUS-T., sars.**,
sec., **SEP., sil.**³, sulph., thuj.⁶,
urt-u.³, verat., visc.¹², xan.¹²,
zinc.

feet, from wet
pieds, les
Füße, nasse
   agn., **all-c., bar-c.**³, bry.³,
   calc.², ³, ⁸, ¹⁶, **camph.**³, caps.³,
   cham., **colch.**³, cupr.³, **dulc.**,
   fl-ac.³, graph.³, ⁶, guaj.³, **lach.**³,
   lob.¹², lem-m.³, **lyc.**³, merc.,
   nat-c., nat-m., nit-ac.³, **nux-m.**,
   NUX-V.³, phos., **PULS., rhus-t.**,
   sep., SIL., stram.³, **sulph.**⁶,
   tub.³, xan.

   am.³
      calad., led., puls.

head, from wet
tête, la
Kopf, von nassem
   bar-c., **BELL.,** hep.³, hyos.³, led.,
   phos.³, **puls.,** rhus-t.¹², **sep.**³

heated, when
s'échauffe, lorsqu'on
erhitzt, wenn
   bell-p.⁹, ¹², rhus-t.¹²

perspiration, during
transpiration, pendant la
Schwitzen, beim
   acon., ant-c.³, ars.³, **bell-p.**³, ¹²,
   bry.³, calc., **clem.**³, colch., con.³,
   dulc., nat-c.³, **nux-m., RHUS-T.,**
   sep., verat-v.²

rooms, in wet²
chambres humides, dans des
Räumen, in feuchten
   aloe, ant-t.⁸, **aran.**³, ⁶⁻⁸, **ARS.**², ⁸,
   ars-i.⁸, atro., **bry., calc.**², ³, ⁶, ⁸,
   calc-p.⁶, calc-sil.⁸, **carb-an.,**
   carb-v.³, caust., **DULC.**¹'⁻³, ⁶, ⁸,
   form., lyc., nat-n.⁶, **NAT-S.**¹', ³, ⁶, ⁸,

nit-ac.⁶, nux-m.⁸, **PULS.**², ³,
rhod.³, **rhus-t.**¹', ³, ⁸, **sel., sep.,**
sil.³, **stram.,** ter.⁸, ¹², **thuj.**³, ⁶,
verat.³

sheets, ailments from wet¹²
draps de lit humides, troubles à la
   suite
Bettüchern, Beschwerden infolge
   von feuchten
   rhus-t.

WHITENESS of parts usually red
PALEUR, blancheur de parties
   habituellement rouges
BLÄSSE, weiße Farbe gewöhnlich
   roter Teile
   ambr., **ars.,** anac.³, ang.³, **BOR., calc.,**
   canth., caust., coloc.³, **ferr., HELL.,**
   kali-c., lac-d.³, lyc., **MERC., merc-c.,**
   nat-c.³, **nit-ac., nux-v., olnd.,** op.,
   petr., phos., **plb.,** puls.³, sabin.³, **sec.,**
   sep., **staph., sul-ac.,** sulph., valer.,
   verat., viol-t.³, **zinc.**

WHOOPING-COUCH, ailments after⁷
COQUELUCHE, troubles après
KEUCHHUSTEN, Beschwerden nach
   sang.

wine see food–wine

winter see seasons–winter

WORMS, ailments from¹²
VERS, troubles à la suite de
WÜRMERN, Beschwerden infolge von
   cina, sabad.

   under the skin, sensation
   sous la peau, sensation de
   unter der Haut, Gefühl von
      COCAIN.

WOUNDS
PLAIES
WUNDEN
   anag.¹², **apis,** arist-cl.⁹, ¹⁰, **arn.,**
   ars.⁶, ¹², bell-p.⁶, ⁹, ¹⁰, bor., bor-ac.¹²,
   bov.¹², bry.¹², bufo⁶, calc-p.⁶,

calen.[1',6,7,10,12], carb-ac.[7], carb-v.,
cham.[10], cic., cist.[6], con., croc.,
echi.[6,10], erig.[12], ery-a.[12], eup-per.[12],
ferr-p.[12], ham.[6,10,12], helia.[7,12],
hell.[12], hep., **hyper.**[6,12], iod.,
kali-p.[12], kreos., **lach.**, lappa[10],
LED., merc., mez., mill.[6,10],
nat-c., nat-m., nit-ac., ph-ac., **phos.**,
phys.[12], plan.[12], plb., **puls.**, rhus-t.,
ruta, sec.[6,8], senec.[12], seneg., sil.,
staph., stront-c.[6], **sul-ac.**, sulph.,
symph.[6,12], zinc., zinc-m.[12]

ailments from[12]
troubles à la suite de
Beschwerden infolge von
    arn., bry., calen., ferr-p., hyper.,
    kali-p., led., phos., plan., senec.

bites[2,4]
morsures
Bißwunden
    acet-ac.[1'], all-s.[2], **arn.**, grind.[12],
    hyper.[2,12], **led.**[1',2,12], **plan.**[2],
    sul-ac.

ailments from[12]
troubles à la suite de
Beschwerden infolge von
    hyper., led.

dogs, of
chiens, de
Hundebisse
    hyper.[1'], **lach.**[2,12], led.[12]
    LYSS.[2,10,12], **ter.**[2]

ailments from[12]
troubles à la suite de
Beschwerden infolge von
    lyss.

rabid[7]
enragés
tollwütiger Hunde
    arist-cl.[9], ars., bell., canth.,
    chr-ac.[2], echi.[12], hyos., **lyss.**[7,10]

poisonous animals, of
venimeux, d'animaux
giftiger Tiere
    am-c.[1',2,4], apis, arn., ars.,

aur., bell., calad., **caust.**[2,4],
cedr., echi., hyper., **lach.**,
LED., lob-p.[7], **lyss.**[2], nat-m.[2,4],
puls.[2,4], **seneg.**[1,7], stram.,
sul-ac.

ailments from[12]
troubles à la suite de
Beschwerden infolge von
    seneg.

snakes, of[7]
serpents, de
Schlangenbisse
    anag.[2,12], **apis.**, arist-cl.[9], arn.,
    ars.[2,7], aur., **bell.**[2,7], calad.,
    camph.[2,12], **cedr.**[2,7,12], **echi.**[7,12],
    gua., gymne.[12], hyper., **LACH.**,
    LED., lob-p.[12], lycps.[12],
    plan.[7,12], seneg.[2,7,12], stram.,
    sul-ac., **thuj.**[1',7], **vip.**

ailments from[12]
troubles à la suite de
Beschwerden infolge von
    lob-p., plan.

chronic sequel[2]
effets chroniques
chronische Folgen
    merc., ph-ac.

tarentula, of[12]
tarentule, de
Tarantel, der
    lycps.

black[2]
noires
schwarze
    chin., lach., trach.[11], vip.[11]

bleeding freely
saignant largement
bluten stark
    acon.[3,4], am-c.[3',7], ant-t.[4], aran.,
    arn., ars.[4], asaf.[4], bell-p.[10],
    bor.[4], both.[11], **carb-v.**, caust.[4],
    cench., **chin.**[3,4], clem.[4], con.[4],
    cop.[2,4], croc., crot-h., **dor.**[7],
    eug.[4], **euphr.**[4], ferr., ferr-p.[3],
    ham.[3,7,8], hep., **HIR.**[7], **hydr.**[1',2],

kreos., **LACH., LAT-M.**[7], led.[1'],
merc., mez.[4], mill., **nat-c.**[4],
nat-m., **NIT-AC.**[3', 4, 7], **nux-m.**[4],
nux-v.[4], **ph-ac.**[1, 7], **PHOS.**, plb.[4],
puls., rhus-t., ruta[4], sec.[2, 3'], sep.[4],
sil.[4], **staph.**[4], sul-ac., **sulph.**, vip.[4],
zinc.

black blood[11]
noirâtre, sang
schwarzes Blut
   vip.

small w.
petites, p.
kleine W.
   am-c., carb-v.[6], hydr.[1'],
   kreos.[1', 6, 7], lach.[1'], ph-ac.[6],
   phos.[1', 16], sul-ac.[6], **zinc.**[6]

bluish[2, 8]
livides
bläuliche
   apis[2], **lach.**, lyss., **vip.**[11]

burning[4]
brûlantes
brennende
   acon., arn., **ars.**, bry., **carb-v.**,
   caust., hyper.[1'], merc., mez., nat-m.,
   rhus-t., **sul-ac., sulph.**, zinc.[7]

cold, become
froides, deviennent
kalt, werden
   led.

constitutional effects of
constitutionnels des, effets
konstitutionelle Folgen der
   arn., carb-v., con., hep., **iod., lach.,**
   LED., nat-m., **nit-ac., phos.**, puls.,
   rhus-t., **staph., sul-ac.**, zinc.

corrosive, gnawing[16]
corrosives, rongeantes
ätzende
   mez.

crushed and lacerated finger-ends
écrasement, bout du doigt dilacéré
   par
Quetsch- und Rißwunden der
   Fingerspitzen
   arist-cl.[9], **carb-ac.**[7], **HYPER.**, led.,
   ruta[3, 7]

cuts
coupures
Schnittwunden
   arn., calen.[1', 2, 7, 8], **carb-v.**[2],
   cic.[2], con.[2], dig.[2], **ham.**[2, 7, 8], hep.[2],
   hyper.[7, 8], kali-m.[12], **lach.**[2], **led.**[1],
   merc., nat-c., **nit-ac.**[2], ph-ac.,
   plan.[12], plb.[2, 3, 4], sil., **STAPH.**,
   sul-ac., sulph.

ailments from[12]
troubles à la suite de
Beschwerden infolge von
   kali-m., plan., staph.

dissecting
dissection, blessures anatomiques,
   par
Sektionsverletzung
   anthraci., **apis, ars.**, crot-h.[7, 8],
   echi.[7, 8], ham.[2], kreos.[8], **lach.**, led.,
   pyrog., ter.[2]

   ptomaine poisoning/ptomaïnes,
      empoisonnement/Ptomaine,
      Vergiftung

   ailments from[12]
   troubles à la suite de
   Beschwerden infolge von
      pyrog.

foreign bodies, from*
étrangers, par corps
Fremdkörper, durch
   arn.[7], **hep.**[1', 2], **lob.**[7, 12], **SIL.**[2, 7, 12]

ailments from[12]
troubles à la suite de
Beschwerden infolge von
   lob., sil.

gangrenous[2, 4]
gangreneuses
Wundgangrän
   acon., am-c., **anthraci.**[2], **ARS., bell.,**
   brom.[2], calen.[7, 8], **carb-v., chin.,**
   eucal.[2], euph., **LACH.**[1', 2, 4],
   sal-ac.[7, 8], sec.[2], **sil.,** sul-ac.[7, 8],
   trach.[11], vip.[11], vip-a.[14]

granulations, proud flesh[2]
granulations, bourgeonnements des
chairs
Granulationen
   alum.[3], **alumn., anac., ant-t., ARS.,**
   calc., calen.[1', 2, 8], carb-v.[3], cund.,
   hep.[3], hydr.[1'], **kali-m.,** kreos.[3],
   lach., merc.[1'], nit-ac.[3, 8], **sabin.**[7, 8],
   SIL.[3, 7, 8], sulph.[4], thuj.[8]

greenish[7]
verdâtres
grünliche
   senec.

gunshot[2, 3, 4]
coup de feu
Schußwunden
   ARN.[2, 3, 4, 7, 8], calen.[7, 8], **euphr.,**
   hyper.[2, 12], **nit-ac.**[2, 3], **plb.,** puls.,
   ruta, **sul-ac.,** sulph., symph.[12]

heal, quick tendency to[2, 10, 12]
guérir vite, tendance à
Heilungstendenz, schnelle
   lyss.

   slow/lente à/langsame
   all-c.[2, 7], alum., alum-p.[1'],
   alum-sil.[1'], am-c., ars.[1'], **bar-c.,**
   bor., both.[11], **calc., carb-v.,** caust.,
   cham., chel., clem.[4], con.,
   cortiso.[14], croc.[4], crot-h., **graph.,**
   hell.[4], **HEP.,** hyper.[1'], kali-c.,
   LACH., lyc., lyss.[10], mag-c.,
   mang., **merc., merc-c.,** mur-ac.,
   nat-c.[4], **NIT-AC.,** nux-v.[4], **PETR.,**
   ph-ac., phos., plb., puls., **rhus-t.,**
   sars.[1'], sep., **SIL.,** squil.[4], **staph.,**
   SULPH., tub.[7]

inflammation see inflammation–
wound

injection, from painful[7]
piqûres médicamenteuses
douloureuses, par
Injektion, durch schmerzhafte
   crot-h., led.

lacerations[7, 8]
lacérations
Rißwunden
   arist-cl.[10], arn., **CALEN.**[1'-3, 6-8, 12],
   CARB-AC., ham.[2, 7, 8],
   hyper.[1', 2, 3, 7, 8], led.,
   staph.[1', 2, 3, 7, 8], sul-ac.,
   symph.

   ailments from[12]
   troubles à la suite de
   Beschwerden infolge von
   calen.

lead colored
plombées
bleifarbige
   lach.[2], vip.[11]

painful
douloureuses
schmerzhafte
   all-c.[7], am-c.[4], **apis,** arist-cl.[9], bell.[4],
   calc.[2], calc-f.[2], calen.[2], cham.[2],
   con.[4], croc.[4], crot-h.[11], eug.[2, 4, 11],
   hep.[4], **HYPER.,** led., nat-c.[2, 8],
   nat-m., **nit-ac.,** nux-v., **ph-ac.**[2, 4],
   STAPH., sulph.

   w.-pulsating/p.-pulsatives/W.-
   klopfende
   w.-stinging/p.-piquantes/W.-
   Stechen

penetrating, punctured
pénétrantes
tiefdringende, punktförmige
   APIS, aran.[12], arn.[3], **carb-v.,** cic.,
   hep., **hyper.,** lach.[12], **LED.,**
   NIT-AC., phase.[7, 8, 12], plan.[3, 12],
   plb., sil., sul-ac.[3], sulph.

   stab/poignard/Stichwunden

ailments from[12]
troubles à la suite de
Beschwerden infolge von
   lach., led., plan.

palms and soles, of
paume de la main et des plantes
   du pied, des
Handteller und Sohlen, der
   HYPER., LED.[1, 7]

poisonous plants, from[7]
plantes vénéneuses, par
Giftpflanzen, durch
   echi.

pulsating[4]
pulsatives
klopfende
   bell., cham., clem., **hep., merc.,**
   mez.[16], **puls., sulph.**

reactionless[3]
sans réaction
reaktionslose
   ars., camph., carb-v., con., laur.,
   op., ph-ac., sulph.

reopening of old[3, 4, 6]
réouverture de vieilles
Wiederaufbrechen alter
   asaf.[1'], **carb-v., caust.**[2, 3, 4, 8], con.,
   croc.[2, 3, 4], **crot-h.**[3, 4], eug.[4],
   fl-ac.[8], **glon.**[3, 4], **graph.**[8], kreos.[3],
   lach., nat-c., **nat-m., nit-ac.**[4],
   nux-v.[4], **PHOS.**[2, 3, 4, 6],
   sil.[1', 3, 4, 6, 8], **sulph., vip.**[3, 6]

   abscesses–recurrent/abcès–
      récidivants/Abszesse-
      rezidivierende

   cicatrices
   Narben
      asaf., **bor.,** calc-p., **carb-an.,**
      carb-v.[16], **caust.,** con., croc.,
      crot-h., fl-ac.[3], glon.[7], **iod., lach.,**
      nat-c., **nat-m., PHOS., SIL.,**
      sulph., **vip.**[6]

scurfiness, with[2]
escarification, avec
Schorfbildung, mit
   calen., **carb-ac., hyper.**

septic[3, 6]
septiques
septische
   ars.

splinters, from
échardes, par
Splitterverletzungen
   acon., **anag.**[2], **apis, arn., carb-v.,**
   CIC., colch., **hep., HYPER.,** lach.,
   led., lob.[12], **nit-ac.,** petr., **plat.,**
   ran-b., **sil., staph.,** sulph.

   w.-foreign bodies/p.-étrangers,
      corps/W.-Fremdkörper

   ailments from[12]
   troubles à la suite d'
   Beschwerden infolge von
      sil.

stab wounds
poignard, instrument piquant, par
Stichwunden
   acet-ac.[7], **all-c.**[2], **apis,** arn., carb-v.,
   cic., con.[3, 4], eug.[4], hep.[3, 4],
   HYPER.[3, 6, 8], lach., **LED.**[1'-3, 6-8],
   nat-m.[4], nit-ac., phase.[8], **phos.**[3],
   plb.[3, 4], **puls.**[3], **rhus-t.**[2], sep.[2, 4], **sil.,**
   staph., sul-ac.[3], sulph.[3, 4, 6]

   penetrating/pénétrantes/
      triefdringende

stinging, in
piquantes, douleurs
Stechen in
   acon., **apis,** arn., bar-c., **bell.**[4],
   bry., caust., chin.[4], clem.[4], **led.,**
   merc., mez.[4], nat-c., **nit-ac.,** sep.[4],
   sil.[4], **staph.,** sulph.

   w.-painful/p.-douloureuses/W.-
      schmerzhafte

suppurating[2]
suppurantes
eiternde
arn.[7], asaf.[2, 4], **bell.**[4], bor.[11], **bufo,**
calc., calc-f., calc-s., **calen.**[2, 7],
caust.[4], **cham., chin.**[4], **croc.**[2, 4],
echi.[7], **hep.,** lach.[4], led.[7], **merc.**[4],
nat-m., plb.[2, 4], **puls.**[2, 4], **sil., sulph.**[4],
vip-a.[14]

abscesses/abcès/Abszesse

swelling of[2, 3, 4]
tuméfaction des
Schwellung der
acon.[2], **arn., bell., bry.,** kali-m.[2],
nux-v., **puls., rhus-t.,** sul-ac.,
sulph., vip.[11]

YAWNING agg.[3]
BAILLEMENT agg.
GÄHNEN agg.
acon., agar., am-c., am-m., anac.,
ant-t., arg-m., **arn.,** ars., aur., bar-c.,

bell., bor., bry., calad., calc., canth.,
caps., carb-an., **caust., chel.,** chin.,
CINA, cocc., croc., cycl., dig., ferr.,
graph., hep., **IGN.,** ip., kali-c.,
KREOS., laur., lyc., mag-c., mag-m.,
mang., **meny.,** mez., **mur-ac.,** nat-c.,
nat-m., **NUX-V., olnd.,** op., par.,
petr., ph-ac., **phos.,** plat., puls.,
RHUS-T., ruta, sabad., **SARS.,** sep.,
sil., stann., **staph., sul-ac., sulph.,**
teucr., thuj., verat., viol-o., zinc.

after, agg.[3]
après, agg.
nach, agg.
am-m., croc., **nux-v.**

am.[3]
chin-s., croc., plat.[4], **staph.**

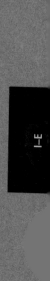

III

INDEX — ENGLISH

(Black type for the column numbers of the headings with additional references and alternating symptoms. **agg.** = ⟨. **am.** = ⟩)

abortion (+ Vol. I index, Vol. III):
  convulsions after 134
  faintness 183
  weakness after 705
adenitis → inflammation 320
alcohol 216–7
  convulsions in drunkards 111
  dropsy from 159
  paralysis after abuse 477
  trembling, dipsomania 649
  twitching, dipsomania 665
  varicose veins, dipsomania 673
  Voal. I: dipsomania **398–400**
  weakness ⟩ + dipsomania 706, 712
alternating states **31**
  change of symptoms **62**
  contradictory, altern. states **95**
  metastasis 369
apoplexy **35–6**
  convulsions after 103
  paralysis after 481
  threatening 36
  weakness 706
arteritis → inflammation 316
arthritis → inflammation 321
asphyxia → death, apparent 152–3
atheroma → tumors, atheroma 660
autumn → seasons 569–570

band → constriction, band 94–5
bandaging → binding up 47
belt → constriction, belt 95
biting nails → children 64
blood → haemorrhage 288–293
  → loss of 352
  → stagnated 602
bones:
  brittle 53
  cancerous affections of 55
  caries of **58**
  constriction of, sensation 93–4
  fistulae of 214
  formication in 284
  inflammation of 317–8
  injuries of 329–330, 581
  necrosis **387–8**
  osteoma 662
  pulsation in 527
  softening **601–2**
  swelling of 622

swollen sensation of 627
  tension of 632
bursitis → inflammation 318

cars → riding 563–4
cartilages, affections **59**
  enchondroma 621
  inflammation of 318
  swelling of 622
  ulcers of 59
cellulitis → inflammation 318
change-weather → weather 751–2
childbed (+ Vol. I index, Vol. III) 63
  convulsions, puerperal 138–9
  faintness, puerperal 201
children, affections **63–4**
  biting nails 64
  chorea, grown too fast **68**
  convulsions in 105–6
  delicate, sickly 64
  dentition, difficult, slow **154–5**
  development, arrested 156
  emaciation in + appetite, ravenous 173
  growing too fast **64–5, 288**
  obesity in 394
  weakness in 708
clear weather → weather 752
climacteric period, during (+ Vol. I index, Vol. III):
  chorea 68
  convulsions 106
  faintness 186
  flushes of heat 300
  obesity 394
  reaction, lack of 557
  trembling 648
  weakness 708
  weariness 748
climbing → mountain sickness 377
cloudy weather → weather 752
coition, during, after + ⟨ (+ Vol. I index, Vol. III) 76–7
  chorea after (woman) 68
  convulsions during, after 107
  faintness during, after 186
  flushes of heat after 300
  interruptus **77**
  lassitude after 342
  orgasm of blood after 398
  paralysis after 478

1

relaxion after, physical 560
trembling after 648
vigor after, increased 607
weakness after 709
weariness after 748
cold dry weather → weather 753
cold, taking 86–7
  faintness from 186
  paralysis after 478
cold-wet weather → weather 753–4
commotion of brain 325
connective tissue → relaxation 559, 90
  lax fibre 89
crowded room → room **566**

dentition difficult (+ Vol. I index) **154–5**
  ailments from 154
  chorea in second 69
  convulsions during 110
  diarrhoea, with 155
  slow 155
  twitching during 665
  weakness in 710
dislocation → injuries 325–6
drinks → food 216–282
dry warm weather → weather 755
dry weather → weather 754–5

ebullition of blood → orgasme 396–401
electric-like → shock 578–580
emissions ⟨+⟩, seminal 174–5
  ailments 175
  chorea with pollutions 72
  faintness after 189
  lassitude from 342
  weakness after 713
  weariness after 748
e*ruptions, suppressed* 618–9
  chorea from 73
  convulsions from 127, 142
  dropsy from 159
  reaction after, lack of **558**
  weakness from 737
exanthemata, suppressed 619
  convulsions from 127
  dropsy from 160
  measles with 364
  scarlet fever with 568

fluids → loss of **352**
foggy weather → weather 755
foot, suppression of perspiration 513
  convulsions after 142
  faintness from 201
  weakness from 729

foreign bodies:
  abscesses, elimination of 18
  wounds from 768
fractures 329–330
  shock from 581
frosty weather → weather 755
full moon 369
  convulsions at 135

glands:
  abscesses of 19
  atrophy of 38
  cancerous affections of 56
  fistulae of 214
  formication in 284
  Hodgkin's disease 311
  indurations of 313–5
  inflammation of 320
  injuries of 330
  itching of 334
  pulsation in 527
  sensitiveness of 575
  swelling of 623–5
  swollen sensation of 627
  tension of 623
  ulcers of 669
growth in length too fast **288**
  children, of **64–5**
  growing pains 432
  weakness after 716
  young people, in 288

hardness → indurations 313–5
horseback → riding 563
hot weather → weather 755–6
hunger ⟨ 311–2
  ailments 312
  faintness from 193
  starving 604
  trembling 652
  weakness from 717

injuries:
  convulsions-i. **131**
  death-i., apparent 153
  shock-i. **581**
  weakness-operation **726**
intoxications, poisonings:
  aluminium 31
  arsenical 36, 487
  bromides 53
  carbon monoxide 152
  china 65
  coal gas 76
  copper fumes, vessels 148
  fish, spoiled 242

2

iodine 331
iron 332
lead **345**, 487
meat, bad 253
medicaments **364–5**
mercury 134, **368**, 487
mushrooms 386
narcotics 387
nicotinism 480, 636
ptomaine, dissecting wounds 521, **768**
purgatives 555
quinine **555**
radiotoxemie 53
sewer-gas 577
silica 592
smoke 601
sulphur 616
vegetable medicaments 365
vegetables, decayed 277

joints:
abscesses of 19
constriction of, sensation 94
dry sensation in 165
fistulae of 214
inflammation of 321–2
jerking in 336
pulsation in 527
swelling of 625–6
tension of 632–3
weakness of 718

loss of blood 351
ailments 289
anaemia after 33
congestion of blood after 91
convulsions with, after 130
faintness from 193, 195
loss of fluids **352**
ailments 352
chorea from 70
emaciation from 174
faintness from 195
nursing **393**
reaction after, lack of 558
weakness from 719
luxation → injuries 325–6
lymphangitis → inflammation 322

marasmus → emaciation 171–4
masturbation, from 363–4
chorea 70
convulsions 133
paralysis 479
weakness 720

mental exertion (+ Vol. I index e.):
convulsions after 134
faintness from meditating 195
flushes of heat from 302
lassitude from 343
trembling from 653
weakness from + ⟩ 722
weariness from 748
mercury, abuse of **368**
convulsions from 134
paralysis from 487
mother milk → suppressed 619
multiple sclerosis → sclerosis 569
muscles:
abscesses of 20
cramps of 150
induration of 315
inflammation of 322
injuries, rupture of 327, 330
jerking of 336–8
myatrophy, progresse spinal 386
relaxion of 559–560
tension of 633
weakness, muscular 723–4
music (+ Vol. I index):
chorea, m. ⟩ 71
faintness on hearing 197
trembling from 653
weakness from 724
myositis → inflammation 322

nerves:
encephaloma 661
ganglion 661
inflammation of 322
injuries of 330
neuroma 662
new moon **370**
chorea during 71
nicotinism 480, 636
nodosites → indurations 313–5
non-union of bones → injuries-bones
329–330
nursing ⟨ **393**
trembling after 653
weakness 725

old people 395–6 (+ Vol. I index)
arteriosclerosis **37**
convulsions 136
emaciation 174
obesity 395
paralysis 480
pulse, hard 540
reaction, lack of 558
weakness 726, 737–8

3

I-FR

(Graissage des numéros de colonnes pour rubriques à indications supplémentaires et symptômes alternants. **agg.** = $\langle$. **am.** = $\rangle$)

convulsions pendant la 110
diarrhée avec 155
faiblesse pendant la 710
lente 155
soubresaut pendant la 665
troubles à la suite de 154

dents, ⟨ , ⟩, en serrant 630
se brossant, ⟨ en 630
descente ⟨ , ⟩, mouvement de 155
déshabillé ⟨, après s'être 671
air, en plein 671

développement arrêté 156

diarrhée ⟩ 156
jaune ⟩ 156

distention, vaisseaux sanguins 156–7
fièvre, pendant la 157
mouvement, au 157

douleurs, troubles **401–477**
amputation, après 405
apparaissent 401–3
articulations, des 408
brûlantes 414–8
cancereuses, dans les affections 407
cartilages, des 407
constrictives **418**–421
coupantes 422–4
crampoïdes 421–2
creusantes 424–5
croissance, de 432
déchirantes 465–473
demi-sommeil, dans le 408
direction 403–5
disparaissent 402–3
échardes, sensation d' 454
écrasé, comme 422
engourdissantes 411
erratiques 475–6
fil, comme un long 473
forantes 412–3
fracturés, comme 413–4
frissons, pendant les 407
glandes, des 407–8
griffure, comme 444–5
intolérables **432**
irradiantes 444
lancinantes 473–4
localisées 410–411
meurtrissantes 445–453
mordicantes 411–412
muscles, des 408–9
ondulantes 475
os, des 406–7
paralysées, des parties 409
paralytiques 434–5
parties, des 409–**410**

périoste, du 410
pinçantes 435–7
piquantes 454–465
pressives 437–444
renvoi ⟩ 407
rongeantes 430–1
saccades, par 432–4
tendons, des 411
tiraillantes 425–430
tordantes 473–4
ulcérantes 474–5
vaisseaux sanguin, des 407

dur, lit paraît 296

eau qui gicle contre, sensation **691**
patauger dans, troubles 692
travaillant dans ⟨, troubles 692
versant de l'e. ⟨, en 692
voir, entendre de l'e. courante ⟨ **691**–2

s'échauffe, ⟨ lorsqu'on 309
ivrognes vieux, chez les 309

éclair, troubles par 351
coup de foudre, troubles 757

éclampsie → convulsions 136

écoulement ⟩ 156

efficience augmentée 170

s'égouttent, sensation de gouttes 658
gouttes chaudes 659

électriques, troubles par états 170

électrochoc, troubles par 170

éléphantiasis 171
Arabes, des 171

empoisonnement par:
aluminium 31
arsenic 36, 487
bromures 53
carbone, monoxyde de 152
champignons 386
cuivre, vapeurs, récipient 148
fer 332
fumée 601
gaz + g. des égoutes 76, 577
iode 331
légumes pourris 277
médicaments **364**–5
médicaments végétaux 365
mercure 134, **368,** 487
narcotiques 387
nicotinisme 480, 636
poisson pourri 242
ptomaines 421, 768
purgatives 555
quinine 555

intermittente 718
joie, par 729
jouer du piano, par 729
lactation, par **725–6**
lait, après ingestion de 722
lavant les pieds, en se 715
lecture, par 730
leucorrhées avec + par 718–9
levant, en se + après **731**
mangé + manger 712–3
manque de sommeil, par 719, 733
marche, par la + 〉 **741–4**
masturbation, par 720
maux des dents, après, avec 739
maux de tête, par + pendant 716
ménopause, pendant 708
menstruation 720–2
monter l'escalier, par 707
mort, comme à l'approche de 710
mortification, par 723
mouvant les bras, en 723
mouvement, par + 〉 723
muscles, des 723–4
musique, par 724
nausée, avec 724
nerveuse 724–5
nuageux, par temps 708
opération, par **726**
palpitations, avec 726
paralytique 726–7
parler, par + conversation des autres **738**
pencher à gauche 〉 718
périodique 728
perte de fluids vitaux, par 719
pertes sémindes, après 713
petit déjeuner + 〉 707
pieds, en se lavant les 735
printemps, au 734
progressive 729
pyrosis, par 716
quinine, abus de 730
rapide **730**
réaction, avec manque de **730**
refroidissement, après 709
regardant en bas, en 719
repos, au + 〉 **730**
reposant 〉, la tète 731
réunion intéressante, par 720
rêve, après 712, 741
réveil, au, après **740–1**
sédentaires, par habitudes 732
selle 735
sexuels, par excès 732
société, en 709
soins donnés aux malades, par 725
sommeil + 〉 + manque de 733

somnambulisme, après 734
somnolence, par 733–4
soulever, par 719
spiritueux 〉 706
sportive 734
stimulants 〉 **734**
subite **736–8**
supprimées, par éruptions 738
syphilis, au cours de 738
tabac, par **738–9**
tempête, avant, pendant 736
thé 〉 738
tiraillantes, après douleurs 712
toux, par + après 728–9
transpiration, par, avec 710
traumatismes, par 717
travail intellectuel, par + 〉 722
tremblante 739
uriner, après 740
vers, avec 745
vertige, avec 740
vin 〈 , 〉 745
vomissement, avec, après 740

faim 〈 311–2
évanoissement par 193
faiblesse par 717
inanition 604
tremblement par 652
troubles 312

fatigue 745–751
air 〉, en plein 747
agg. 747
s'asseoir, désir de 749
assis, étant 750
coït, après 748
conversation, par 748
debout, étant 750
diarrhée, après 748
exercise physique 〉 749
jouer du piano, par 749
leucorrhée, avec, après 749
lire, par 749
mangé + mangeant 748
marchant + marche 750–1
ménopause, pendant 748
menstruation 749
monter l'escalier, par 748
parler, par 750
pertes sémindes, après 748
réveil, au 750
sexuelle, par excitation 749
travail intellectuel, par **748**

femmes, mal des 212–3
fer, abus de 332
fièvre 〈, avant, pendant, après 213
fils, sensation des **635**

faiblesse par humidité 710
paralysie après 487
mollesse, sensation 215
  interne 215
  parties dures, des 215
montagne → mal de **376**–7
monter ⟨ , ⟩ 37–**38**
  haut ⟨ 38
  troubles 38
monter à cheval + ⟨ , ⟩ 563
  aller en voiture, train + ⟨ , ⟩ 563–4
  voyage par mer, troubles 564
mort apparente, état de 152–3
  carbone, par monoxyde de **152**
  coupe de foudre, après 153
  gelées, des personnes 152
  hémorrhagies, après 152
  nouveau-nés, des 153
  noyés, des 152
  pendues, étranglés, des personnes 153
  traumatismes, après 153
morve 287
se moiller, troubles par 762–4
  chorée après humidité 74
  convulsions en se m. 147
  évanouissement après 210
  faiblesse par humidité 710
  paralysie après 487
mourir de faim, sensation de 604
mouvement ⟨ , ⟩ 370–2
  affectées ⟨ , ⟩, des parties 373
  air ⟨, en plein 375
  après le m. ⟨ 373
  aversion 374
  continu ⟩ 375
  au début de m. ⟨ **374**
  de descente ⟨ + ⟩ 155
  désir 375
  lent ⟨ , ⟩ 376
  rapide ⟩ 376
  violent ⟨ , ⟩ 376
muqueuse, hypersécrétion + ⟩ 377–386
  acide, goût 383
  acre 378
  albumoïde 378
  amer, goût 378
  aqueuse 385
  blanche 385
  bleuâtre 379
  brûlante 379
  brunâtre 379
  chaude 381
  corrosive 380
  douce 378
  douceâtre, goût 383
  dure 381

épaisse 384
excoriante 380
fétide 382
floconneuse 380
fluide 384
froide 380
gélatineuse 380
grise 380
grumeleuse 381
jaunâtre-verte 386
jaune 385–6
laiteuse 381
métallique, goût 381
miel, comme du 381
moisie, odeur 382
purulente 382
salé, goût 383
sanguinolante 378–9
spumeuse 380
supprimée 383
tenace, visqueuse 382–3
transparente 384
urine, odeur d' 384
verdâtre 381
vicariante 385
muscles, des:
  abcès 220
  amyotrophie spinale progressive 386
  crampes 150
  faiblesse 723–4
  indurations 315
  inflammations 322
  relaxion 559–560
  tension 633
  traumatismes + rupture 327, 330
  tressaillement 336–8
musique (+ Vol. I index):
  chorée ⟩ 71
  évanouissement en entendant 197
  faiblesse par 724
  tremblement par 653
myxoedème 386

nanisme 166
narcotiques, ⟨ par 387
  désir **387**
  troubles 387
nécrose des os **387**–8
neige ⟨, temps de 601
  troubles 601
neige brillante, troubles 601
nerfs:
  encéphalome 661
  ganglion 661
  inflammations des 322
  neurogliome 662

traumatismes, douleurs névritiques 330
neurasthémie → faiblesse-nerveuse **724**–5
nicotinisme 480, 636
noirceur, externes **47**–8
   chaude 48
   diabétique 48
   froide 47
   moite 48
   sénile 48
   traumatique 48
nombreuses symptômes 363
nourrissons, maladies 393
«noué» intérieurement **338**
nuit + 〉 12–16
   air de la nuit 〈 13
   minuit, avant, après 14–16
   une nuit sur deux 14

obésité 393–5
   enfants, chez 394
   jambes maigres, avec 394
   jeunes, chez 395
   ménopause, pendant 394
   vieillesse, dans 395
obscurité 〈 , 〉 151–2
oedème → hydropisie externe 160
onanisme → masturbation 363–4
opération:
   évanouissement en entendant parler
      d' 198
   faiblesse par 726
   fistules, après 214
   troubles par 326–7
orgasme sanguin 396–401
   agitation, avec 400
   anxiété avec 398
   assis, étant 400
   brûlantes, mains; peau 398
   coït, après 398
   couché, côté gauche 399
   désagréables nouvelles, par 398
   émotions, après 399
   s'endormant, en 399
   évanouissement, avec 399
   fumant du tabac, en 400
   mangenant, en + 〉 398
   marche, après + longue 400–1
   menstruation 399
   montant des escaliers, en 398
   mouvement ou parler 〉 399
   nervosité, par 400
   palpitations, avec 400
   sensorielles, par impressions 400
   tout bougeait, comme 399
   vertige, pendant 400
   vexations, après 400

vin, après 401
vomissement, après 400
os, des:
   cancéreuses, affections 55
   carie osseuse 58
   constriction, sensation de 93–4
   enflé, sensation 627
   fistules 214
   formication dans 284
   fragiles, os 53
   inflammations 377–8
   nécrose **387**–8
   ostéomalacie **661**–2
   ostéome 662
   pulsations dans 527
   tension 632
   traumatisme 329–330, 581
   tuméfaction 622
os fragiles 53
ostéomalacie 601–2
ovulation, à l' 401

paralysie 477–487
   accouchement, après 485
   agitante 477
   alcool, par 477
   ascendante aiguë 479
   atrophie, avec 477
   bain froid 〉 + par 478, 486
   bas, vers le 478
   changement, au froid humide 477
   choc mental, par 479
   coït, par 478
   colère, après 477
   couché sur un sol humide 479
   douloureuse **484**
   empoisonnement (ars, merc., plb.) 487
   excitation émotionelle, par 479
   exercice physique, après 478
   frayeur, par 478
   graduellement, apparaît 478
   haut, vers le 478
   indolore 485
   inférieure du corps, de la partie 479
   interne 479
   intermittente, après fièvre 478
   isolées, de parties 486
   masturbation, par 479
   mouillé, après 487
   muscles extenseurs, fléchisseurs 479–480
   névralgies, avec 480
   nicotinisme, par 480
   organes, des 484
   paraplégie 485
   poliomyélite 485–6
   post-diphtérique 486

(Fettdruck der Spaltennummern bei Rubriken mit Hinweisen und abwechselnden Symptomen. **agg.** = ⟨. **am.** = ⟩)

10

Erkältung, durch 186
Erregung, durch 190
Erwachen, beim 208
Essen, vor, nach **189**
Fallen, mit 190–1
Fasten ⟩ 191
Fieber, vor, im, nach 191
Fieberfrost, vor, im 185
Fluor, mit 194
Freien, im + ⟩ 183
Frösteln mit 186
Frühstück, vor, nach 185
Gehen, beim, nach + ⟩ 208–9
Gehirnerschütterung, durch 194
geistige Anstrengung, durch 195
Geräusche, durch 197
Gerüche, durch **198**
Gesichtsfarbe blaß, blau, rot 190
Gewitter, vor 207
Haemoptysis, nach 192
häufig 191
Heben der Arme, des Kopfes 202
Herzdruck, mit **193**
Herzklopfen, bei 200
Herzleiden, bei 185
hinaufläuft, wenn Treppen 203
Hitze, mit, durch 193
Hitzewallungen, mit 193
Hunger, durch 193
Husten, bei 187
hysterische 193
kalter Haut, mit 187
kaltes Wasser ⟩ 187
kaltes Wetter, durch 187
Kindbett, im 201
Kirche, in der **186**
Kleidung, durch enge 186
Kleinigkeiten, bei 208
Klimakterium, im 186
Knien in Kirche, beim **194**
Koitus, beim, nach 186
Konvulsionen, nach 187
Kopfschmerzen, bei 192–3
Kummer, durch 192
lang anhaltende 201
Lesen, beim, nach 202
Lichter, durch viele 194
Liegen, im + ⟩, nach 195
Magen aufsteigt, wie etwas vom 206
Magenerkrankungen, bei **192**
Meningites, bei 196
Menses + unterdrückte 196
Metrorrhagen, mit 196
Mittagessen, beim, nach 188
Musik, beim Hören von 197
Mydriasis, mit 197

Nachwehe, nach jeder 183
Nasenbluten, durch, vor, mit 189
Naßwerden, nach 198
neurasthenische 197
Obst ⟩, saures 192
Operationen, beim Gespräch über 198
periodische 200
plötzliche 207
Puls-Störungen 201–2
qualvoller Angst, nach 184
Rauchen, beim, nach 204–5
Retten, beim, nach dem 202
Rückwärtsbeugen des Kopfes ⟩ 184
Ruhelosigkeit, nach 202
Säfteverluste, durch 195
Samenverlust, nach 189
Schelte, durch 203
Schlaf, gefolgt von, nach 204
Schlafen auf li. Seite, beim 204
Schlafmangel, durch 204
Schläfen, beim Reiben der 207
Schläfrigkeit, mit 188
Schmerzen, durch **198**–200
Schnarchen, mit 205
schnell vorübergehende 207
Schock, durch 203
Schreck, durch 191
Schreiben, nach 210
Schwäche, aus **210**
Schwangerschaft, in 201
Schweiß, bei, ⟩, nach 200–1
  Unterdrückung von Fußschw. 190
Sehen, durch angestrengtes 195
sexuellen Ausschweifungen, nach 203
Sitzen, beim 203–4
Sommerhitze, durch 207
Sprechen, durch 205
Stehen, beim 205
Steigen (Berg, Hügel, Treppen) 184
Stuhlgang 206
Sturm, vor 205
Taubheit, mit 198
Tendenz zur 207
tetanischen Spasmus, vor, nach 207
Tiefatmen ⟩ 185
Übelkeit, vor, bei, nach 197
überfüllten Zimmer, im **187**
Urinieren, beim, nach 208
Uteruserkrankung, bei 208
Verletzungsschock, mit **194**
warmen Zimmer, im 209
warmes Bad, durch 209
Wasser ⟩, Bespritzen 210
Wein ⟨ 210
Wunden, durch kleine 210
Zittern, mit 207